Nursing Diagnosis Handbook

A Guide to Planning Care

Nursing Diagnosis Handbook

A Guide to Planning Care

THIRD EDITION

BETTY J. ACKLEY, MSN, EdS, RN

GAIL B. LADWIG, MSN, RN

with 4 Consultants and 38 Contributors

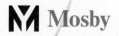 Mosby

St. Louis Baltimore Boston Carlsbad Chicago Naples New York Philadelphia Portland
London Madrid Mexico City Singapore Sydney Tokyo Toronto Wiesbaden

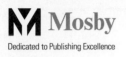
Mosby

Dedicated to Publishing Excellence

A Times Mirror Company

Vice President and Publisher: Nancy L. Coon
Editor: Loren S. Wilson
Developmental Editor: Brian Dennison
Project Manager: Linda McKinley
Production Editor: Catherine Bricker
Cover Designer: Elizabeth Fett
Manufacturing Manager: Don Carlisle

Third Edition

Copyright © 1997 by Mosby–Year Book, Inc.

Previous editions copyrighted 1993, 1995

Printed in the United States of America
Composition by Top Graphics
Printing/binding by R.R. Donnelley and Sons

Mosby–Year Book, Inc.
11830 Westline Industrial Drive
St. Louis, Missouri 63146

Library of Congress Cataloging in Publication Data

Nursing diagnosis handbook: a guide to planning care / [edited by]
  Betty J. Ackley, Gail B. Ladwig; and 38 contributors, with 4
  consultants.—3rd ed.
    p.   cm.
  Includes bibliographical references and index.
  ISBN 0-8151-0912-1 (pbk.)
  1. Nursing diagnosis—Handbooks, manuals, etc.   2. Nursing care
plans—Handbooks, manuals, etc.   I. Ackley, Betty J.   II. Ladwig,
Gail B.
  [DNLM: 1. Nursing Diagnosis—handbooks.   2. Patient Care Planning—
handbooks.   WY 49 N9745 1997]
RT48.6.A35   1997
610.73—dc21
DNLM/DLC
for Library of Congress   96-47933
                                                          CIP

97 98 99 00 01 / 9 8 7 6 5 4 3 2 1

Contributors

Betty J. Ackley, MSN, EdS, RN
Professor of Nursing,
Jackson Community College,
Jackson, Michigan;
Staff Nurse—Stepdown Cardiac Care,
W.A. Foote Memorial Hospital,
Jackson, Michigan

Victoria L. Cole-Schonlau, DNSc, MPA, RN
House Supervisor,
North Cancer Hospital,
Los Angeles, California

Sandra K. Cunningham, MS, RN, CCRN, CS
Clinical Nurse Specialist,
Edward J. Hines, Jr. Hospital,
Department of Veterans Affairs,
Hines, Illinois

Jane Maria Curtis, MSN, CNA, RN
Consultant in Nursing,
Santa Fe, New Mexico

Gwethalyn B. Edwards, MSN, RN
Director of Nursing Education,
W.A. Foote Memorial Hospital,
Jackson, Michigan

Pamela M. Emery, BS, RNFA, CNOR, RN
Coordinator of Clinical Practice,
    Operating Room,
North Oakland Medical Centers,
Pontiac, Michigan

Nancy English, PhD, RN
Consultant in Nursing Education,
Denver, Colorado

Roslyn Fine, MS, CCC, SLP
Speech Language Pathologist,
Sundance Rehabilitation Corporation,
Southfield, Michigan

Mary A. Fuerst-DeWys, BS, RN
Infant Developmental Specialist,
Devos Children's Hospital at Butterworth,
Grand Rapids, Michigan

Mikel Gray, PhD, CUNP, CCCN, FAAN
Associate Professor of Nursing;
Nurse Practitioner,
Department of Urology,
University of Virginia,
Charlottesville, Virginia;
Adjunct Professor of Nursing,
Bellarmine College, Lansing School of Nursing,
Louisville, Kentucky

J. Keith Hampton, MSN, RN, CS
Nurse Manager, Dialysis Services,
University of Minnesota Hospital and Clinic;
Adjunct Faculty,
School of Nursing,
University of Minnesota,
Minneapolis, Minnesota

Mary Henrikson, MN, RNC, ARNP
Director of Nursing, Maternal,
Salem Hospital,
Salem, Oregon

Kathie D. Hesnan, BSN, RN, CETN
Continence Nursing;
Enterstomal Therapist Nurse,
VNA of Greater Philadelphia,
Langhorne, Pennsylvania

Leslie Kalbach, MN, RN, CNRN
Clinical Nurse Specialist,
Group Health Cooperative of Puget Sound,
Seattle, Washington

Helen Kelley, MSN, RN
Psychiatric Nurse Consultant,
University of Michigan Medical Center,
Ann Arbor, Michigan

Diane Krasner, MS, RN, CETN
Enterstomal Therapist Nurse Consultant;
Doctoral Student,
University of Maryland School of Nursing,
Baltimore, Maryland

Gail B. Ladwig, MSN, RN
Associate Professor of Nursing;
Consultant in Guided Imagery,
Jackson Community College;
Healing Touch Practitioner,
Jackson, Michigan

Marcia LaHaie, BSN, RN, OCN
Oncology Education Coordinator,
St. Joseph Mercy Hospital,
Ann Arbor, Michigan

Margaret Lunney, PhD, RN, CS
Associate Professor of Nursing,
Hunter-Bellevue School of Nursing,
New York, New York

Carroll A. Lutz, MA, BSN, RN
Consultant in Nutrition,
Jackson, Michigan

Leslie Lysaght, MS, RN, CCRN, CS
Clinical Nurse Specialist,
Critical Care, Pulmonary,
St. Joseph Mercy Hospital,
Ann Arbor, Michigan

Marty J. Martin, MSN, RN
Associate Professor of Nursing,
Jackson Community College,
Jackson, Michigan;
Staff Nurse, Mental Health,
St. Lawrence Hospital,
Lansing, Michigan

Margo McCaffery, MS, RN, FAAN
Consultant in Nursing Care of Patients with Pain,
Los Angeles, California

Vicki E. McClurg, MN, RN
Assistant Professor of Nursing,
Seattle Pacific University,
Seattle, Washington

Pamela H. Mitchell, PhD, RN, CNRN, FAAN
Elizabeth S. Soule Distinguished Professor of Nursing
    and Health Promotion;
Professor of Biobehavioral Nursing and Health
    Systems,
University of Washington School of Nursing,
Seattle, Washington

Christine L. Pasero, BSN, RN
Consultant in Pain Management,
Rocklin, California

Beverly Pickett, MA, BS, RN
Certification in Holistic Health;
Laboratory Assistant,
Department of Nursing,
Jackson Community College;
Healing Touch Practitioner;
Consultant in Guided Imagery;
Jackson, Michigan

Nancee B. Radtke, MSN, RN
Administrative Director,
Ambulatory Care Department,
W.A. Foote Hospital,
Jackson, Michigan

Judith S. Rizzo, MS, RN, CS
Clinical Nurse Specialist,
Psychiatric Emergency Services,
University of Michigan Medical Center,
Ann Arbor, Michigan

Pam B. Schweitzer, MS, RN, CS
Clinical Nurse Specialist,
Anxiety Disorders Program,
University of Michigan Psychiatric Hospitals,
Ann Arbor, Michigan

Suzanne Skowronski, MSN, RN
Lecturer in Nursing,
Wayne State University,
College of Nursing,
Detroit, Michigan

Teepa Snow, MS, OTRIL, FAOTA
Program Director,
Occupational Therapy Assistant Program,
Durham Technical Community College,
Durham, North Carolina

Martha A. Spies, MSN, RN
Assistant Professor,
Deaconess College of Nursing,
St. Louis, Missouri

Linda L. Straight, MA, CES, RN
Manager Cardiac and Pulmonary Rehabilitation,
W.A. Foote Memorial Hospital,
Jackson, Michigan

Terry VandenBosch, MS, RN, CS
Research Specialist,
St. Joseph Mercy Hospital,
Ann Arbor, Michigan

Catherine Vincent, MSN, RN
Assistant Professor,
School of Nursing,
Oakland University,
Rochester, Michigan

Virginia R. Wall, MN, RN, IBCLC
Lactation Specialist,
University of Washington Medical Center,
Seattle, Washington

Peggy Wetsch, MSN, RN, CNA
Systems Administrator,
Information Resources Group,
Subsidiary of Silver Platter,
Pasadena, California;
Consultant in Nursing Information and Education,
Los Angeles, California

Linda Williams, MSN, RN, C, CS
Professor of Nursing;
Gerontological Clinical Nurse Specialist,
Jackson Community College;
Staff Nurse, PACU,
W.A. Foote Hospital,
Jackson, Michigan

Kathy Wyngarden, MSN, RN
Director of Clinical Practice Model,
Butterworth Hospital,
Grand Rapids, Michigan

Consultants in Nursing Research Utilization

Ann F. Jacobson, PhD, RN
Assistant Professor,
School of Nursing,
Kent State University,
Kent, Ohio

Brenda J. Wagner, PhD, RN
Licensed Psychologist,
Scottish Rite Children's Medical Center,
Atlanta, Georgia

Elizabeth H. Winslow, PhD, RN, FAAN
Research Consultant,
Presbyterian Hospital of Dallas,
Dallas, Texas

Consultant in Home Care—Contributor of Home Care Interventions

Elizabeth L. Foster, MS, RN
Staff Development Specialist,
University Medical Center of Tucson,
Tucson, Arizona

To

Dale Ackley, the greatest guy in the world without whose support this book would have never happened; Dawn Ackley, who with Dale has been the joy of my life

Jerry Ladwig, my wonderful husband who after 32 years is still supportive and patient—I couldn't have done it without him; my children and their spouses and my grandchildren—Jerry, Kathy, Alexandra, and Elizabeth; Chrissy, John, and Sean; Jenny, Jim and Abby; and Amy—the greatest family anyone could ever hope for

A special thank you to our research assistants, Amy Ladwig and Scott Bertram, and our nursing faculty colleagues—friends are one of life's most precious gifts

Preface

Nursing Diagnosis Handbook: A Guide to Planning Care is a convenient reference to help the practicing nurse or nursing student make a nursing diagnosis and write a care plan with ease and confidence. This handbook helps nurses correlate nursing diagnoses with known information about clients on the basis of assessment findings, established medical or psychiatric diagnoses, and the current treatment plan.

Making a nursing diagnosis and planning care are complex processes that involve diagnostic reasoning and critical thinking skills. Nursing students and practicing nurses cannot possibly memorize the more than 1000 defining characteristics, related factors, and risk factors for the 129 diagnoses approved by the North American Nursing Diagnosis Association (NANDA). This book correlates suggested nursing diagnoses with what nurses know about clients and offers a care plan for each nursing diagnosis.

Section I, Nursing Diagnosis and the Nursing Process, explains how the nurse formulates a nursing diagnosis statement using assessment findings and other data. In Section II, Guide to Nursing Diagnoses, the nurse can look up symptoms and problems and their suggested nursing diagnoses for more than 1000 client symptoms, medical and psychiatric diagnoses, diagnostic procedures, surgical interventions, and clinical states. In Section III, Guide to Planning Care, the nurse can find care plans for all nursing diagnoses suggested in Section II. In this edition, we have included the suggested nursing interventions from the Nursing Interventions Classification (NIC) by the Iowa Intervention Project as well as a listing of all NIC interventions in Appendix E. We are excited about this work and believe it is a significant addition to the nursing process to further define nursing practice.

Nursing Diagnosis Handbook: A Guide to Planning Care includes medical diagnoses because nurses find them useful in suggesting appropriate nursing diagnoses. For example, under the medical diagnosis of **AIDS,** the nurse will find the nursing diagnosis **Body image disturbance** related to (r/t) chronic contagious illness, cachexia. The nurse needs to determine whether this suggested nursing diagnosis relates to the client.

New special features of the third edition of *Nursing Diagnosis Handbook: A Guide to Planning Care* include the following:

- Addition of Home Care Interventions written by Elizabeth L. Foster, a specialist in home care
- Inclusion of suggested NIC interventions for each nursing diagnosis
- Inclusion of a complete list of NIC Interventions in Appendix E
- Increased depth of the nursing research base utilizing three consultants in nursing research: Ann F. Jacobson, PhD, RN; Brenda J. Wagner, PhD, RN; and Elizabeth H. Winslow, PhD, RN
- Addition of two contributors who are nationally known specialists in their fields: Dr.

Mikel Gray, writing on problems with urology, and Dr. Pamela H. Mitchell, writing on intracranial pressure

The following features of *Nursing Diagnosis Handbook: A Guide to Planning Care* are included from the second edition:

- Suggested nursing diagnoses for more than 1000 clinical entities including 300 signs and symptoms, 300 medical diagnoses, 120 surgeries, 200 maternal-child disorders, 100 mental health disorders, and 50 geriatric disorders
- Rationales for nursing interventions that are based on nursing research and literature
- Nursing references identified for each care plan
- Major clinical practice guidelines of the Agency for Health Care Policy and Research (AHCPR) used in appropriate care plans
- Nursing care plans that contain many holistic interventions
- Care plans for **Pain** written by national experts on pain, Margo McCaffery and Christine L. Pasero
- Care plans for **Skin integrity** written by national expert Diane Krasner who has lectured and written extensively on the topic
- Care plans for **Community** written by national expert Dr. Margaret Lunney
- A format that facilitates analyzing signs and symptoms by the process already known by nurses, which is using defining characteristics of nursing diagnoses to make a diagnosis
- Use of NANDA terminology and approved diagnoses
- Inclusion of two additional nursing diagnoses, **Grieving** and **Altered comfort**
- An alphabetical format for Section II, Guide to Nursing Diagnoses, and Section III, Guide to Planning Care, which allows rapid access to information
- Nursing care plans for all nursing diagnoses listed in Section II
- Specific geriatric interventions in appropriate plans of care
- Specific client/family teaching interventions in each plan of care

- Inclusion of commonly used abbreviations (e.g., AIDS, MI, CHF) and cross-references to the complete term in Section II
- Contributions by 44 nurse experts from throughout the United States who together represent all of the major nursing specialties and have extensive experience with nursing diagnoses and the nursing process

We acknowledge the work of NANDA, which is used extensively throughout this text. In some cases the authors and contributors have modified the NANDA work to increase ease of use. The original NANDA work can be found in *NANDA Nursing Diagnoses: Definitions and Classification 1997-1998.*

Several contributors are the original authors of the nursing diagnoses established by NANDA. These contributors include the following:

Mary A. Fuerst–DeWys
Disorganized infant behavior
Potential for enhanced organized infant behavior
Risk for disorganized behavior

Dr. Nancy English
Impaired environmental interpretation syndrome

Dr. Margaret Lunney
Effective management of therapeutic regimen
Ineffective community coping
Ineffective management of therapeutic regimen
Ineffective management of therapeutic regimen: community
Ineffective management of therapeutic regimen: families
Potential for enhanced community coping

Vicki E. McClurg, Mary Henrikson, and Virginia R. Wall
Effective breast-feeding
Ineffective breast-feeding
Interrupted breast-feeding

Dr. Pamela H. Mitchell
Decreased adaptive capacity: intracranial

Kathy Wyngarden
Risk for altered parent/infant/child attachment

We and the consultants and contributors trust that nurses will find this third edition of *Nursing Diagnosis Handbook: A Guide to Planning Care* to be a valuable tool that simplifies the process of diagnosing clients and planning for their care and thus allows nurses more time to provide care that speeds each client's recovery.

ACKNOWLEDGMENTS

We would like to thank the following people at Mosby: Loren Wilson, Nursing Editor, who supported us with this third edition of the text with intelligence and kindness; Brian Dennison, Developmental Editor, who was a continual support and constant source of wise advice, and all of the people in the production editing department who finalized this edition, especially Cathy Bricker.

We acknowledge with gratitude the nursing students and graduates of Jackson Community College who made us think and shared a very special time with us; the nurses at W. A. Foote Memorial Hospital, Doctors Hospital in Jackson, and Community Mental Health and the Community Nursing Agencies who have helped us educate students and served as role models for excellence in nursing care; and finally, each other, for perseverance, patience, and friendship.

Betty J. Ackley
Gail B. Ladwig

Contents

Nursing Diagnosis and the Nursing Process

The nursing process is an organizing framework for professional nursing practice. Components of the process include performing a nursing assessment; making nursing diagnoses; planning: writing outcome/goal statements, determining appropriate nursing interventions; implementing care; and evaluating the nursing care that has been given. An essential part of this process is the nursing diagnosis:

> A nursing diagnosis is a clinical judgment about individual, family, or community responses to actual or potential health problems or life processes. Nursing diagnoses provide the basis for selection of nursing interventions to achieve outcomes for which the nurse is accountable (NANDA, 1990).

ASSESSMENT

Before determining appropriate nursing diagnoses, the nurse must perform a thorough holistic nursing assessment of the client. The nurse may use the assessment format adopted by the facility in which the practice is situated. Several organizational approaches to assessment are available, including Gordon's Functional Health Patterns and head-to-toe and body systems approaches. Regardless of the approach used, the nurse assesses for client symptoms to help formulate a nursing diagnosis.

To elicit as many symptoms as possible, the nurse uses open-ended rather than yes/no questions during the assessment. The nurse also obtains information via physical assessment and diagnostic test results. If the client is critically ill or unable to respond verbally, the nurse obtains most of the data from physical assessment and diagnostic test results and possibly from the client's significant others. The nurse can use data from each of these sources to formulate a nursing diagnosis.

NURSING DIAGNOSTIC STATEMENT

A working nursing diagnostic statement has three parts:
1. The nursing diagnosis
2. "Related to" phrase or etiology
3. Defining characteristics phrase

Nursing Diagnosis

The nurse makes a nursing diagnosis by categorizing symptoms as common patterns of response to actual or potential health problems. After completing the assessment, the nurse lists all identified symptoms and clusters similar symptoms together. For example, the following symptoms may be identified in the assessment of a client with an admitting medical diagnosis of asthma: dyspnea, anxiety, hypertension, respiratory rate of 28, temperature of 99° F. Of these signs and symptoms, dyspnea and respiratory rate of 28 (tachypnea) would be clustered because they are related. Using Section II: Guide to Nursing Diagnoses, the nurse can then look up dyspnea or tachypnea and find the nursing diagnosis **Ineffective breathing pattern** suggested for each symptom.

To validate that the diagnosis **Ineffective breathing pattern** is appropriate for the client, the nurse then turns to Section III: Guide to Planning Care and reads through its definition and its list of defining characteristics. The definition should describe the condition that the nurse is observing in the client. Many of the nursing diagnoses in Section III differentiate between major and minor defining characteristics or specify critical defining characteristics. For a diagnosis to be accurate, NANDA suggests that the client should have most of the major or critical defining characteristics.

To help verify the diagnoses made on the basis of client signs and symptoms, the nurse may look up the client's medical diagnoses in Section II: Guide to Nursing Diagnoses. For example, one of the nursing diagnoses listed under the medical diagnosis asthma is **Ineffective breathing pattern.**

The process of identifying significant symptoms, clustering them into logical patterns, and then choosing an appropriate nursing diagnosis involves diagnostic reasoning skills (critical thinking) that must be learned in the process of becoming a nurse. Our text serves as a tool to help the nurse in this process.

"Related to" Phrase or Etiology

The second part of the nursing diagnosis statement is the "related to" (r/t) phrase. This phrase states what may be causing or contributing to the nursing diagnosis, or the etiology. Pathophysiological and psychosocial changes, such as developmental age and cultural and environmental situations, may be causative factors.

Ideally, the etiology, or cause, of the nursing diagnosis is something the nurse can treat. A carefully written, individualized r/t statement enables the nurse to plan nursing interventions that will assist the client in accomplishing goals and returning to a state of optimum health.

For each suggested nursing diagnosis, the nurse should refer to the statements listed under the heading "Related Factors (r/t)" in Section III. These r/t factors may or may not be appropriate for the individual client. If they are not appropriate, the nurse should write an appropriate r/t statement.

Defining Characteristics Phrase

The third part of the nursing diagnostic statement consists of defining characteristics (signs and symptoms) that the nurse has gathered during the assessment phase. The phrase "as evidenced by" (aeb) may be used to connect the etiology (r/t) and defining characteristics. The use of defining characteristics is similar to the process the physician uses when making a medical diagnosis. For example, for the medical diagnosis of asthma the physician may observe the following signs and symptoms: wheezing, chest retractions, and pulmonary function testing abnormalities. The nurse uses the same process.

Examples of Writing a Nursing Diagnostic Statement

To write a nursing diagnostic statement for a client with the symptom of alopecia, the nurse should use Section II. Listed under the heading **Alopecia** is the following information:

Alopecia
Body image disturbance (nursing diagnosis) r/t loss of hair, change in appearance (etiology)

To the information found in Section II, the defining characteristics phrase is added: aeb verbalization of fear of rejection by others because of hair loss.

With the preceding information, the nurse is able to make the following nursing diagnosis statement:

Body image disturbance r/t loss of hair, change in appearance aeb verbalization of fear of rejection by others because of hair loss.

To use Section II to write a nursing diagnostic statement for a client who has peritonitis, the nurse should look up the diagnosis **Peritonitis.** Listed under this medical diagnosis is the following information:

Peritonitis
Fluid volume deficit (nursing diagnosis) r/t retention of fluid in the bowel with loss of circulating blood volume (etiology).

To the information in Section II, the defining characteristics phrase is added: aeb dry mucous membranes, poor skin turgor.

With the preceding information, the nurse is able to make the following nursing diagnostic statement:

Fluid volume deficit r/t retention of fluid in the bowel with loss of circulating blood volume aeb dry mucous membranes, poor skin turgor.

PLANNING

For most clients the nurse will make more than one nursing diagnosis. Therefore the next step in the nursing process is to determine the priority for care from the list of nursing diagnoses. The nurse can determine the highest priority nursing diagnoses by using Maslow's Hierarchy of Needs. In this hierarchy, highest priority is generally given to immediate problems that may be life threatening. For example, **Ineffective airway clearance** would have a higher priority than **Ineffective individual coping.** Refer to Appendix A, "Nursing Diagnoses Arranged by Maslow's Hierarchy of Needs" for assistance in prioritizing nursing diagnoses.

Outcomes/Goals

After determining the appropriate priority of the nursing diagnoses, the nurse writes client outcome/goal statements. Section III lists suggested choices of outcomes/goals for each nursing diagnosis. If at all possible, the nurse involves the client in determining appropriate outcomes/goals. After a discussion with the client, the nurse plans nursing care that will assist the client in accomplishing the outcome/goal.

After the client's outcomes/goals are selected, the nurse establishes a means to accomplish the outcomes/goals. The usual means are by nursing interventions.

INTERVENTIONS

Interventions are like road maps directing the best ways to provide nursing care. The more clearly a nurse writes an intervention, the easier it will be to complete the journey and arrive at the destination of successful client outcomes/goals.

This text includes suggested Nursing Interventions Classification (NIC) interventions for each nursing diagnosis. The NIC interventions are a comprehensive, standardized classification of treatments that nurses perform. The classification includes both physiological and psychosocial interventions and covers all nursing specialities. See Appendix E for a listing of the NIC interventions. For further information on NIC, see McCloskey JC, Bulechek GM: *Nursing interventions classification (NIC),* ed 2, St Louis, 1996, Mosby.

Section III supplies choices of interventions for each nursing diagnosis. The nurse may choose the ones appropriate for the client and individualize them accordingly or determine additional interventions.

Putting It All Together—Writing the Care Plan

The final planning phase is writing the actual care plan, including prioritized nursing diagnostic statements, outcomes/goals, and interventions. The care plan must be written and shared with all health care personnel caring for the client to ensure continuity of care.

IMPLEMENTATION

The implementation phase of the nursing process is the actual initiation of the nursing care plan. Client outcomes/goals are achieved by the performance of the nursing interventions. During this phase the nurse continues to assess the client to determine whether the interventions are effective. An important part of this phase is documentation. The nurse should use the facility's tool for documentation and record the results of implementing nursing interventions. Documentation is also necessary for legal reasons because in a legal dispute, "If it wasn't charted, it wasn't done."

EVALUATION

Although the evaluation is listed as the last phase of the nursing process, it is actually an integral part of each phase that the nurse does continuously. When the evaluation is performed as the last phase, the nurse refers to the client's outcomes/goals and determines whether they were met. If the outcomes/goals were not met, the nurse begins again with assessment and determines why they were not met. Were the goals attainable? Was the wrong nursing diagnosis made? Should the interventions be changed? At this point the nurse can look up any new symptoms or conditions that have been identified in the client and then adjust the care plan as needed.

Many health care providers are using critical pathways to plan nursing care. The use of nursing diagnoses should be an integral part of any critical pathway to ensure that nursing care needs are being assessed and appropriate nursing interventions are planned and implemented.

The use of nursing diagnoses ensures that nurses are speaking a common language when taking care of client problems. This system is also easily computerized for easier documentation and analysis of patterns of care. Nursing diagnosis is the essence of nursing to ensure that clients receive excellent, holistic nursing care.

Section II

Guide to Nursing Diagnoses

A

Abdominal Distention

Altered nutrition: less than body requirements r/t
nausea, vomiting
Constipation r/t decreased activity, decreased fluid
intake, pathological process
Pain r/t retention of air and gastrointestinal secretions

Abdominal Hysterectomy

See Hysterectomy

Abdominal Pain

Altered nutrition: less than body requirements r/t
unresolved pain
Pain r/t injury, pathological process
See cause of Abdominal Pain

Abdominal Perineal Resection

Risk for perioperative positioning injury r/t
prolonged surgery and lithotomy position
See Abdominal Surgery; Colostomy

Abdominal Surgery

Altered health maintenance r/t knowledge deficit
regarding self-care after surgery
Altered nutrition: less than body requirements r/t
high metabolic needs, decreased ability to digest
food
Constipation r/t decreased activity, decreased fluid
intake, anesthesia, narcotics
Pain r/t surgical procedure
Risk for altered tissue perfusion: peripheral r/t
immobility and abdominal surgery resulting in stasis
of blood flow
Risk for infection r/t invasive procedure
See Surgery

Abortion—Induced

Altered health maintenance r/t knowledge deficit
regarding self-care following abortion
Health-seeking behaviors r/t desire to control fertility
Ineffective family coping: compromised r/t
unresolved feelings about decision
Risk for infection r/t open uterine blood vessels,
dilated cervix
Self-esteem disturbance r/t feelings of guilt
Spiritual distress r/t perceived moral implications of
decision

Abortion—Spontaneous

Altered family processes r/t unmet expectations for
pregnancy and childbirth
Altered health maintenance r/t knowledge deficit
regarding self-care following abortion
Body image disturbance r/t perceived inability to
carry pregnancy, produce child
Fear r/t implications for future pregnancies
Ineffective family coping: disabling r/t unresolved
feelings about loss
Ineffective individual coping r/t personal
vulnerability
Pain r/t uterine contractions, surgical intervention
Risk for dysfunctional grieving r/t loss of fetus
Risk for fluid volume deficit r/t hemorrhage
Risk for infection r/t septic or incomplete abortion of
products of conception, open uterine blood vessels,
dilated cervix
Self-esteem disturbance r/t feelings of failure, guilt

Abruptio Placenta >36 weeks

Altered family processes r/t unmet expectations for
pregnancy/childbirth
Altered health maintenance r/t knowledge deficit
regarding self-care with disorder
Anxiety r/t unknown outcome, change in birth plans
Fear r/t threat to well-being of self and fetus
Impaired gas exchange (placental) r/t decreased
uteroplacental area
Pain r/t irritable uterus, hypertonic uterus
Risk for altered tissue perfusion (fetal) r/t
uteroplacental insufficiency
Risk for fluid volume deficit r/t hemorrhage
Risk for impaired tissue integrity (maternal) r/t
possible uterine rupture
Risk for infection r/t partial separation of the placenta

Abscess Formation

Altered health maintenance r/t knowledge deficit
regarding self-care with an abscess
Altered protection r/t inadequate nutrition, abnormal
blood profile, drug therapy or treatment
Impaired tissue integrity r/t altered circulation,
nutritional deficit/excess

Abuse, Child

See Child Abuse

Abuse—Spouse, Parent, or Significant Other

Altered family process: alcoholism r/t inadequate
coping skills
Anxiety r/t threat to self-concept, situational crisis of
abuse

Caregiver role strain r/t chronic illness, self-care deficits, lack of respite care, extent of caregiving required

Defensive coping r/t low self-esteem

Impaired verbal communication r/t psychological barriers of fear

Ineffective family coping: compromised r/t abusive patterns

Post-trauma response r/t history of abuse

Powerlessness r/t life-style of helplessness

Risk for violence: self-directed r/t history of abuse

Self-esteem disturbance r/t negative family interactions

Sleep pattern disturbance r/t psychological stress

Accessory Muscle Use (to Breathe)

Ineffective breathing pattern r/t neuromuscular impairment, pain, musculoskeletal impairment, perception/cognitive impairment, anxiety, decreased energy, fatigue

See COPD; Asthma; Bronchitis; Respiratory Infections, Acute, Childhood

Accident Prone

Acute confusion r/t altered level of consciousness

Ineffective individual coping r/t personal vulnerability, situational crises

Risk for injury r/t history of accidents

Achalasia

Impaired swallowing r/t neuromuscular impairment

Ineffective individual coping r/t chronic disease

Pain r/t stasis of food in the esophagus

Risk for aspiration r/t nocturnal regurgitation

Acidosis, Metabolic

Altered nutrition: less than body requirements r/t inability to ingest, absorb nutrients

Altered thought processes r/t central nervous system depression

Decreased cardiac output r/t dysrhythmias from hyperkalemia

Impaired memory r/t electrolyte imbalance

Pain: headache r/t neuromuscular irritability

Risk for injury r/t disorientation, weakness, stupor

Acidosis, Respiratory

Activity intolerance r/t imbalance between oxygen supply and demand

Altered thought processes r/t central nervous system depression

Impaired gas exchange r/t ventilation perfusion imbalance

Impaired memory r/t hypoxia

Risk for decreased cardiac output r/t arrhythmias associated with respiratory acidosis

Acquired Immune Deficiency Disorder

See AIDS

Activity Intolerance

Activity intolerance r/t bedrest/immobility, generalized weakness, sedentary life-style, imbalance between oxygen supply/demand, pain

Activity Intolerance, Potential to Develop

Risk for activity intolerance r/t deconditioned status, presence of circulatory/respiratory problems, inexperience with activity

Acute Abdomen

Fluid volume deficit r/t fluids trapped in bowel, inability to drink

Pain r/t pathological process

See cause of Acute Abdomen

Acute Back

Altered health maintenance r/t knowledge deficit regarding self-care with painful back

Anxiety r/t situational crisis, back injury

Colonic constipation r/t decreased activity

Impaired physical mobility r/t pain

Ineffective individual coping r/t situational crisis, back injury

Pain r/t back injury

Acute Confusion

Acute confusion r/t being more than 60 years of age, dementia, alcohol abuse, drug abuse, delirium

Adams-Stokes Syndrome

See Dysrhythmia

Addiction

See Alcoholism; Drug Abuse

Addison's Disease

Activity intolerance r/t weakness, fatigue

Altered health maintenance r/t knowledge deficit

Altered nutrition: less than body requirements r/t chronic illness

Fluid volume deficit r/t failure of regulatory mechanisms

Risk for injury r/t weakness

Adenoidectomy

Altered comfort r/t effects of anesthesia, nausea and vomiting

Altered health maintenance r/t knowledge deficit of postoperative care

Ineffective airway clearance r/t hesitation/reluctance to cough secondary to pain

Pain r/t surgical incision

Risk for altered nutrition: less than body requirements r/t hesitation/reluctance to swallow

Risk for aspiration/suffocation r/t postoperative drainage and impaired swallowing

Risk for fluid volume deficit r/t decreased intake secondary to painful swallowing, effects of anesthesia

Adhesions, Lysis of

See Abdominal Surgery

Adjustment Disorder

Anxiety r/t inability to cope with psychosocial stressor

Impaired adjustment r/t assault to self-esteem

Personal identity disturbance r/t psychosocial stressor (specific to individual)

Situational low self-esteem r/t change in role function

Adjustment Impairment

Impaired adjustment r/t disability requiring change in life-style, inadequate support systems, impaired cognition, sensory overload, assault to self-esteem, altered locus of control, incomplete grieving

Adolescent, Pregnant

Altered family processes r/t unmet expectations for adolescent, situational crisis

Altered growth and development r/t pregnancy

Altered health maintenance r/t knowledge deficit with denial of pregnancy, desire to keep pregnancy secret, fear

Altered nutrition: less than body requirements r/t lack of knowledge of nutritional needs during pregnancy and as a growing adolescent

Altered role performance r/t pregnancy

Anxiety r/t situational and maturational crisis, pregnancy

Body image disturbance r/t pregnancy superimposed on developing body

Decisional conflict: keeping child vs giving up child vs abortion r/t lack of experience with decision making, interference with decision-making, multiple or divergent sources of information, lack of support system

Family coping: disabling r/t highly ambivalent family relationships, chronically unresolved feelings of guilt, anger, or despair

Fear r/t labor and delivery

Health-seeking behaviors r/t desire for optimal maternal and fetal outcome

Impaired social interaction r/t self-concept disturbance

Ineffective denial r/t fear of consequences of pregnancy becoming known

Ineffective individual coping r/t situational and maturational crisis, personal vulnerability

Noncompliance r/t denial of pregnancy

Situational low self-esteem r/t feelings of shame and guilt about becoming and being pregnant

Adoption, Giving Child up for

Decisional conflict r/t unclear personal values or beliefs, perceived threat to value system, support system deficit

Grieving r/t loss of child, loss of role of parent

Potential for enhanced spiritual well-being r/t harmony with self regarding final decision

Adrenal Crisis

Altered protection r/t inability to tolerate stress

See Addison's Disease; Shock

Adult Respiratory Distress Syndrome

See ARDS

Advance Directives

Anticipatory grieving r/t possible loss of self, significant other

Decisional conflict r/t unclear personal values or beliefs, perceived threat to value system, support system deficit

Potential for enhanced spiritual well-being r/t harmonious interconnectedness with self, others, and higher power/God

Affective Disorders

Altered health maintenance r/t lack of ability to make good judgments regarding ways to obtain help

Chronic low self-esteem r/t repeated unmet expectations

Colonic constipation r/t inactivity, decreased fluid intake

Dysfunctional grieving r/t lack of previous resolution of former grieving response

Fatigue r/t psychological demands

Hopelessness r/t feeling of abandonment, long-term stress

Ineffective individual coping r/t dysfunctional grieving

Risk for loneliness r/t pattern of social isolation and feelings of low self-esteem

Risk for violence: self-directed r/t panic state

Self-care deficit: specify r/t depression, cognitive impairment

Sexual dysfunction r/t loss of sexual desire

Sleep pattern disturbance r/t inactivity

Social isolation r/t ineffective coping

See specific disorder: Depression; Dysthymic Disorder; Manic Disorder, Bipolar I

Aggressive Behavior

Risk for violence: self-directed or directed at others r/t antisocial character, battered woman, catatonic excitement, child abuse, manic excitement, organic brain syndrome, panic states, rage reactions, suicidal behavior, temporal lobe epilepsy, toxic reactions to medication

Agitation

Acute confusion r/t side effects of medication, alcohol abuse or withdrawal, substance abuse or withdrawal, sensory deprivation, sensory overload

Agoraphobia

Anxiety r/t real or perceived threat to physical integrity

Fear r/t leaving home and going out in public places

Impaired social interaction r/t disturbance in self-concept

Ineffective individual coping r/t inadequate support systems

Social isolation r/t altered thought process

Agranulocytosis

Altered health maintenance r/t knowledge deficit of protective measures to prevent infection

Altered protection r/t abnormal blood profile

AIDS (Acquired Immune Deficiency Syndrome)

Altered family processes r/t distress about diagnosis of human immunodeficiency virus (HIV) infection

Altered health maintenance r/t knowledge deficit regarding transmission of infection, lack of exposure to information, misinterpretation of information

Altered nutrition: less than body requirements r/t decreased ability to eat and absorb nutrients secondary to anorexia, nausea, or diarrhea

Altered protection r/t risk for infection secondary to inadequate immune system

Anticipatory grieving: family/parental r/t potential/impending death of loved one

Anticipatory grieving: individual r/t loss of physio-psychosocial well-being

Body image disturbance r/t chronic contagious illness, cachexia

Caregiver role strain r/t unpredictable illness course, presence of situation stressors

Chronic pain r/t tissue inflammation and destruction

Diarrhea r/t inflammatory bowel changes

Energy field disturbance r/t chronic illness

Fatigue r/t disease process, stress, poor nutritional intake

Fear r/t powerlessness, threat to well-being

Hopelessness r/t deteriorating physical condition

Risk for altered oral mucous membranes r/t immunological deficit

Risk for altered thought processes r/t infection in brain

Risk for fluid volume deficit r/t diarrhea, vomiting, fever, bleeding

Risk for impaired skin integrity r/t immunological deficit or diarrhea

Risk for infection r/t inadequate immune system

Risk for loneliness r/t social isolation

Situational low self-esteem r/t crisis of chronic contagious illness

Social isolation r/t self-concept disturbance, therapeutic isolation

Spiritual distress r/t challenged beliefs or moral system

See Cancer; Pneumonia; AIDS in Child

AIDS in Child

Altered parenting r/t congenital acquisition of infection secondary to intravenous (IV) drug use, multiple sexual partners, history of contaminated blood transfusion

See AIDS; Hospitalized Child; Child with Chronic Condition; Terminally Ill Child

AIDS Dementia

Impaired environmental interpretation syndrome r/t viral invasion of nervous system

Airway Obstruction/Secretions

Ineffective airway clearance r/t decreased energy; fatigue; tracheobronchial infection, obstruction, or secretions; perceptual/cognitive impairment; trauma; decreased force of cough because of aging

Alcohol Withdrawal

Acute confusion r/t effects of alcohol withdrawal

Altered health maintenance r/t knowledge deficit regarding chronic illness or effects of alcohol consumption

Altered nutrition: less than body requirements r/t poor dietary habits

Altered thought processes r/t potential delirium tremors

Alcoholism

Anxiety r/t situational crisis, withdrawal
Chronic low self-esteem r/t repeated unmet
  expectations
Ineffective individual coping r/t personal
  vulnerability
Risk for fluid volume deficit r/t excessive diaphoresis,
  agitation, decreased fluid intake
Risk for violence r/t substance withdrawal
Sensory/perceptual alterations; visual, auditory,
  kinesthetic, tactile, olfactory r/t neurochemical
  imbalance in brain
Sleep pattern disturbance r/t effect of depressants,
  alcohol withdrawal, anxiety

Alcoholism

Acute confusion r/t alcohol abuse
Altered family process: alcoholism r/t alcohol abuse
Altered nutrition: less than body requirements r/t
  anorexia
Altered protection r/t malnutrition, sleep deprivation
Anxiety r/t loss of control
Compromised/dysfunctional family coping r/t
  codependency issues
Coping, Defensive r/t alcoholism
Denial, Ineffective r/t refusal to deny alcoholism
Impaired environmental interpretation syndrome r/t
  neurological effects of chronic alcohol intake
Impaired home maintenance management r/t
  memory deficits, fatigue
Impaired memory r/t alcohol abuse
Ineffective individual coping r/t use of alcohol to
  cope with life events
Powerlessness r/t alcohol addiction
Risk for injury r/t alteration in sensory/perceptual
  function
Risk for loneliness r/t unacceptable social behavior
Risk for violence r/t reactions to substances used,
  impulsive behavior, disorientation, impaired
  judgment
Self-esteem disturbance r/t failure at life events
Sleep pattern disturbance r/t irritability, nightmares,
  tremors
Social isolation r/t unacceptable social behavior,
  values

Alkalosis

See Metabolic Alkalosis

Allergies

Altered health maintenance r/t knowledge deficit
  regarding allergies

Alopecia

Body image disturbance r/t loss of hair, change in
  appearance

Alzheimer Type Dementia

Altered health maintenance r/t knowledge deficit of
  caregiver regarding appropriate care
Altered thought processes r/t chronic organic
  disorder
Caregiver role strain r/t duration and extent of
  caregiving required
Chronic confusion r/t Alzheimer's disease
Fear r/t loss of self
Hopelessness r/t deteriorating condition
Impaired environmental interpretation syndrome r/t
  Alzheimer's disease
Impaired home maintenance management r/t
  impaired cognitive function, inadequate support
  systems
Impaired memory r/t neurological disturbance
Impaired physical mobility r/t severe neurological
  dysfunction
Ineffective family coping: compromised r/t altered
  family processes
Powerlessness r/t deteriorating condition
Risk for injury r/t confusion
Risk for loneliness r/t potential social isolation
Risk for violence: directed at others r/t frustration,
  fear, anger
Self-care deficit: specify r/t psychological-
  physiological impairment
Sleep pattern disturbance r/t neurological impairment
  and daytime naps
Social isolation r/t fear of disclosure of memory loss
See Dementia

Amenorrhea

Risk for sexual dysfunction r/t altered body function
See Sexuality, Adolescent

Amnesia

Impaired memory r/t excessive environmental
  disturbance, neurological disturbance
Post-trauma response r/t history of abuse,
  catastrophic illness, disaster, or accident

Amniocentesis

Anxiety r/t threat to self and fetus and unknown future
Decisional conflict r/t choice of treatment pending
  results of test
Risk for infection r/t invasive procedure

Amnionitis

See Chorioamnionitis

Amniotic Membrane Rupture

See Premature Rupture of Membranes

Amputation

Altered health maintenance r/t knowledge deficit of care of stump, rehabilitation

Altered tissue perfusion: peripheral r/t impaired arterial circulation

Body image disturbance r/t negative effects of amputation, response from others

Grieving r/t loss of body part and future life-style changes

Impaired physical mobility r/t musculoskeletal impairment and limited movement

Impaired skin integrity r/t poor healing, prosthesis rubbing

Pain r/t surgery, phantom limb sensation

Risk for fluid volume deficit: hemorrhage r/t vulnerable surgical site

Amyotrophic Lateral Sclerosis

Decisional conflict: ventilator therapy r/t unclear personal values or beliefs, lack of relevant information

Impaired swallowing r/t weakness of muscles involved in swallowing

Impaired verbal communication r/t weakness of muscles of speech, knowledge deficit of ways to compensate and alternative communication devices

Inability to sustain spontaneous ventilation r/t weakness of muscles of respiration

Risk for aspiration r/t impaired swallowing

See Neurological Disorders

Anal Fistula

See Hemorrhoidectomy

Anaphylactic Shock

Inability to maintain spontaneous ventilation r/t acute airway obstruction

See Shock

Anasarca

Fluid volume excess r/t excessive fluid intake, cardiac/renal dysfunction, loss of plasma proteins

Risk for impaired skin integrity r/t impaired circulation to skin

See cause of Anasarca

Anemia

Altered health maintenance r/t knowledge deficit regarding nutritional and medical treatment of anemia

Altered protection r/t bleeding disorder

Anxiety r/t cause of disease

Fatigue r/t decreased oxygen supply to the body and increased cardiac workload

Impaired memory r/t anemia

Risk for injury r/t alteration in peripheral sensory perception

Anemia in Pregnancy

Altered health maintenance r/t knowledge deficit regarding nutrition in pregnancy

Anxiety r/t concerns about health of self and fetus

Fatigue r/t decreased oxygen supply to the body and increased cardiac workload

Risk for infection r/t reduction in the oxygen-carrying capacity of the blood

Anemia, Sickle Cell

See Sickle Cell Anemia/Crisis; Anemia

Anencephaly

See Neurotube Defects

Aneurysm, Abdominal Surgery

Risk for altered tissue perfusion: peripheral r/t impaired arterial circulation

Risk for fluid volume deficit: hemorrhage r/t potential abnormal blood loss

Risk for infection r/t invasive procedure

See Abdominal Surgery

Aneurysm, Cerebral

See Craniectomy/Craniotomy; Subarachnoid Hemorrhage (if aneurysm has ruptured)

Anger

Anxiety r/t situational crisis

Fear r/t environmental stressor, hospitalization

Grieving r/t significant loss

Impaired adjustment r/t assault to self-esteem, disability requiring change in life-style, inadequate support system

Powerlessness r/t health care environment

Risk for violence r/t history of violence, rage reaction

Angina Pectoris

Activity intolerance r/t acute pain, arrhythmias

Altered health maintenance r/t knowledge deficit of care of angina condition

Altered sexuality pattern r/t disease process, medications, loss of libido

Anxiety r/t situational crisis

Decreased cardiac output r/t myocardial ischemia, medication effect, arrhythmia

Grieving r/t pain and life-style changes

Ineffective individual coping r/t personal
vulnerability to situational crisis of new diagnosis,
deteriorating health
Pain r/t myocardial ischemia

Angiocardiography (Cardiac Catheterization)

See Cardiac Catheterization

Angioplasty, Coronary Balloon

Altered health maintenance r/t knowledge deficit
regarding care following procedures, measures to
limit coronary artery disease
Fear r/t possible outcome of interventional procedure
Risk for altered tissue perfusion:
peripheral/cardiopulmonary r/t vasospasm,
hematoma formation
Risk for decreased cardiac output r/t ventricular
ischemia, dysrhythmias
Risk for fluid volume deficit r/t possible damage to
coronary artery, hematoma formation, hemorrhage

Anomaly, Fetal/Newborn (Parent Dealing with)

Altered family processes r/t unmet expectations for
perfect baby, lack of adequate support systems
Altered parenting r/t interruption of bonding process
Anxiety r/t threat to role functioning, situational crisis
Decisional conflict: interventions for fetus/newborn
r/t lack of relevant information, spiritual distress,
threat to value system
Fear r/t real or imagined threat to baby, implications
for future pregnancies, powerlessness
Hopelessness r/t long-term stress, deteriorating
physical condition of child, lost spiritual belief
Ineffective family coping: disabling r/t chronically
unresolved feelings about loss of perfect baby
Ineffective individual coping r/t personal
vulnerability in situational crisis
Knowledge deficit r/t limited exposure to situation
Parental role conflict r/t separation from newborn,
intimidation with invasive or restrictive modalities,
specialized care center policies
Powerlessness r/t complication threatening
fetus/newborn
Risk for altered parent/infant/child attachment r/t
ill infant who is unable to effectively initiate parental
contact as a result of altered behavioral organization
Risk for altered parenting r/t interruption of bonding
process; unrealistic expectations for self, infant, or
partner; perceived threat to own emotional survival;
severe stress; lack of knowledge
Risk for dysfunctional grieving r/t loss of perfect
child

Self-esteem disturbance r/t perceived inability to
produce a perfect child
Spiritual distress r/t test of spiritual beliefs

Anorexia

Altered nutrition: less than body requirements r/t
loss of appetite, nausea, vomiting
Fluid volume deficit r/t inability to drink

Anorexia Nervosa

Activity intolerance r/t fatigue, weakness
Altered nutrition: less than body requirements r/t
inadequate food intake
Altered patterns of sexuality r/t loss of libido from
malnutrition
Altered thought processes r/t anorexia
Body image disturbance r/t misconception of actual
body appearance
Chronic low self-esteem r/t repeated unmet
expectations
Constipation r/t lack of adequate food, fluid intake
Defensive coping r/t psychological impairment, eating
disorder
Diarrhea r/t laxative abuse
Ineffective denial r/t fear of consequences of therapy
and possible weight gain
Ineffective family coping: disabling r/t highly
ambivalent family relationships
Ineffective management of therapeutic regimen:
families r/t family conflict, excessive demands on
family r/t complexity of condition and treatment
Risk for infection r/t malnutrition resulting in
depressed immune system
See Maturational Issues, Adolescent

Anosmia—Loss of Smell

Sensory/perceptual alteration: olfactory r/t altered
sensory reception, transmission, and/or integration

Antepartum Period

See Prenatal Care—Normal; Pregnancy—Normal

Anterior Repair—Anterior Colporrhaphy

Risk for perioperative positioning injury
See Vaginal Hysterectomy

Anticoagulant Therapy

Altered health maintenance r/t knowledge deficit
regarding precautions to take with anticoagulant
therapy
Altered protection r/t altered clotting function from
anticoagulant
Anxiety r/t situational crisis

Risk for fluid volume deficit: hemorrhage r/t altered
 clotting mechanism

Antisocial Personality Disorder

Impaired social interaction r/t sociocultural conflict,
 chemical dependence, inability to form relationships
Ineffective individual coping r/t frequently violating
 the norms and rules of society
Ineffective management of therapeutic regimen:
 families r/t excessive demands on family
Risk for altered parenting r/t inability to function as a
 parent or guardian, emotional instability
Risk for loneliness r/t inability to interact
 appropriately with others
Risk for violence directed at others r/t history of
 violence

Anuria

See Renal Failure

Anxiety

Anxiety r/t unconscious conflict about essential values
 or goals of life, threat to self-concept, threat of death,
 threat to or change in health status, threat to or
 change in role functioning, threat to or change in
 environment, threat to or change in interaction
 patterns, situational or maturational crises,
 interpersonal transmission/contagion, unmet needs

Anxiety Disorder

Altered thought processes r/t anxiety
Anxiety r/t unmet security and safety needs
Decisional conflict r/t low self-esteem, fear of making
 a mistake
Energy field disturbance r/t hopelessness,
 helplessness, fear
Ineffective family coping: disabling r/t ritualistic
 behavior, actions
Ineffective individual coping r/t inability to express
 feelings appropriately
Powerlessness r/t life-style of helplessness
Self-care deficit r/t ritualistic behavior, activities
Sleep pattern disturbance r/t psychological
 impairment, emotional instability

Aortic Aneurysm Repair
(Abdominal Surgery)

See Aneurysm, Abdominal Surgery; Abdominal Surgery

Aortic Valvular Stenosis

See Congenital Heart Disease/Cardiac Anomalies

Aphasia

Altered health maintenance r/t knowledge deficit
 regarding information on aphasia and alternative
 communication techniques
Anxiety r/t situational crisis of aphasia
Impaired verbal communication r/t decrease in
 circulation to brain
Ineffective individual coping r/t loss of speech

Apnea in Infancy

See SIDS; Premature Infant

Apneustic Respirations

Impaired breathing pattern r/t perception/cognitive
 impairment, neurological impairment
See cause of Apneustic Respirations

Appendectomy

Altered health maintenance r/t knowledge deficit
 regarding self-care following appendectomy
Fluid volume r/t fluid restriction, hypermetabolic state,
 nausea and vomiting
Pain r/t surgical incision
Risk for infection r/t perforation/rupture of appendix,
 surgical incision, peritonitis
See Surgery; Hospitalized Child

Appendicitis

Fluid volume deficit r/t anorexia, nausea, and
 vomiting
Pain r/t inflammation
Risk for infection r/t possible perforation of appendix

Apprehension

Anxiety r/t threat to self-concept, threat to health
 status, situational crisis

ARDS (Adult Respiratory Distress
Syndrome)

Impaired gas exchange r/t damage to alveolar-
 capillary membrane, change in lung compliance
Inability to sustain spontaneous ventilation r/t
 damage to the alveolar capillary membrane
Ineffective airway clearance r/t excessive
 tracheobronchial secretions
See Ventilator Client; Child with Chronic Condition

Arrhythmia

See Dysrhythmia

Arterial Insufficiency

Altered tissue perfusion: peripheral r/t interruption
 of arterial flow

A

Arthritis

Activity intolerance r/t chronic pain, fatigue, weakness

Altered health maintenance r/t knowledge deficit regarding care of arthritis

Body image disturbance r/t ineffective coping with joint abnormalities

Chronic pain r/t progression of joint deterioration

Impaired physical mobility r/t musculoskeletal impairment

Self-care deficit: specify r/t pain, musculoskeletal impairment

See Rheumatoid Arthritis, Juvenile

Arthrocentesis

Pain r/t invasive procedure

Arthroplasty—Total Hip Replacement

Constipation r/t immobility

Impaired physical mobility r/t decreased muscle strength, surgery

Pain r/t tissue trauma associated with surgery

Risk for infection r/t invasive surgery, foreign object in body, anesthesia, immobility with stasis of respiratory secretions

Risk for injury r/t interruption of arterial blood flow, dislocation of prosthesis

Risk for perioperative positioning injury r/t immobilization, muscle weakness

Risk for peripheral neurovascular dysfunction r/t orthopedic surgery

See Surgery

Arthroscopy

Altered health maintenance r/t knowledge deficit regarding procedure, postoperative restrictions

Ascites

Altered health maintenance r/t knowledge deficit of care with condition of ascites

Altered nutrition: less than body requirements r/t loss of appetite

Chronic pain r/t altered body function

Ineffective breathing pattern r/t increased abdominal girth

See cause of Ascites; Cirrhosis; Cancer

Asphyxia, Birth

Altered (cerebral) tissue perfusion r/t poor placental perfusion or cord compression resulting in lack of oxygen to the brain

Fear (parental) r/t concern over safety of infant

Impaired gas exchange r/t poor placental perfusion or lack of initiation of breathing by newborn

Inability to sustain spontaneous ventilation r/t brain injury

Ineffective breathing pattern r/t depression of breathing reflex secondary to anoxia

Risk for injury r/t lack of oxygen to brain

Aspiration, Danger of

Risk for aspiration r/t reduced level of consciousness; depressed cough or gag reflexes; presence of tracheostomy or endotracheal tube; incomplete lower esophageal sphincter; presence of gastrointestinal tubes or tube feedings; medication administration; situations hindering elevation of upper body; increased intragastric pressure; increased gastric residual; decreased gastrointestinal motility; delayed gastric emptying; impaired swallowing; facial, oral, or neck surgery or trauma; wired jaws

Assault Victim

Post-trauma response r/t assault

Rape-trauma syndrome r/t rape

Assaultive Client

Altered thought process r/t use of hallucinogenic substance, psychological disorder

Ineffective individual coping r/t lack of control of impulsive actions

Risk for injury r/t confused thought process and impaired judgment

Risk for violence r/t paranoid ideation

Asthma

Activity intolerance r/t fatigue, energy shift to meet muscle needs for breathing to overcome airway obstruction

Altered health maintenance r/t knowledge deficit regarding physical triggers, medications, treatment of early warning signs

Anxiety r/t inability to breathe effectively, fear of suffocation

Body image disturbance r/t decreased participation in physical activities

Impaired home maintenance management r/t knowledge deficit regarding control of environmental triggers

Ineffective airway clearance r/t tracheobronchial narrowing, excessive secretions

Ineffective breathing pattern r/t anxiety

Ineffective individual coping r/t personal vulnerability to a situational crisis

See Child with Chronic Condition; Hospitalized Child

Ataxia

Anxiety r/t change in health status

Body image disturbance r/t staggering gait
Impaired physical mobility r/t neuromuscular impairment
Risk for injury r/t gait alteration

Atelectasis

Impaired gas exchange r/t decreased alveolar-capillary surface
Ineffective breathing pattern r/t loss of functional lung tissue, depression of respiratory function or hypoventilation because of pain

Athlete's Foot

Altered health maintenance r/t knowledge deficit regarding treatment and prevention of athlete's foot
Impaired skin integrity r/t effects of fungal agent

Atrial Septal Defect

See Congenital Heart Disease/Cardiac Anomalies

Attention Deficit Disorder

Risk for altered parenting r/t lack of knowledge of factors contributing to child's behavior
Risk for loneliness r/t social isolation
Self-esteem disturbance r/t difficulty in participating in expected activities
Social isolation r/t unacceptable social behavior

Autism

Altered growth and development r/t inability to develop relations with other human beings, inability to identify own body as separate from those of other people, inability to integrate concept of self
Altered thought processes r/t inability to perceive self or others, cognitive dissonance, perceptual dysfunction
Identity disturbance r/t inability to distinguish between self and environment, inability to identify own body as separate from those of other people, inability to integrate concept of self
Impaired social interaction r/t communication barriers, inability to relate to others
Impaired verbal communication r/t speech and language delays
Ineffective family coping: compromised/disabling r/t parental guilt over etiology of disease, inability to accept or adapt to child's condition, inability to help child and other family members seek treatment
Personal identity disturbance r/t inability to distinguish between self and environment, inability to identify own body as separate from those of other people, inability to integrate concept of self
Risk for self-mutilation r/t autistic state
Risk for violence: self- and other-directed r/t frequent destructive rages towards self or others secondary to

extreme response to changes in routine, fear of harmless things
See Mental Retardation; Child with Chronic Condition

Autonomic Hyperreflexia

Dysreflexia r/t bladder distention, bowel distention, other noxious stimuli

B

Back Pain

Altered health maintenance r/t knowledge deficit regarding prevention of further injury, proper body mechanics
Anxiety r/t situational crisis, back injury
Impaired physical mobility r/t pain
Ineffective individual coping r/t situational crisis, back injury
Pain r/t back injury
Risk for colonic constipation r/t decreased activity
Risk for disuse syndrome r/t severe pain

Barrel Chest

Can also be associated with aging
See COPD

Bathing/Hygiene Problems

Bathing/hygiene self-care deficit r/t intolerance to activity, decreased strength and endurance, pain, discomfort, perceptual or cognitive impairment, neuromuscular impairment, musculoskeletal impairment, depression, severe anxiety

Battered Child Syndrome

Altered family process: alcoholism r/t inadequate coping skills
Altered growth and development: regression vs delayed r/t diminished/absent environmental stimuli, inadequate caretaking, inconsistent responsiveness by caretaker
Altered nutrition: less than body requirements r/t inadequate caretaking
Anxiety/fear r/t threat of punishment for perceived wrongdoing
Chronic low self-esteem r/t lack of positive feedback or excessive negative feedback
Diversional activity deficit r/t diminished/absent environmental or personal stimuli
Impaired skin integrity r/t altered nutritional state, physical abuse
Pain r/t physical injuries

Post-trauma response r/t physical abuse, incest, rape, molestation

Risk for poisoning r/t inadequate safeguards, lack of proper safety precautions, accessibility of illicit substances secondary to impaired home maintenance management

Risk for self-mutilation r/t feelings of rejection, dysfunctional family

Risk for suffocation/aspiration r/t propped bottle, unattended child

Risk for trauma r/t inadequate precautions, cognitive or emotional difficulties

Sleep pattern disturbance r/t hypervigilance, anxiety

Social isolation: family imposed r/t fear of disclosure of family dysfunction and abuse

Battered Person

See Abuse—Spouse, Parent, or Significant Other

Bedbugs, Infestation

Impaired home maintenance management r/t knowledge deficit regarding prevention of bedbug infestation

Impaired skin integrity r/t bites of bedbugs

Bedrest, Prolonged

Disuse syndrome r/t prolonged immobility

Bedsores

See Pressure Ulcer

Bedwetting

See Enuresis

Benign Prostatic Hypertrophy

See BPH; Prostatic Hypertrophy

Bereavement

Grieving r/t loss of significant person

Biliary Atresia

Altered comfort r/t pruritis, nausea

Altered nutrition: less than body requirements r/t decreased absorption of fat and fat-soluble vitamins, poor feeding

Anxiety/fear r/t surgical intervention, possible liver transplantation

Risk for impaired skin integrity r/t pruritis

Risk for ineffective breathing patterns r/t enlarged liver, development of ascites

Risk for injury: bleeding r/t vitamin K deficiency, altered clotting mechanisms

See Hospitalized Child; Child with Chronic Condition; Terminally Ill Child; Cirrhosis (as complication)

Biliary Calculus

See Cholelithiasis

Biliary Obstruction

See Jaundice

Biopsy

Altered health maintenance r/t knowledge deficit regarding biopsy site, further needed health care

Fear r/t outcome of biopsy

Bipolar Disorder I (Most Recent Episode, Depressed or Manic)

Altered health maintenance r/t lack of ability to make good judgments regarding ways to obtain help

Chronic low self-esteem r/t repeated unmet expectations

Dysfunctional grieving r/t lack of previous resolution of former grieving response

Fatigue r/t psychological demands

Ineffective individual coping r/t dysfunctional grieving

Self-care deficit: specify r/t depression, cognitive impairment

Social isolation r/t ineffective coping

See Depression; Manic Disorder, Bipolar I

Birth Asphyxia

See Asphyxia, Birth

Bladder Cancer

Urinary retention r/t clots obstructing urethra

See TURP; Cancer

Bladder Distention

Urinary retention r/t high urethral pressure caused by weak detrusor, inhibition of reflex arc, blockage, strong sphincter

Bladder Training

Altered health maintenance r/t knowledge deficit regarding incontinence self-care

Functional incontinence r/t altered environment; sensory, cognitive, or mobility deficit

Stress incontinence r/t degenerative change in pelvic muscles and structural supports

Urge incontinence r/t decreased bladder capacity, increased urine concentration, overdistention of bladder

Bleeding Tendency

Altered protection r/t abnormal blood profile, drug therapies

Blepharoplasty

Altered health maintenance r/t knowledge deficit regarding postoperative care of surgical area
Body image disturbance r/t effects of surgery

Blindness

Sensory perceptual alteration: visual r/t altered sensory reception, transmission and/or integration

Blood Disorder

Altered protection r/t abnormal blood profile
See cause of Blood Disorder

Blood Pressure Alteration

See Hypertension; Hypotension

Blood Transfusion

Anxiety r/t possibility of harm from transfusion
See Anemia

Body Image Change

Body image disturbance r/t chronic illness, loss of body part, change in body appearance

Body Temperature, Altered

Risk for altered body temperature r/t extremes of age or weight, exposure to cold or hot environment, dehydration, change in activity, effects of medication, dysfunction of body temperature regulation center

Bone Marrow Biopsy

Altered health maintenance r/t knowledge deficit of expectations following procedure, disease treatment following biopsy
Fear r/t unknown outcome of results of biopsy
Pain r/t bone marrow aspiration
See disease necessitating Bone Marrow Biopsy (e.g., Leukemia)

Borderline Personality Disorder

Altered thought process r/t poor reality testing
Anxiety r/t perceived threat to self-concept
Defensive coping r/t difficulty with relationships, inability to accept blame for own behavior
Disturbance in self-concept r/t unmet dependency needs
Ineffective individual coping r/t use of maladjusted defense mechanisms (e.g., projection, denial)
Ineffective management of therapeutic regimen: families r/t manipulative behavior of client
Powerlessness r/t life-style of helplessness
Risk for caregiver role strain r/t inability of care receiver to accept criticism, care receiver taking advantage of others to meet own needs or having unreasonable expectations
Risk for self-mutilation r/t ineffective coping, feelings of self-hatred
Risk for violence: self-directed r/t feelings of need to punish self, manipulative behavior
Social isolation r/t immature interests

Boredom

Diversional activity deficit r/t environmental lack of diversional activity

Botulism

Altered health maintenance r/t knowledge deficit regarding prevention of botulism, care following episode
Fluid volume deficit r/t profuse diarrhea

Bowel Incontinence

Bowel incontinence r/t decreased awareness of need to defecate, loss of sphincter control, fecal impaction

Bowel Obstruction

Altered nutrition: less than body requirements r/t nausea, vomiting
Constipation r/t decreased motility, intestinal obstruction
Fluid volume deficit r/t inadequate fluid volume intake, fluid loss in bowel
Pain r/t pressure from distended abdomen

Bowel Resection

See Abdominal Surgery

Bowel Sounds, Absent or Diminished

Constipation r/t decreased or absent peristalsis
Fluid volume deficit r/t inability to ingest fluids, loss of fluids in bowel

Bowel Sounds, Hyperactive

Diarrhea r/t increased gastrointestinal motility

Bowel Training

Altered health maintenance r/t knowledge deficit regarding treatment of bowel incontinence
Bowel incontinence r/t loss of control of rectal sphincter

BPH (Benign Prostatic Hypertrophy)

Altered health maintenance r/t knowledge deficit regarding self-care with prostatic hypertrophy
Risk for infection r/t urinary residual postvoiding, bacterial invasion of bladder

Bradycardia

Sleep pattern disturbance r/t nocturia
Urinary retention r/t obstruction

Bradycardia

Altered health maintenance r/t knowledge deficit of
condition, effects of cardiac medications
Altered tissue perfusion: cerebral r/t decreased
cardiac output secondary to bradycardia
Decreased cardiac output r/t slow heart rate supplying
inadequate amount of blood for body function
Risk for injury r/t decreased cerebral tissue perfusion

Bradypnea

Ineffective breathing pattern r/t neuromuscular
impairment, pain, musculoskeletal impairment,
perception/cognitive impairment, anxiety,
fatigue/decreased energy, effects of drugs
See cause of Bradypnea

Brain Injury

See Intracranial Pressure, Increased

Brain Surgery

See Craniectomy/Craniotomy

Brain Tumor

Altered thought processes r/t altered circulation or
destruction of brain tissue
Anticipatory grieving r/t potential loss of
physiosocial-psychosocial well-being
Decreased adaptive capacity: intracranial r/t
presence of brain tumor
Fear r/t threat to well-being
Pain r/t neurological injury
Risk for injury r/t sensory-perceptual alterations,
weakness
Sensory/perceptual alteration: specify r/t tumor
growth compressing brain tissue
See Craniectomy/Craniotomy; Cancer; Chemotherapy;
Radiation Therapy; Hospitalized Child; Child with
Chronic Condition; Terminally Ill Child

Braxton Hicks Contractions

Activity intolerance r/t increased perception of
contractions with increased gestation
Altered sexuality patterns r/t fear of contractions
Anxiety r/t uncertainty about beginning labor
Fatigue r/t lack of sleep
Sleep pattern disturbance r/t contractions when lying
down
Stress incontinence r/t increased pressure on bladder
with contractions

Breast Biopsy

Altered health maintenance r/t knowledge deficit
regarding appropriate postoperative care of breasts
Fear r/t potential for diagnosis of cancer

Breast Cancer

Fear r/t diagnosis of cancer
Ineffective individual coping r/t treatment and
prognosis
Sexual dysfunction r/t loss of body part, partner's
reaction to loss
See Cancer; Chemotherapy; Mastectomy; Radiation

Breast-Feeding, Effective

Effective breast-feeding r/t basic breast-feeding
knowledge, normal breast structure, normal infant
oral structure, infant gestational age greater than 34
weeks, support sources or maternal confidence

Breast-Feeding, Ineffective

Ineffective breast-feeding r/t prematurity, infant
anomaly, maternal breast anomaly, previous breast
surgery, previous history of breast-feeding failure,
infant receiving supplemental feedings with artificial
nipple, poor infant sucking reflex, nonsupportive
partner/family, knowledge deficit, interruption in
breast-feeding, maternal anxiety or ambivalence
See Painful Breasts—Engorgement; Painful Breasts—
Cracked Nipples

Breast-Feeding, Interrupted

Interrupted breast-feeding r/t maternal or infant
illness, prematurity, maternal employment,
contraindications to breast-feeding (e.g., drugs, true
breast milk jaundice), need to abruptly wean infant

Breast Lumps

Altered health maintenance r/t knowledge deficit
regarding appropriate care of breasts
Fear r/t potential for diagnosis of cancer

Breast Pumping

Altered health maintenance r/t knowledge deficit
regarding breast milk expression and storage
Anxiety r/t interrupted breast-feeding
Body image disturbance r/t individual response to
breast-feeding process
Decisional conflict r/t infant feeding method
Risk for impaired skin integrity r/t high suction
Risk for infection r/t contaminated breast pump parts,
incomplete emptying of breast

Breath Sounds, Decreased or Absent

See Atelectasis; Pneumothorax

Breathing Pattern Alteration

Ineffective breathing pattern r/t neuromuscular impairment, pain, musculoskeletal impairment, perception/cognitive impairment, anxiety, decreased energy/fatigue

Breech Birth

Altered cerebral tissue perfusion r/t compressed umbilical cord

Anxiety (maternal) r/t threat to self and infant

Impaired gas exchange: fetal r/t compressed umbilical cord

Risk for aspiration: fetal r/t birth of body before head

Risk for impaired tissue integrity: fetal r/t difficult birth

Risk for impaired tissue integrity: maternal r/t difficult birth

Bronchitis

Altered health maintenance r/t knowledge deficit regarding care of condition

Anxiety r/t potential chronic condition

Health-seeking behavior r/t wish to stop smoking

Ineffective airway clearance r/t excessive thickened mucus secretion

Bronchopulmonary Dysplasia

Activity intolerance r/t imbalance between oxygen supply and demand

Altered nutrition: less than body requirements r/t poor feeding, increased caloric needs secondary to increased work of breathing

Fluid volume excess r/t sodium and water retention

See Respiratory Conditions of the Neonate; Child with Chronic Condition; Hospitalized Child

Bronchoscopy

Risk for aspiration r/t temporary loss of gag reflex

Risk for injury r/t complication of pneumothorax, laryngeal edema, hemorrhage (if biopsy done)

Bruits, Carotid

Altered tissue perfusion: cerebral r/t interruption of carotid blood flow

Risk for injury r/t loss of motor, sensory, or visual function

Bryant's Traction

See Traction and Casts

Buck's Traction

See Traction and Casts

Buerger's Disease

See Peripheral Vascular Disease

Bulimia

Altered nutrition: less than body requirements r/t induced vomiting

Chronic low self-esteem r/t lack of positive feedback

Defensive coping r/t eating disorder

Disturbance in body image r/t misperception about actual appearance and body weight

Fear r/t food ingestion and weight gain

Ineffective family coping r/t chronically unresolved feelings of guilt, anger, and hostility

Noncompliance r/t negative feelings toward treatment regimen

Powerlessness r/t urge to purge self after eating

See Maturational Issues, Adolescent

Bunion

Altered health maintenance r/t knowledge deficit regarding appropriate care of feet

Bunionectomy

Altered health maintenance r/t knowledge deficit regarding postoperative care of feet

Impaired physical mobility r/t sore foot

Risk for infection r/t surgical incision, advanced age

Burns

Altered nutrition: less than body requirements r/t increased metabolic needs, anorexia, protein and fluid loss

Altered tissue perfusion: peripheral r/t circumferential burns, impaired arterial/venous circulation

Anticipatory grieving r/t loss of bodily function, loss of future hopes and plans

Anxiety/fear r/t pain from treatments, possible permanent disfigurement

Body image disturbance r/t altered physical appearance

Diversional activity deficit r/t long-term hospitalization

Hypothermia r/t impaired skin integrity

Impaired physical mobility r/t pain, musculoskeletal impairment, contracture formation

Impaired skin integrity r/t injury of skin

Pain r/t injury and treatments

Post-trauma response r/t life-threatening event

Risk for fluid volume deficit r/t loss from skin surface, fluid shift

Risk for ineffective airway clearance r/t potential tracheobronchial obstruction, edema

Risk for infection r/t loss of intact skin, trauma, invasive sites

Risk for peripheral neurovascular dysfunction r/t eschar formation with circumferential burn

See Safety, Childhood; Hospitalized Child

Bursitis

Impaired physical mobility r/t inflammation in joint

Pain r/t inflammation in joint

Bypass Graft

See Coronary Artery Bypass Grafting

C

Cachexia

Altered nutrition: less than body requirements r/t inability to ingest food because of biological factors

Altered protection r/t inadequate nutrition

Calcium Alteration

See Hypercalcemia; Hypocalcemia

Cancer

Activity intolerance r/t side effects of treatment, weakness from cancer

Altered health maintenance r/t knowledge deficit regarding prescribed treatment

Altered nutrition: less than body requirements r/t loss of appetite, difficulty swallowing, side effects of chemotherapy, obstruction by tumor

Altered oral mucous membranes r/t chemotherapy, oral pH changes, decreased/altered oral flora

Altered protection r/t cancer suppressing immune system

Altered role performance r/t change in physical capacity, inability to resume prior role

Anticipatory grieving r/t potential loss of significant others, high risk for infertility

Body image disturbance r/t side effects of treatment, cachexia

Chronic pain r/t metastatic cancer

Colonic constipation r/t side effects of medication, altered nutrition, decreased activity

Decisional conflict r/t selection of treatment choices, continuation/discontinuation of treatment, "do not resuscitate" decision

Fear r/t serious threat to well-being

Hopelessness r/t loss of control, terminal illness

Impaired physical mobility r/t weakness, neuromusculoskeletal impairment, pain

Impaired skin integrity r/t immunological deficit, immobility

Ineffective denial r/t dysfunctional grieving process

Ineffective family coping: compromised r/t prolonged disease or disability progression that exhausts the supportive ability of significant others

Ineffective individual coping r/t personal vulnerability in situational crisis, terminal illness

Potential for enhanced spiritual well-being r/t desire for harmony with self, others, and higher power/God when faced with serious illness

Powerlessness r/t treatment, progression of disease

Risk for disuse syndrome r/t severe pain, change in level of consciousness

Risk for impaired home maintenance management r/t lack of familiarity with community resources

Risk for infection r/t inadequate immune system

Risk for injury r/t bleeding secondary to bone marrow depression

Self-care deficit: specify r/t pain, intolerance to activity, decreased strength

Sleep pattern disturbance r/t anxiety, pain

Social isolation r/t hospitalization, life-style changes

Spiritual distress r/t test of spiritual beliefs

See Chemotherapy; Child with Chronic Condition; Hospitalized Child; Terminally Ill Child

Candidiasis, Oral

Altered health maintenance r/t knowledge deficit regarding care of infected mouth

Altered oral mucous membranes r/t overgrowth of infectious agent, depressed immune function

Capillary Refill Time, Prolonged

Altered tissue perfusion: peripheral r/t interruption of arterial or venous flow

Impaired gas exchange r/t ventilation perfusion imbalance

Risk for peripheral neurovascular dysfunction r/t vascular obstruction

See Shock

Cardiac Catheterization

Altered comfort r/t postprocedure restrictions, invasive procedure

Altered health maintenance r/t knowledge deficit regarding procedure, postprocedure care, and treatment and prevention of coronary artery disease

Anxiety/fear r/t invasive procedure, uncertainty of outcome of procedure

Risk for altered tissue perfusion r/t impaired arterial or venous circulation

Risk for decreased cardiac output r/t ventricular ischemia, dysrhythmias

Risk for injury: hematoma r/t invasive procedure

Risk for peripheral neurovascular dysfunction r/t vascular obstruction

Cardiac Disorders

Decreased cardiac output r/t cardiac disorder
See specific disorder

Cardiac Disorders in Pregnancy

Activity intolerance r/t cardiac pathophysiology, increased demand secondary to pregnancy, weakness, fatigue

Altered family processes r/t hospitalization, maternal incapacitation, changes in role

Altered health maintenance r/t knowledge deficit regarding treatment, restrictions with cardiac disorder

Altered role performance r/t changes in life-style, expectations secondary to disease process with superimposed pregnancy

Anxiety r/t unknown outcomes of pregnancy, family well-being

Fatigue r/t metabolic demands, psychological-emotional demands

Fear r/t potential maternal effects, potential poor fetal/maternal outcome

Ineffective family coping: compromised r/t prolonged hospitalization/maternal incapacitation that exhausts supportive capacity of significant others

Ineffective individual coping r/t personal vulnerability

Powerlessness r/t illness-related regimen

Risk for altered fetal tissue perfusion r/t poor maternal oxygenation

Risk for fluid volume excess r/t compromised regulatory mechanism with increased afterload, preload, and/or circulating blood volume

Risk for impaired gas exchange r/t pulmonary edema

Situational low self-esteem r/t situational crisis, pregnancy

Social isolation r/t limitations of activity, bedrest/hospitalization, separation from family and friends

Cardiac Dysrhythmia

See Dysrhythmia

Cardiac Output Decrease

Decreased cardiac output r/t cardiac dysfunction

Cardiac Tamponade

Decreased cardiac output r/t fluid in pericardial sac
See Pericarditis

Cardiogenic Shock

Decreased cardiac output r/t decreased myocardial contractility, dysrhythmia
See Shock

Caregiver Role Strain

Caregiver role strain r/t pathophysiological factors, developmental factors, psychosocial factors, situational factors

Risk for caregiver role strain r/t pathophysiological factors, developmental factors, psychosocial factors, situational factors

Carious Teeth

See Cavities in Teeth

Carotid Endarterectomy

Altered health maintenance r/t knowledge deficit regarding postoperative care

Fear r/t surgery in vital area

Risk for altered tissue perfusion: cerebral r/t hemorrhage, clot formation

Risk for ineffective airway clearance r/t hematoma compressing trachea

Risk for injury r/t possible hematoma formation

Carpal Tunnel Syndrome

Impaired physical mobility r/t neuromuscular impairment
Pain r/t unrelieved pressure on median nerve

Carpopedal Spasm

See Hypocalcemia

Casts

Altered health maintenance r/t knowledge deficit regarding cast care, personal care with cast

Diversional activity deficit r/t physical limitations from the cast

Impaired physical mobility r/t limb immobilization

Risk for impaired skin integrity r/t unrelieved pressure on skin

Risk for peripheral neurovascular dysfunction r/t mechanical compression from cast

Cataract Extraction

Altered health maintenance r/t knowledge deficit regarding postoperative restrictions

Anxiety r/t threat of permanent vision loss, surgical procedure

Risk for injury r/t increased intraocular pressure, accommodation to new visual field

Sensory/perceptual alteration: vision r/t edema from surgery

Cataracts

Sensory/perceptual alteration: vision r/t altered sensory input

Catatonic Schizophrenia

Altered nutrition: less than body requirements r/t decrease in outside stimulation, loss of perception of hunger, resistance to instructions to eat

Impaired memory r/t cognitive impairment

Impaired physical mobility r/t cognitive impairment, maintenance of rigid posture, inappropriate/bizarre postures

Impaired verbal communication r/t muteness

Social isolation r/t inability to communicate, immobility

See Schizophrenia

Catheterization, Urinary

Altered health maintenance r/t knowledge deficit of normal sensation of catheter in place, care of catheter

Risk for infection r/t invasive procedure

Cavities in Teeth

Altered health maintenance r/t lack of knowledge regarding prevention of dental disease secondary to high-sugar diet, giving infants/toddlers with erupted teeth bottles of milk at bedtime, lack of fluoride treatments, inadequate or improper brushing of teeth

Cellulitis

Altered tissue perfusion: peripheral r/t edema

Impaired skin integrity r/t inflammatory process damaging skin

Pain r/t inflammatory changes in tissues from infection

Cellulitis, Periorbital

Hyperthermia r/t infectious process

Impaired skin integrity r/t inflammation/infection of skin/tissues

Pain r/t edema and inflammation of skin/tissues

Sensory/perceptual alterations: visual r/t decreased visual fields secondary to edema of eyelids

See Hospitalized Child

Central Line Insertion

Altered health maintenance r/t knowledge deficit regarding precautions to take when central line in place

Risk for infection r/t invasive procedure

Cerebral Aneurysm

See Craniectomy/Craniotomy; Intracranial Pressure, Increased; Subarachnoid Hemorrhage

Cerebral Palsy

Altered nutrition: less than body requirements r/t spasticity, feeding or swallowing difficulties

Diversional activity deficit r/t physical impairments, limitations on ability to participate in recreational activities

Impaired physical mobility r/t spasticity, neuromuscular impairment/weakness

Impaired social interaction r/t impaired communication skills, limited physical activity, perceived differences from peers

Impaired verbal communication r/t impaired ability to articulate/speak words secondary to facial muscle involvement

Risk for injury/trauma r/t muscle weakness, inability to control spasticity

Self-care deficit: specify r/t neuromuscular impairments, sensory deficits

See Child with Chronic Condition

Cerebrovascular Accident

See CVA

Cervixitis

Altered health maintenance r/t knowledge deficit regarding care and prevention of condition

Altered pattern of sexuality r/t abstinence during acute stage

Risk for infection r/t spread of infection, recurrence of infection

Cesarean Delivery

Alteration in comfort: nausea, vomiting, pruritis r/t side effects of systemic or epidural narcotics

Altered family processes r/t unmet expectations for childbirth

Altered health maintenance r/t knowledge deficit regarding postoperative care

Altered role performance r/t unmet expectations for childbirth

Anxiety r/t unmet expectations for childbirth, unknown outcome of surgery

Body image disturbance r/t surgery, unmet expectations for childbirth

Fear r/t perceived threat to own well-being

Impaired physical mobility r/t pain

Pain r/t surgical incision, decreased or absent peristalsis secondary to anesthesia, manipulation of abdominal organs during surgery, immobilization, restricted diet

Risk for aspiration r/t positioning for general anesthesia

Risk for fluid volume deficit r/t increased blood loss secondary to surgery

Risk for infection r/t surgical incision, stasis of respiratory secretions secondary to general anesthesia

Risk for urinary retention r/t regional anesthesia

Situational low self-esteem r/t inability to deliver child vaginally

Chemical Dependence

See Alcoholism; Drug Abuse

Chemotherapy

Altered comfort: nausea and vomiting r/t effects of chemotherapy

Altered health maintenance r/t knowledge deficit regarding action, side effects, and way to integrate chemotherapy into life-style

Altered nutrition: less than body requirements r/t side effects of chemotherapy

Altered oral mucous membranes r/t effects of chemotherapy

Altered protection r/t suppressed immune system, decreased platelets

Body image disturbance r/t loss of weight, loss of hair

Fatigue r/t disease process, anemia, drug effects

Risk for altered tissue perfusion r/t anemia

Risk for fluid volume deficit r/t vomiting, diarrhea

Risk for infection r/t immunosuppression

See Cancer

Chest Pain

Fear r/t potential threat of death

Pain r/t myocardial injury, ischemia

Risk for decreased cardiac output r/t ventricular ischemia

See Angina Pectoris; MI

Chest Tubes

Impaired gas exchange r/t decreased functional lung tissue

Ineffective breathing pattern r/t asymmetrical lung expansion secondary to pain

Pain r/t presence of chest tubes, injury

Risk for injury r/t presence of invasive chest tube

Cheyne-Stokes Respiration

Ineffective breathing pattern r/t critical illness

See cause of Cheyne-Stokes Respiration

CHF (Congestive Heart Failure)

Activity intolerance r/t weakness, fatigue

Altered health maintenance r/t knowledge deficit regarding care of disease

Constipation r/t activity intolerance

Decreased cardiac output r/t impaired cardiac function

Fatigue r/t disease process

Fear r/t threat to one's own well-being

Fluid volume excess r/t impaired excretion of sodium and water

Impaired gas exchange r/t excessive fluid in interstitial space of lungs, alveoli

See Congenital Heart Disease/Cardiac Anomalies; Hospitalized Child; Child with Chronic Condition

Chickenpox

See Communicable Diseases, Childhood

Child Abuse

Altered family process: alcoholism r/t inadequate coping skills

Altered growth and development: regression vs delayed r/t diminished/absent environmental stimuli, inadequate caretaking, inconsistent responsiveness by caretaker

Altered nutrition: less than body requirements r/t inadequate caretaking

Altered parenting r/t psychological impairment, physical or emotional abuse of parent, substance abuse, unrealistic expectations of child

Anxiety/fear r/t threat of punishment for perceived wrongdoing

Chronic low self-esteem r/t lack of positive feedback or excessive negative feedback

Diversional activity deficit r/t diminished or absent environmental/personal stimuli

Impaired skin integrity r/t altered nutritional state, physical abuse

Ineffective management of therapeutic regimen: community r/t deficits in community regarding prevention of child abuse

Pain r/t physical injuries

Post-trauma response r/t physical abuse, incest, rape, molestation

Risk for poisoning r/t inadequate safeguards, lack of proper safety precautions, accessibility of illicit substances secondary to impaired home maintenance management

Risk for suffocation/aspiration r/t propped bottle, unattended child

Risk for trauma r/t inadequate precautions, cognitive or emotional difficulties

Sleep pattern disturbance r/t hypervigilance, anxiety

Social isolation: family imposed r/t fear of disclosure of family dysfunction and abuse

Childbirth

See Labor—Normal; Postpartum, Normal Care

Child Neglect

See Child Abuse; Failure to Thrive

Child with Chronic Condition

Activity intolerance r/t fatigue associated with chronic illness

Altered family processes r/t intermittent situational crisis of illness, disease, and hospitalization

Altered growth and development r/t regression or lack of progression toward developmental milestones secondary to frequent or prolonged hospitalization, inadequate or inappropriate stimulation, cerebral insult, chronic illness, effects of physical disability, prescribed dependence

Altered health maintenance r/t exhausting family resources (finances, physical energy, support systems)

Altered nutrition: less than body requirements r/t anorexia, fatigue secondary to physical exertion

Altered nutrition: more than body requirements r/t effects of steroid medications on appetite

Altered sexuality patterns: parental r/t disrupted relationship with sexual partner

Chronic low self-esteem r/t actual or perceived differences; peer acceptance; decreased ability to participate in physical, school, and social activities

Chronic pain r/t physical, biological, chemical, or psychological factors

Decisional conflict r/t treatment options, conflicting values

Diversional activity deficit r/t immobility, monotonous environment, frequent/lengthy treatments, reluctance to participate, self-imposed social isolation

Family coping: potential for growth r/t impact of crisis on family values, priorities, goals, or relationships; changes in family choices to optimize wellness

Hopelessness: child r/t prolonged activity restriction, long-term stress, lack of involvement in or passively allowing care secondary to parental overprotection

Impaired home maintenance management r/t overtaxed family members (e.g., exhausted, anxious)

Impaired social interaction r/t developmental lag/delay, perceived differences

Ineffective family coping: disabling r/t prolonged disease or disability progression that exhausts supportive capacity of significant people

Ineffective family coping: compromised r/t prolonged overconcern for child; distortion of reality regarding child's health problem, including extreme denial about its existence or severity

Ineffective individual coping: child r/t situational or maturational crises

Knowledge deficit: potential for enhanced health maintenance r/t knowledge/skill acquisition regarding health practices, acceptance of limitations, promotion of maximal potential of child and self-actualization of rest of family

Parental role conflict r/t separation from child due to chronic illness, home care of child with special needs, interruptions of family life due to home care regimen

Powerlessness: child r/t health care environment, illness-related regimen, life-style of learned helplessness

Risk for altered parenting r/t impaired/disrupted bonding, caring for child with perceived overwhelming care needs

Risk for infection r/t debilitating physical condition

Risk for noncompliance r/t complex or prolonged home care regimens; expressed intent to not comply secondary to value systems, health beliefs, and cultural/religious practices

Sleep pattern disturbance: child or parent r/t time-intensive treatments, exacerbation of condition, 24-hour care needs

Social isolation: family r/t actual or perceived social stigmatization, complex care requirements

Chills

Hyperthermia r/t infectious process

Chlamydia Infection

See Sexually Transmitted Disease

Choking/Coughing with Feeding

Impaired swallowing r/t neuromuscular impairment

Risk for aspiration r/t depressed cough and gag reflexes

Cholasma

Body image disturbance r/t change in skin color

Cholecystectomy

Altered health maintenance r/t knowledge deficit regarding postoperative care

Altered nutrition: less than body requirements r/t high metabolic needs, decreased ability to digest fatty foods

Pain r/t recent surgery

Risk for fluid volume deficit r/t restricted intake, nausea, vomiting

Risk for ineffective breathing pattern r/t proximity of incision to lungs resulting in pain with deep breathing

See Abdominal Surgery

Cholelithiasis

Altered health maintenance r/t knowledge deficit regarding care of disease

Altered nutrition: less than body requirements r/t anorexia, nausea, vomiting

Pain r/t obstruction of bile flow, inflammation in gallbladder

Chorioamnionitis

Anticipatory grieving r/t guilt about potential loss of ideal pregnancy and birth

Anxiety r/t threat to self and infant

Hyperthermia r/t infectious process

Risk for altered growth and development r/t risk of preterm birth

Risk for infection transmission from mother to fetus r/t infection in fetal environment

Situational low self-esteem r/t guilt about threat to infant's health

Chovstek's Sign

See Hypocalcemia

Chronic Lymphocytic Leukemia

See Leukemia

Chronic Obstructive Pulmonary Disease

See COPD

Chronic Pain

See Pain, Chronic

Chronic Renal Failure

See Renal Failure

Circumcision

Altered health maintenance r/t knowledge deficit (parental) regarding care of surgical area

Pain r/t surgical intervention

Risk for fluid volume deficit r/t hemorrhage

Risk for infection r/t surgical wound

Cirrhosis

Altered health maintenance r/t knowledge deficit regarding correlation between life-style habits and disease process

Altered nutrition: less than body requirements r/t loss of appetite, nausea, vomiting

Altered thought processes r/t chronic organic disorder with increased ammonia levels or substance abuse

Chronic low self-esteem r/t chronic illness

Chronic pain r/t liver enlargement

Diarrhea r/t dietary changes, medications

Fatigue r/t malnutrition

Ineffective management of therapeutic regimen r/t denial of severity of illness

Risk for altered oral mucous membranes r/t altered nutrition

Risk for fluid volume deficit: hemorrhage r/t abnormal bleeding from esophagus

Risk for injury r/t substance intoxication, potential delirium tremors

Cleft Lip/Cleft Palate

Altered health maintenance r/t lack of parental knowledge regarding feeding techniques, wound care, use of elbow restraints

Altered nutrition: less than body requirements r/t inability to feed with normal techniques

Altered oral mucous membranes r/t surgical correction

Fear: parental r/t special care needs, surgery

Grieving r/t loss of perfect child, birth of child with congenital defect

Impaired physical mobility r/t imposed restricted activity, use of elbow restraints

Impaired skin integrity r/t incomplete joining of lip, palate ridges

Impaired verbal communication r/t inadequate palate function and possible hearing loss from infected eustachian tubes

Ineffective airway clearance r/t common feeding and breathing passage, postoperative laryngeal and/or incisional edema

Ineffective breast-feeding r/t infant anomaly

Ineffective infant feeding pattern r/t cleft lip, cleft palate

Pain r/t surgical correction, elbow restraints

Risk for aspiration r/t common feeding and breathing passage

Risk for body image disturbance r/t disfigurement, speech impediment

Risk for infection r/t invasive procedure, disruption of eustachian tube development, aspiration

Clotting Disorder

Altered health maintenance r/t knowledge deficit regarding treatment of disorder

Altered protection r/t clotting disorder

Anxiety/fear r/t threat to well-being

Risk for fluid volume deficit r/t uncontrolled bleeding
See Hemophilia; Anticoagulant Therapy; DIC

Coarctation of the Aorta

See Congenital Heart Disease/Cardiac Anomalies

Cocaine Abuse

Altered thought processes r/t excessive stimulation of
nervous system by cocaine
Ineffective breathing pattern r/t drug effect on
respiratory center
Ineffective individual coping r/t inability to deal with
life stresses
See Substance Abuse

Cocaine Baby

See Crack Baby

Codependency

Caregiver role strain r/t codependency
Decisional conflict r/t support system deficit
Denial r/t unmet self-needs
Impaired verbal communication r/t psychological
barriers
Ineffective individual coping r/t inadequate support
systems
Powerlessness r/t life-style of helplessness

Cognitive Deficit

Altered thought processes r/t neurological impairment

Cold, Viral

Altered comfort: sore throat, aching, nasal
discomfort r/t viral infection
Altered health maintenance r/t knowledge deficit
regarding care of viral condition, prevention of
further infections

Colectomy

Altered health maintenance r/t knowledge deficit
regarding procedure, postoperative care
Altered nutrition: less than body requirements r/t
high metabolic needs, decreased ability to
ingest/digest food
Constipation r/t decreased activity, decreased fluid
intake
Pain r/t recent surgery
Risk for infection r/t invasive procedure
See Abdominal Surgery

Colitis

Diarrhea r/t inflammation in colon
Fluid volume deficit r/t frequent stools
Pain r/t inflammation in colon

See Ulcerative Colitis; Crohn's Disease; Inflammatory
Bowel Syndrome

Collagen Disease

See specific disease (e.g., Lupus Erythematosus;
Rheumatoid Arthritis, Juvenile)

Colostomy

Altered health maintenance r/t knowledge deficit
regarding care of stoma, integrating colostomy care
into life-style
Body image disturbance r/t presence of stoma, daily
care of fecal material
Risk for altered sexuality pattern r/t altered body
image, self-concept
Risk for constipation/diarrhea r/t inappropriate diet
Risk for impaired skin integrity r/t irritation from
bowel contents
Risk for social isolation r/t anxiety about appearance
of stoma and possible leakage

Colporrhaphy, Anterior

See Vaginal Hysterectomy

Coma

Altered family processes r/t illness/disability of family
member
Altered thought processes r/t neurological changes
Ineffective management of therapeutic regimen:
families r/t complexity of therapeutic regimen
Risk for altered oral mucous membranes r/t dry
mouth
Risk for aspiration r/t impaired swallowing, loss of
cough/gag reflex
Risk for disuse syndrome r/t altered level of
consciousness impairing mobility
Risk for impaired skin integrity r/t immobility
Risk for injury r/t potential seizure activity
Self-care deficit: specify r/t neuromuscular impairment
Total incontinence r/t neurological dysfunction
See cause of Coma

Comfort, Loss of

Altered comfort r/t injury agent

Communicable Diseases, Childhood (Measles, Mumps, Rubella, Chickenpox, Scabies, Lice, Impetigo)

Altered comfort r/t hyperthermia secondary to
infectious disease process, pruritis secondary to skin
rash or subdermal organisms
Altered health maintenance r/t nonadherence to
appropriate immunization schedules, lack of
prevention of transmission of infection

Diversional activity deficit r/t imposed isolation from peers, disruption in usual play activities, fatigue, activity intolerance

Pain r/t impaired skin integrity, edema

Risk for infection: transmission to others r/t contagious organisms

See Meningitis/Encephalitis; Respiratory Infections, Acute Childhood; Reye's Syndrome

Communication Problems

Impaired verbal communication r/t decrease in circulation to brain, brain tumor, physical barrier (tracheostomy, intubation), anatomical defect, cleft palate, psychological barriers, cultural differences, developmental lag

Community Coping

Ineffective community coping r/t deficits in social support, inadequate resources for problem solving powerlessness

Potential for enhanced community coping r/t available social supports, available resources for problem solving, community's sense of power to manage stressors

Community Management of Therapeutic Regimen

Ineffective management of therapeutic regimen: community r/t inadequate community resources

Compartment Syndrome

Altered tissue perfusion: peripheral r/t increased pressure within compartment

Fear r/t possible loss of limb, damage to limb

Compulsion

See Obsessive-Compulsive Disorder

Conduction Disorders (Cardiac)

See Dysrhythmia

Confusion, Acute

Acute confusion r/t process causing delirium

Confusion, Chronic

Altered thought processes r/t organic mental disorder, disruption of cerebral arterial blood flow, chemical imbalance, intoxication

Chronic confusion r/t Alzheimer's disease, Korsakoff's psychosis, multiinfarct dementia, cerebral vascular accident, head injury

Congenital Heart Disease/ Cardiac Anomalies

Acyanotic

Patent ductus arteriosus, atrial/ventricular septal defect, pulmonary stenosis, endocardial cushion defect, aortic valvular stenosis, coarctation of the aorta

Cyanotic

Tetralogy of Fallot, tricuspid atresia, transposition of the great vessels, truncus arteriosus, total anomalous pulmonary venous return, hypoplastic left lung

Activity intolerance r/t fatigue, generalized weakness, lack of adequate oxygenation

Altered family processes r/t ill child

Altered growth and development r/t inadequate oxygen and nutrients to tissues

Altered nutrition: less than body requirements r/t fatigue, generalized weakness, inability of infant to suck and feed, increased caloric requirements

Decreased cardiac output r/t cardiac dysfunction

Fluid volume excess r/t cardiac defect, side effects of medication

Impaired gas exchange r/t cardiac defect, pulmonary congestion

Ineffective breathing patterns r/t pulmonary vascular disease

Risk for disorganized infant behavior r/t invasive procedures

Risk for fluid volume deficit r/t side effects of diuretics

Risk for ineffective thermoregulation r/t neonatal age

Risk for poisoning r/t potential toxicity of cardiac medications

See Hospitalized Child; Child with Chronic Illness

Congestive Heart Failure

See CHF

Conjunctivitis

Pain r/t inflammatory process

Risk for injury r/t change in visual acuity

Sensory/perceptual alteration r/t change in visual acuity resulting from inflammation

Consciousness, Altered Level of

Altered thought processes r/t neurological changes

Altered tissue perfusion: cerebral r/t increased intracranial pressure, decreased cerebral perfusion

Decreased adaptive capacity: intracranial r/t brain injury

Disuse syndrome r/t impaired mobility resulting from altered level of consciousness

Impaired memory r/t neurological disturbances

Risk for altered oral mucous membranes r/t dry mouth

Risk for aspiration r/t impaired swallowing, loss of cough/gag reflex

Risk for impaired skin integrity r/t immobility

Self-care deficit: specify r/t neuromuscular impairment

Total incontinence r/t neurological dysfunction

See cause of Altered Level of Consciousness

Constipation

Constipation r/t decreased fluid intake, decreased intake of foods containing bulk, inactivity, immobility, knowledge deficit of appropriate bowel routine, lack of privacy for defecation

Constipation, Colonic with Hard, Dry Stool

Colonic constipation r/t less than adequate fluid and/or dietary intake

Constipation, Perceived

Perceived constipation r/t cultural or family health beliefs, faulty appraisal, impaired thought processes

Continent Ileostomy (Kock Pouch)

Altered health maintenance r/t knowledge deficit regarding postoperative care

Altered nutrition: less than body requirements r/t malabsorption

Ineffective individual coping r/t stress of disease and exacerbations related to stress

Risk for injury r/t failure of valve, stomal cyanosis, intestinal obstruction

See Abdominal Surgery

Contraceptive Method

Decisional conflict: method of contraception r/t unclear personal values or beliefs, lack of experience or interference with decision-making, lack of relevant information, support system deficit

Conversion Disorder

Altered role performance r/t physical conversion system

Anxiety r/t unresolved conflict

Hopelessness r/t long-term stress

Impaired physical mobility r/t physical conversion symptom

Impaired social interaction r/t altered thought process

Ineffective individual coping r/t personal vulnerability

Powerlessness r/t life-style of helplessness

Risk for injury r/t physical conversion symptom

Self-esteem disturbance r/t unsatisfactory or inadequate interpersonal relationships

Convulsions

Altered health maintenance r/t knowledge deficit regarding need for medication and care during seizure activity

Anxiety r/t concern over controlling convulsions

Impaired memory r/t neurological disturbance

Risk for altered thought processes r/t seizure activity

Risk for aspiration r/t impaired swallowing

Risk for injury r/t seizure activity

See Seizure Disorders

COPD (Chronic Obstructive Pulmonary Disease)

Activity intolerance r/t imbalance between oxygen supply and demand

Altered family process r/t role changes

Altered health maintenance r/t knowledge deficit regarding care of disease

Altered nutrition: less than body requirements r/t decreased intake because of dyspnea, unpleasant taste in mouth left by medications

Anxiety r/t breathlessness, change in health status

Chronic low self-esteem r/t chronic illness

Health-seeking behavior r/t wish to stop smoking

Impaired gas exchange r/t ventilation-perfusion inequality

Impaired social interaction r/t social isolation secondary to oxygen use, activity intolerance

Ineffective airway clearance r/t bronchoconstriction, increased mucus, ineffective cough, infection

Noncompliance r/t reluctance to accept responsibility for changing detrimental health practices

Powerlessness r/t progressive nature of the disease

Risk for infection r/t stasis of respiratory secretions

Self-care deficit: specify r/t fatigue secondary to increased work of breathing

Sleep pattern disturbance r/t dyspnea, effects of medications

Coping Problems

Defensive coping r/t superior attitude toward others, difficulty establishing or maintaining relationships, hostile laughter or ridicule of others, difficulty in reality-testing perceptions, lack of follow-through or participation in treatment or therapy

Ineffective individual coping r/t situational crises, maturational crises, personal vulnerability

See Family Problems; Community Coping

Corneal Reflex, Absent

Risk for injury r/t accidental corneal abrasion, drying of cornea

Coronary Artery Bypass Grafting

Altered health maintenance r/t knowledge deficit regarding postprocedure care, life-style adjustment after surgery

Decreased cardiac output r/t dysrhythmia, depressed cardiac function, increased systemic vascular resistance

Fear r/t outcome of surgical procedure

Fluid volume deficit r/t intraoperative fluid loss, use of diuretics in surgery

Pain r/t traumatic surgery

Risk for perioperative positioning injury r/t hypothermia, extended supine position

Costovertebral Angle Tenderness

See Kidney Stone; Pyelonephritis

Cough, Effective/Ineffective

Ineffective airway clearance r/t decreased energy, fatigue, normal aging changes

See Bronchitis; COPD; Pulmonary Edema

Crack Abuse

See Cocaine Abuse

Crack Baby

Altered growth and development r/t effects of maternal use of drugs, neurological impairment, decreased attentiveness to environmental stimuli

Altered nutrition: less than body requirements r/t feeding problems; uncoordinated/ineffective suck and swallow; effects of diarrhea, vomiting, colic

Altered parenting r/t impaired/lack of attachment behaviors, inadequate support systems

Altered protection r/t effects of maternal substance abuse

Diarrhea r/t effects of withdrawal, increased peristalsis secondary to hyperirritability

Disorganized infant behavior r/t prematurity, pain, lack of attachment

Ineffective airway clearance r/t pooling of secretions secondary to lack of adequate cough reflex

Ineffective infant feeding r/t prematurity, neurological impairment

Risk for infection (skin, meningeal, respiratory) r/t effects of withdrawal

Sensory-perceptual alteration r/t hypersensitivity to environmental stimuli

Sleep pattern disturbance r/t hyperirritability, hypersensitivity to environmental stimuli

Crackles in Lungs, Coarse

Ineffective airway clearance r/t excessive secretions in airways, ineffective cough

See cause of Coarse Crackles

Crackles in Lungs, Fine

Ineffective breathing pattern r/t fatigue, surgery, decreased energy

See CHF (cardiac in origin); Infection; Bronchitis or Pneumonia (if from pulmonary infection)

Craniectomy/Craniotomy

Altered tissue perfusion: cerebral r/t cerebral edema, decreased cerebral perfusion, increased intracranial pressure

Decreased adaptive capacity: intracranial r/t brain injury, intracranial hypertension

Fear r/t threat to well-being

Impaired memory r/t neurological surgery

Pain r/t recent surgery, headache

Risk for altered thought processes r/t neurophysiological changes

Risk for injury r/t potential confusion

See Coma (if relevant)

Crepitation, Subcutaneous

See Pneumothorax

Crisis

Anticipatory grieving r/t potential significant loss

Anxiety r/t threat to/change in environment, health status, interaction patterns, situation, self-concept, or role-functioning; threat of death of self or significant other

Energy field disturbance r/t disharmony caused by crisis

Fear r/t crisis situation

Ineffective family coping: compromised r/t situational or developmental crisis

Ineffective individual coping r/t situational or maturational crisis

Situational low self-esteem r/t perception of inability to handle crisis

Spiritual distress r/t intense suffering

Crohn's Disease

Altered health maintenance r/t knowledge deficit regarding management of the disease

Altered nutrition: less than body requirements r/t diarrhea, altered ability to digest and absorb food

Anxiety r/t change in health status

Diarrhea r/t inflammatory process

Ineffective individual coping r/t repeated episodes of diarrhea

Pain r/t increased peristalsis
Powerlessness r/t chronic disease
Risk for fluid volume deficit r/t abnormal fluid loss
    with diarrhea

Croup

See Respiratory Infections, Acute Childhood

Cryosurgery for Retinal Detachment

See Retinal Detachment

Cushing's Syndrome

Activity intolerance r/t fatigue, weakness
Altered health maintenance r/t knowledge deficit
    regarding needed care
Body image disturbance r/t change in appearance
    from disease process
Fluid volume excess r/t failure of regulatory
    mechanisms
Risk for infection r/t suppression of the immune
    system secondary to increased cortisol
Risk for injury r/t decreased muscle strength,
    osteoporosis
Sexual dysfunction r/t loss of libido

CVA (Cerebrovascular Accident)

Altered family process r/t illness, disability of family
    member
Altered health maintenance r/t knowledge deficit
    regarding self-care following CVA
Altered thought processes r/t neurophysiological
    changes
Anxiety r/t situational crisis, change in physical or
    emotional condition
Body image disturbance r/t chronic illness, paralysis
Caregiver role strain r/t cognitive problems of care
    receiver, need for significant home care
Chronic confusion r/t neurological changes
Constipation r/t decreased activity
Grieving r/t loss of health
Impaired home maintenance management r/t
    neurological disease affecting ability to do activities
    of daily living (ADLs)
Impaired memory r/t neurological disturbances
Impaired physical mobility r/t loss of balance and
    coordination
Impaired social interaction r/t limited physical
    mobility, limited ability to communicate
Impaired swallowing r/t neuromuscular dysfunction
Impaired verbal communication r/t pressure damage,
    decreased circulation to the brain in speech center
    informational sources
Ineffective individual coping r/t disability

Reflex incontinence r/t loss of feeling to void
Risk for aspiration r/t impaired swallowing, loss of
    gag reflex
Risk for disuse syndrome r/t paralysis
Risk for impaired skin integrity r/t immobility
Risk for injury r/t sensory-perceptual alteration
Self-care deficit: specify r/t decreased strength and
    endurance, paralysis
Sensory/perceptual alteration: visual, tactile,
    kinesthetic r/t neurological deficit
Total incontinence r/t neurological dysfunction
Unilateral neglect r/t disturbed perception from
    neurological damage

Cyanosis, Central with Cyanosis of Oral Mucous Membranes

Impaired gas exchange r/t alveolar-capillary
    membrane changes

Cyanosis, Peripheral with Cyanosis of Nailbeds

Altered tissue perfusion r/t interruption of arterial
    flow, severe vasoconstriction, cold temperatures
Risk for peripheral neurovascular dysfunction r/t
    condition causing disruption in circulation

Cystic Fibrosis

Activity intolerance r/t imbalance between oxygen
    supply and demand
Altered nutrition: less than body requirements r/t
    anorexia; decreased absorption of nutrients, fat;
    increased work of breathing
Anxiety r/t dyspnea, oxygen deprivation
Body image disturbance r/t changes in physical
    appearance, treatment of chronic lung disease
    (clubbing, barrel chest, home oxygen therapy)
Impaired gas exchange r/t ventilation-perfusion
    imbalance
Impaired home maintenance management r/t
    extensive daily treatment, medications necessary for
    health, mist/oxygen tents
Ineffective airway clearance r/t increased production
    of thick mucus
Risk for caregiver role strain r/t illness severity of
    care receiver, unpredictable course of illness
Risk for fluid volume deficit r/t decreased fluid intake
    and increased work of breathing
Risk for infection r/t thick, tenacious mucus;
    harboring of bacterial organisms; debilitated state
See Child with Chronic Condition; Hospitalized Child;
Terminally Ill Child

Cystitis

Altered health maintenance r/t knowledge deficit regarding methods to treat and prevent urinary tract infections

Altered urinary elimination: frequency r/t urinary tract infection

Pain: dysuria r/t inflammatory process in bladder

Cystocele

Altered health maintenance r/t knowledge deficit regarding personal care, Kegel's exercises to strengthen perineal muscles

Stress incontinence r/t prolapsed bladder

Urge incontinence r/t prolapsed bladder

Cystoscopy

Altered health maintenance r/t knowledge deficit regarding postoperative care

Risk for infection r/t invasive procedure

Urinary retention r/t edema in urethra obstructing flow of urine

D

Deafness

Impaired verbal communication r/t impaired hearing

Sensory perceptual alteration: olfactory r/t alteration in sensory reception, transmission, and/or integration

Death, Oncoming

Anticipatory grieving r/t loss of significant other

Fear r/t threat of death

Ineffective family coping: compromised r/t client's inability to provide support to family

Ineffective individual coping r/t personal vulnerability

Potential for enhanced spiritual well-being r/t desire of client and family to be in harmony with each other and higher power/God

Powerlessness r/t effects of illness, oncoming death

Social isolation r/t altered state of wellness

Spiritual distress r/t intense suffering

See Terminally Ill Child

Decisons, Difficulty Making

Decisional conflict r/t unclear personal values or beliefs, perceived threat to value system, lack of experience or interference with decision-making, lack of relevant information, support system deficit, multiple or divergent sources of information

Decubitus Ulcer

See Pressure Ulcer

Deep Vein Thrombosis

See DVT

Defensive Behavior

Defensive coping r/t nonacceptance of blame, denial of problems or weakness

Dehiscence, Abdominal

Fear r/t threat of death, severe dysfunction

Impaired skin integrity r/t altered circulation, malnutrition, opening in incision

Impaired tissue integrity r/t exposure of abdominal contents to external environment

Pain r/t stretching of abdominal wall

Risk for infection r/t loss of skin integrity

Dehydration

Altered health maintenance r/t knowledge deficit regarding treatment and prevention of dehydration

Altered oral mucous membranes r/t decreased salivation and fluid deficit

Fluid volume deficit r/t active fluid volume loss

See cause of Dehydration

Delirium

Acute confusion r/t effects of medication, response to hospitalization, alcohol abuse, substance abuse, sensory deprivation or overload

Altered thought processes r/t head trauma, altered metabolic state, substance abuse, sleep deprivation, sensory deprivation or overload

Delirium Tremens (DT)

See Alcohol Withdrawal

Delivery

See Labor—Normal

Delusions

Altered thought processes r/t mental disorder

Anxiety r/t content of intrusive thoughts

Impaired verbal communication r/t psychological impairment, delusional thinking

Ineffective individual coping r/t distortion and insecurity of life events

Risk for violence: self-directed or directed at others r/t delusional thinking

Dementia

Altered family process r/t disability of family member

Altered nutrition: less than body requirements r/t psychological impairment

Chronic confusion r/t neurological dysfunction

Impaired environmental interpretation syndrome r/t dementia

Impaired home maintenance management r/t inadequate support system

Impaired physical mobility r/t neuromuscular impairment

Risk for caregiver role strain r/t number of caregiving tasks, duration of caregiving required

Risk for impaired skin integrity r/t altered nutritional status, immobility

Risk for injury r/t confusion, decreased muscle coordination

Self-care deficit: specify r/t psychological or neuromuscular impairment

Sleep pattern disturbance r/t neurological impairment, naps during the day

Total incontinence r/t neuromuscular impairment

Denial of Health Status

Ineffective denial r/t lack of perception about health status effects of illness

Ineffective management of therapeutic regimen r/t denial of seriousness of health situation

Dental Caries

Altered health maintenance r/t lack of knowledge regarding prevention of dental disease secondary to high-sugar diet, giving infants or toddlers with erupted teeth bottles of milk at bedtime, lack of fluoride treatments, inadequate or improper brushing of teeth

Depression (Major Depressive Disorder)

Altered health maintenance r/t lack of ability to make good judgments regarding ways to obtain help

Chronic low self-esteem r/t repeated unmet expectations

Colonic constipation r/t inactivity, decreased fluid intake

Dysfunctional grieving r/t lack of previous resolution of former grieving response

Energy field disturbance r/t disharmony

Fatigue r/t psychological demands

Hopelessness r/t feeling of abandonment, long-term stress

Impaired environmental interpretation syndrome r/t severe mental functional impairment

Ineffective individual coping r/t dysfunctional grieving

Powerlessness r/t pattern of helplessness

Risk for violence: self-directed r/t panic state

Self-care deficit: specify r/t depression, cognitive impairment

Sexual dysfunction r/t loss of sexual desire

Sleep pattern disturbance r/t inactivity

Social isolation r/t ineffective coping

Dermatitis

Altered comfort: pruritis r/t inflammation of skin

Altered health maintenance r/t knowledge deficit regarding methods to decrease inflammation

Anxiety r/t situational crisis imposed by illness

Impaired skin integrity r/t side effect of medication, allergic reaction

Despondency

Hopelessness r/t long-term stress

See Depression

Destructive Behavior toward Others

Ineffective individual coping r/t situational crises, maturational crises, personal vulnerability

Diabetes in Pregnancy

See Gestational Diabetes

Diabetes Insipidus

Altered health maintenance r/t knowledge deficit regarding care of disease, importance of medications

Fluid volume deficit r/t inability to conserve fluid

Diabetes Mellitus

Altered health maintenance r/t knowledge deficit regarding care of diabetic condition

Altered nutrition: less than body requirements r/t inability to use glucose (type I diabetes)

Altered nutrition: more than body requirements r/t excessive intake of nutrients (type II diabetes)

Altered tissue perfusion: peripheral r/t impaired arterial circulation

Ineffective management of therapeutic regimen r/t complexity of therapeutic regimen

Noncompliance r/t restrictive life-style; changes in diet, medication, and exercise

Powerlessness r/t perceived lack of personal control

Risk for altered thought processes r/t hypoglycemia, hyperglycemia

Risk for impaired skin integrity r/t loss of pain perception in extremities

Risk for infection r/t hyperglycemia, impaired healing, circulatory changes

Risk for injury: hypoglycemia or hyperglycemia r/t
   failure to consume adequate calories, failure to take
   insulin

Sensory/perceptual alteration r/t altered tissue
   perfusion

Sexual dysfunction r/t neuropathy associated with
   disease

Diabetes Mellitus, Juvenile (IDDM Type I)

Altered health maintenance r/t parental/child
   knowledge deficit regarding dietary management,
   medication administration, physical activity, and
   interaction between the three; daily changes in diet,
   medications, and activity related to child's growth
   spurts and needs; need to instruct other caregivers
   and teachers regarding signs and symptoms of
   hypoglycemia or hyperglycemia and treatment

Altered nutrition: less than body requirements r/t
   inability of body to adequately metabolize and use
   glucose and nutrients, increased caloric needs of
   child to promote growth and physical activity
   participation with peers

Body image disturbance r/t imposed deviations from
   biophysical and psychosocial norm, perceived
   differences from peers

Impaired adjustment r/t inability to participate in
   normal childhood activities

Pain r/t insulin injections, peripheral blood glucose
   testing

Risk for noncompliance r/t body image disturbance
   and impaired adjustment secondary to adolescent
   maturational crises

See Diabetes Mellitus; Child with Chronic Illness;
Hospitalized Child

Diabetic Coma

Altered thought processes r/t hyperglycemia,
   presence of excessive metabolic acids

Fluid volume deficit r/t hyperglycemia resulting in
   polyuria

Ineffective management of therapeutic regimen r/t
   lack of understanding of preventive measures and
   adequate blood sugar control

Risk for infection r/t hyperglycemia, changes in
   vascular system

See Diabetes Mellitus

Diabetic Ketoacidosis

See Ketoacidosis

Diabetic Retinopathy

Altered health maintenance r/t knowledge deficit
   regarding preserving vision with treatment if
   possible, use of low vision aids

Grieving r/t loss of vision

Sensory–perceptual alteration: visual r/t change in
   sensory reception

Dialysis

See Hemodialysis; Peritoneal Dialysis

Diaphoresis

Altered comfort r/t excessive sweating

Diaphragmatic Hernia

See Hiatus Hernia

Diarrhea

Diarrhea r/t infection, change in diet, gastrointestinal
   disorders, stress, medication effect, impaction

DIC (Disseminated Intravascular Coagulation)

Altered protection r/t abnormal clotting mechanism

Fear r/t threat to well-being

Fluid volume deficit: hemorrhage r/t depletion of
   clotting factors

Risk for altered tissue perfusion: peripheral r/t
   hypovolemia from profuse bleeding, formation of
   microemboli in vascular system

Digitalis Toxicity

Decreased cardiac output r/t drug toxicity affecting
   cardiac rhythm, rate

Ineffective management of therapeutic regimen r/t
   knowledge deficit regarding action, appropriate
   method of administration of digitalis

Dilation and Curretage (D & C)

Altered health maintenance r/t knowledge deficit
   regarding postoperative self-care

Pain r/t uterine contractions

Risk for altered sexuality patterns r/t painful coitus,
   fear associated with surgery on genital area

Risk for fluid volume deficit: hemorrhage r/t
   excessive blood loss during or after the procedure

Risk for infection r/t surgical procedure

Discharge Planning

Altered health maintenance r/t lack of material
   sources

Knowledge deficit r/t lack of exposure to information
   for home care

Impaired home maintenance management r/t family
   member's disease or injury interfering with home
   maintenance

Discomforts of Pregnancy

Alteration in comfort r/t hormonal changes (nausea, ptyalism, leukorrhea, urinary frequency), enlarged uterus (shortness of breath, abdominal distention, pruritus, reduced bladder capacity), and increased vascularization (nasal stuffiness, varicosities)

Body image disturbance r/t pregnancy-induced body changes

Constipation r/t decreased gastrointestinal tract motility, pressure from enlarged uterus, supplementary iron

Fatigue r/t hormonal, metabolic, and body changes

Pain: indigestion and heartburn r/t decreased gastrointestinal tract motility, relaxed cardiac sphincter, enlarged uterus

Hemorrhoids r/t enlarged uterus, constipation, pelvic venous stasis, decreased gastrointestinal tract motility

Joint and backache r/t enlarged uterus, relaxation of joints

Leg cramps r/t nerve compression and calcium/phosphorus/potassium imbalance

Headache r/t vascular and hormonal changes

Risk for injury r/t faintness and/or syncope secondary to vasomotor lability or postural hypotension, venous stasis in lower extremities

Sleep pattern disturbance r/t psychological stress, fetal movement, muscular cramping, urinary frequency, shortness of breath

Stress incontinence r/t enlarged uterus and fetal movement

Dissecting Aneurysm

Fear r/t threat to own well-being
See Aneurysm; Abdominal Surgery

Disseminated Intravascular Coagulation

See DIC

Dissociative Disorder (Not Otherwise Specified)

Alteration in thought processes r/t repressed anxiety

Anxiety r/t psychosocial stress

Disturbance in self-concept r/t childhood trauma, childhood abuse

Impaired memory r/t altered state of consciousness

Ineffective individual coping r/t personal vulnerability in crisis of accurate self-perception

Personal identity disturbance r/t inability to distinguish self caused by multiple personality disorder, depersonalization, or disturbance in memory

Sensory/perceptual alteration: kinesthetic r/t underdeveloped ego

Distress

Anxiety r/t situational crises, maturational crises

Disuse Syndrome, Potential to Develop

Risk for disuse syndrome r/t paralysis, mechanical immobilization, prescribed immobilization, severe pain, altered level of consciousness

Diversional Activity, Lack of

Diversional activity deficit r/t environmental lack of diversional activity

Diverticulitis

Altered nutrition: less than body requirements r/t loss of appetite

Constipation r/t dietary deficiency of fiber and roughage

Diarrhea r/t increased intestinal motility secondary to inflammation

Knowledge deficit r/t diet needed to control disease, medication regimen

Pain r/t inflammation of bowel

Risk for fluid volume deficit r/t diarrhea

Dizziness

Altered tissue perfusion: cerebral r/t interruption of cerebral arterial blood flow

Decreased cardiac output r/t dysfunctional electrical conduction

Impaired physical mobility r/t dizziness

Risk for injury r/t difficulty maintaining balance

Down Syndrome

See Mental Retardation; Child with Chronic Illness

Dress Self (Inability to)

Dressing/grooming self-care deficit r/t intolerance to activity, decreased strength and endurance, pain, discomfort, perceptual or cognitive impairment, neuromuscular impairment, musculoskeletal impairment, depression, severe anxiety

Dribbling of Urine

Stress incontinence r/t degenerative changes in pelvic muscles and structural supports

Drooling

Impaired swallowing r/t neuromuscular impairment, mechanical obstruction

Drug Abuse

Altered nutrition: less than the body requirements r/t poor eating habits

Anxiety r/t threat to self-concept, lack of control of drug use

Ineffective individual coping r/t situational crisis

Noncompliance r/t denial of illness

Risk for injury r/t hallucinations, drug effects

Risk for violence r/t poor impulse control

Sensory/perceptual alterations: specify r/t substance intoxication

Sleep pattern disturbance r/t effects of drugs and/or medications

Drug Withdrawal

Acute confusion r/t effects of substance withdrawal

Altered nutrition: less than body requirements r/t poor eating habits

Anxiety r/t physiological withdrawal

Ineffective individual coping r/t situational crisis, withdrawal

Noncompliance r/t denial of illness

Risk for injury r/t hallucinations

Risk for violence r/t poor impulse control

Sensory/perceptual alterations: specify r/t substance intoxication

Sleep pattern disturbance r/t effects of drugs and/or medications

DTs (Delirium Tremens)

See Alcohol Withdrawal

DVT—Deep Vein Thrombosis

Altered health maintenance r/t knowledge deficit regarding self-care needs, treatment regimen, outcome

Altered tissue perfusion: peripheral r/t interruption of venous blood flow

Colonic constipation r/t inactivity, bedrest

Impaired physical mobility r/t pain in extremity, forced bedrest

Pain r/t vascular inflammation, edema

See Anticoagulant Therapy

Dying Client

See Terminally Ill Adult

Dysfunctional Eating Pattern

Risk for altered nutrition: more than body requirements r/t observed use of food as a reward or comfort measure

See Anorexia Nervosa; Bulimia

Dysfunctional Family Unit

See Family Problems

Dysfunctional Grieving

Dysfunctional grieving r/t actual or perceived loss

Dysfunctional Ventilatory Weaning

Dysfunctional ventilatory weaning response r/t physical, psychological, or situational factors

Dysmenorrhea

Altered health maintenance r/t knowledge deficit regarding prevention and treatment of painful menstruation

Pain r/t cramping from hormonal effects

Dyspareunia

Sexual dysfunction r/t lack of lubrication during intercourse, alteration in reproductive organ function

Dyspepsia

Altered health maintenance r/t knowledge deficit regarding treatment of disease

Anxiety r/t pressures of personal role

Pain r/t gastrointestinal disease, consumption of irritating foods

Dysphagia

Impaired swallowing r/t neuromuscular impairment

Risk for aspiration r/t loss of gag or cough reflex

Dysphasia

Impaired social interaction r/t difficulty in communicating

Impaired verbal communication r/t decrease in circulation to the brain

Dyspnea

Activity intolerance r/t imbalance between oxygen supply and demand

Fear r/t threat to state of well-being, potential death

Impaired gas exchange r/t alveolar-capillary damage

Ineffective airway clearance r/t decrease energy, fatigue

Ineffective breathing pattern r/t decreased lung expansion, neurological impairment affecting respiratory center, extreme anxiety

Sleep pattern disturbance r/t difficulty breathing, positioning required for effective breathing

Dysreflexia

Dysreflexia r/t bladder distention, bowel distention, noxious stimuli

Dysrhythmia

Activity intolerance r/t decreased cardiac output

Altered health maintenance r/t knowledge deficit regarding self-care with disease

Altered tissue perfusion: cerebral r/t interruption of cerebral arterial flow secondary to decreased cardiac output

Anxiety/fear r/t threat of death, change in health status

Decreased cardiac output r/t altered electrical conduction

Dysthymic Disorder

Altered health maintenance r/t inability to make good judgments regarding ways to obtain help

Altered sexual pattern r/t loss of sexual desire

Chronic low self-esteem r/t repeated unmet expectations

Ineffective individual coping r/t impaired social interaction

Sleep pattern disturbance r/t anxious thoughts

Social isolation r/t ineffective coping

Dystocia

Anxiety r/t difficult labor and knowledge deficit regarding normal labor pattern

Fatigue r/t prolonged labor

Grieving r/t loss of ideal labor experience

Ineffective individual coping r/t situational crisis

Pain r/t difficult labor and medical interventions

Powerlessness r/t perceived inability to control outcome of labor

Risk for altered tissue perfusion: cerebral (fetal) r/t difficult labor and birth

Risk for fluid volume deficit r/t hemorrhage secondary to uterine atony

Risk for impaired tissue integrity: maternal and fetal r/t difficult labor

Risk for infection r/t prolonged rupture of membranes

Situational low self-esteem r/t perceived inability to have normal labor and delivery

Dysuria

Altered urinary elimination r/t urinary tract infection

E

Ear Surgery

Altered health maintenance r/t knowledge deficit regarding postoperative restrictions, expectations, and care

Pain r/t edema in ears from surgery

Risk for injury r/t dizziness from excessive stimuli to vestibular apparatus

Sensory/perceptual alteration: hearing r/t invasive surgery of ears, dressings

See Hospitalized Child

Earache

Pain r/t trauma, edema

Sensory perceptual alteration: auditory r/t altered sensory reception, transmission, and/or integration

Eating Disorder

See Anorexia Nervosa; Bulimia; Obesity

Eclampsia

Altered family processes r/t unmet expectations for pregnancy and childbirth

Fear r/t threat of well-being to self and fetus

Risk for altered fetal tissue perfusion r/t uteroplacental insufficiency

Risk for aspiration r/t seizure activity

Risk for fluid volume excess r/t decreased urine output secondary to renal dysfunction

Risk for injury: maternal r/t seizure activity

ECT (Electroconvulsive Therapy)

Decisional conflict r/t lack of relevant information

Fear r/t real or imagined threat to well-being

Impaired memory r/t effects of treatment

See Depression

Ectopic Pregnancy

Altered role performance r/t loss of pregnancy

Body image disturbance r/t negative feelings about the body and reproductive functioning

Fear r/t threat to self, surgery, implications for future pregnancy

Fluid volume deficit r/t loss of blood

Pain r/t stretching or rupture of implantation site

Risk for altered family processes r/t situational crisis

Risk for ineffective individual coping r/t loss of pregnancy

Risk for infection r/t traumatized tissue and blood loss

Risk for spiritual distress r/t grief process

Situational low self-esteem r/t loss of pregnancy, inability to carry pregnancy to term

Eczema

Altered health maintenance r/t knowledge deficit regarding how to decrease inflammation and prevent further outbreaks

Body image disturbance r/t change in appearance from inflamed skin

Impaired skin integrity r/t side effect of medication, allergic reaction

Pain: pruritis r/t inflammation of skin

Edema

Altered health maintenance r/t knowledge deficit regarding treatment of edema

Fluid volume excess r/t excessive fluid intake, cardiac dysfunction, renal dysfunction, loss of plasma proteins

Risk for impaired skin integrity r/t impaired circulation, fragility of skin

See cause of Edema

Elderly Abuse

See Abuse; Spouse, Parent, or Significant Other

Electroconvulsive Therapy

See ECT

Emaciated Person

Altered nutrition: less than body requirements r/t inability to ingest food, digest food, or absorb nutrients because of biological, psychological, or economic factors

Embolectomy

Fear r/t threat of great body harm from embolus

Risk for fluid volume deficit: hemorrhage r/t postoperative complication, surgical area

Risk for peripheral neurovascular dysfunction r/t decreased circulation to extremity

See Surgery—Postoperative Care

Emboli

See Pulmonary Embolism

Emesis

See Vomiting

Emotional Problems

See Coping Problems

Emphysema

See COPD

Encephalitis

See Meningitis/Encephalitis

Endocardial Cushion Defect

See Congenital Heart Disease/Cardiac Anomalies

Endocarditis

Activity intolerance r/t reduced cardiac reserve and prescribed bedrest

Altered health maintenance r/t knowledge deficit regarding treatment of disease, preventive measures against further incidence of disease

Altered tissue perfusion: cardiopulmonary/ peripheral r/t high risk for development of emboli

Decreased cardiac output r/t inflammation of lining of heart and change in structure in valve leaflets, increased myocardial workload

Pain r/t biological injury and inflammation

Risk for alteration in nutrition: less than body requirements r/t fever, hypermetabolic state associated with fever

Endometriosis

Altered health maintenance r/t knowledge deficit about disease condition, medications, and other treatments

Anticipatory grieving r/t possible infertility

Pain r/t onset of menses with distention of endometrial tissue

Sexual dysfunction r/t painful coitus

Endometritis

Altered health maintenance r/t knowledge deficit regarding condition, treatment, and antibiotic regimen

Anxiety r/t prolonged hospitalization, fear of unknown

Hyperthermia r/t infectious process

Pain r/t infectious process in reproductive tract

Energy Field Disturbance

Energy field disturbance r/t disruption in flow of energy as a result of pain, depression, fatigue, anxiety, or stress

Enuresis

Altered health maintenance r/t unachieved developmental task, neuromuscular immaturity, diseases of the urinary system, infections or illnesses such as diabetes mellitus or insipidus, regression in developmental stage secondary to hospitalization or stress, parental knowledge deficit regarding involuntary urination at night after age 6, fluid intake at bedtime, lack of control during sound sleep, male gender

See Toilet Training

Environmental Interpretation Problems

Impaired environmental interpretation syndrome r/t dementia, Parkinson's disease, Huntington's disease, depression, alcoholism

Epididymitis

Altered health maintenance r/t knowledge deficit regarding treatment for pain and infection

Altered pattern of sexuality r/t edema of epididymis and testes

Anxiety r/t situational crisis, pain, threat to future fertility

Pain r/t inflammation in scrotal sac

Epiglottitis

See Respiratory Infections, Acute Childhood

Epilepsy

Altered health maintenance r/t knowledge deficit regarding seizures and seizure control
Anxiety r/t threat to role functioning
Impaired memory r/t seizure activity
Risk for altered thought processes r/t excessive, uncontrolled neurological stimuli
Risk for aspiration r/t impaired swallowing, excessive secretions
Risk for injury r/t environmental factors during seizure
See Seizure Disorders

Episiotomy

Anxiety r/t fear of pain
Body image disturbance r/t fear of resuming sexual relations
Impaired physical mobility r/t pain, swelling, and tissue trauma
Impaired skin integrity r/t perineal incision
Pain r/t tissue trauma
Risk for infection r/t tissue trauma
Sexual dysfunction r/t altered body structure and tissue trauma

Epistaxis

Fear r/t large amount of blood loss
Risk for fluid volume deficit r/t excessive fluid loss

Epstein-Barr Virus

See Mononucleosis

Esophageal Varices

Fear r/t threat of death
Fluid volume deficit: hemorrhage r/t portal hypertension, distended variceal vessels that can easily rupture
See Cirrhosis

Esophagitis

Altered health maintenance r/t knowledge deficit regarding treatment of disease
Pain r/t inflammation of esophagus

ETOH Withdrawal

See Alcohol Withdrawal

Evisceration

See Dehiscence

Exposure to Hot or Cold Environment

Risk for altered body temperature r/t exposure

External Fixation

Body image disturbance r/t trauma and change to affected part
Risk for infection r/t pressure of pins on skin surface
See Fracture

Eye Surgery

Altered health maintenance r/t knowledge deficit regarding postoperative activity, medications, and eye care
Anxiety r/t possible loss of vision
Risk for injury r/t impaired vision
Self-care deficit r/t impaired vision
Sensory/perceptual alteration: visual r/t surgical procedure
See Hospitalized Child

F

Failure to Thrive, Nonorganic

Altered growth and development r/t parental knowledge deficit, lack of stimulation, nutritional deficit, long-term hospitalization
Altered nutrition: less than body requirements r/t inadequate type/amounts of food for infant, inappropriate feeding techniques
Altered parenting r/t lack of parenting skills, inadequate role modeling
Chronic low self-esteem: parental r/t feelings of inadequacy, support system deficiencies, inadequate role model
Disorganized infant behavior r/t lack of boundaries
Risk for altered parent/infant attachment r/t inability of parents to meet infant's needs
Sleep pattern disturbance r/t inconsistency of caretaker, lack of quiet environment
Social isolation r/t limited support systems, self-imposed situation

Family Problems

Altered family process r/t situation transition and/or crises, developmental transition and/or crises
Family coping: potential for growth r/t needs sufficiently gratified and adaptive tasks effectively addressed to enable goals of self-actualization to surface
Ineffective family coping: compromised r/t inadequate or incorrect information or understanding by a primary person; temporary preoccupation by a significant person who is trying to manage emotional conflicts and personal suffering and is unable to perceive or act effectively in regard to client's needs;

temporary family disorganization and role changes; other situational or developmental crises the significant person may be facing; little support provided by client, in turn for primary person; prolonged disease or disability progression that exhausts supportive capacity of significant people

Ineffective family coping: disabling r/t significant person with chronically unexpressed feelings such as guilt, anxiety, hostility, despair, dissonant discrepancy of coping styles for dealing with adaptive tasks by significant person and client or among significant people; highly ambivalent family relationships; arbitrary handling of family's resistance to treatment, which tends to solidify defensiveness as it fails to deal adequately with underlying anxiety

Ineffective management of therapeutic regimen: families r/t complexity of health care system, complexity of therapeutic regimen, decisional conflicts, economic difficulties, excessive demands made on individual or family, family conflict

Fatigue

Energy field disturbance r/t disharmony

Fatigue r/t decreased or increased metabolic energy production, overwhelming psychological or emotional demands, increased energy requirements to perform ADLs, excessive social and/or role demands, states of discomfort, altered body chemistry

Fear

Fear r/t identifiable physical or psychological threat to person

Febrile Seizures

See Seizure Disorders, Childhood

Fecal Impaction

See Impaction of Stool

Fecal Incontinence

Bowel incontinence r/t neurological impairment, gastrointestinal disorders, anorectal trauma

Feeding Problems—Newborn

Ineffective breast-feeding r/t prematurity, infant anomaly, maternal breast anomaly, previous breast surgery, previous history of breast-feeding failure, infant receiving supplemental feedings with artificial nipple, poor infant sucking reflex, nonsupportive partner and family, knowledge deficit, maternal anxiety or ambivalence

Ineffective infant feeding pattern r/t prematurity, neurological impairment or delay, oral hypersensitivity, prolonged NPO

Interrupted breast-feeding r/t maternal or infant illness, prematurity, maternal employment, contraindications to breast-feeding, need to abruptly wean infant

Femoral Popliteal Bypass

Anxiety r/t threat to or change in health status

Pain r/t surgical trauma and edema in surgical area

Risk for altered tissue perfusion: peripheral r/t impaired arterial circulation

Risk for fluid volume deficit: hemorrhage r/t abnormal blood loss

Risk for infection r/t invasive procedure

Risk for neurovascular dysfunction r/t vascular surgery, emboli

Fetal Alcohol Syndrome

See Infant of Substance-Abusing Mother

Fetal Distress/Nonreassuring Fetal Heart Rate Pattern

Altered tissue perfusion: fetal r/t interruption of umbilical cord blood flow

Altered tissue perfusion: placental r/t small or old placenta, interference with gas exchange transplacentally

Fear r/t threat to fetus

Fever

Hyperthermia r/t infectious process, damage to hypothalamus, exposure to hot environment, medications, anesthesia, inability or decreased ability to perspire

Fibrocystic Breast Disease

See Breast Lumps

Filthy Home Environment

Impaired home maintenance management r/t individual or family member disease or injury, insufficient family organization or planning, impaired cognitive or emotional functioning, lack of knowledge, economic factors

Financial Crisis in the Home Environment

Impaired home maintenance management r/t insufficient finances

Fistulectomy

See Hemorrhoidectomy (same nursing care)

Flashbacks

Post-trauma response r/t catastrophic event

Flat Affect

Hopelessness r/t prolonged activity restriction creating isolation, failing or deteriorating physiological condition, long-term stress, abandonment, lost belief in transcendent values or God

Risk for loneliness r/t social isolation, lack of interest in surroundings

Fluid Volume Deficit

Fluid volume deficit r/t active fluid loss, failure of regulatory mechanisms

Fluid Volume Excess

Fluid volume excess r/t compromised regulatory mechanism, excess sodium intake

Foreign Body Aspiration

Altered health maintenance r/t parental knowledge deficit regarding small toys, pieces of toys, nuts, balloons

Impaired home maintenance management r/t insufficient family organization or planning, lack of resources or support systems, inability to maintain orderly and clean surroundings

Ineffective airway clearance r/t obstruction of airway

Risk for suffocation r/t inhalation of small object

See Safety, Childhood

Formula Feeding

Altered health maintenance r/t maternal knowledge deficit regarding formula feeding

Decisional conflict: maternal r/t multiple or divergent sources of information, values conflict, support system deficit

Grieving: maternal r/t loss of desired breast-feeding experience

Risk for altered nutrition: more than body requirements r/t composition of formula and bottle feeding, overuse of food for reward or comfort measures

Risk for constipation: infant r/t iron-fortified formula

Risk for infection: infant r/t lack of passive maternal immunity and supine feeding position

Fractured Hip

See Hip Fracture

Fracture

Altered health maintenance r/t knowledge deficit regarding care of fracture

Diversional activity deficit r/t immobility

Impaired physical mobility r/t limb immobilization

Pain r/t muscle spasm, edema, and trauma

Risk for altered tissue perfusion r/t immobility, presence of cast

Risk for impaired skin integrity r/t immobility, presence of cast

Risk for peripheral neurovascular impairment r/t mechanical compression, treatment of fracture

Frequency of Urination

Altered urinary elimination r/t anatomical obstruction, sensory motor impairment, urinary tract infection

Stress incontinence r/t degenerative change in pelvic muscles and structural support

Urge incontinence r/t decreased bladder capacity, irritation of bladder stretch receptors causing spasm, alcohol, caffeine, increased fluids, increased urine concentration, overdistended bladder

Urinary retention r/t high urethral pressure caused by weak detrusor, inhibition of reflex arc, strong sphincter, blockage

Frostbite

Impaired skin integrity r/t freezing of skin

Pain r/t decreased circulation from prolonged exposure to cold

See Hypothermia

Frothy Sputum

See Pulmonary Edema; CHF; Seizure Disorders

Fusion, Lumbar

Altered health maintenance r/t knowledge deficit regarding postoperative mobility restrictions, body mechanics

Anxiety r/t fear of surgical procedure and possible recurring problems

Impaired physical mobility r/t limitations related to surgical procedure, presence of brace

Pain r/t discomfort at bone donor site

Risk for injury r/t improper body mechanics

Risk for perioperative positioning injury r/t immobilization

G

Gag Reflex, Depressed or Absent

Impaired swallowing r/t neuromuscular impairment

Risk for aspiration r/t depressed cough/gag reflex

Gallop Rhythm

Decreased cardiac output r/t decreased contractility of heart

Gallstones

See Cholelithiasis

Gangrene

Altered tissue perfusion: peripheral r/t obstruction of arterial flow

Fear r/t possible loss of extremity

Gas Exchange, Impaired

Impaired gas exchange r/t ventilation-perfusion imbalance

Gastric Surgery

Risk for injury r/t inadvertent insertion of nasogastric tube through gastric incision line

See Abdominal Surgery

Gastric Ulcer

See Ulcer, Peptic

Gastritis

Altered nutrition: less than body requirements r/t vomiting, inadequate intestinal absorption of nutrients, restricted dietary regimen

Pain r/t inflammation of gastric mucosa

Risk for fluid volume deficit r/t excessive loss from gastrointestinal tract secondary to vomiting, decreased intake

Gastroenteritis

Altered health maintenance r/t knowledge deficit regarding treatment of disease

Altered nutrition: less than body requirements r/t vomiting, inadequate intestinal absorption of nutrients, restricted dietary intake

Diarrhea r/t infectious process involving intestinal tract

Fluid volume deficit r/t excessive loss from gastrointestinal tract secondary to diarrhea, vomiting

Pain r/t increased peristalsis causing cramping

See Gastroenteritis—Child

Gastroenteritis—Child

Altered health maintenance r/t lack of parental knowledge regarding fluid and dietary changes

Impaired skin integrity (diaper rash) r/t acidic excretions on perineal tissues

See Gastroenteritis; Hospitalized Child

Gastroesophageal Reflux

Altered health maintenance r/t knowledge deficit regarding antireflux regimen (e.g., positioning, oral or enteral feeding techniques, medications), possible home apnea monitoring

Altered nutrition: less than body requirements r/t poor feeding, vomiting

Anxiety/fear: parental r/t possible need for surgical intervention (Nissen fundoplication, gastrostomy tube)

Fluid volume deficit r/t persistent vomiting

Ineffective airway clearance r/t reflux of gastric contents into esophagus and tracheal or bronchial tree

Pain r/t irritation of esophagus from gastric acids

Risk for altered parenting r/t disruption in bonding secondary to irritable or inconsolable infant

Risk for aspiration r/t entry of gastric contents in tracheal or bronchial tree

See Hospitalized Child; Child with Chronic Condition

Gastrointestinal Hemorrhage

See GI Bleed

Gastroschisis/Omphalocele

Altered bowel elimination pattern r/t effects of congenital herniated abdominal contents

Anticipatory grieving r/t threatened loss of infant, loss of perfect birth or infant secondary to serious medical condition

Impaired gas exchange r/t effects of anesthesia and subsequent atelectasis

Ineffective airway clearance r/t complications of anesthetic effects

Risk for fluid volume deficit r/t inability to feed secondary to condition and subsequent electrolyte imbalance

Risk for infection r/t disrupted skin integrity with exposure of abdominal contents

Risk for injury r/t disrupted skin integrity and altered protection

See Hospitalized Child; Premature Infant

Gastrostomy

Risk for impaired skin integrity r/t presence of gastric contents on skin

See Tube Feeding

Gestational Diabetes (Diabetes in Pregnancy)

Altered fetal nutrition: more than body requirements r/t excessive glucose uptake

Altered health maintenance: maternal r/t knowledge deficit regarding care of diabetic condition in pregnancy

Altered maternal nutrition: less than body

requirements r/t decreased insulin production and glucose uptake in cells

Anxiety r/t threat to self and/or fetus

Powerlessness r/t lack of control over outcome of pregnancy

Risk for altered tissue integrity: fetal r/t macrosomia, congenital defects, and birth injury

Risk for impaired tissue integrity (maternal) r/t delivery of large infant

See Diabetes Mellitus

GI Bleed (Gastrointestinal Bleeding)

Altered nutrition: less than body requirements r/t nausea, vomiting

Fatigue r/t loss of circulating blood volume, decreased ability to transport oxygen

Fear r/t threat to well-being, potential death

Fluid volume deficit r/t gastrointestinal bleeding

Pain r/t irritated mucosa from acid secretion

Risk for ineffective individual coping r/t personal vulnerability in a crisis, bleeding, hospitalization

Gingivitis

Altered oral mucous membranes r/t ineffective oral hygiene

Glaucoma

Sensory/perceptual alteration: visual r/t increased intraocular pressure

Glomerulonephritis

Altered health maintenance r/t knowledge deficit regarding care of disease

Altered nutrition: less than body requirements r/t anorexia, restrictive diet

Fluid volume excess r/t renal impairment

Pain r/t edema of kidney

Gonorrhea

Altered health maintenance r/t knowledge deficit regarding treatment and prevention of disease

Pain r/t inflammation of reproductive organs

Risk for infection r/t spread of organism throughout reproductive organs

Gout

Altered health maintenance r/t knowledge deficit regarding medications and home care

Impaired physical mobility r/t musculoskeletal impairment

Pain r/t inflammation of affected joint

Grand Mal Seizure

See Seizure Disorders

Grandiosity

Defensive coping r/t inaccurate perception of self and abilities

Graves' Disease

See Hyperthyroidism

Grieving

Anticipatory grieving r/t anticipated significant loss

Dysfunctional grieving r/t actual or perceived significant loss

Grieving r/t actual significant loss; change in life status, style, or function

Groom Self (Inability to)

Dressing/grooming self-care deficit r/t intolerance to activity, decreased strength and endurance pain, discomfort, perceptual or cognitive impairment, neuromuscular impairment, musculoskeletal impairment, depression, severe anxiety

Growth and Development Lag

Altered growth and development r/t inadequate caretaking, indifference, inconsistent responsiveness, multiple caretakers, separation from significant others, environmental and stimulation deficiencies, effects of physical disability, prescribed dependence

Guillain-Barré Syndrome

Inability to sustain spontaneous ventilation r/t weak respiration muscles

See Neurological Disorders

Guilt

Anticipatory grieving r/t potential loss of significant person, animal, or prized material possession

Dysfunctional grieving r/t actual loss of significant person, animal, or prized material possession

Potential for enhanced spiritual well-being r/t desire to be in harmony with self, others, and higher power/God

Self-esteem disturbance r/t unmet expectations of self

H

Hair Loss

Altered nutrition: less than body requirements r/t inability to ingest food because of biological, psychological, or economic factors

Body image disturbance r/t psychological reaction to loss of hair

Halitosis

Altered oral mucous membranes r/t ineffective oral hygiene

Hallucinations

Altered thought processes r/t inability to control bizarre thoughts

Anxiety r/t threat to self-concept

Risk for self-mutilation r/t command hallucinations

Risk for violence: self-directed or directed at others r/t catatonic excitement, manic excitement, rage/panic reactions, response to violent internal stimuli

Head Injury

Altered thought processes r/t pressure damage to brain

Altered tissue perfusion: cerebral r/t effects of increased intracranial pressure

Decreased adaptive capacity: intracranial r/t brain injury

Ineffective breathing patterns r/t pressure damage to breathing center in brain stem

Sensory/perceptual alteration r/t pressure damage to sensory centers in brain

See Neurological Disorders

Headache

Energy field disturbance r/t disharmony

Pain: headache r/t lack of knowledge of pain control techniques or methods to prevent headaches

Health Maintenance Problems

Altered health maintenance r/t significant alteration in communication skills, lack of ability to make deliberate and thoughtful judgments, perceptual or cognitive impairment, ineffective individual coping, dysfunctional grieving, unachieved developmental tasks, ineffective family coping, disabling spiritual distress, lack of material resources

Health-Seeking Person

Health-seeking behavior r/t expressed desire for increased control of own personal health

Hearing Impairment

Impaired verbal communication r/t inability to hear own voice

Sensory/perceptual alteration: auditory r/t altered state of auditory system

Social isolation r/t difficulty with communication

Heartburn

Altered health maintenance r/t knowledge deficit regarding information about factors that cause esophageal reflex

Pain: heartburn r/t gastroesophageal reflux

Risk for altered nutrition: less than body requirements r/t pain after eating

Heart Failure

See CHF

Heart Surgery

See Coronary Artery Bypass Grafting

Heat Stroke

Altered thought processes r/t hyperthermia, increased oxygen needs

Fluid volume deficit r/t profuse diaphoresis

Hyperthermia r/t vigorous activity, hot environment

Helplessness

Hopelessness r/t prolonged activity restriction creating isolation, failing or deteriorating physiological condition, long-term stress, abandonment, lost belief in transcendent values or God

Hematemesis

See GI Bleed

Hematological Disorder

Altered protection r/t abnormal blood profile

See cause of Hematological Disorder

Hematuria

Risk for fluid volume deficit r/t excessive loss of blood through urinary system

Hemianopsia

Anxiety r/t change in vision

Sensory/perceptual alteration r/t altered sensory reception, transmission, and/or integration

Unilateral neglect r/t effects of disturbed perceptual abilities

Hemiplegia

Anxiety r/t change in health status

Body image disturbance r/t functional loss of one side of body

Impaired physical mobility r/t loss of neurological control of involved extremities

Risk for impaired skin integrity r/t alteration in sensation, immobility

Risk for injury r/t impaired mobility

Risk for unilateral neglect r/t neurological impairment; loss of sensation, vision, and/or movement

Self-care deficit: specify r/t neuromuscular impairment

Unilateral neglect r/t effects of disturbed perceptual abilities
See CVA

Hemodialysis

Altered family processes r/t changes in role responsibilities due to therapy regimen
Altered health maintenance r/t knowledge deficit regarding hemodialysis procedure, restrictions, blood access care
Fluid volume excess r/t renal disease with minimal urine output
Ineffective individual coping r/t situational crisis
Noncompliance: dietary restrictions r/t denial of chronic illness
Powerlessness r/t treatment regimen
Risk for caregiver role strain r/t complexity of care receiver treatment
Risk for fluid volume deficit r/t excessive removal fluid during dialysis
Risk for infection r/t exposure to blood products and risk for developing hepatitis B or C
Risk for injury: clotting of blood access r/t abnormal surface for blood flow
See Renal Failure; Renal Failure Acute/Chronic—Child

Hemodynamic Monitoring

Risk for infection r/t invasive procedure
Risk for injury r/t inadvertent wedging of catheter, dislodgment of catheter, disconnection of catheter with embolism

Hemolytic Uremic Syndrome

Altered comfort: nausea/vomiting r/t effects of uremia
Fluid volume deficit r/t vomiting and diarrhea
Risk for impaired skin integrity r/t diarrhea
Risk for injury r/t decreased platelet count, seizure activity
See Renal Failure, Acute/Chronic—Child; Hospitalized Child

Hemophilia

Altered health maintenance r/t knowledge and skill acquisition regarding home administration of intravenous clotting factors, protection from injury
Altered protection r/t deficient clotting factors
Fear r/t high risk for AIDS secondary to contaminated blood products
Impaired physical mobility r/t pain from acute bleeds, imposed activity restrictions
Pain r/t bleeding into body tissues
Risk for injury r/t deficient clotting factors, child's developmental level, age-appropriate play, inappropriate use of toys or sports equipment

See Hospitalized Child; Child with Chronic Condition; Maturational Issues, Adolescent

Hemoptysis

Fear r/t serious threat to well-being
Risk for fluid volume deficit r/t excessive loss of blood
Risk for ineffective airway clearance r/t obstruction of airway with blood and mucus

Hemorrhage

Fear r/t threat to well-being
Fluid volume deficit r/t massive blood loss
See cause of Hemorrhage; Hypovolemic Shock

Hemorrhoidectomy

Altered health maintenance r/t knowledge deficit regarding pain relief, use of stool softeners, dietary changes
Anxiety r/t embarrassment, need for privacy
Colonic constipation r/t fear of pain with defecation
Pain r/t surgical procedure
Risk for fluid volume deficit: hemorrhage r/t inadequate clotting
Urinary retention r/t pain, anesthetic effect

Hemorrhoids

Altered health maintenance r/t knowledge deficit regarding care of condition
Constipation r/t painful defecation, poor bowel habits
Pain: pruritis r/t inflammation of hemorrhoids

Hemothorax

Fluid volume deficit r/t blood in pleural space
See Pneumothorax

Hepatitis

Activity intolerance r/t weakness or fatigue secondary to infection
Altered health maintenance r/t knowledge deficit regarding disease process and home management
Altered nutrition: less than body requirements r/t anorexia, impaired use of proteins and carbohydrates
Diversional activity deficit r/t isolation
Fatigue r/t infectious process, altered body chemistry
Pain r/t edema of liver, bile irritating skin
Risk for fluid volume deficit r/t excessive loss of fluids via vomiting and diarrhea
Social isolation r/t treatment-imposed isolation

Hernia

See Inguinal Hernia Repair; Hiatus Hernia

Herniated Disk

See Low Back Pain

Herniorrhapy

See Inguinal Hernia Repair

Herpes in Pregnancy

Altered health maintenance r/t knowledge deficit regarding treatment of disease, protection of fetus

Altered urinary elimination r/t pain with urination

Fear r/t threat to fetus, impending surgery

Impaired tissue integrity r/t active herpes lesion

Pain r/t active herpes lesion

Risk for infection transmission r/t transplacental transfer during primary herpes, exposure to active herpes during birth process

Situational low self-esteem r/t threat to fetus secondary to disease process

Herpes Simplex I

Altered oral mucous membranes r/t inflammatory changes in mouth

Herpes Simplex II

Altered health maintenance r/t knowledge deficit regarding treatment, prevention of spread of disease

Altered urinary elimination r/t pain with urination

Impaired tissue integrity r/t active herpes lesion

Pain r/t active herpes lesion

Situational low self-esteem r/t expressions of shame or guilt

Hiatus Hernia

Altered health maintenance r/t knowledge deficit regarding care of disease

Altered nutrition: less than body requirements r/t pain after eating

Pain: heartburn r/t gastroesophageal reflux

Hip Fracture

Acute confusion r/t sensory overload, sensory deprivation, medication side effects

Colonic constipation r/t immobility, narcotics, anesthesia

Fear r/t outcome of treatment, future mobility, and present helplessness

Impaired physical mobility r/t surgical incision and temporary absence of weight bearing

Pain r/t injury, surgical procedure

Powerlessness r/t health care environment

Risk for fluid volume deficit: hemorrhage r/t postoperative complication, surgical blood loss

Risk for impaired skin integrity r/t immobility

Risk for infection r/t invasive procedure

Risk for injury r/t dislodged prosthesis, unsteadiness when ambulating

Risk for perioperative positioning injury r/t immobilization, muscle weakness, emaciation

Self-care deficit: specify r/t musculoskeletal impairment

Hip Replacement

See Total Joint Replacement

Hirschsprung's Disease

Altered health maintenance r/t parental knowledge deficit regarding temporary stoma care, dietary management, treatment for constipation or diarrhea

Altered nutrition: less than body requirements r/t anorexia, pain from distended colon

Constipation (bowel obstruction) r/t inhibited peristalsis secondary to congenital absence of parasympathetic ganglion cells in the distal colon

Grieving r/t loss of perfect child, birth of child with congenital defect even though child expected to be normal within 2 years

Impaired skin integrity r/t stoma, potential skin care problems associated with stoma

Pain r/t distended colon, incisional postoperative pain

See Hospitalized Child

Hirsutism

Body image disturbance r/t excessive hair

Hitting Behavior

Acute confusion r/t dementia, alcohol abuse, drug abuse, delirium

Risk for violence: directed at others r/t antisocial character, catatonic or manic excitement, organic brain syndrome, panic states, rage reactions, temporal lobe epilepsy, toxic reactions to drugs

HIV (Human Immunodeficiency Virus)

Altered protection r/t depressed immune system

Fear r/t possible death

See AIDS

Hodgkin's Disease

See Cancer; Anemia

Home Maintenance Problems

Impaired home maintenance management r/t individual or family member disease or injury, insufficient family organization or planning, insufficient finances, unfamiliarity with neighborhood resources, impaired cognitive or emotional functioning, lack of knowledge, lack of role modeling, inadequate support systems

Homelessness

Impaired home maintenance management r/t impaired cognitive or emotional functioning, inadequate support system, insufficient finances

Hopelessness

Hopelessness r/t prolonged activity restriction creating isolation, failing or deteriorating physiological condition, long-term stress, abandonment, lost belief in transcendent values or God

Hospitalized Child

Activity intolerance r/t fatigue associated with acute illness

Altered family processes r/t situational crisis of illness, disease and hospitalization

Altered growth and development r/t regression or lack of progression toward developmental milestones secondary to frequent or prolonged hospitalization, inadequate or inappropriate stimulation, cerebral insult, chronic illness, effects of physical disability, prescribed dependence

Anxiety: separation (child) r/t familiar surroundings and separation from family and friends

Diversional activity deficit r/t immobility, monotonous environment, frequent or lengthy treatments, reluctance to participate, therapeutic isolation, separation from peers

Family coping: potential for growth r/t impact of crisis on family values, priorities, goals, or relationships in family

Fear r/t knowledge deficit or maturational level with fear of unknown, mutilation, painful procedures, surgery

Hopelessness (child) r/t prolonged activity restriction and/or uncertain prognosis

Ineffective family coping: compromised r/t possible prolonged hospitalization that exhausts supportive capacity of significant people

Ineffective individual coping (parent) r/t possible guilt regarding hospitalization of child, parental inadequacies

Pain r/t treatments, diagnostic or therapeutic procedures

Powerlessness: child r/t health care environment, illness-related regimen

Risk for altered growth and development: regression r/t disruption of normal routine, unfamiliar environment or caregivers, developmental vulnerability of young children

Risk for altered nutrition: less than body requirements r/t anorexia, absence of familiar foods, cultural preferences

Risk for altered parent/child attachment r/t separation

Risk for injury r/t unfamiliar environment, developmental age, lack of parental knowledge regarding safety (e.g., side rails, IV site/pole)

Sleep pattern disturbance: child or parent r/t 24-hour care needs of hospitalization

Hostile Behavior

Risk for violence: self-directed or directed at others r/t antisocial personality disorder

HTN (Hypertension)

Altered health maintenance r/t knowledge deficit regarding treatment and control of disease process

Altered nutrition: more than body requirements r/t lack of knowledge of relationship between diet and disease process

Noncompliance r/t side effects of treatments, lack of understanding regarding importance of controlling hypertension

Pain: headache r/t cerebral vascular changes

Hydrocele

Altered sexuality pattern r/t recent surgery on area of scrotum

Pain r/t severely enlarged hydrocele

Hydrocephalus

Altered family processes r/t situational crisis

Altered growth and development r/t sequelae of increased intracranial pressure

Altered nutrition: less than body requirements r/t inadequate intake secondary to anorexia, nausea, and/or vomiting; feeding difficulties

Altered tissue perfusion: cerebral r/t interrupted flow and/or hypervolemia of cerebral ventricles

Decisional conflict: cerebral ventricles r/t unclear or conflicting values regarding selection of treatment modality

Fluid volume excess: cerebral ventricles r/t compromised regulatory mechanism

Impaired skin (tissue) integrity r/t impaired physical mobility, mechanical irritation

Risk for infection r/t sequelae of invasive procedure (shunt placement)

See Premature Infant; Child with Chronic Condition; Hospitalized Child; Mental Retardation (if appropriate)

Hygiene, Inability to Provide Own

Bathing/hygiene self-care deficit r/t intolerance to activity, decreased strength and endurance, pain, discomfort, perceptual or cognitive impairment,

neuromuscular impairment, musculoskeletal
impairment, depression, severe anxiety

Hyperactive Syndrome

Altered role performance: parent r/t stressors
associated with dealing with hyperactive child,
perceived or projected blame for causes of child's
behavior, unmet needs for support or care, lack of
energy to provide for those needs

Decisional conflict r/t multiple or divergent sources of
information regarding education, nutrition, and
medication regimens; willingness to change own
food habits; limited resources

Impaired social interaction r/t impulsive and
overactive behaviors, concomitant emotional
difficulties, distractibility and excitability

Ineffective family coping: compromised r/t
unsuccessful strategies to control excessive activity,
behaviors, frustration, and anger

Parental role conflict: when siblings present r/t
increased attention toward hyperactive child

Risk for altered parenting r/t disruptive or
uncontrollable behaviors of child

Risk for violence: parent or child r/t frustration with
disruptive behavior, anger, unsuccessful
relationship(s)

Self-esteem disturbance/chronic low self-esteem r/t
inability to achieve socially acceptable behaviors;
frustration; frequent reprimands, punishment, or
scoldings secondary to uncontrolled activity and
behaviors; mood fluctuations and restlessness;
inability to succeed academically; lack of peer
support

Hyperalimentation

See TPN

Hyperbilirubinemia

Altered nutrition: less than body requirements:
infant r/t disinterest in feeding because of jaundice-
related lethargy

Anxiety: parents r/t threat to infant and unknown
future

Parental role conflict r/t interruption of family life
because of care regimen

Risk for altered body temperature: infant r/t
phototherapy

Risk for injury: infant r/t kernicterus, phototherapy
lights

Sensory/perceptual alteration: visual (infant) r/t use
of eye patches for protection of eyes during
phototherapy

Hypercalcemia

Altered nutrition: less than body requirements r/t
gastrointestinal manifestations of hypercalcemia
(nausea, anorexia, ileus)

Altered thought processes r/t elevated calcium levels
that cause paranoia

Decreased cardiac output r/t bradydysrhythmia

Impaired physical mobility r/t decreased tone in
smooth and striated muscle

Pain r/t activity

Risk for trauma r/t risk for fractures

Hypercapnea

Fear r/t difficulty breathing

Impaired gas exchange r/t ventilation perfusion
imbalance

Hyperemesis Gravidarum

Altered comfort: nausea r/t hormonal changes of
pregnancy

Altered nutrition: less than body requirements r/t
vomiting

Anxiety r/t threat to self and infant, hospitalization

Fluid volume deficit r/t vomiting

Impaired home maintenance management r/t
chronic nausea, inability to function

Powerlessness r/t health care regimen

Social isolation r/t hospitalization

Hyperglycemia

Ineffective management of therapeutic regimen r/t
complexity of therapeutic regimen, decisional
conflicts, economic difficulties, nonsupportive
family, insufficient cues to action, knowledge
deficits, mistrust, lack of acknowledgement of
seriousness of condition

See Diabetes Mellitus

Hyperkalemia

Risk for activity intolerance r/t muscle weakness

Risk for decreased cardiac output r/t possible
dysrhythmia

Risk for fluid volume excess r/t untreated renal failure

Hypernatremia

Risk for fluid volume deficit r/t abnormal water loss,
inadequate water intake

Hyperosmolar Nonketotic Coma

Altered thought processes r/t dehydration, electrolyte
imbalance

Fluid volume deficit r/t polyuria, inadequate fluid
intake

Risk for injury: seizures r/t hyperosmolar state, electrolyte imbalance
See Diabetes

Hypersensitivity to Slight Criticism

Defensive coping r/t situational crisis, psychological impairment, substance abuse

Hypertension

Altered health maintenance r/t knowledge deficit regarding treatment and control of disease process
Altered nutrition: more than body requirements r/t lack of knowledge of relationship between diet and disease process
Noncompliance r/t side effects of treatment
Pain: headache r/t cerebral vascular changes

Hyperthermia

Hyperthermia r/t exposure to hot environment, vigorous activity, medications, anesthesia, inappropriate clothing, increased metabolic rate, illness, trauma, dehydration, inability or decreased ability to perspire

Hyperthyroidism

Activity intolerance r/t increased oxygen demands from increased metabolic rate
Altered health maintenance r/t knowledge deficit regarding medications, methods of coping with stress
Altered nutrition: less than body requirements r/t increased metabolic rate, increased gastrointestinal activity
Anxiety r/t increased stimulation, loss of control
Diarrhea r/t increased gastric motility
Risk for injury: eye damage r/t exophthalmos
Sleep pattern disturbance r/t anxiety, excessive sympathetic discharge

Hyperventilation

Ineffective breathing pattern r/t anxiety, acid-base imbalance

Hypocalcemia

Activity intolerance r/t neuromuscular irritability
Altered nutrition: less than body requirements r/t effects of vitamin D deficiency, renal failure, malabsorption, laxative use
Ineffective breathing pattern r/t laryngospasm

Hypoglycemia

Altered health maintenance r/t knowledge deficit regarding disease process, self-care

Altered nutrition: less than body requirements r/t imbalance of glucose and insulin level
Altered thought processes r/t insufficient blood glucose to brain
See Diabetes

Hypokalemia

Activity intolerance r/t muscle weakness
Decreased cardiac output r/t possible dysrhythmia from electrolyte imbalance

Hypomania

Sleep pattern disturbance r/t psychological stimulus
See Manic Disorder

Hyponatremia

Altered thought processes r/t electrolyte imbalance
Fluid volume excess r/t excessive intake of hypotonic fluids

Hypoplastic Left Lung

See Congenital Heart Disease/Cardiac Anomalies

Hypotension

Altered thought processes r/t decreased oxygen supply to brain
Altered tissue perfusion: cardiopulmonary/ peripheral r/t hypovolemia, decreased contractility, decreased afterload
Decreased cardiac output r/t decreased preload, decreased contractility
Risk for fluid volume deficit r/t excessive fluid loss
See cause of Hypotension

Hypothermia

Hypothermia r/t exposure to cold environment, illness, trauma, damage to hypothalamus, malnutrition, aging

Hypothyroidism

Activity intolerance r/t muscular stiffness, shortness of breath on exertion
Altered health maintenance r/t knowledge deficit regarding disease process and self-care
Altered nutrition: more than body requirements r/t decreased metabolic process
Altered thought processes r/t altered metabolic process
Colonic constipation r/t decreased gastric motility
Impaired gas exchange r/t possible respiratory depression
Impaired skin integrity r/t edema, dry or scaly skin

Hypovolemic Shock

See Shock

Hypoxia

Altered thought processes r/t decreased oxygen supply to brain

Fear r/t breathlessness

Impaired gas exchange r/t altered oxygen supply, inability to transport oxygen

Impaired memory r/t hypoxia

Ineffective airway clearance r/t decreased energy and fatigue, increased secretions

Hysterectomy

Altered health maintenance r/t knowledge deficit regarding precautions and self-care following surgery

Anticipatory grieving r/t change in body image, loss of reproductive status

Constipation r/t narcotics, anesthesia, bowel manipulation during surgery

Ineffective individual coping r/t situational crisis of surgery

Pain r/t surgical injury

Risk for altered tissue perfusion r/t thrombo-embolism

Risk for fluid volume deficit r/t abnormal blood loss, hemorrhage

Risk for urinary retention r/t edema in area, anesthesia, narcotics, pain

Sexual dysfunction r/t disturbance in self-concept

See Surgery

I

IBS (Irritable Bowel Syndrome)

Altered health maintenance r/t knowledge deficit regarding self-care with IBS

Constipation r/t low-residue diet, stress

Diarrhea r/t increased motility of intestines associated with stress

Ineffective management of therapeutic regimen r/t knowledge deficit, powerlessness

Pain r/t spasms, increased motility of bowel

ICD (Internal Cardioverter Defibrillator)

Preoperative

Anxiety r/t surgical procedure

Knowledge deficit r/t purpose and function of ICD

Postoperative

Altered health maintenance r/t knowledge deficit regarding self-care and care of internal cardiac defibrillator

Risk for decreased cardiac output r/t possible dysrhythmia

Risk for infection r/t invasive surgical procedure

See Coronary Artery Bypass Grafting

IDDM (Insulin-Dependent Diabetes)

See Diabetes Mellitus

Identity Disturbance

Personal identity disturbance r/t situational crisis, psychological impairment, chronic illness, pain

Idiopathic Thrombocytopenia Purpura

See ITP

Ileal Conduit

Altered sexuality pattern r/t altered body function and structure

Body image disturbance r/t presence of stoma

Ineffective management of therapeutic regimen r/t new skills required to care for appliance and self

Knowledge deficit r/t care of stoma

Risk for impaired skin integrity r/t difficulty obtaining tight seal of appliance

Social isolation r/t alteration in physical appearance, fear of accidental spill of ostomy contents

Ileostomy

Altered sexuality pattern r/t altered body function and structure

Body image disturbance r/t presence of stoma

Constipation/diarrhea r/t dietary changes, change in intestinal motility

Ineffective management of therapeutic regimen r/t new skills required to care for appliance and self

Knowledge deficit r/t limited practice of stoma care, dietary modifications

Risk for impaired skin integrity r/t difficulty obtaining tight seal of appliance, caustic drainage

Social isolation r/t alteration in physical appearance, fear of accidental spill of ostomy contents

Ileus

Constipation r/t decreased gastric motility

Fluid volume deficit r/t loss of fluids from vomiting, fluids trapped in bowel

Pain r/t pressure, abdominal distention

Immobility

Altered thought process r/t sensory deprivation from immobility

Altered tissue perfusion: peripheral r/t interruption of venous flow

Constipation r/t immobility

Disuse syndrome r/t immobilization

Impaired physical mobility r/t medically imposed bedrest

Ineffective breathing pattern r/t inability to deep breathe in supine position

Powerlessness r/t forced immobility from health care environment

Risk for impaired skin integrity r/t pressure on immobile parts, shearing forces when moving

Immunosuppression

Altered protection r/t medications/treatments suppressing immune system function

Risk for infection r/t immunosuppression

Impaction of Stool

Colonic constipation r/t decreased fluid intake, less than adequate amounts of fiber and bulk-forming foods in diet, immobility

Imperforate Anus

Altered health maintenance r/t parental knowledge deficit regarding care of impetigo

Anxiety r/t ability to care for newborn

Knowledge deficit r/t home care for newborn

Risk for impaired skin integrity r/t presence of stool at surgical repair site

Impaired skin integrity r/t pruritis

Impetigo

See Communicable Diseases, Childhood

Impotence

Self-esteem disturbance r/t physiological crisis, inability to practice usual sexual activity

Sexual dysfunction r/t altered body function

Inactivity

Impaired physical mobility r/t intolerance to activity, decreased strength and endurance, depression, severe anxiety, musculoskeletal impairment, perceptual or cognitive impairment, neuromuscular impairment, pain, discomfort

Incompetent Cervix

See Premature Dilation of the Cervix

Incontinence of Stool

Bowel incontinence r/t decreased awareness of need to defecate, loss of sphincter control

Knowledge deficit r/t lack of information on normal bowel elimination

Risk for impaired skin integrity r/t presence of stool

Self-care deficit r/t toileting needs

Situational low self-esteem r/t inability to control elimination of stool

Incontinence of Urine

Functional incontinence r/t altered environment; sensory, cognitive, or mobility deficits

Reflex incontinence r/t neurological impairment

Risk for impaired skin integrity r/t presence of urine

Self-care deficit: toileting r/t toileting needs

Situational low self-esteem r/t inability to control passage of urine

Stress incontinence r/t degenerative change in pelvic muscles and structural supports associated with increased age, high intraabdominal pressure (e.g., from obesity, gravid uterus), incompetent bladder outlet, overdistention between voidings, weak pelvic muscles and structural supports

Total incontinence r/t neuropathy preventing transmission of reflex indicating bladder fullness, neurological dysfunction causing triggering of micturation at unpredictable times, independent contraction of detrusor reflex due to surgery, trauma or disease affecting spinal cord nerves, anatomical fistula

Urge incontinence r/t decreased bladder capacity (i.e., history of pelvic inflammatory disease, abdominal surgeries, indwelling urinary catheter); irritation of bladder stretch receptors, causing spasm (e.g., bladder infection); alcohol; caffeine; increased fluids; increased urine concentration; overdistention of bladder

Indigestion

Altered comfort r/t burning, bloating, heaviness, unpleasant sensations experienced when eating

Altered nutrition: less than body requirements r/t discomfort when eating

Induction of Labor

Anxiety r/t medical interventions

Decisional conflict r/t perceived threat to idealized birth

Ineffective individual coping r/t situational crisis of medical intervention in birthing process

Risk for injury: maternal and fetal r/t hypertonic uterus, potential prematurity of newborn

Self-esteem disturbance r/t inability to carry out normal labor

Infant Apnea

See Premature Infant; Respiratory Conditions of the Neonate; SIDS

Infant Feeding Pattern, Ineffective

Ineffective infant feeding pattern r/t prematurity, neurological impairment or delay, oral hypersensitivity, prolonged NPO

Infant of Diabetic Mother

Altered growth and development r/t prolonged and severe postnatal hypoglycemia

Altered nutrition: less than body requirements r/t hypotonia, lethargy, poor sucking, postnatal metabolic changes from hyperglycemia to hypoglycemia and hyperinsulinism

Fluid volume deficit r/t increased urinary excretion and osmotic diuresis

Risk for decreased cardiac output r/t increased incidence of cardiomegaly

Risk for impaired gas exchange r/t increased incidence of cardiomegaly, prematurity

See Premature Infant; Respiratory Conditions of Neonate

Infant Behavior

Disorganized infant behavior r/t pain, oral/motor problems, feeding intolerance, environmental overstimulation, lack of containment/boundaries, prematurity, invasive/painful procedures

Potential for enhanced organized infant behavior r/t prematurity, pain

Risk for disorganized infant behavior r/t pain, oral/motor problems, environmental overstimulation, lack of containment/boundaries

Infant of Substance-Abusing Mother (Fetal Alcohol Syndrome, Crack Baby, Other Drug Withdrawal Infants)

Altered growth and development r/t effects of maternal use of drugs, effects of neurological impairment, decreased attentiveness to environmental stimuli or inadequate stimuli

Altered nutrition: less than body requirements r/t feeding problems; uncoordinated or ineffective suck and swallow; effects of diarrhea, vomiting, or colic associated with maternal substance abuse

Altered parenting r/t impaired or absent attachment behaviors, inadequate support systems

Altered protection r/t effects of maternal substance abuse

Diarrhea r/t effects of withdrawal, increased peristalsis secondary to hyperirritability

Ineffective airway clearance r/t pooling of secretions secondary to lack of adequate cough reflex, effects of viral or bacterial lower airway infection secondary to altered protective state

Ineffective infant feeding pattern r/t uncoordinated or ineffective sucking reflex

Interrupted breast-feeding r/t use of drugs or alcohol by mother

Risk for infection: skin, meningeal, respiratory r/t effects of withdrawal

Sensory-perceptual alteration r/t hypersensitivity to environmental stimuli

Sleep pattern disturbance r/t hyperirritability/hypersensitivity to environmental stimuli

See Failure to Thrive, Nonorganic; SIDS; Hospitalized Child; Cerebral Palsy; Hyperactive Syndrome

Infantile Spasms

See Seizure Disorders, Childhood

Infection

Altered protection r/t inadequate nutrition, abnormal blood profiles, drug therapies, treatments

Hyperthermia r/t increased metabolic rate

Infection, Potential for

Risk for infection r/t inadequate primary defenses (e.g., broken skin, traumatized tissue, decrease in ciliary action, stasis of body fluids, change in pH secretions, altered peristalsis), inadequate secondary defenses (e.g., decreased hemoglobin, leukopenia suppressed inflammatory response), immuno-suppression, inadequate acquired immunity, tissue destruction and increased environmental exposure, chronic disease, invasive procedures, malnutrition, pharmaceutical agents, trauma, rupture of amniotic membranes, insufficient knowledge to avoid exposure to pathogens

Inflammatory Bowel Disease (Child and Adult)

Altered nutrition: less than body requirements r/t anorexia, decreased absorption of nutrients from gastrointestinal tract

Diarrhea r/t effects of inflammatory changes of the bowel

Fluid volume deficit r/t frequent and loose stools

Impaired skin integrity r/t frequent stools, development of anal fissures

Ineffective individual coping r/t repeated episodes of diarrhea

Pain r/t abdominal cramping and anal irritation
Social isolation r/t diarrhea
See Crohn's Disease; Hospitalized Child; Child with
Chronic Condition; Maturational Issues, Adolescent

Influenza

Altered health maintenance r/t knowledge deficit
regarding self-care
Fluid volume deficit r/t inadequate fluid intake
Hyperthermia r/t infectious process
Ineffective management of therapeutic regimen r/t
lack of knowledge regarding preventive
immunizations
Pain r/t inflammatory changes in joints

Inguinal Hernia Repair

Impaired physical mobility r/t pain at surgical site and
fear of causing hernia to "break open"
Pain r/t surgical procedure
Risk for infection r/t surgical procedure
Urinary retention r/t possible edema at surgical site

Injury

Risk for injury r/t environmental conditons interacting
with client's adaptive and defensive resources

Insomnia

Anxiety r/t actual or perceived loss of sleep
Sleep pattern disturbance r/t sensory alterations,
internal factors, external factors

Insulin Shock

See Hypoglycemia

Intermittent Claudication

Altered tissue perfusion: peripheral r/t interruption
of arterial flow
Knowledge deficit r/t lack of knowledge of cause and
treatment of peripheral vascular diseases
Pain r/t decreased circulation to extremities with
activity
Risk for injury r/t tissue hypoxia
Risk for peripheral neurovascular dysfunction r/t
disruption in arterial flow
See Peripheral Vascular Disease

Internal Cardioverter Defibrillator

See ICD

Internal Fixation

Risk for infection r/t traumatized tissue, broken skin
See Fracture

Interstitial Cystitis

Altered urinary elimination r/t inflammation of
bladder
Pain r/t inflammatory process
Risk for infection r/t suppressed inflammatory
response

Intervertebral Disk Excision

See Laminectomy

Intestinal Obstruction

See Ileus

Intoxication

Acute confusion r/t alcohol abuse
Altered thought process r/t effect of substance on
central nervous sytem
Anxiety r/t loss of control of actions
Ineffective individual coping r/t use of mind-altering
substances as a means of coping
Risk for violence r/t inability to control thoughts and
actions
Sensory/perceptual alterations: visual, auditory,
kinesthetic, tactile, olfactory r/t neurochemical
imbalance in brain

Intraaortic Balloon Counterpulsation

Anxiety r/t device providing cardiovascular assistance
Decreased cardiac output r/t failing heart needing
counterpulsation
Impaired physical mobility r/t restriction of movement
because of mechanical device
Risk for peripheral neurovascular dysfunction r/t
vascular obstruction of balloon catheter, thrombus
formation, emboli, edema

Intracranial Pressure, Increased

Acute confusion r/t increased intracranial pressure
Altered thought processes r/t pressure damage to
brain
Altered tissue perfusion: cerebral r/t effects of
increased intracranial pressure
Decreased adaptive capacity: intracranial r/t
sustained increase in intracranial pressure (10 to 15
mm Hg)
Ineffective breathing patterns r/t pressure damage to
breathing center in brain stem
Sensory/perceptual alteration r/t pressure damage to
sensory centers in brain
See cause of Increased Intracranial Pressure

Intrauterine Growth Retardation

Altered growth and development r/t insufficient
supply of oxygen and nutrients

Altered nutrition: less than body requirements r/t
insufficient placenta
Anxiety: maternal r/t threat to fetus
Impaired gas exchange r/t insufficient placental
perfusion
Ineffective individual coping: maternal r/t situational
crisis, threat to fetus
Risk for injury r/t insufficient supply of oxygen and
nutrients
Situational low self-esteem: maternal r/t guilt about
threat to fetus

Intubation—Endotracheal or Nasogastric

Altered nutrition: less than body requirements r/t
inability to ingest food due to presence of tubes
Altered oral mucous membranes r/t presence of tubes
Body image disturbance r/t altered appearance with
mechanical devices
Impaired verbal communication r/t endotracheal tube

Irregular Pulse

See Dysrhythmia

Irritable Bowel Syndrome

See IBS

Isolation

Risk for loneliness r/t lack of affection, physical
isolation, cathectic deprivation, social isolation
Social isolation r/t factors contributing to absence of
satisfying personal relationships, such as delay in
accomplishing developmental tasks, immature
interests, alterations in mental status, unacceptable
social behavior, unacceptable social values, altered
state of wellness, inadequate personal resources,
inability to engage in satisfying personal
relationships

Itching

Altered comfort r/t irritation of the skin
Risk for infection r/t potential break in skin

ITP (Idiopathic Thrombocytopenia Purpura)

Altered protection r/t decreased platelet count
Diversional activity deficit r/t activity restrictions,
safety precautions
Impaired home health maintenance r/t parental lack
of ability to follow through with safety precautions
secondary to child's developmental stage (active
toddler)
Risk for injury r/t decreased platelet count,
developmental level, age-appropriate play
See Hospitalized Child

J

Jaundice

Altered comfort: pruritis r/t toxic metabolites
excreted in the skin
Altered thought processes r/t toxic blood metabolites
Risk for impaired skin integrity r/t pruritis, itching
See Cirrhosis

Jaw Surgery

Altered nutrition: less than body requirements r/t
jaws being wired closed
Impaired swallowing r/t edema from surgery
Knowledge deficit r/t emergency care for wired jaw
(e.g., cutting bands and wires), oral care
Pain r/t surgical procedure
Risk for aspiration r/t wired jaw

Jittery

Anxiety r/t unconscious conflict about essential values
and goals, threat to or change in health status

Joint Replacement

Risk for peripheral neurovascular dysfunction r/t
orthopedic surgery
See Total Joint Replacement

JRA (Juvenile Rheumatoid Arthritis)

See Rheumatoid Arthritis, Juvenile

K

Kaposi's Sarcoma

See AIDS

Kawasaki Syndrome (Formerly called "Mucocutaneous Lymph Node Syndrome")

Altered nutrition: less than body requirements r/t
altered oral mucous membranes
Altered oral mucous membranes r/t inflamed mouth
and pharynx; swollen lips that become dry, cracked,
and fissured
Anxiety: parental r/t progression of disease,
complications of arthritis and cardiac involvement
Hyperthermia r/t inflammatory disease process
Impaired skin integrity r/t inflammatory skin changes
Pain r/t enlarged lymph nodes; erythematous skin rash
that progresses to desquamation, peeling, and
denuding of skin
See Hospitalized Child

Kegel's Exercise

Health-seeking behavior r/t desire for information to relieve incontinence

Stress incontinence r/t degenerative change in pelvic muscles

Urge incontinence r/t decreased bladder capacity

Ketoacidosis

Altered nutrition: less than body requirements r/t body's inability to use nutrients

Fluid volume deficit r/t excess excretion of urine, nausea, vomiting, increased respiration

Impaired memory r/t fluid and electrolyte imbalance

Ineffective management of therapeutic regimen r/t denial of illness, lack of understanding of preventive measures and adequate blood sugar control

Noncompliance (with diabetic regimen) r/t ineffective coping with chronic disease

See Diabetes Mellitus

Kidney Failure

See Renal Failure

Kidney Stone

Altered patterns of urinary elimination: frequency, urgency r/t anatomical obstruction, irritation caused by stone

Knowledge deficit r/t fluid requirements and dietary restrictions

Pain r/t obstruction from renal calculi

Risk for fluid volume deficit r/t nausea, vomiting

Risk for infection r/t obstruction of urinary tract with stasis of urine

Knee Replacement

See Total Joint Replacement

Knowledge Deficit

Altered health maintenance r/t lack of or significant alteration in communication skills (written, verbal, and/or gestural)

Knowledge deficit r/t lack of exposure, lack of recall, information misinterpretation, cognitive limitation, lack of interest in learning, unfamiliarity with information resources

Kock Pouch

See Continent Ileostomy

Korsakoff's Syndrome

Acute confusion r/t alcohol abuse

Impaired memory r/t neurological changes

Risk for altered nutrition r/t lack of adequate balanced intake

Risk for injury r/t sensory dysfunction, lack of coordination when ambulating

L

Labor, Induction of

See Induction of Labor

Labor—Normal

Anxiety r/t fear of the unknown, situational crisis

Fatigue r/t childbirth

Health-seeking behaviors r/t healthy outcome of pregnancy, prenatal care, and childbirth education

Knowledge deficit r/t lack of preparation for labor

Impaired tissue integrity r/t passge of infant through birth canal, episiotomy

Pain r/t uterine contractions, stretching of cervix and birth canal

Risk for fluid volume deficit r/t excessive loss of blood

Risk for infection r/t multiple vaginal examinations, tissue trauma, prolonged rupture of membranes

Risk for injury: fetal r/t hypoxia

Laminectomy

Anxiety r/t change in health status, surgical procedure

Impaired physical mobility r/t neuromuscular impairment

Knowledge deficit r/t appropriate postoperative and postdischarge activities

Pain r/t localized inflammation and edema

Risk for impaired tissue perfusion r/t edema, hemorrhage, or embolism

Risk for perioperative positioning injury r/t prone position

Sensory/perceptual alteration: tactile r/t possible edema or nerve injury

Urinary retention r/t competing sensory impulses, effects of narcotics/anesthesia

See Surgery; Scoliosis

Laparotomy

See Abdominal Surgery

Laparoscopic Laser Cholecystectomy

See Cholecystectomy; Laser Surgery

Laryngectomy

Alteration in family process r/t surgery, serious condition of family member, difficulty communicating

Alteration in nutrition: less than body requirements r/t absence of oral feeding, difficulty swallowing, increased need for fluids

Alteration in oral mucous membranes r/t absence of oral feeding

Altered health maintenance r/t knowledge deficit regarding self-care with laryngectomy

Anticipatory grieving r/t loss of voice, fear of death

Body image disturbance r/t change in body structure and function

Impaired swallowing r/t edema, laryngectomy tube

Impaired verbal communication r/t removal of larynx

Ineffective airway clearance r/t surgical removal of glottis, decreased humidification of air

Risk for infection r/t invasive procedure, surgery

Laser Surgery

Constipation r/t laser intervention in vulval and perianal areas

Knowledge deficit r/t preoperative and postoperative care associated with laser procedure

Pain r/t heat from laser

Risk for infection r/t delayed heating reaction of tissue exposed to laser

Risk for injury r/t accidental exposure to laser beam

Laxative Abuse

Perceived constipation r/t health belief, faulty appraisal, impaired thought processes

Lens Implant

See Cataract Extraction

Lethargy/Listlessness

Altered tissue perfusion: cerebral r/t lack of oxygen supply to brain

Fatigue r/t decreased metabolic energy production

Sleep pattern disturbance r/t internal or external stressors

See cause of Lethargy/Listlessness

Leukemia

Altered protection r/t abnormal blood profile

Risk for fluid volume deficit r/t nausea, vomiting, bleeding, side effects of treatment

Risk for infection r/t ineffective immune system

See Chemotherapy; Cancer

Leukopenia

Risk for infection r/t low white blood cell count

Level of Consciousness, Decreased

See Confusion

Lice

See Communicable Diseases, Childhood

Limb Reattachment Procedures

Anticipatory grieving r/t unknown outcome of reattachment procedure

Anxiety r/t unknown outcome of reattachment procedure, use and appearance of limb

Body image disturbance r/t unpredictability of function and appearance of reattached body part

Risk for fluid volume deficit: hemorrhage r/t severed vessels

Risk for perioperative positioning injury r/t immobilization

Risk for peripheral neurovascular dysfunction r/t trauma, orthopedic and neurovascular surgery, compression of nerves and blood vessels

See Surgery, Postoperative Care

Liver Biopsy

Anxiety r/t procedure and results

Risk for fluid volume deficit r/t hemorrhage from biopsy site

Liver Disease

See Cirrhosis; Hepatitis

Living Will

See Advanced Directives

Lobectomy

See Thoracotomy

Loneliness

Risk for loneliness r/t lack of affection, physical isolation, cathectic deprivation, social isolation

Loose Stools

Diarrhea r/t increased gastric motility

See cause of Loose Stools

Low Back Pain

Altered health maintenance r/t knowledge deficit regarding self-care with back pain

Chronic pain r/t degenerative processes, musculotendinous strain, injury, inflammation, congenital deformities

Impaired physical mobility r/t back pain

Urinary retention r/t possible spinal cord compression

Lumbar Puncture

Anxiety r/t invasive procedure and unknown results

Knowledge deficit r/t information about procedure

Pain: headache r/t possible loss of cerebrospinal fluid
Risk for infection r/t invasive procedure

Lung Cancer

See Cancer; Thoracotomy

Lupus Erythematosus

Altered health maintenance r/t knowledge deficit
regarding medication, diet, and activity
Body image disturbance r/t change in skin, rash,
lesions, ulcers, mottled erythema
Fatigue r/t increased metabolic requirements
Pain r/t inflammatory process
Powerlessness r/t unpredictability of course of disease
Risk for impaired skin integrity r/t chronic
inflammation, edema, altered circulation
Spiritual distress r/t chronicity of disease, unknown
etiology

Lyme Disease

Fatigue r/t increased energy requirements
Knowledge deficit r/t lack of information concerning
disease, prevention, and treatment
Pain r/t inflammation of joints, urticaria, rash
Risk for decreased cardiac output r/t dysrhythmia

Lymphedema

Fluid volume excess r/t compromised regulatory
system; inflammation, obstruction, or removal of
lymph glands
Knowledge deficit r/t management of condition

Lymphoma

See Cancer

M

Magnetic Resonance Imaging

See MRI

Major Depressive Disorder

See Depression

Malabsorption Syndrome

Alteration in nutrition: less than body requirements
r/t inability of body to absorb nutrients because of
biological factors
Diarrhea r/t lactose intolerance, gluten sensitivity,
resection of small bowel
Knowledge deficit r/t lack of information about diet
and nutrition
Risk for fluid volume deficit r/t diarrhea

Maladaptive Behavior

See Crisis; Suicide Attempt

Malnutrition

Altered nutrition: less than body requirements r/t
inability to ingest food, digest food, or absorb
nutrients because of biological, psychological, or
economic factors; institutionalization (i.e., lack of
menu choices)
Altered protection r/t inadequate nutrition
Ineffective management of therapeutic regimen r/t
economic difficulties
Knowledge deficit r/t misinformation about normal
nutrition, social isolation, lack of food preparation
facilities

Manic Disorder, Bipolar I

Altered family processes r/t family member's illness
Altered nutrition: less than body requirements r/t
lack of time and motivation to eat, constant
movement
Altered role performance r/t impaired social
interactions
Altered thought processes r/t mania
Anxiety r/t change in role function
Fluid volume deficit r/t decreased intake
Impaired home maintenance management r/t altered
psychological state, inability to concentrate
Ineffective denial r/t fear of inability to control
behavior
Ineffective individual coping r/t situational crisis
Ineffective management of therapeutic regimen r/t
lack of social supports
**Ineffective management of therapeutic regimen:
families** r/t unpredictability of client, excessive
demands on family, chronicity of condition
Noncompliance r/t denial of illness
Risk for caregiver role strain r/t unpredictability of
condition, mood swings
Risk for violence: self-directed or directed at others
r/t hallucinations, delusions
Sleep pattern disturbance r/t constant anxious
thoughts

Manipulative Behavior

Defensive coping r/t superior attitude toward others
Impaired social interaction r/t self-concept
disturbance
Ineffective individual coping r/t inappropriate use of
defense mechanisms
Risk for loneliness r/t inability to interact
appropriately with others

Risk for self-mutilation r/t inability to cope with increased psychological or physiological tension in a healthy manner

Marasmus

See Failure to Thrive, Nonorganic

Marshall-Marchetti-Krantz Operation

Preoperative

Stress incontinence r/t weak pelvic muscles and pelvic supports

Postoperative

Knowledge deficit r/t lack of exposure to information regarding care after surgery and at home

Pain r/t manipulation of organs, surgical incision

Risk for infection r/t presence of urinary catheter

Urinary retention r/t swelling of urinary meatus

Mastectomy

Body image disturbance r/t loss of sexually significant body part

Fear r/t change in body image, prognosis

Knowledge deficit r/t self-care activities

Pain r/t surgical procedure

Risk for impaired physical mobility r/t nerve or muscle damage, pain

Sexual dysfunction r/t change in body image, fear of loss of feminism

See Cancer; Surgery

Mastitis

Altered role performance r/t change in capacity to function in expected role

Anxiety r/t threat to self and concern over safety of milk for infant

Ineffective breast-feeding r/t breast pain, conflicting advice from health care providers

Knowledge deficit r/t antibiotic regimen and comfort measures

Pain r/t infectious disease process and swelling of breast tissue

Maternal Infection

Altered protection r/t invasive procedures, traumatized tissue, stress of recent childbirth

See Postpartum Normal Care

Maturational Issues, Adolescent

Altered family processes r/t developmental crises of adolescence secondary to challenge of parental authority and values, situational crises secondary to change in parental marital status

Impaired social interaction r/t ineffective, unsuccessful, or dysfunctional interaction with peers

Ineffective individual coping r/t maturational crises

Knowledge deficit: potential for enhanced health maintenance r/t information misinterpretation, lack of education regarding age-related factors

Risk for injury/trauma r/t thrill-seeking behaviors

Social isolation r/t perceived alteration in physical appearance, social values not accepted by dominant peer group

See Sexuality, Adolescent; Substance Abuse (if relevant)

Measles (Rubeola)

See Communicable Diseases, Childhood

Meconium Aspiration

See Respiratory Conditions of the Neonate

Melanoma

Altered health maintenance r/t knowledge deficit regarding self-care and treatment of melanoma

Body image disturbance r/t altered pigmentation, surgical incision

Fear r/t threat to well-being

Pain r/t surgical incision

See Cancer

Melena

Fear r/t presence of blood in feces

Risk for fluid volume deficit r/t hemorrhage

See GI Bleed

Memory Deficit

Impaired memory r/t acute or chronic hypoxia, anemia, decreased cardiac output, fluid and electrolyte imbalance, neurological disturbance, excessive environmental disturbances

Meningitis/Encephalitis

Altered comfort: nausea and vomiting r/t central nervous system inflammation

Altered comfort: photophobia r/t increased sensitivity to external stimuli secondary to central nervous system inflammation

Altered growth and development r/t brain damage secondary to infectious process, increased intracranial pressure

Altered thought processes r/t inflammation of brain, fever

Altered tissue perfusion: cerebral r/t inflamed cerebral tissues and meninges, increased intracranial pressure

Decreased adaptive capacity: intracranial r/t sustained increase in intracranial pressure (10 to 15 mm Hg)

Fluid volume excess r/t increased intracranial pressure, syndrome of inappropriate secretion of antidiuretic hormone (SIADH)

Impaired mobility r/t neuromuscular or central nervous system insult

Ineffective airway clearance r/t seizure activity

Pain r/t neck (nuchal) rigidity, inflammation of meninges, headache, kinesthetic sensory-perceptual alteration (i.e. pain felt when skin touched), fever, earache

Risk for aspiration r/t seizure activity

Risk for injury r/t seizure activity

Sensory/perceptual alteration: hearing r/t CNS infection, ear infection

Sensory/perceptual alteration: kinesthetic r/t CNS infection

Sensory-perceptual alteration: visual r/t photophobia secondary to CNS infection

See Hospitalized Child

Meningocele

See Neurotube Defects

Menopause

Altered sexuality patterns r/t altered body structure, lack of physiological lubrication, lack of knowledge of artificial lubrication

Effective management of therapeutic regimen r/t verbalized desire to manage menopause

Health-seeking behavior r/t menopause, therapies associated with change in hormonal levels

Ineffective thermoregulation r/t changes in hormonal levels

Risk for altered nutrition: more than body requirements r/t change in metabolic rate caused by fluctuating hormone levels

Menorrhagia

Fear r/t loss of large amounts of blood

Risk for fluid volume deficit r/t excessive loss of menstrual blood

Mental Illness

Altered thought process r/t head injury, mental disorder, personality disorder, organic mental disorder, substance abuse, severe interpersonal conflict, sleep deprivation, sensory deprivation or overload, impaired cerebral perfusion

Defensive coping r/t psychological impairment, substance abuse

Ineffective denial r/t refusal to acknowledge abuse problem, fear of the social stigma of disease

Ineffective family coping: compromised r/t lack of available support from client

Ineffective family coping: disabling r/t chronically unexpressed feelings of guilt, anxiety, hostility, or despair

Ineffective individual coping r/t situational crisis, coping with mental illness

Ineffective management of therapeutic regimen: community r/t inadequate services to care for mentally ill clients, lack of information regarding how to access services

Ineffective management of therapeutic regimen: families r/t chronicity of condition, unpredictability of client, unknown prognosis

Risk for loneliness r/t social isolation

Mental Retardation

Altered family processes r/t crisis of diagnosis and situational transition

Altered growth and development r/t cognitive or perceptual impairment, developmental delay

Chronic low self-esteem r/t perceived differences

Family coping: potential for growth r/t adaptation and acceptance of child's condition and needs

Grieving r/t loss of perfect child; birth of child with congenital defect or subsequent head injury

Impaired home maintenance management r/t insufficient support systems

Impaired social interaction r/t developmental lag or delay, perceived differences

Impaired swallowing r/t neuromuscular impairment

Impaired verbal communication r/t developmental delay

Parental role conflict r/t home care of child with special needs

Risk for self-mutilation r/t separation anxiety, depersonalization

Self-care deficit: bathing/hygiene, dressing/grooming, feeding, toileting r/t perceptual or cognitive impairment

See Safety, Childhood; Child with Chronic Condition

Metabolic Acidosis

See Ketoacidosis

Metabolic Alkalosis

Fluid volume deficit r/t fluid volume loss, vomiting, gastric suctioning, failure of regulatory mechanisms

MI (Myocardial Infarction)

Altered family processes r/t crisis, role change

Altered health maintenance r/t knowledge deficit regarding self-care and treatment

Altered sexuality pattern r/t fear of chest pain, possibility of heart damage

Anxiety r/t threat of death, possible change in role status

Colonic constipation r/t decreased peristalsis from decreased physical activity, medication effect, change in diet

Decreased cardiac output r/t ventricular damage, ischemia, dysrhythmias

Fear r/t threat to well-being

Ineffective denial r/t fear, knowledge deficit about heart disease

Ineffective family coping r/t spouse or significant other's fear of partner loss

Pain r/t myocardial tissue damage from inadequate blood supply

Situational low self-esteem r/t crisis of MI

Midlife Crisis

Ineffective individual coping r/t inability to deal with changes associated with aging

Potential for enhanced spiritual well-being r/t desire to find purpose and meaning to life

Powerlessness r/t lack of control over life situation

Spiritual distress r/t questioning belief/value system

Migraine Headache

Altered health maintenance r/t knowledge deficit regarding prevention and treatment of headaches

Pain: headache r/t vasodilation of cerebral and extracerebral vessels

Miscarriage

See Pregnancy Loss

Mitral Stenosis

Activity intolerance r/t imbalance between oxygen supply and demand

Altered health maintenance r/t knowledge deficit regarding self-care with disorder

Anxiety r/t possible worsening of symptoms, activity intolerance, fatigue

Decreased cardiac output r/t incompetent heart valves, abnormal forward or backward blood flow, flow into a dilated chamber, flow through an abnormal passage between chambers

Fatigue r/t reduced cardiac output

Mitral Valve Prolapse

Altered health maintenance r/t knowledge deficit regarding methods to relieve pain and treat dysrhythmia and shortness of breath, need for prophylactic antibiotics before invasive procedures

Altered tissue perfusion: cerebral r/t postural hypotension

Anxiety r/t symptoms of condition: palpitations, chest pain

Fatigue r/t abnormal catecholamine regulation, decreased intravascular volume

Fear r/t lack of knowledge about mitral valve prolapse, feelings of having a heart attack

Pain r/t mitral valve regurgitation

Risk for infection r/t invasive procedures

Mobility, Impaired Physical

Impaired physical mobility r/t intolerance to activity, decreased strength and endurance, pain, discomfort, perceptual or cognitive impairment, neuromuscular impairment, musculoskeletal impairment, depression, severe anxiety

Modified Radical Mastectomy

Decisional conflict r/t treatment of choice

See Mastectomy

Mononucleosis

Activity intolerance r/t generalized weakness

Altered health maintenance r/t knowledge deficit concerning transmission and treatment of disease

Hyperthermia r/t infectious process

Impaired swallowing r/t irritation of oropharyngeal cavity

Pain r/t enlargement of lymph nodes, irritation of oropharyngeal cavity

Risk for injury r/t possible rupture of spleen

Mood Disorders

Caregiver role strain r/t symptoms associated with disorder of care receiver

Impaired adjustment r/t hopelessness, altered locus of control

Social isolation r/t alterations in mental status

See specific disorder: Depression; Dysthymic Disorder; Manic Disorder; Hypomania

Moon Face

Body image disturbance r/t change in appearance from disease to medication

See Cushing's Syndrome

Mottling of Peripheral Skin

Altered tissue perfusion: peripheral r/t interruption of arterial flow, decreased circulating blood volume

Mouth Lesions

See Mucous Membranes, Altered Oral

M

MRI (Magnetic Resonance Imaging)

MRI (Magnetic Resonance Imaging)

Anxiety r/t fear of being in closed spaces
Knowledge deficit r/t preparation for examination, contraindications to test, especially presence of any metal in body

Mucocutaneous Lymph Node Syndrome

See Kawasaki Syndrome

Mucous Membranes, Altered Oral

Altered oral mucous membranes r/t pathological conditions—oral cavity (radiation to head or neck), dehydration, chemical trauma (e.g., acidic foods, drugs, noxious agents, alcohol), mechanical trauma (e.g., ill-fitting dentures, braces, endotracheal or nasogastric tubes, surgery in oral cavity), NPO for more than 24 hours, ineffective oral hygiene, mouth breathing, malnutrition, infection, lack of or decreased salivation, medication

Multiinfarct Dementia

See Dementia

Multiple Gestation

Altered nutrition: less than body requirements r/t physiological demands of a multifetal pregnancy
Anxiety r/t uncertain outcome of pregnancy
Fatigue r/t physiological demands of a multifetal pregnancy and/or care of more than one infant
Impaired home maintenance management r/t fatigue
Impaired physical mobility r/t increased uterine size
Knowledge deficit r/t caring for more than one infant
Risk for ineffective breast-feeding r/t lack of support, physical demands of feeding more than one infant
Sleep pattern disturbance r/t discomforts of multiple gestation or care of infants
Stress incontinence r/t increased pelvic pressure

Multiple Personality Disorder (Dissociative Identity Disorder)

Anxiety r/t loss of control of behavior and feelings
Body image disturbance r/t feelings of powerlessness with personality changes
Chronic low self-esteem r/t inability to deal with life events, history of abuse
Defensive coping r/t unresolved past traumatic events, severe anxiety
Hopelessness r/t long-term stress
Ineffective individual coping r/t history of abuse
Personal identity disturbance r/t severe child abuse
Risk for self-mutilation r/t need to act out to relieve stress
See Dissociative Disorder

Multiple Sclerosis (MS)

Anticipatory grieving r/t risk for loss of normal body functioning
Disuse syndrome r/t physical immobility
Energy field disturbance r/t disruption in energy flow resulting from disharmony between mind and body
Impaired physical mobility r/t neuromuscular impairment
Ineffective airway clearance r/t decreased energy/fatigue
Potential for enhanced spiritual well-being r/t struggling with chronic debilitating condition
Powerlessness r/t progressive nature of disease
Risk for altered nutrition: less than body requirements r/t impaired swallowing, depression
Risk for injury r/t altered mobility, sensory dysfunction
Self-care deficit: specify r/t neuromuscular impairment
Sensory/perceptual alteration: specify r/t pathology in sensory tracts
Sexual dysfunction r/t biopsychosocial alteration of sexuality
Spiritual distress r/t perceived hopelessness of diagnosis
Urinary retention r/t inhibition of the reflex arc
See Neurological Disorders

Mumps

See Communicable Diseases, Childhood

Murmurs

Decreased cardiac output r/t incompetent heart valves, abnormal forward or backward blood flow, flow into a dilated chamber, flow through an abnormal passage between chambers

Muscular Atrophy/Weakness

Risk for disuse syndrome r/t impaired physical mobility

Muscular Dystrophy (MD)

Activity intolerance r/t fatigue
Altered nutrition: less than body requirements r/t impaired swallowing or chewing
Altered nutrition: more than body requirements r/t inactivity
Constipation r/t immobility
Decreased cardiac output r/t effects of congestive heart failure
Disuse syndrome r/t complications of immobility
Fatigue r/t increased energy requirements to perform activities of daily living
Impaired mobility r/t muscle weakness and development of contractures

Ineffective airway clearance r/t muscle weakness and decreased ability to cough

Risk for aspiration r/t impaired swallowing

Risk for impaired gas exchange r/t ineffective airway clearance and ineffective breathing patterns secondary to muscle weakness

Risk for impaired skin integrity r/t immobility, braces or adaptive devices

Risk for ineffective breathing patterns r/t muscle weakness

Risk for infection r/t pooling of pulmonary secretions secondary to immobility and muscle weakness

Risk for injury r/t muscle weakness and unsteady gait

Self-care deficits: feeding, bathing, dressing, toileting r/t muscle weakness and fatigue

See Hospitalized Child; Child with Chronic Condition; Terminally Ill Child

MVA (Motor Vehicle Accident)

See Injury; Head Injury; Fracture; Pneumothorax

Myasthenia Gravis

Altered family process r/t crisis of dealing with diagnosis

Altered nutrition: less than body requirements r/t difficulty eating and swallowing

Fatigue r/t paresthesia, aching muscles

Impaired physical mobility r/t defective transmission of nerve impulses at the neuromuscular junction

Impaired swallowing r/t neuromuscular impairment

Ineffective airway clearance r/t decreased ability to cough and swallow

Ineffective management of therapeutic regimen r/t lack of knowledge of treatment, uncertainty of outcome

Risk for caregiver role strain r/t severity of illness of client

See Neurological Disorders

Mycoplasma Pneumonia

See Pneumonia

Myelocele

See Neurotube Defects

Myelogram, Contrast

Pain r/t irritation of nerve roots

Risk for altered tissue perfusion: cerebral r/t hypotension, loss of cerebrospinal fluid

Risk for fluid volume deficit r/t possible dehydration, loss of cerebrospinal fluid

Urinary retention r/t pressure on spinal nerve roots

Myelomeningocele

See Neurotube Defects

Myocardial Infarction

See MI

Myocarditis

Activity intolerance r/t reduced cardiac reserve and prescribed bedrest

Decreased cardiac output r/t impaired contractility of ventricles

Knowledge deficit r/t treatment of disease

See CHF (if appropriate)

Myringotomy

Altered health maintenance r/t knowledge deficit regarding self-care following surgery

Fear r/t hospitalization, surgical procedure

Risk for infection r/t invasive procedure

Pain r/t surgical procedure

Sensory/perceptual alteration r/t possible hearing impairment

Myxedema

See Hypothyroidism

N

Narcissistic Personality Disorder

Decisional conflict r/t lack of realistic problem-solving skills

Defensive coping r/t grandiose sense of self

Impaired social interaction r/t self-concept disturbance

Risk for loneliness r/t inability to interact appropriately with others

Narcolepsy

Anxiety r/t fear of lack of control over falling asleep

Risk for trauma r/t falling asleep during potentially dangerous activity

Sleep pattern disturbance r/t uncontrollable desire to sleep

Nasogastric Suction

Altered comfort r/t presence of nasogastric tube

Altered oral mucous membranes r/t presence of nasogastric tube

Risk for fluid volume deficit r/t loss of gastrointestinal fluids without adequate replacement

Nausea

Altered comfort: nausea r/t alteration in gastrointestinal function

Risk for altered nutrition: less than body requirements r/t nausea (specify cause)

Risk for fluid volume deficit r/t inadequate fluid intake secondary to nausea

Near-Drowning

Altered health maintenance r/t parental knowledge deficit regarding safety measures appropriate for age

Anticipatory/dysfunctional grieving r/t potential death of child, unknown sequelae, guilt about accident

Aspiration r/t aspiration of fluid into the lungs

Fear: parental r/t possible death of child, possible permanent and debilitating sequelae

Hypothermia r/t central nervous system injury, prolonged submersion in cold water

Impaired gas exchange r/t laryngospasm, holding breath, aspiration

Ineffective airway clearance/ineffective breathing pattern r/t aspiration, impaired gas exchange

Potential for enhanced spiritual well-being r/t struggle with survival of life-threatening situation

Risk for altered growth and development r/t hypoxemia, cerebral anoxia

Risk for infection r/t aspiration, invasive monitoring

See Safety—Childhood; Hospitalized Child; Child with Chronic Condition; Terminally Ill Child/Death of Child

Neck Vein Distention

Decreased cardiac output r/t decreased contractility of heart and resulting increased payload

Fluid volume excess r/t excess fluid intake, compromised regulatory mechanisms

See CHF

Necrotizing Enterocolitis (NEC)

Altered nutrition: less than body requirements r/t decreased ability to absorb nutrients, decreased perfusion to gastrointestinal tract

Altered tissue perfusion: gastrointestinal r/t shunting of blood away from mesenteric circulation and toward vital organs secondary to perinatal stress, hypoxia

Fluid volume deficit r/t vomiting, gastrointestinal bleeding

Ineffective breathing pattern r/t abdominal distention, hypoxia

Risk for infection r/t bacterial invasion of gastrointestinal tract, invasive procedures

See Premature Infant; Hospitalized Child

Negative Feelings about Self

Chronic low self-esteem r/t long-standing negative self-evaluation

Self-esteem disturbance r/t inappropriate learned negative feelings about self

Neglect, Unilateral

See Unilateral Neglect of One Side of Body

Neglectful Care of Family Member

Altered family processes r/t situational transition or crisis

Caregiver role strain r/t care demands of family member, lack of social or financial support

Ineffective family coping: disabling r/t highly ambivalent family relationships, lack of respite care

Ineffective management of therapeutic regimen: community r/t deficits in community for support of caregivers and detection of client neglect

Knowledge deficit r/t care needs

Neoplasm

Fear r/t possible malignancy

See Cancer

Nephrectomy

Alteration in urinary elimination r/t loss of kidney

Anxiety r/t surgical recovery, prognosis

Constipation r/t lack of return of peristalsis

Ineffective breathing pattern r/t location of surgical incision

Pain r/t incisional discomfort

Risk for fluid volume deficit r/t vascular losses, decreased intake

Risk for infection r/t invasive procedure, lack of deep breathing because of location of surgical incision

Nephrostomy, Percutaneous

Altered urinary elimination r/t nephrostomy tube

Pain r/t invasive procedure

Risk for infection r/t invasive procedure

Nephrotic Syndrome

Activity intolerance r/t generalized edema

Altered comfort r/t edema

Altered nutrition: less than body requirements r/t anorexia, protein loss

Altered nutrition: more than body requirements r/t increased appetite secondary to steroid therapy

Body image disturbance r/t edematous appearance and side effects of steroid therapy

Fluid volume excess r/t edema secondary to oncotic fluid shift resulting from serum protein loss and renal retention of salt and water

Risk for impaired skin integrity r/t edema

Risk for infection r/t altered immune mechanisms secondary to disease and effects of steroids

Risk for noncompliance r/t side effects of home steroid therapy

Social isolation r/t edematous appearance

See Hospitalized Child; Child with Chronic Condition

Nerve Entrapment

See Carpal Tunnel Syndrome

Neuritis

Activity intolerance r/t pain with movement

Altered health maintenance r/t knowledge deficit regarding self-care with neuritis

Pain r/t stimulation of affected nerve endings, inflammation of sensory nerves

Neurogenic Bladder

Reflex incontinence r/t neurological impairment

Urinary retention r/t interruption in the lateral spinal tracts

Neurological Disorders

Acute confusion r/t dementia, alcohol abuse, drug abuse, delirium

Altered family process r/t situational crisis, illness or disability of family member

Altered nutrition: less than body requirements r/t impaired swallowing, depression, difficulty feeding self

Anticipatory grieving r/t loss of usual body functioning

Impaired home maintenance management r/t client's or family member's disease

Impaired memory r/t neurological disturbance

Impaired physical mobility r/t neuromuscular impairment

Impaired swallowing r/t neuromuscular dysfunction

Ineffective airway clearance r/t perceptual or cognitive impairment, decreased energy, fatigue

Ineffective individual coping r/t disability requiring change in life-style

Powerlessness r/t progressive nature of disease

Risk for disuse syndrome r/t physical immobility, neuromuscular dysfunction

Risk for impaired skin integrity r/t altered sensation, altered mental status, paralysis

Risk for injury r/t altered mobility, sensory dysfunction, cognitive impairment

Self-care deficit: specify r/t neuromuscular dysfunction

Sexual dysfunction r/t biopsychosocial alteration of sexuality

Social isolation r/t altered state of wellness

Neurotube Defects (Meningocele, Myelomeningocele, Spina Bifida, Anencephaly)

Altered growth and development r/t physical impairments, possible cognitive impairment

Chronic low self-esteem r/t perceived differences, decreased ability to participate in physical and social activities at school

Colonic constipation r/t immobility or less than adequate mobility

Family coping: potential for growth r/t effective adaptive response by family members

Grieving r/t loss of perfect child, birth of child with congenital defect

Impaired mobility r/t neuromuscular impairment

Impaired skin integrity r/t incontinence

Reflex incontinence r/t neurogenic impairment

Risk for altered nutrition: more than body requirements r/t diminished, limited, or impaired physical activity

Risk for impaired skin integrity: lower extremities r/t decreased sensory perception

Sensory/perceptual alteration: visual r/t altered reception secondary to strabismus

Total incontinence r/t neurogenic impairment

Urge incontinence r/t neurogenic impairment

See Premature Infant; Child with Chronic Condition

Newborn, Normal

Altered protection r/t immature immune system

Effective breast-feeding r/t normal oral structure and gestational age greater than 34 weeks

Ineffective thermoregulation r/t immaturity of neuroendocrine system

Potential for enhanced organized infant behavior r/t appropriate environmental stimuli

Risk for infection r/t open umbilical stump

Risk for injury r/t immaturity, need for caretaking

Newborn, Postmature

Hypothermia r/t depleted stores of subcutaneous fat

Impaired skin integrity r/t cracked and peeling skin secondary to decreased vernix

Risk for ineffective airway clearance r/t meconium aspiration

Risk for injury r/t hypoglycemia secondary to depleted glycogen stores

Newborn, Small for Gestational Age (SGA)

Altered nutrition: less than body requirements r/t history of placental insufficiency

Ineffective thermoregulation r/t decreased brown fat, subcutaneous fat

Risk for injury r/t hypoglycemia, perinatal asphyxia, meconium aspiration

Nicotine Addiction

Altered health maintenance r/t lack of ability to make a judgment about smoking cessation

Powerlessness r/t perceived lack of control over ability to give up nicotine

NIDDM (Non–Insulin-Dependent Diabetes Mellitus)

Health–seeking behaviors r/t desiring information on exercise and diet to manage diabetes

See Diabetes Mellitus

Nightmares

Energy field disturbance r/t disharmony of body and mind

Post–trauma response r/t disaster, war, epidemic, rape, assault, torture, catastrophic illness or accident

Rape–trauma syndrome: compound reaction/silent reaction r/t forced violent sexual penetration against the victim's will and consent

Nipple Soreness

Pain r/t injury to nipples

See Painful Breasts—Sore Nipples

Nocturia

Altered urinary elimination r/t sensory motor impairment, urinary tract infection

Total incontinence r/t neuropathy preventing transmission of reflex indicating bladder fullness, neurological dysfunction causing triggering of micturition at unpredictable times, independent contraction of detrusor reflex as result of surgery, trauma or disease affecting spinal cord nerves, anatomical fistula

Urge incontinence r/t decreased bladder capacity, irritation of bladder stretch receptors causing spasm, alcohol, caffeine, increased fluids, increased urine concentration, overdistention of bladder

Nocturnal Paroxysmal Dyspnea

See PND

Noncompliance

Noncompliance r/t client value system, health beliefs, cultural influences, spiritual values, client-provider relationships, knowledge deficit

Non–Insulin-Dependent Diabetes Mellitus (NIDDM)

See Diabetes Mellitus

Nutrition, Altered

Altered nutrition: high risk for more than body requirements r/t obesity in parents, use of food as reward or comfort measure, dysfunctional eating pattern, eating in response to cues other than hunger

Altered nutrition: less than body requirements r/t inability to ingest or digest food or absorb nutrients because of biological, psychological, or economic factors

Altered nutrition: more than body requirements r/t excessive intake in relation to metabolic need

O

Obesity

Altered nutrition: more than body requirements r/t caloric intake exceeding energy expenditure

Body image disturbance r/t eating disorder, excess weight

Chronic low self–esteem r/t ineffective individual coping, overeating

Obsessive-Compulsive Disorder

Altered thought process r/t persistent thoughts, ideas, and impulses that seem irrelevant and will not relent

Anxiety r/t threat to self-concept, unmet needs

Decisional conflict r/t inability to make a decision for fear of reprisal

Ineffective family coping: disabling r/t family process being disrupted by client's ritualistic activities

Ineffective individual coping r/t expression of feelings in an unacceptable way, ritualistic behavior

Powerlessness r/t unrelenting repetitive thoughts to perform irrational activities

Obstruction, Bowel

See Bowel Obstruction

Oligohydramnios

Anxiety: maternal r/t fear of unknown and threat to fetus

Risk for injury: fetal r/t decreased umbilical cord blood flow secondary to compression

Oliguria

Fluid volume deficit r/t active fluid loss, failure of regulatory mechanism

See Renal Failure; Shock; Cardiac Output Decrease

Omphalocele

See Gastroschisis/Omphalocele

Oophorectomy

Risk for altered sexuality patterns r/t altered body function

See Surgery

Open Reduction of Fracture with Internal Fixation (Femur)

Anxiety r/t outcome of corrective procedure

Impaired physical mobility r/t postoperative position, abduction of leg, avoidance of acute flexion

Powerlessness r/t loss of control, unanticipated change in life-style

Risk for perioperative positioning injury r/t immobilization

Risk for peripheral neurovascular dysfunction r/t mechanical compression, orthopedic surgery, immobilization

See Surgery, Postoperative Care

Opportunistic Infection

Altered infection r/t abnormal blood profiles

See AIDS

Oral Mucous Membrane, Altered

Altered oral mucous membrane r/t pathological conditions—oral cavity (radiation to head or neck), dehydration, chemical trauma (e.g., acidic foods, drugs, noxious agents, alcohol), mechanical trauma (e.g., ill-fitting dentures, braces, endotracheal and nasogastric tubes, surgery in oral cavity), NPO for more than 24 hours, ineffective oral hygiene, mouth breathing, malnutrition, infection, lack of or decreased salivation, medication

Organic Mental Disorders

Impaired social interaction r/t altered thought processes

Risk for injury r/t disorientation to time, place, and person

See Dementia

Orthopedic Traction

Altered role performance r/t limited physical mobility

Impaired social interaction r/t limited physical mobility

See Traction and Casts

Orthopnea

Decreased cardiac output r/t inability of heart to meet demands of body

Ineffective breathing pattern r/t inability to breathe with the head of the bed flat

Orthostatic Hypotension

See Dizziness

Osteoarthritis

Activity intolerance r/t pain after exercise or use of joint

Pain r/t movement

See Arthritis

Osteomyelitis

Altered health maintenance r/t continued immobility at home, possible extensive casts, continued antibiotics

Diversional activity deficit r/t prolonged immobilization and hospitalization

Fear: parental r/t concern regarding possible growth plate damage secondary to infection, concern that infection may become chronic

Hyperthermia r/t infectious process

Impaired physical mobility r/t imposed immobility secondary to infected area

Pain r/t inflammation in affected extremity

Risk for colonic constipation r/t immobility

Risk for impaired skin integrity r/t irritation from splint/cast

Risk for spread of infection r/t inadequate primary and secondary defenses

See Hospitalized Child

Osteoporosis

Altered nutrition: less than body requirements r/t inadequate intake of calcium and vitamin D

Effective management of therapeutic regimen: individual r/t appropriate choices for diet and exercise to prevent and manage condition

Impaired physical mobility r/t pain, skeletal changes

Knowledge deficit r/t diet, exercise, need to abstain from alcohol and nicotine

Pain r/t fracture, muscle spasms

Risk for injury: fracture r/t lack of activity, risk of falling resulting from environmental hazards, neuromuscular disorders, diminished senses, cardiovascular responses, responses to drugs

Ostomy

See Colostomy; Ileostomy; Ileal Conduit; Child with Chronic Condition

Otitis Media

Pain r/t inflammation, infectious process

Risk for infection r/t eustachian tube obstruction, traumatic eardrum perforation, infectious disease process

Sensory/perceptual alteration: auditory r/t incomplete resolution of otitis media, presence of excess drainage in middle ear

Ovarian Carcinoma

Altered health maintenance r/t knowledge deficit regarding self-care and treatment of condition

Fear r/t unknown outcome, possible poor prognosis

See Hysterectomy; Chemotherapy; Radiation Therapy

P

Pacemaker

Anxiety r/t change in health status, presence of pacemaker

Knowledge deficit r/t self-care program, when to seek medical attention

Pain r/t surgical procedure

Risk for decreased cardiac output r/t malfunction of pacemaker

Risk for infection r/t invasive procedure, presence of foreign body (catheter and generator)

Paget's Disease

Body image disturbance r/t possible enlarged head, bowed tibias, kyphosis

Knowledge deficit r/t appropriate diet of high protein and high calcium, mild exercise

Risk for trauma: fracture r/t excessive bone destruction

Pain

Energy field disturbance r/t unbalanced energy field

Pain r/t injury agents (biological, chemical, physical, psychological)

Pain, Chronic

Chronic pain r/t chronic physical or psychosocial disability

Painful Breasts—Engorgement

Altered role performance r/t change in physical capacity to assume role of breast-feeding mother

Impaired tissue integrity r/t excessive fluid in breast tissues

Pain r/t distention of breast tissue

Risk for ineffective breast-feeding r/t pain and infant's inability to latch on to engorged breast

Risk for infection r/t milk stasis

Painful Breasts—Sore Nipples

Altered role performance r/t change in physical capacity to assume role of breast-feeding mother

Impaired skin integrity r/t mechanical factors involved in suckling and breast-feeding management

Ineffective breast-feeding r/t pain

Pain r/t cracked nipples

Risk for infection r/t break in skin

Pallor of Extremities

Altered tissue perfusion: peripheral r/t interruption of vascular flow

Pancreatic Cancer

Anticipatory grieving r/t shortened life span

Fear r/t poor prognosis of the disease

Ineffective family coping r/t poor prognosis

Knowledge deficit r/t disease-induced diabetes, home management

Spiritual distress r/t poor prognosis

See Cancer; Radiation Therapy; Surgery

Pancreatitis

Altered health maintenance r/t knowledge deficit concerning diet, alcohol use, medication

Altered nutrition: less than body requirements r/t inadequate dietary intake, increased nutritional needs secondary to acute illness, increased metabolic needs caused by increased body temperature

Diarrhea r/t decrease in pancreatic secretions resulting in steatorrhea

Fluid volume deficit r/t vomiting, decreased fluid intake, fever, diaphoresis, fluid shifts

Ineffective breathing pattern r/t splinting from severe pain

Ineffective denial r/t ineffective coping, alcohol use

Pain r/t irritation and edema of the inflamed pancreas

Panic Disorder

Anxiety r/t situational crisis

Ineffective individual coping r/t personal vulnerability

Post-trauma response r/t previous catastrophic event

Risk for loneliness r/t inability to socially interact because of fear of losing control

Social isolation r/t fear of lack of control

Paralysis

Altered health maintenance r/t knowledge deficit regarding self-care with paralysis

Body image disturbance r/t biophysical changes, loss of movement, immobility

Colonic constipation r/t effects of spinal cord disruption, diet inadequate in fiber

Disuse syndrome r/t paralysis

Impaired home maintenance management r/t
physical disability

Impaired physical mobility r/t neuromuscular
impairment

Pain r/t prolonged immobility

Powerlessness r/t illness-related regimen

Reflex incontinence r/t neurological impairment

Risk for impaired skin integrity r/t altered circulation,
altered sensation, and immobility

Risk for injury r/t altered mobility, sensory dysfunction

Self-care deficit: specify r/t neuromuscular
impairment

Sexual dysfunction r/t loss of sensation,
biopsychosocial alteration

See Child with Chronic Condition; Hospitalized Child;
Neurotube Defects; Hemiplegia; Spinal Cord Injury

Paralytic Ileus

Altered oral mucous membranes r/t presence of
nasogastric tube

Constipation r/t decreased gastric motility

Fluid volume deficit r/t loss of fluids from vomiting,
retention of fluid in the bowels

Pain r/t pressure, abdominal distention

Paranoid Personality Disorder

Altered thought processes r/t psychological conflicts

Anxiety r/t uncontrollable intrusive, suspicious
thoughts

Chronic low self-esteem r/t inability to trust others

Risk for loneliness r/t social isolation

Risk for violence: directed at others r/t being
suspicious of others and others' actions

Sensory/perceptual alteration: specify r/t
psychological dysfunction, suspicious thoughts

Social isolation r/t inappropriate social skills

Paraplegia

See Spinal Cord Injury

Parathyroidectomy

Anxiety r/t surgery

Risk for impaired verbal communication r/t possible
laryngeal damage, edema

Risk for ineffective airway clearance r/t edema or
hematoma formation, airway obstruction

Risk for infection r/t surgical procedure

See Hypocalcemia

Parent Attachment

Risk for altered parent/infant/child attachment r/t
inability of parents to meet personal needs; anxiety
associated with parental role; substance abuse;
premature infant; ill infant/child who is unable to
effectively initiate parental contact as a result of
altered behavioral organization, separation, physical
barriers, or lack of privacy

Parental Role Conflict

Parental role conflict r/t separation from child
because of chronic illness, intimidation with invasive
or restrictive modalities (e.g., isolation, intubation),
specialized care center policies, home care of a child
with special needs (e.g., apnea monitoring, postural
drainage, hyperalimentation), change in marital
status, interruptions of family life because of home
care regimen (e.g., treatments, caregivers, lack of
respite)

Parenting, Altered

Altered parenting r/t lack of available role model;
ineffective role model; physical and psychosocial
abuse of nurturing figure; lack of support between
and from significant other(s); unmet social,
emotional, or maturational needs of parenting
figures; interruption in bonding process, (e.g.,
maternal, paternal, other); unrealistic expectations
for self, infant, partner; physical illness; presence of
stress (e.g., financial, legal, recent crisis, cultural
move); lack of knowledge; limited cognitive
functioning; lack of role identity; lack or
inappropriate response of child to relationship;
multiple pregnancies

Parenting, Risk for Altered

Risk for altered parenting r/t lack of available role
model; ineffective role model; physical and
psychosocial abuse of nurturing figure; lack of
support between or from significant other(s); unmet
social, emotional, or maturational needs of parenting
figures; interruption in bonding process (e.g.,
maternal, paternal, other); unrealistic expectations
for self, infant, partner; physical illness; presence of
stress (e.g., financial, legal, recent crisis, cultural
move); lack of knowledge; limited cognitive
functioning; lack of role identity; lack of
inappropriate response of child to relationship;
multiple pregnancies

Paresthesia

Sensory/perceptual alteration: tactile r/t altered
sensory reception, transmission, or integration

Parkinson's Disease

Altered nutrition: less than body requirements r/t
tremor, slowness in eating, difficulty in chewing and
swallowing

Constipation r/t weakness of defecation muscles, lack
of exercise, inadequate fluid intake, decreased
autonomic nervous system activity

Impaired verbal communication r/t decreased speech
volume, slowness of speech, impaired facial muscles

Risk for injury r/t tremors, slow reactions, altered gait

See Neurological Disorders

Paroxysmal Nocturnal Dyspnea

See PND

Patent Ductus Arteriosus (PDA)

See Congenital Heart Disease/Cardiac Anomalies

Patient-Controlled Analgesia

See PCA

Patient Education

Effective management of therapeutic regimen r/t
verbalized desire to manage illness and prevent
complications

Health–seeking behaviors r/t expressed or observed
desire to seek a higher level of wellness or control of
health practices

Knowledge deficit r/t lack of exposure to information,
information misinterpretation, unfamiliarity with
information resources

Potential for enhanced spiritual well–being r/t desire
to reach harmony with self, others, and higher
power/God

PCA (Patient-Controlled Analgesia)

Altered comfort: pruritis, nausea, vomiting r/t side
effects of medication

Effective management of therapeutic regimen r/t
ability to manage pain with appropriate use of
patient-controlled analgesia

Knowledge deficit r/t self-care of pain control

Risk for injury r/t possible complications associated
with PCA

Pelvic Inflammatory Disease

See PID

Penile Prosthesis

Altered sexuality pattern r/t use of penile prosthesis

Health–seeking behavior r/t information regarding use
and care of prosthesis

Risk for infection r/t invasive surgical procedure

Risk for situational low self-esteem r/t altered
sexuality pattern

Peptic Ulcer

See Ulcer

Percutaneous Transluminal Coronary Angioplasty (PTCA)

See Angioplasty, Coronary Balloon

Pericardial Friction Rub

Decreased cardiac output r/t inflammation in
pericardial sac, fluid accumulation compressing heart

Pain r/t inflammation, effusion

Pericarditis

Activity intolerance r/t reduced cardiac reserve and
prescribed bedrest

Altered tissue perfusion: cardiopulmonary/
peripheral r/t risk for development of emboli

Knowledge deficit r/t unfamiliarity with information
sources

Pain r/t biological injury, inflammation

Risk for altered nutrition: less than body
requirements r/t fever, hypermetabolic state
associated with fever

Risk for decreased cardiac output r/t inflammation in
pericardial sac, fluid accumulation compressing heart
function

Perioperative Positioning

Risk for perioperative positioning injury r/t
disorientation; immobilization; muscle weakness;
sensory/perceptual disturbances resulting from
anesthesia, obesity, emaciation, edema

Peripheral Neurovascular Dysfunction, Risk for

Risk for peripheral neurovascular dysfunction r/t
fractures, mechanical compression, orthopedic
surgery, trauma, immobilization, burns, vascular
obstruction

Peripheral Vascular Disease

Activity intolerance r/t imbalance between peripheral
oxygen supply and demand

Altered health maintenance r/t knowledge deficit
regarding self-care and treatment of disease

Altered tissue perfusion: peripheral r/t interruption
of vascular flow

Chronic pain: intermittent claudication r/t ischemia

Risk for impaired skin integrity r/t altered circulation
or sensation

Risk for injury r/t tissue hypoxia, altered mobility,
altered sensation

Risk for peripheral neurovascular dysfunction r/t
possible vascular obstruction

Peritoneal Dialysis

Impaired home maintenance management r/t complex home treatment of client

Knowledge deficit r/t treatment procedure, self-care with peritoneal dialysis

Pain r/t instillation of dialysate, temperature of dialysate

Risk for fluid volume excess r/t retention of dialysate

Risk for ineffective breathing pattern r/t pressure from the dialysate

Risk for ineffective individual coping r/t disability requiring change in life-style

Risk for infection: peritoneal r/t invasive procedure, presence of catheter, dialysate

See Renal Failure; Renal Failure, Acute/Chronic—Child; Hospitalized Child; Child with Chronic Condition

Peritonitis

Altered nutrition: less than body requirements r/t nausea, vomiting

Constipation r/t decreased oral intake, decrease of peristalsis

Fluid volume deficit r/t retention of fluid in bowel with loss of circulating blood volume

Ineffective breathing pattern r/t pain, increased abdominal pressure

Pain r/t inflammation and stimulation of somatic nerves

Persistent Fetal Circulation

See Congenital Heart Disease/Cardiac Anomalies

Personal Identity Problems

Personal identity disturbance r/t situational crisis, psychological impairment, chronic illness, pain

Personality Disorder

Chronic low self-esteem r/t inability to set and achieve goals

Decisional conflict r/t low self-esteem, feelings that choices will always be wrong

Impaired adjustment r/t ambivalent behavior toward others, testing of others' loyalty

Impaired social interaction r/t knowledge or skill deficit regarding ways to interact effectively with others, self-concept disturbances

Ineffective family coping: compromised r/t inability of client to provide positive feedback to family, chronicity exhausting family

Personal identity disturbance r/t lack of consistent positive self-image

Risk for loneliness r/t inability to interact appropriately with others

Spiritual distress r/t lack of identifiable values, lack of meaning to life

See Antisocial Personality Disorder; Borderline Personality Disorder

Pertussis (Whooping Cough)

See Respiratory Infections, Acute Childhood

Petechiae

See Clotting Disorder

Pharyngitis

See Sore Throat

Pheochromocytoma

Altered health maintenance r/t knowledge deficit regarding treatment and self-care

Anxiety r/t symptoms from increased catecholamines—headache, palpitations, sweating, nervousness, nausea, vomiting, syncope

Risk for altered tissue perfusion: cardiopulmonary and renal r/t episodes of hypertension

Sleep pattern disturbance r/t high levels of catecholamines

See Surgery

Phobia (Specific)

Anxiety r/t inability to control emotions when dreaded object or situation is encountered

Fear r/t presence or anticipation of specific object or situation

Ineffective individual coping r/t transfer of fears from self to dreaded object situation

Powerlessness r/t anxiety about encountering unknown or known entity

See Anxiety; Panic Disorder

Photosensitivity

Altered health maintenance r/t knowledge deficit regarding medications inducing photosensitivity

Risk for impaired skin integrity r/t exposure to sun

Physical Abuse

See Abuse

PID (Pelvic Inflammatory Disease)

Altered health maintenance r/t knowledge deficit regarding self-care and treatment of disease

Altered sexuality patterns r/t medically imposed abstinence from sexual activities until acute infection subsides, change in reproductive potential

Risk for infection r/t insufficient knowledge to avoid exposure to pathogens; proper hygiene, nutrition, and other health habits

Pain r/t biological injury; inflammation, edema, and congestion of pelvic tissues
See Maturational Issues, Adolescent

PIH (Pregnancy-Induced Hypertension/Preeclampsia)

Altered family processes r/t situational crisis
Altered parenting r/t bedrest
Altered role performance r/t change in physical capacity to assume role of pregnant woman or resume other roles
Anxiety r/t fear of the unknown, threat to self and infant, change in role functioning
Diversional activity deficit r/t bedrest
Fluid volume excess r/t decreased renal function
Impaired home maintenance management r/t bedrest
Impaired physical mobility r/t medically prescribed limitations
Impaired social interaction r/t imposed bedrest
Knowledge deficit r/t lack of experience with situation
Powerlessness r/t complication threatening pregnancy and medically prescribed limitations
Risk for injury: fetal r/t decreased uteroplacental perfusion, seizures
Risk for injury: maternal r/t vasospasm, high blood pressure
Situational low self-esteem r/t loss of idealized pregnancy

Piloerection

Hypothermia r/t exposure to cold environment

Placenta Previa

Altered family processes r/t maternal bedrest or hospitalization
Altered role performance r/t maternal bedrest or hospitalization
Altered tissue perfusion: placental r/t dilation of cervix, loss of placental implantation site
Body image disturbance r/t negative feelings about body and reproductive ability, feelings of helplessness
Diversional activity deficit r/t long-term hospitalization
Fear r/t threat to self and fetus, unknown future
Impaired home maintenance management r/t maternal bedrest or hospitalization
Impaired physical mobility r/t medical protocol, maternal bedrest
Ineffective individual coping r/t threat to self and fetus
Risk for altered parenting r/t maternal bedrest or hospitalization
Risk for fluid volume deficit r/t maternal blood loss

Risk for injury: fetal and maternal r/t threat to uteroplacental perfusion, hemorrhage
Situational low self-esteem r/t situational crisis
Spiritual distress r/t inability to participate in usual religious rituals, situational crisis

Pleural Effusion

Fluid volume excess r/t compromised regulatory mechanisms; heart, liver, or kidney failure
Hyperthermia r/t increased metabolic rate secondary to infection
Ineffective breathing pattern r/t pain
Pain r/t inflammation, fluid accumulation

Pleural Friction Rub

Ineffective breathing pattern r/t pain
Pain r/t inflammation, fluid accumulation
See cause of Pleural Friction Rub

Pleurisy

Ineffective breathing pattern r/t pain
Pain r/t pressure on pleural nerve endings associated with fluid accumulation or inflammation
Risk for impaired gas exchange r/t ventilation perfusion imbalance
Risk for impaired physical mobility r/t activity intolerance, inability to "catch breath"
Risk for ineffective airway clearance r/t increased secretions, ineffective cough because of pain

PMS (Premenstrual Tension Syndrome)

Effective management of therapeutic regimen: individual r/t desire for information to manage and prevent symptoms
Fatigue r/t hormonal changes
Fluid volume excess r/t alterations of hormonal levels inducing fluid retention
Knowledge deficit r/t methods to deal with and prevent syndrome
Pain r/t hormonal stimulation of gastrointestinal structures

PND (Paroxysmal Nocturnal Dyspnea)

Anxiety r/t inability to breathe during sleep
Decreased cardiac output r/t failure of the left ventricle
Ineffective breathing pattern r/t increase in carbon dioxide levels, decrease in oxygen levels
Sleep pattern disturbance r/t suffocating feeling from fluid in lungs on awakening from sleep

Pneumonia

Activity intolerance r/t imbalance between oxygen supply and demand

Altered health maintenance r/t knowledge deficit regarding self-care and treatment of disease

Altered nutrition: less than body requirements r/t loss of appetite

Altered oral mucous membranes r/t dry mouth from mouth breathing, decreased fluid intake

Hyperthermia r/t dehydration, increased metabolic rate, illness

Impaired gas exchange r/t decreased functional lung tissue

Ineffective airway clearance r/t inflammation and presence of secretions

Knowledge deficit r/t risk factors predisposing person to pneumonia, treatment

Risk for fluid volume deficit r/t inadequate intake of fluids

See Respiratory Infections, Acute Childhood (for child)

Pneumothorax

Fear r/t threat to own well-being, difficulty breathing

Impaired gas exchange r/t ventilation-perfusion imbalance

Pain r/t recent injury, coughing, deep breathing

Risk for injury r/t possible complications associated with closed chest drainage system

Poisoning, Risk for

Internal

Risk for poisoning r/t reduced vision, verbalization of occupational settings without adequate safeguards, lack of safety or drug education, lack of proper precaution, cognitive or emotional difficulties, insufficient finances

External

Risk for poisoning r/t large supplies of drugs in house, medicine stored in unlocked cabinets accessible to children or confused persons, dangerous products placed or stored within the reach of children or confused persons, availability of illicit drugs potentially contaminated by poisonous additives, flaking or peeling paint or plaster in presence of young children, chemical contamination of food and water, unprotected contact with heavy metals or chemicals, paint or lacquer used in poorly ventilated areas or without effective protection, presence of poisonous vegetation, presence of atmospheric pollutants

Polydipsia

See Diabetes Mellitus

Polyphagia

See Diabetes Mellitus

Polyuria

See Diabetes Mellitus

Postoperative Care

See Surgery, Postoperative

Postpartum, Normal Care

Altered role performance r/t new responsibilities of parenting

Altered urinary elimination r/t effects of anesthesia or tissue trauma

Anxiety r/t change in role functioning, parenting

Constipation r/t hormonal effects on smooth muscles, fear of straining with defecation, effects of anesthesia

Effective breast-feeding r/t basic breast-feeding knowledge, support of partner and health care provider

Family coping: potential for growth r/t adaptation to new family member

Fatigue r/t childbirth, new responsibilities of parenting, body changes

Health-seeking behaviors r/t postpartum recovery and adaptation

Impaired skin integrity r/t episiotomy, lacerations

Ineffective breast-feeding r/t lack of knowledge, lack of support, lack of motivation

Knowledge deficit: infant care r/t lack of preparation for parenting

Pain r/t episiotomy, lacerations, bruising, breast engorgement, headache, sore nipples, epidural or IV site, hemorrhoids

Risk for altered parenting r/t lack of role models, knowledge deficit

Risk for infection r/t tissue trauma, blood loss

Sexual dysfunction r/t fear of pain or pregnancy

Sleep pattern disturbance r/t care of infant

Postpartum Blues

Altered parenting r/t hormone-induced depression

Altered role performance r/t new responsibilities of parenting

Anxiety r/t new responsibilities of parenting

Body image disturbance r/t normal postpartum recovery

Fatigue r/t childbirth, postpartum state

Impaired adjustment r/t lack of support systems

Impaired home maintenance management r/t fatigue, care of newborn

Impaired social interaction r/t change in role functioning

Ineffective individual coping r/t hormonal changes, maturational crisis

Knowledge deficit r/t life-style changes

Sexual dysfunction r/t fear of another pregnancy, postpartum pain and lochia flow

Sleep pattern disturbance r/t new responsibilities of parenting

Postpartum Hemorrhage

Activity intolerance r/t anemia from loss of blood

Altered tissue perfusion r/t hypovolemia

Body image disturbance r/t loss of ideal childbirth

Decreased cardiac output r/t hypovolemia

Fear r/t threat to self, unknown future

Fluid volume deficit r/t uterine atony, loss of blood

Impaired home maintenance management r/t lack of stamina

Interrupted breast-feeding r/t separation from infant for medical treatment

Knowledge deficit r/t lack of exposure to situation

Pain r/t nursing and medical interventions to control bleeding

Risk for altered parenting r/t weakened maternal condition

Risk for infection r/t loss of blood, depressed immunity

Post-Trauma Response

Post-trauma response r/t disaster, war, epidemic, rape, assault, torture, catastrophic illness or accident

Post-Traumatic Stress Disorder

Altered thought process r/t sense of reliving the experience (flashbacks)

Anxiety r/t exposure to internal or external cues that symbolize or resemble an aspect of the traumatic event

Energy field disturbance r/t disharmony of mind, body, and spirit

Ineffective breathing pattern r/t hyperventilation associated with anxiety

Ineffective individual coping r/t extreme anxiety

Post-trauma response r/t exposure to a traumatic event

Potential for enhanced spiritual well-being r/t desire for harmony after stressful event

Risk for violence r/t fear of self or others

Sensory/perceptual alteration r/t psychological stress

Sleep pattern disturbance r/t recurring nightmares

Spiritual distress r/t feelings of detachment or estrangement from others

Potassium, Increase or Decrease

See Hyperkalemia or Hypokalemia

Powerlessness

Powerlessness r/t prolonged activity restriction

creating isolation, failing or deteriorating physiological condition, long-term stress, abandonment, lost belief in transcendent values or God

Preeclampsia

See PIH

Pregnancy—Cardiac Disorders

See Cardiac Disorders in Pregnancy

Pregnancy—Induced Hypertension/Preeclampsia

See PIH

Pregnancy—Normal

Altered family process r/t developmental transition of pregnancy

Altered nutrition: less than body requirements r/t growing fetus, nausea

Altered nutrition: more than body requirements r/t knowledge deficit regarding nutritional needs of pregnancy

Body image disturbance r/t altered body function and appearance

Family coping: potential for growth r/t satisfying partner relationship, attention to gratification of needs, effective adaptation to developmental tasks of pregnancy

Fear r/t labor and delivery

Health-seeking behaviors r/t desire to promote optimal fetal and maternal health

Ineffective individual coping r/t personal vulnerability, situational crisis

Knowledge deficit r/t primiparity

Sexual dysfunction r/t altered body function, self-concept, and body image with pregnancy

Sleep pattern disturbance r/t sleep deprivation secondary to uncomfortable pregnant state

See Discomforts of Pregnancy

Pregnancy Loss

Altered role performance r/t inability to assume parenting role

Altered sexuality patterns r/t self-esteem disturbance resulting from pregnancy loss and anxiety about future pregnancies

Anxiety r/t threat to role functioning, health status, situational crisis

Ineffective family coping: compromised r/t lack of support by significant other because of personal suffering

Ineffective individual coping r/t situational crisis

Pain r/t surgical intervention

Potential for enhanced spiritual well-being r/t desire
for acceptance of loss

Risk for altered sexuality patterns r/t self-esteem
disturbance, anxiety, grief

Risk for dysfunctional grieving r/t loss of pregnancy

Risk for fluid volume deficit r/t blood loss

Risk for infection r/t retained products of conception

Spiritual distress r/t intense suffering

Premature Dilation of the Cervix (Incompetent Cervix)

Altered role performance r/t inability to continue
usual patterns of responsibility

Anticipatory grieving r/t potential loss of infant

Diversional activity deficit r/t bedrest

Fear r/t potential loss of infant

Impaired physical mobility r/t imposed bedrest to
prevent preterm birth

Impaired social interaction r/t bedrest

Ineffective individual coping r/t bedrest, threat to fetus

Knowledge deficit r/t treatment regimen, prognosis for
pregnancy

Powerlessness r/t inability to control outcome of
pregnancy

Risk for infection r/t invasive procedures to prevent
preterm birth

Risk for injury: fetal r/t preterm birth, use of
anesthetics

Risk for injury: maternal r/t surgical procedures to
prevent preterm birth (e.g., cerclage)

Sexual dysfunction r/t fear of harm to fetus

Situational low self-esteem r/t inability to complete
normal pregnancy

Premature Infant (Child)

Altered growth and development: developmental
lag r/t prematurity, environmental and stimulation
deficiencies, multiple caretakers

Altered nutrition: less than body requirements r/t
delayed or understimulated rooting reflex, easy
fatigue during feeding, diminished endurance

Disorganized infant behavior r/t prematurity

Impaired gas exchange r/t effects of cardiopulmonary
insufficiency

Impaired swallowing r/t decreased or absent gag
reflex, fatigue

Ineffective thermoregulation r/t large body
surface/weight ratio, immaturity of thermal
regulation, state of prematurity

Potential for enhanced organized infant behavior r/t
prematurity

Risk for infection r/t inadequate, immature, or
undeveloped acquired immune response

Risk for injury r/t prolonged mechanical ventilation,
retrolental fibroplasia (RLF) secondary to 100%
oxygen environment

Sensory/perceptual alteration r/t noxious stimuli,
noisy environment

Sleep pattern disturbance r/t noisy and noxious
intensive care environment

Premature Infant (Parent)

Anticipatory grieving r/t loss of perfect child possibly
leading to dysfunctional grieving

Dysfunctional grieving (prolonged) r/t unresolved
conflicts

Decisional conflict r/t support system deficit, multiple
sources of information

Ineffective breast-feeding r/t disrupted establishment
of effective pattern secondary to prematurity or
insufficient opportunities

Ineffective family coping: compromised r/t disrupted
family roles and disorganization, prolonged
condition exhausting supportive capacity of
significant people

Parental role conflict r/t expressed concerns,
expressed inability to care for child's physical,
emotional, or developmental needs

Risk for altered parent/infant/child attachment r/t
separation, physical barriers, lack of privacy

Spiritual distress r/t challenged belief or value systems
regarding moral or ethical implications of treatment
plans

See Hospitalized Child; Child with Chronic Condition

Premature Rupture of Membranes

Anticipatory grieving r/t potential loss of infant

Anxiety r/t threat to infant's health status

Body image disturbance r/t inability to carry
pregnancy to term

Ineffective individual coping r/t situational crisis

Risk for infection r/t rupture of membranes

Risk for injury: fetal r/t risk of premature birth

Situational low self-esteem r/t inability to carry
pregnancy to term

Premenstrual Tension Syndrome

See PMS

Prenatal Care—Normal

Altered family processes r/t developmental transition

Altered nutrition: less than body requirements r/t
nausea from normal hormonal changes

Altered urinary elimination r/t frequency caused by
increased pelvic pressure and hormonal stimulation

Anxiety r/t unknown future, threat to self secondary to
pain of labor

Constipation r/t decreased gastrointestinal motility
  secondary to hormonal stimulation
Fatigue r/t increased energy demands
Health-seeking behaviors r/t consistent prenatal care
  and education
Ineffective breathing pattern r/t increased
  intrathoracic pressure and decreased energy
  secondary to enlarged uterus
Knowledge deficit r/t lack of experience with
  pregnancy and care
Risk for activity intolerance r/t enlarged abdomen,
  increased cardiac workload
Risk for injury: maternal r/t change in balance and
  center of gravity secondary to enlarged abdomen
Risk for sexual dysfunction r/t enlarged abdomen,
  fear of harm to infant
Sleep pattern disturbance r/t discomforts of
  pregnancy and fetal activity

Prenatal Testing

Anxiety r/t unknown outcome, delayed test results
Pain r/t invasive procedures
Risk for infection r/t invasive procedures during
  amniocentesis or chorionic villi sampling
Risk for injury: fetal r/t invasive procedures

Preoperative Teaching

Knowledge deficit r/t preoperative regimens,
  postoperative precautions, expectations of role of
  client during preoperative or postoperative time
See Surgery, Preoperative Care

Pressure Ulcer

Altered nutrition: less than body requirements r/t
  limited access to food, inability to absorb nutrients
  because of biological factors, anorexia
Impaired skin integrity: stage I or II pressure ulcer
  r/t physical immobility, mechanical factors, altered
  circulation, skin irritants
Impaired tissue integrity: stage III or IV pressure
  ulcer r/t altered circulation, impaired physical
  mobility
Pain r/t tissue destruction, exposure of nerves
Risk for infection r/t physical immobility, mechanical
  factors (shearing forces, pressure, restraint, altered
  circulation, skin irritants)
Total incontinence r/t neurological dysfunction

Preterm Labor

Altered role performance r/t inability to carry out
  normal roles secondary to bedrest or hospitalization,
  change in expected course of pregnancy
Anticipatory grieving r/t loss of idealized pregnancy,
  potential loss of fetus

Anxiety r/t threat to fetus, change in role functioning,
  change in environment and interaction patterns, use
  of tocolytic drugs
Diversional activity deficit r/t long-term
  hospitalization
Impaired home maintenance management r/t
  medical restrictions
Impaired physical mobility r/t medically imposed
  restrictions
Impaired social interaction r/t prolonged bedrest or
  hospitalization
Ineffective individual coping r/t situational crisis,
  preterm labor
Risk for injury: fetal r/t premature birth, immature
  body systems
Risk for maternal injury r/t use of tocolytic drugs
Sexual dysfunction r/t actual or perceived limitation
  imposed by preterm labor and/or prescribed
  treatment, separation from partner because of
  hospitalization
Situational low self-esteem r/t threatened ability to
  carry pregnancy to term
Sleep pattern disturbance r/t change in usual pattern
  secondary to contractions, hospitalization, or
  treatment regimen

Problem-Solving Ability

Defensive coping r/t situational crisis
Impaired adjustment r/t altered locus of control
Ineffective individual coping r/t situational crisis
Potential for enhanced spiritual well-being r/t desire
  to draw on inner strength and find meaning and
  purpose to life

Projection

Anxiety r/t threat to self-concept
Chronic low self-esteem r/t failure
Defensive coping r/t inability to acknowledge that own
  behavior may be a problem, blaming others
Impaired social interaction r/t self-concept
  disturbance, confrontational communication style
Risk for loneliness r/t blaming others for problems

Prolapsed Umbilical Cord

Altered tissue perfusion: fetal r/t interruption in
  umbilical blood flow
Fear r/t threat to fetus, impending surgery
Risk for injury: fetal r/t cord compression, altered
  tissue perfusion
Risk for injury: maternal r/t emergency surgery

Prolonged Gestation

Altered nutrition: less than body requirements:
  fetal r/t aging of placenta

Anxiety r/t potential change in birthing plans, need for increased medical intervention, unknown outcome for fetus

Defensive coping r/t underlying feeling of inadequacy regarding ability to give birth normally

Powerlessness r/t perceived lack of control over outcome of pregnancy

Situational low self-esteem r/t perceived inadequacy of body functioning

Prostatectomy

See TURP

Prostatic Hypertrophy

Altered health maintenance r/t knowledge deficit regarding self-care and prevention of complications

Risk for infection r/t urinary residual postvoiding, bacterial invasion of bladder

Sleep pattern disturbance r/t nocturia

Urinary retention r/t obstruction

Prostatitis

Altered health maintenance r/t knowledge deficit regarding treatment

Altered protection r/t depressed immune system

Risk for urge incontinence r/t irritation of bladder

Protection, Altered

Altered protection r/t extremes of age, inadequate nutrition, alcohol abuse, abnormal blood profiles (leukopenia, thrombocytopenia, anemia, coagulation), drug therapies (antineoplastic, corticosteroid, immune, anticoagulant, thrombolytic), treatments (surgery, radiation), diseases (e.g., cancer, immune disorders)

Pruritis

Altered comfort: pruritis r/t inflammation in tissues

Knowledge deficit r/t methods to treat and prevent itching

Risk for impaired skin integrity r/t scratching from pruritis

Psoriasis

Altered health maintenance r/t knowledge deficit regarding treatment modalities

Body image disturbance r/t lesions on body

Impaired skin integrity r/t lesions on body

Powerlessness r/t lack of control over condition with frequent exacerbations and remissions

Psychosis

Alteration in family process r/t inability to express feelings, impaired communication

Alteration in nutrition: less than body requirements r/t lack of awareness of hunger, disinterest toward food

Alteration in thought process r/t inaccurate interpretations of environment

Altered health maintenance r/t cognitive impairment, ineffective individual and family coping

Anxiety r/t unconscious conflict with reality

Fear r/t altered contact with reality

Impaired home maintenance management r/t impaired cognitive or emotional functioning, inadequate support systems

Impaired social interaction r/t impaired communication patterns, self-concept disturbance, altered thought process

Impaired verbal communication r/t psychosis, inaccurate perceptions, hallucinations, delusions

Ineffective individual coping r/t inadequate support systems, unrealistic perceptions, altered thought processes, impaired communication

Risk for violence: self-directed or directed at others r/t lack of trust, panic, hallucinations, delusional thinking

Self-care deficit r/t loss of contact with reality, impairment in perception

Self-esteem disturbance r/t excessive use of defense mechanisms (e.g., projection, denial, rationalization)

Sleep pattern disturbance r/t sensory alterations contributing to fear and anxiety

Social isolation r/t lack of trust, regression, delusional thinking, repressed fears

See Schizophrenia

PTCA (Percutaneous Transluminal Coronary Angioplasty)

See Angioplasty

Pulmonary Edema

Altered health maintenance r/t knowledge deficit regarding treatment regimen

Anxiety r/t fear of suffocation

Impaired gas exchange r/t ambulation of extravascular fluid in lung tissues and alveoli

Ineffective breathing pattern r/t presence of tracheobronchial secretions

See CHF

Pulmonary Embolism

Altered tissue perfusion: pulmonary r/t interruption of pulmonary blood flow secondary to lodged embolus

Fear r/t severe pain, possible death

Impaired gas exchange r/t altered blood flow to alveoli secondary to lodged embolus

Knowledge deficit r/t activities to prevent embolism, self-care after diagnosis of embolism

Pain r/t biological injury, lack of oxygen to cells

Risk for altered cardiac output r/t right ventricular failure secondary to obstructed pulmonary artery

See Anticoagulant Therapy

Pulmonary Stenosis

See Congenital Heart Disease/Cardiac Anomalies

Pulse Deficit

Decreased cardiac output r/t dysrhythmia

See Dysrhythmia

Pulse Oximetry

Knowledge deficit r/t use of oxygen-monitoring equipment

See Hypoxia

Pulse Pressure, Increased

See Intracranial Pressure, Increased

Pulse Pressure, Narrowed

See Shock

Pulses, Absent or Diminished Peripheral

Altered tissue perfusion: peripheral r/t interruption of arterial flow

Risk for peripheral neurovascular dysfunction r/t fractures, mechanical compression, orthopedic surgery trauma, immobilization, burns, vascular obstruction

See Cause of Absent or Diminished Peripheral Pulses

Purpura

See Clotting Disorder

Pyelonephritis

Altered comfort r/t chills and fever

Altered health maintenance r/t knowledge deficit regarding self-care, treatment of disease, prevention of further urinary tract infections

Altered urinary elimination r/t irritation of urinary tract

Pain r/t inflammation and irritation of urinary tract

Sleep pattern disturbance r/t urinary frequency

Pyloric Stenosis

Altered health maintenance r/t parental knowledge deficit regarding home care feeding regimen, wound care

Altered nutrition: less than body requirements r/t vomiting secondary to pyloric sphincter obstruction

Fluid volume deficit r/t vomiting, dehydration

Pain r/t surgical incision

See Hospitalized Child

Q

Quadriplegia

Anticipatory grieving r/t loss of normal life-style, severity of disability

Ineffective breathing pattern r/t inability to use intercostal muscles

Risk for dysreflexia r/t bladder distention, bowel distention, skin irritation, lack of client and caregiver knowledge

See Spinal Cord Injury

R

Rabies

Altered health maintenance r/t knowledge deficit regarding care of wound, isolation and observation of infected animal

Health-seeking behaviors r/t prophylactic immunization of domestic animals, avoidance of contact with wild animals

Hopelessness r/t poor prognosis

Pain r/t multiple immunization injections

Radiation Therapy

Activity intolerance r/t fatigue from possible anemia

Altered nutrition: less than body requirements r/t anorexia, nausea, vomiting, irradiation of areas of pharynx and esophagus

Alteration in oral mucous membranes r/t irradiation effects

Altered protection r/t suppression of bone marrow

Body image disturbance r/t change in appearance, hair loss

Diarrhea r/t irradiation effects

Knowledge deficit r/t what to expect with radiation therapy

Risk for impaired skin integrity r/t irradiation effects

Social isolation r/t possible limitations on time exposure of caregivers and significant others to client

Radical Neck Dissection

See Laryngectomy

Rage

Risk for violence: directed at others r/t panic state, manic excitement, organic brain syndrome
Risk for self-mutilation r/t command hallucinations

Rape-Trauma Syndrome

Rape-trama syndrome r/t forced, violent sexual penetration against the victim's will and consent
Rape-trauma syndrome: compound reaction r/t forced and violent sexual penetration against the victim's will and consent, activation of previous health disruptions (e.g., physical illness, psychiatric illness, substance abuse)
Rape-trauma syndrome: silent reaction r/t forced and violent sexual penetration against the victim's will and consent, demonstration of repression of the incident

Rash

Altered comfort: pruritis r/t inflammation in skin
Impaired skin integrity r/t mechanical trauma
Risk for infection r/t traumatized tissue, broken skin

Rationalization

Defensive coping r/t situational crisis, inability to accept blame for consequences of own behavior
Ineffective denial r/t fear of consequences, actual or perceived loss
Potential for enhanced spiritual well-being r/t possibility of seeking harmony with self, others, and higher power/God

Rats, Rodents in the Home

Impaired home maintenance management r/t lack of knowledge, insufficient finances

Raynaud's Disease

Altered tissue perfusion: peripheral r/t transient reduction of blood flow
Knowledge deficit r/t lack of information about disease process, possible complications, self-care needs regarding disease process and medication

RDS (Respiratory Distress Syndrome)

See Respiratory Conditions of the Neonate

Rectal Fullness

Constipation r/t decreased activity level, decreased fluid intake, inadequate fiber in diet, decreased peristalsis, side effects from antidepressant or antipsychotic therapy

Rectal Pain/Bleeding

Constipation r/t pain on defecation
Knowledge deficit r/t possible causes of rectal bleeding, pain, treatment modalities
Pain r/t pressure of defecation
Risk for fluid volume deficit: bleeding r/t untreated rectal bleeding

Rectal Surgery

See Hemorrhoidectomy

Rectocele Repair

Altered health maintenance r/t knowledge deficit of postoperative care of surgical site, dietary measures, exercise to prevent constipation
Colonic constipation r/t painful defecation
Pain r/t surgical procedure
Risk for infection r/t surgical procedure and possible contamination of site with feces
Urinary retention r/t edema related to surgery

Reflex Incontinence

Reflex incontinence r/t neurological impairment

Regression

Altered role performance r/t powerlessness over health status
Anxiety r/t threat to or change in health status
Defensive coping r/t denial of obvious problems or weaknesses
Powerlessness r/t health care environment
See Hospitalized Child; Separation Anxiety

Regretful

Anxiety r/t situational or maturational crises

Rehabilitation

Altered comfort r/t difficulty in performing rehabilitation tasks
Impaired physical mobility r/t injury, surgery, or psychosocial condition warranting rehabilitation
Ineffective individual coping r/t loss of normal function
Self-care deficit r/t impaired physical mobility

Relaxation Techniques

Anxiety r/t energy field disturbance
Health-seeking behaviors r/t requesting information about ways to relieve stress

Religious Concern

Potential for enhanced spiritual well-being r/t desire for increased spirituality

Spiritual distress r/t separation from religious or cultural ties

Relocation Stress Syndrome

Relocation stress syndrome r/t past, concurrent, and recent losses; losses involved with decision to move; feeling of powerlessness; lack of adequate support system; little or no preparation for the impending move; moderate to high degree of environmental change; history and types of previous transfers; impaired psychosocial health status; decreased physical health status; advanced age

Renal Failure

Activity intolerance r/t effects of anemia and congestive heart failure

Altered comfort: pruritis r/t effects of uremia

Altered nutrition: less than body requirements r/t anorexia, nausea, vomiting, altered taste sensation, dietary restrictions

Altered oral mucous membranes r/t irritation from nitrogenous waste products

Altered urinary elimination r/t effects of disease, need for dialysis

Decreased cardiac output r/t effects of congestive heart failure, elevated potassium levels interfering with conduction system

Fatigue r/t effects of chronic uremia and anemia

Fluid volume excess r/t decreased urine output, sodium retention, inappropriate fluid intake

Ineffective individual coping r/t depression secondary to chronic disease

Risk for altered oral mucous membranes r/t dehydration, effects of uremia

Risk for infection r/t altered immune functioning

Risk for injury r/t bone changes, neuropathy, muscle weakness

Risk for noncompliance r/t complex medical therapy

Spiritual distress r/t dealing with chronic illness

Renal Failure, Acute/Chronic—Child

Body image disturbance r/t growth retardation, bone changes, visibility of dialysis access devices (shunt, fistula), edema

Diversional activity deficit r/t immobility during dialysis

See Renal Failure; Hospitalized Child; Child with Chronic Illness

Renal Failure, Nonoliguric

Anxiety r/t change in health status

Risk for fluid volume deficit r/t loss of large volumes of urine

See Renal Failure

Renal Transplantation, Donor

Decisional conflict r/t harvesting of kidney from traumatized donor

Family coping: potential for growth r/t decision to allow organ donation

Potential for enhanced spirituality r/t inner peace resulting from allowance of organ donation

Spiritual distress r/t anticipatory grieving from loss of significant person

See Nephrectomy

Renal Transplantation, Recipient

Altered protection r/t immunosuppression therapy

Alteration in urinary elimination r/t possible impaired renal function

Anxiety r/t possible rejection, procedure

Impaired health maintenance r/t long-term home treatment after transplantation, diet, signs of rejection, use of medications

Knowledge deficit r/t specific nutritional needs, possible paralytic ileus, fluid or sodium restrictions

Risk for infection r/t use of immunosuppressive therapy to control rejection

Spiritual distress r/t obtaining transplanted kidney from someone's traumatic loss

Respiratory Acidosis

See Acidosis, Respiratory

Respiratory Conditions of the Neonate (Respiratory Distress Syndrome [RDS], Meconium Aspiration, Diaphragmatic Hernia)

Fatigue r/t increased energy requirements and metabolic demands

Impaired gas exchange r/t decreased surfactant, immature lung tissue

Ineffective airway clearance r/t sequelae of attempts to breathe in utero resulting in meconium aspiration

Ineffective breathing patterns r/t prolonged ventilator dependence

Risk for infection r/t tissue destruction or irritation secondary to aspiration of meconium fluid

See Hospitalized Child; Premature Infant; Bronchopulmonary Dysplasia

Respiratory Distress

See Dyspnea

Respiratory Distress Syndrome (RDS)

See Respiratory Conditions of the Neonate

Respiratory Infections, Acute Childhood (Croup, Epiglotitis, Pertussis, Pneumonia, Respiratory Syncytial Virus)

Activity intolerance r/t generalized weakness, dyspnea, fatigue, poor oxygenation

Altered nutrition: less than body requirements r/t anorexia, fatigue, generalized weakness, poor sucking and breathing coordination, dyspnea

Anxiety/fear r/t oxygen deprivation, difficulty breathing

Fluid volume deficit r/t insensible losses (fever, diaphoresis), inadequate oral fluid intake

Hyperthermia r/t infectious process

Impaired gas exchange r/t insufficient oxygenation secondary to inflammation or edema of epiglottis, larynx, or bronchial passages

Ineffective airway clearance r/t excess tracheobronchial secretions

Ineffective breathing patterns r/t inflamed bronchial passages, coughing

Risk for aspiration r/t inability to coordinate breathing, coughing, and sucking

Risk for infection: transmission to others r/t virulent infectious organisms

Risk for injury (to pregnant others) r/t exposure to aerosolized medications (e.g., ribavirin, pentamidine), and resultant potential fetal toxicity

Risk for suffocation r/t inflammation of larynx or epiglottis

See Hospitalized Child

Respiratory Syncytial Virus

See Respiratory Infections, Acute Childhood

Retching

Altered comfort r/t visceral disorders

Altered nutrition: less than body requirements r/t inability to ingest food

Retinal Detachment

Anxiety r/t change in vision, threat of loss of vision

Knowledge deficit r/t symptoms, need for early intervention to prevent permanent damage

Risk for impaired home maintenance management r/t postoperative care, activity limitations, care of affected eye

Sensory perceptual alteration: visual r/t changes in vision, sudden flashes of light, floating spots, blurring of vision

Reye's Syndrome

Altered health maintenance r/t knowledge deficit regarding use of salicylates during viral illness of child

Altered nutrition: less than body requirements r/t effects of liver dysfunction, vomiting

Altered thought processes r/t degenerative changes in fatty brain tissue

Anticipatory grieving r/t uncertain prognosis and sequelae

Fluid volume deficit r/t vomiting, hyperventilation

Fluid volume excess: cerebral r/t cerebral edema

Impaired gas exchange r/t hyperventilation, sequelae of increased intracranial pressure

Impaired skin integrity r/t effects of decorticate or decerebrate posturing, seizure activity

Ineffective breathing patterns r/t neuromuscular impairment

Ineffective family coping: compromised r/t acute situational crisis

Risk for injury r/t combative behavior, seizure activity

Sensory/perceptual alteration r/t cerebral edema

Situational low self-esteem: family r/t negative perceptions of self, perceived inability to manage family situation, expressions of guilt

See Hospitalized Child

Rh Factor Incompatibility

Anxiety r/t unknown outcome of pregnancy

Health-seeking behaviors r/t prenatal care, compliance with diagnostic and treatment regimen

Knowledge deficit r/t treatment regimen from lack of experience with situation

Powerlessness r/t perceived lack of control over outcome of pregnancy

Risk for fetal injury r/t intrauterine destruction of red blood cells, transfusions

Rheumatic Fever

See Endocarditis

Rheumatoid Arthritis, Juvenile (JRA)

Altered growth and development r/t effects of physical disability, chronic illness

Fatigue r/t chronic inflammatory disease

Impaired physical mobility r/t pain, restricted joint movement

Pain r/t swollen or inflamed joints, restricted movement, physical therapy

Risk for impaired skin integrity r/t splints, adaptive devices

Risk for injury r/t impaired physical mobility, splints, adaptive devices, increased bleeding potential secondary to antiinflammatory medications

Self-care deficits: feeding, bathing/hygiene, dressing/grooming, toileting r/t restricted joint movement, pain

See Child with Chronic Condition; Hospitalized Child

Rib Fracture

Ineffective breathing pattern r/t fractured ribs
Pain r/t movement, deep breathing
See Ventilator Client (if relevant)

Ridicule of Others

Defensive coping r/t situational crisis, psychological
impairment, substance abuse

Roaches, Invasion of Home with

Impaired home maintenance management r/t lack of
knowledge, insufficient finances

Role Performance, Altered

Altered role performance r/t inability to perform role
as anticipated

RSV (Respiratory Synctical Virus)

See Respiratory Infection, Acute Childhood

Rubella

See Communicable Diseases, Childhood

Rubor of Extremities

Altered tissue perfusion: peripheral r/t interruption
of arterial flow
See Peripheral Vascular Disease

S

Sadness

Dysfunctional grieving r/t actual or perceived loss
Potential for enhanced spiritual well-being r/t desire
for harmony following actual or perceived loss
Spiritual distress r/t intense suffering

Safety, Childhood

Health-seeking behaviors: enhanced parenting r/t
adequate support systems, appropriate requests for
help, desire and request for safety information,
requests for information or assistance regarding
parenting skills
Knowledge deficit: potential for enhanced health
maintenance r/t parental knowledge and skill
acquisition regarding appropriate safety measures
Risk for altered health maintenance r/t parental
knowledge deficit regarding appropriate safety needs
per developmental stage, childproofing house, infant
and child car restraints, water safety, teaching of
child the way to avoid molestation

Risk for altered parenting r/t lack of available and
effective role model, lack of knowledge,
misinformation from other family members ("old
wives' tales")
Risk for aspiration and/or suffocation r/t pillow or
propped bottle placed in infant's crib; sides of
playpen/crib being wide enough for child to get head
through; child left in car with engine running;
enclosed areas; plastic bags or small objects used as
toys; toys with small, breakaway parts; refrigerators
or freezers with doors left accessible as play areas
for children; children left unattended in or near
bathtubs, pools, or spas; low clotheslines; electric
garage doors without automatic stop/reopen; pacifier
being hung around infant's neck; food not cut into
small, bite-size, and age-appropriate pieces;
balloons, hot dogs, nuts, or popcorn given to infants
or young children (especially less than 1 year of
age); use of baby powder
Risk for injury/trauma r/t developmental age, altered
home maintenance management (house not
childproofed), altered parenting, hot liquids within
child's reach, no infant or child car restraints, no
gates at top of stairs, lack of immunizations for age,
no fences or pool or spa covers, leaving of child in
car unattended with closed windows in hot weather,
firearms loaded and within child's reach
Risk for poisoning r/t use of lead-based paint,
presence of asbestos or radon gas, drugs not locked
in cabinet, household products left in accessible area
(bleach, detergent, drain cleaners, household
cleaners), alcohol and perfume within reach of child,
presence of poisonous plants, atmospheric pollutants

Salmonella

See Gastroenteritis

Salpingectomy

Anticipatory grieving r/t possible loss due to tubal
pregnancy
Decisional conflict r/t sterilization procedure
Risk for altered urinary elimination r/t trauma to
ureter during surgery
See Hysterectomy; Surgery

Sarcoidosis

Altered health maintenance r/t knowledge deficit
regarding home care and medication regimen
Anxiety r/t change in health status
Impaired gas exchange r/t ventilation-perfusion
imbalance
Pain r/t possible disease affecting the joints
Risk for decreased cardiac output r/t dysrhythmias

SBE (Self Breast Examination)

Health–seeking behaviors r/t desire to have information about self breast examination

Scabies

See Communicable Diseases, Childhood

Scared

Anxiety r/t threat of death, threat to or change in health status

Fear r/t hospitalization, real or imagined threat to own well-being

Schizophrenia

Alteration in family process r/t inability to express feelings, impaired communication

Altered nutrition: less than body requirements r/t fear of eating, unaware of hunger, disinterest toward food

Altered thought process r/t inaccurate interpretations of environment

Altered health maintenance r/t cognitive impairment, ineffective individual and family coping, lack of material resources

Anxiety r/t unconscious conflict with reality

Diversional activity deficit r/t social isolation, possible regression

Fear r/t altered contact with reality

Impaired home maintenance management r/t impaired cognitive or emotional functioning, insufficient finances, inadequate support systems

Impaired social interaction r/t impaired communication patterns, self-concept disturbance, altered thought process

Impaired verbal communication r/t psychosis, disorientation, inaccurate perception, hallucinations, delusions

Ineffective individual coping r/t inadequate support systems, unrealistic perceptions, inadequate coping skills, altered thought processes, impaired communication

Ineffective management of therapeutic regimen: families r/t chronicity and unpredictability of condition

Risk for caregiver role strain r/t bizarre behavior of client, chronicity of condition

Risk for loneliness r/t inability to interact socially

Risk for violence: self–directed or directed at others r/t lack of trust, panic, hallucinations, delusional thinking

Self–care deficit r/t loss of contact with reality, impairment in perception

Self–esteem disturbance r/t excessive use of defense mechanisms (e.g., projection, denial, rationalization)

Sleep pattern disturbance r/t sensory alterations contributing to fear and anxiety

Social isolation r/t lack of trust, regression, delusional thinking, repressed fears

Scoliosis

Altered health maintenance r/t knowledge deficit regarding treatment modalities, restrictions, home care, postoperative activities

Body image disturbance r/t use of therapeutic braces, postsurgery scars, restricted physical activity

Impaired adjustment r/t lack of developmental maturity to comprehend long-term consequences of noncompliance with treatment procedures

Impaired gas exchange r/t restricted lung expansion secondary to severe presurgery curvature of spine, immobilization

Impaired physical mobility r/t restricted movement, dyspnea secondary to severe curvature of spine

Impaired skin integrity r/t braces, casts, surgical correction

Ineffective breathing patterns r/t restricted lung expansion secondary to severe curvature of spine

Pain r/t musculoskeletal restrictions, surgery, reambulation with cast or spinal rod

Risk for infection r/t surgical incision

Risk for perioperative positioning injury r/t prone position

See Hospitalized Child; Maturational Issues, Adolescent

Sedentary Life-Style

Activity intolerance r/t sedentary life-style

Seizure Disorders, Adult

Acute confusion r/t postseizure state

Altered health maintenance r/t lack of knowledge regarding anticonvulsive therapy

Impaired memory r/t seizure activity

Risk for altered thought processes r/t effects of anticonvulsant medications

Risk for ineffective airway clearance r/t accumulation of secretions during seizure

Risk for injury r/t uncontrolled movements during seizure, falls, drowsiness secondary to anticonvulsants

Social isolation r/t unpredictability of seizures, community-imposed stigma

See Epilepsy

Seizure Disorders, Childhood (Epilepsy, Febrile Seizures, Infantile Spasms)

Altered health maintenance r/t lack of knowledge regarding anticonvulsive therapy, fever reduction (febrile seizures)

Risk for altered growth and development r/t effects of seizure disorder, parental overprotection

Risk for altered thought processes r/t effects of anticonvulsant medications

Risk for ineffective airway clearance r/t accumulation of secretions during seizure

Risk for injury r/t uncontrolled movements during seizure, falls, drowsiness secondary to anticonvulsants

Social isolation r/t unpredictability of seizures, community-imposed stigma

See Epilepsy

Self Breast Examination

See SBE

Self-Care Deficit, Bathing/Hygiene

Self-care deficit: dressing/grooming r/t intolerance to activity, decreased strength and endurance, pain, discomfort, perceptual or cognitive impairment, neuromuscular impairment, musculoskeletal impairment, depression, severe anxiety

Self-Care Deficit, Dressing/Grooming

Self-care deficit: dressing/grooming r/t intolerance to activity, decreased strength and endurance, pain, discomfort, perceptual or cognitive impairment, neuromuscular impairment, musculoskeletal impairment, depression, severe anxiety

Self-Care Deficit, Feeding

Self-care deficit: feeding r/t intolerance to activity, decreased strength and endurance, pain, discomfort, perceptual or cognitive impairment, neuromuscular impairment, musculoskeletal impairment, depression, severe anxiety

Self-Care Deficit, Toileting

Self-care deficit: toileting r/t impaired transfer ability, impaired mobility status, intolerance to activity, decreased strength and endurance, pain, discomfort, perceptual or cognitive impairment, neuromuscular impairment, musculoskeletal impairment, depression, severe anxiety

Self-Destructive Behavior

Post-trauma response r/t unresolved feelings related to traumatic event

Risk for self-mutilation r/t feelings of depression, rejection, self-hatred, or depersonalization; command hallucinations

Risk for violence: self-directed r/t panic state, history of child abuse, toxic reaction to medication

S

Self-Esteem, Chronic Low

Chronic low self-esteem r/t long-standing negative self-evaluation

Self-Esteem, Situational Low

Situational low self-esteem r/t situational crisis

Self-Esteem Disturbance

Self-esteem disturbance r/t inappropriate and learned negative feelings about self

Self-Mutilation, Risk for

Risk for self-mutilation r/t inability to cope with increased psychological or physiological tension in a healthy manner; feelings of depression, rejection, self-hatred, separation anxiety, guilt, and depersonalization; fluctuating emotions; command hallucinations; need for sensory stimuli; parental emotional deprivation; dysfunctional family

Senile Dementia

See Dementia

Sensory/Perceptual Alterations

Sensory/perceptual alterations: visual, auditory, kinesthetic, gustatory, tactile, olfactory r/t altered, excessive, or insufficient environmental stimuli; altered sensory reception, transmission, and/or integration; endogenous (electrolyte) or exogenous (e.g., drugs) chemical alterations; psychological stress

Separation Anxiety

Ineffective individual coping r/t maturational and situational crises, vulnerability secondary to developmental age, hospitalization, separation from family and familiar surroundings, multiple caregivers

See Hospitalized Child

Sepsis—Child

Altered comfort: increased sensitivity to environmental stimuli r/t sensory-perceptual alterations: visual, auditory, kinesthetic

Altered nutrition: less than body requirements r/t anorexia, generalized weakness, poor sucking reflex

Altered tissue perfusion: cardiopulmonary, peripheral r/t arterial or venous blood flow exchange problems, septic shock

Ineffective thermal regulation r/t infectious process, septic shock

Risk for impaired skin integrity r/t desquamation secondary to disseminated intravascular coagulation (DIC)

See Hospitalized Child; Premature Infant

Septicemia

Altered nutrition: less than body requirements r/t anorexia, generalized weakness

Altered tissue perfusion r/t decreased systemic vascular resistance

Fluid volume deficit r/t vasodilation of peripheral vessels, leaking of capillaries

See Sepsis—Child; Shock; Shock, Septic

Sexual Dysfunction

Sexual dysfunction r/t biopsychosocial alteration of sexuality, ineffectual or absent role models, physical abuse or harmful relationships, vulnerability, conflicting values, lack of privacy, lack of significant others, altered body structure or function (pregnancy, recent childbirth, drug use, surgery, anomalies, disease process, trauma, radiation), misinformation or lack of knowledge

Sexuality, Adolescent

Body image disturbance r/t anxiety secondary to unachieved developmental milestone (puberty) or knowledge deficit regarding reproductive maturation as manifested by amenorrhea or expressed concerns regarding lack of growth of secondary sex characteristics

Decisional conflict: sexual activity r/t undefined personal values or beliefs, multiple or divergent sources of information, lack of relevant information

Knowledge deficit: potential for enhanced health maintenance r/t multiple or divergent sources of information or lack of relevant information regarding sexual transmission of disease, contraception, and prevention of toxic shock syndrome

Risk for rape-trauma syndrome r/t date rape, campus rape, insufficient knowledge regarding self-protection mechanisms

See Maturational Issues, Adolescent

Sexuality Patterns, Altered

Altered sexuality patterns r/t knowledge or skill deficit regarding alternative responses to health-related transitions, altered body function or structure, illness or medical problems, lack of privacy, lack of significant other, ineffective or absent role models, fear of pregnancy or acquiring a sexually transmitted disease, impaired relationship with a significant other

Sexually Transmitted Disease

See STD

Shakiness

Anxiety r/t situational or maturational crisis, threat of death

Shame

Self-esteem disturbance r/t inability to deal with past traumatic events, blaming of self for events not responsible for

Shivering

Hypothermia r/t exposure to cool environment

Shock

Altered tissue perfusion: cardiopulmonary, peripheral r/t arterial/venous blood flow exchange problems

Fear r/t serious threat to health status

Risk for injury r/t prolonged shock resulting in multiple organ failure, death

See Shock, Cardiogenic; Shock, Hypovolemic; Shock, Septic

Shock, Cardiogenic

Decreased cardiac output r/t decreased myocardial contractility, dysrhythmia

See Shock

Shock, Hypovolemic

Fluid volume deficit r/t abnormal loss of fluid

See Shock

Shock, Septic

Altered protection r/t inadequately functioning immune system

Fluid volume deficit r/t abnormal loss of fluid through capillaries, pooling of blood in peripheral circulation

See Shock; Sepsis, Child; Septicemia

Shoulder Repair

Risk for perioperative positioning injury r/t immobility

Self-care deficit: bathing/hygiene, dressing/grooming, feeding r/t immobilization of affected shoulder

See Surgery; Total Joint Replacement

Sickle Cell Anemia/Crisis

Activity intolerance r/t fatigue, effects of chronic anemia

Fluid volume deficit r/t decreased intake, increased fluid requirements during sickle cell crisis, decreased ability of kidneys to concentrate urine

Impaired physical mobility r/t pain, fatigue

Pain r/t viscous blood, tissue hypoxia

Risk for altered tissue perfusion (renal, cerebral, cardiac, gastrointestinal, peripheral) r/t effects of red cell sickling, infarction of tissues

Risk for infection r/t alterations in splenic function

See Hospitalized Child; Child with Chronic Condition

SIDS

Altered family processes r/t stress secondary to special care needs of infant with apnea

Anticipatory grieving r/t potential loss of infant

Anxiety/fear: parental r/t life-threatening event

Knowledge deficit: potential for enhanced health maintenance r/t knowledge or skill acquisition of CPR and home apnea monitoring

Sleep pattern disturbance: parental/infant r/t home apnea monitoring

See Terminally Ill Child/Death of Child

Situational Crisis

Altered family processes r/t situational crisis

Ineffective individual coping r/t situational crisis

Potential for enhanced spiritual well-being r/t desire for harmony following crisis

Skin Cancer

Altered health maintenance r/t knowledge deficit regarding self-care with skin cancer

Impaired skin integrity r/t abnormal cell growth in skin, treatment of skin cancer

Skin Disorders

External

Impaired skin integrity r/t hyperthermia, hypothermia, chemical substances, mechanical factors (shearing forces, pressure, restraint), radiation, physical immobilization, humidity

Internal

Impaired skin integrity r/t medication, altered nutritional state (obesity, emaciation), altered metabolic state, altered circulation, altered sensation, altered pigmentation, skeletal prominence, developmental factors, immunological deficit, alterations in turgor (change in elasticity)

Skin Integrity, Risk for Impaired

Risk for impaired skin integrity r/t internal or external factors that are potentially harmful to skin

Skin Turgor, Change in Elasticity

Fluid volume deficit r/t active fluid loss

NOTE: Decreased skin turgor can be normal finding in the elderly.

Sleep Apnea

See PND

Sleep Deprivation

Altered sensory perception r/t lack of sleep

Fatigue r/t lack of sleep

Sleep Pattern Disorders

Sleep pattern disorders r/t sensory alterations, internal factors (illness, psychological stress), external factors (environmental changes, social cues)

Sleep Pattern Disturbance, Parent/Child

Sleep pattern disturbance: child r/t anxiety or apprehension secondary to parental deprivation (see **Suspected Child Abuse and Neglect),** fear, night terrors, enuresis, inconsistent parental responses to child's requests to alter bedtime rules, frequent nighttime awakening, inability to wean from parents' bed, hypervigilance

Sleep pattern disturbance: parental r/t time-intensive home treatments, increased caretaker demands

Slurring of Speech

Impaired verbal communication r/t decrease in circulation to brain, brain tumor, anatomical defect, cleft palate

Situational low self-esteem r/t speech impairment

Small Bowel Resection

See Abdominal Surgery

Smell, Loss of

Sensory/perceptual alteration: olfactory r/t altered sensory reception, transmission, or integration

Smoking Behavior

Altered health maintenance r/t denial of effects of smoking, lack of effective support for smoking withdrawal

Social Interaction, Impaired

Social interaction: impaired r/t knowledge or skill deficit about ways to enhance mutuality, communication barriers, self-concept disturbance, absence of available significant others or peers, limited physical mobility, therapeutic isolation, sociocultural dissonance, environmental barriers, altered thought processes

Social Isolation

Social isolation r/t factors contributing to the absence of satisfying personal relationships, such as delay in accomplishing developmental tasks, immature interests, alterations in physical appearance, alterations in mental status, unaccepted social behavior, unaccepted social values, altered state of wellness, inadequate personal resources, inability to engage in satisfying personal relationships, fear

Sociopath

See Antisocial Personality Disorder

Sodium, Decrease/Increase

See Hyponatremia, Hypernatremia

Somatoform Disorder

Anxiety r/t unresolved conflicts being channeled into physical complaints or conditions

Chronic pain r/t unexpressed anger, multiple physical disorders, depression

Ineffective individual coping r/t lack of insight into underlying conflicts

Sore Nipples: Breast-Feeding

Ineffective breast-feeding r/t knowledge deficit regarding correct feeding procedure

See Painful Breasts—Sore Nipples

Sore Throat

Altered oral mucous membranes r/t inflammation or infection of oral cavity

Impaired swallowing r/t irritation of oropharyngeal cavity

Knowledge deficit r/t treatment, relieving discomfort

Pain r/t inflammation, irritation, dryness

Sorrow

Anticipatory grieving r/t impending loss of significant person or object

Grieving r/t loss of significant person, object, or role

Potential for enhanced spiritual well-being r/t desire to find purpose and meaning of loss

Speech Disorders

Anxiety r/t difficulty with communication

Impaired verbal communication r/t anatomical defect, cleft palate, psychological barriers, decrease in circulation to brain

Spina Bifida

See Neurotube Defects

Spinal Cord Injury

Altered health maintenance r/t knowledge deficit regarding self-care with spinal cord injury

Body image disturbance r/t change in body function

Constipation r/t immobility, loss of sensation

Diversional activity deficit r/t long-term hospitalization, frequent lengthy treatments

Dysfunctional grieving r/t loss of usual body function

Fear r/t powerlessness over loss of body function

Impaired home maintenance r/t change in health status, insufficient family planning or finances, knowledge deficit, inadequate support systems

Impaired physical mobility r/t neuromuscular impairment

Reflex incontinence r/t spinal cord lesion interfering with conduction of cerebral messages

Risk for disuse syndrome r/t paralysis

Risk for dysreflexia r/t bladder or bowel distention, skin irritation, knowledge deficits of patient and caregiver

Risk for impaired skin integrity r/t immobility, paralysis

Risk for ineffective breathing pattern r/t neuromuscular impairment

Risk for infection r/t chronic disease, stasis of body fluids

Risk for loneliness r/t physical immobility

Self-care deficit r/t neuromuscular impairment

Sexual dysfunction r/t altered body function

Urinary retention r/t inhibition of reflex arc

See Hospitalized Child; Child with Chronic Condition; Neurotube Defects

Spiritual Distress

Spiritual distress r/t separation from religious or cultural ties, challenged belief and value system resulting from moral or ethical implications of therapy or from intense suffering

Spiritual Well-Being

Potential for enhanced spiritual well-being r/t desire for harmonious interconnectedness, desire to find purpose and meaning to life

Splenectomy

See Abdominal Surgery

Stapedectomy

Altered sensory perception: auditory r/t hearing loss related to edema from surgery

Pain r/t headache

Risk for infection r/t invasive procedure

Risk for injury: falling r/t dizziness

Stasis Ulcer

Impaired tissue integrity r/t chronic venous congestion

See Varicose Veins

STD (Sexually Transmitted Disease)

Altered health maintenance r/t knowledge deficit regarding transmission, symptoms, and treatment of sexually transmitted disease

Altered sexuality patterns r/t illness, altered body function

Fear r/t altered body function, risk for social isolation, fear of incurable illness

Pain r/t biological or psychological injury

Risk for infection/spread of infection r/t lack of knowledge concerning transmission of disease

Social isolation r/t fear of contracting or spreading disease

See Maturational Issues, Adolescent

Stertorous Respirations

Ineffective airway clearance r/t pharyngeal obstruction

Stillbirth

See Pregnancy Loss

Stoma

See Ostomy

Stomatitis

Altered oral mucous membranes r/t pathological conditions of oral cavity

Stone, Kidney

See Kidney Stone

Stool; Hard, Dry

Colonic constipation r/t inadequate fluid intake, inadequate fiber intake, decreased activity level, decreased gastric motility

Straining with Defecation

Colonic constipation r/t less than adequate fluid intake, less than adequate dietary intake

Risk for decreased cardiac output r/t vagal stimulation with dysrhythmia secondary to Valsalva's maneuver

Stress

Anxiety r/t feelings of helplessness, feelings of being threatened

Energy field disturbance r/t low energy level, feelings of hopelessness

Fear r/t powerlessness over feelings

Ineffective individual coping r/t ineffective use of problem-solving process, feelings of apprehension or helplessness

Potential for enhanced spiritual well-being r/t desire for harmony and peace in stressful situation

Self-esteem disturbance r/t inability to deal with life events

Stress Incontinence

Stress incontinence r/t degenerative change in pelvic muscles

See Incontinence of Urine

Stridor

Ineffective airway clearance r/t obstruction, tracheobronchial infection, trauma

Stroke

See CVA

Stuttering

Impaired verbal communication r/t anxiety, psychological problems

Subarachnoid Hemorrhage

Altered tissue perfusion: cerebral r/t bleeding from cerebral vessel

Pain: headache r/t irritation of meninges from blood, increased intracranial pressure

See Intracranial Pressure, Increased

Substance Abuse

Altered family process: alcohol r/t inadequate coping skills

Altered nutrition: less than body requirements r/t anorexia

Altered protection r/t malnutrition, sleep deprivation

Anxiety r/t loss of control

Compromised/dysfunctional family coping r/t codependency issues

Defensive coping r/t substance abuse

Ineffective denial r/t refusal to acknowledge substance abuse problem

Ineffective individual coping r/t use of substances to cope with life events

Powerlessness r/t substance addiction

Risk for altered parent/infant/child attachment r/t substance abuse

Risk for injury r/t alteration in sensory perception

Risk for violence r/t reactions to substances used, impulsive behavior, disorientation, impaired judgment

Self-esteem disturbance r/t failure at life events

Sleep pattern disturbance r/t irritability, nightmares, tremors

Social isolation r/t unacceptable social behavior or values

See Maturational Issues, Adolescent

Substance Abuse, Adolescent

See Alcohol Withdrawal; Substance Abuse; Maturational Issues, Adolescent

Substance Abuse in Pregnancy

Altered health maintenance r/t addiction

Defensive coping r/t denial of situation, differing value system

Knowledge deficit r/t lack of exposure to information about effects of substance abuse in pregnancy

Noncompliance r/t differing value system, cultural influences, addiction

Risk for altered parenting r/t lack of ability to meet infant's needs

Risk for fetal injury r/t effects of drugs on fetal growth and development

Risk for infection r/t intravenous drug use, life-style

Risk for maternal injury r/t drug use

See Substance Abuse

Sucking Reflex

Effective breast-feeding r/t regular and sustained suckling and swallowing at the breast

Sudden Infant Death Syndrome, Near Miss (Infant Apnea)

See SIDS

Suffocation, Risk for

Internal

Risk for Suffocation r/t reduced olfactory sensation, reduced motor abilities, lack of safety education, lack of safety precautions, cognitive or emotional difficulties, disease or injury process

External

Risk for Suffocation r/t pillow placed in infant's crib, propped bottle placed in infant's crib, vehicle warming in closed garage, children playing with plastic bags, children inserting small objects into their mouths or noses, discarded or unused refrigerators or freezers with doors, children left unattended in or near bathtubs/pools/hot tubs, low clotheslines, pacifier being hung around infant's neck, eating of large mouthfuls of food

Suicide Attempt

Hopelessness r/t perceived or actual loss, substance abuse, low self-concept, inadequate support systems

Ineffective individual coping r/t anger, dysfunctional grieving

Post-trauma response r/t history of traumatic events, abuse, rape, incest, war, torture

Potential for enhanced spiritual well-being r/t desire for harmony and inner strength to help redefine purpose for life

Risk for violence: self-directed r/t suicidal ideation, feelings of hopelessness or worthlessness, lack of impulse control, feelings of anger or hostility (self-directed)

Self-esteem disturbance r/t guilt, inability to trust, feelings of worthlessness or rejection

Social isolation r/t inability to engage in satisfying personal relationships

Spiritual distress r/t hopelessness, despair

Support System

Family coping: potential for growth r/t ability to adapt to tasks related to care, support of significant other during health crisis

Suppression of Labor

See Preterm Labor; Tocolytic Therapy

Surgery, Postoperative Care

Activity intolerance r/t pain, surgical procedure

Altered nutrition: less than body requirements r/t anorexia, nausea, vomiting, decreased peristalsis

Anxiety r/t change in health status, hospital environment

Knowledge deficit r/t postoperative expectations, life-style changes

Pain r/t inflammation or injury in surgical area

Risk for altered tissue perfusion: peripheral r/t hypovolemia, circulatory stasis, obesity, prolonged immobility, decreased coughing, decreased deep breathing

Risk for colonic constipation r/t decreased activity, decreased food or fluid intake, anesthesia, pain medication

Risk for fluid volume deficit r/t hypermetabolic state, fluid loss during surgery, presence of indwelling tubes

Risk for ineffective breathing pattern r/t pain, location of incision, effects of anesthesia/narcotics

Risk for infection r/t invasive procedure, pain, anesthesia, location of incision, weakened cough due to aging

Urinary retention r/t anesthesia, pain, fear, unfamiliar surroundings, client's position

Surgery, Preoperative Care

Anxiety r/t threat to or change in health status, situational crisis, fear of unknown

Knowledge deficit r/t preoperative procedures, postoperative expectations

Sleep pattern disturbance r/t anxiety about upcoming surgery

Suspected Child Abuse and Neglect (SCAN)—Child

Altered growth and development: regression vs delayed r/t diminished or absent environmental stimuli, inadequate caretaking, inconsistent responsiveness by caretaker

Altered nutrition: less than body requirements r/t inadequate caretaking

Anxiety/fear: child r/t threat of punishment for perceived wrongdoing

Chronic low self-esteem r/t lack of positive feedback, excessive negative feedback

Diversional activity deficit r/t diminished or absent environmental or personal stimuli

Impaired skin integrity r/t altered nutritional state, physical abuse

Pain r/t physical injuries

Post-trauma response r/t physical abuse, incest, rape, molestation

Potential for enhanced community coping r/t obtaining of resources to prevent child abuse and neglect

Rape-trauma syndrome: compound/silent reaction r/t altered life-style secondary to abuse and changes in residence

Risk for poisoning r/t inadequate safeguards, lack of proper safety precautions, accessibility of illicit substances secondary to impaired home maintenance management

Risk for suffocation: secondary to aspiration r/t propped bottle, unattended child

Risk for trauma r/t inadequate precautions, cognitive or emotional difficulties

Sleep pattern disturbance r/t hypervigilance, anxiety

Social isolation: family imposed r/t fear of disclosure of family dysfunction and abuse

See Hospitalized Child; Maturational Issues, Adolescent

Suspected Child Abuse and Neglect (SCAN)—Parent

Altered family process: alcoholism r/t inadequate coping skills

Altered health maintenance r/t knowledge deficit of parenting skills secondary to unachieved developmental tasks

Altered parenting r/t unrealistic expectations of child; lack of effective role model; unmet social, emotional, or maturational needs of parents; interruption in bonding process

Chronic low self-esteem r/t lack of successful parenting experiences

Impaired home maintenance management r/t disorganization, parental dysfunction, neglect of safe and nurturing environment

Ineffective family coping: disabling r/t dysfunctional family, underdeveloped nurturing parental role, lack of parental support systems or role models

Powerlessness r/t inability to perform parental role responsibilities

Risk for violence toward child r/t inadequate coping mechanisms, unresolved stressors, unachieved maturational level by parent

Suspicion

Impaired social interaction r/t altered thought process, paranoid delusions, hallucinations

Powerlessness r/t repetitive paranoid thinking

Risk for violence: directed at self or others r/t inability to trust

Swallowing Difficulties

Impaired swallowing r/t neuromuscular impairment (e.g., decreased or absent gag reflex, decreased strength or excursion of muscles involved in mastication), perceptual impairment, facial paralysis, mechanical obstruction (e.g., edema, tracheostomy tube, tumor), fatigue, limited awareness, reddened or irritated oropharyngeal cavity, improper feeding or positioning

Syncope

Altered tissue perfusion: cerebral r/t interruption of blood flow

Anxiety r/t fear of falling

Decreased cardiac output r/t dysrhythmia

Impaired physical mobility r/t fear of falling

Risk for injury r/t altered sensory perception, transient loss of consciousness, risk for falls

Social isolation r/t fear of falling

Syphilis

See STD

Systemic Lupus Erythematosus

See Lupus Erythematosus

T

T & A (Tonsil & Adenoidectomy)

Altered comfort r/t effects of anesthesia (nausea and vomiting)

Ineffective airway clearance r/t hesitation or reluctance to cough secondary to pain

Knowledge deficit: potential for enhanced health maintenance r/t insufficient knowledge regarding postoperative nutritional and rest requirements, signs and symptoms of complications, positioning

Pain r/t surgical incision

Risk for altered nutrition: less than body requirements r/t hesitation or reluctance to swallow

Risk for aspiration/suffocation r/t postoperative drainage and impaired swallowing

Risk for fluid volume deficit r/t decreased intake secondary to painful swallowing, effects of anesthesia (nausea, vomiting), hemorrhage

Tachycardia

See Dysrhythmia

Tachypnea

Ineffective breathing pattern r/t pain, anxiety

See cause of Tachypnea

Taste Abnormality

Sensory/perceptual alteration: gustatory r/t medication side effects; altered sensory reception, transmission, and/or integration; aging changes

TBI (Traumatic Brain Injury)

Acute confusion r/t brain injury

Altered family process r/t traumatic injury to family member

Altered thought processes r/t pressure damage to brain

Altered tissue perfusion: cerebral r/t effects of increased intracranial pressure

Decreased adaptive capacity: intracranial r/t brain injury

Ineffective breathing patterns r/t pressure damage to breathing center in brain stem

Sensory/perceptual alteration: specify r/t pressure damage to sensory centers in brain

Temperature, Decreased

Hypothermia r/t exposure to cold environment

Temperature, Increased

Hyperthermia r/t dehydration, illness, trauma

Temperature Regulation, Impaired

Ineffective thermoregulation r/t trauma, illness

Tension

Anxiety r/t threat to or change in health status, situational crisis

Energy field disturbance r/t change in health status, discouragement, pain

Terminally Ill Child—Adolescent

Altered body image r/t effects of terminal disease, already critical feelings of group identity and self-image

Impaired social interaction/social isolation r/t forced separation from peers

Ineffective individual coping r/t inability to establish personal and peer identity secondary to threat of being different or "not being," inability to achieve maturational tasks

See Hospitalized Child; Child with Chronic Condition

Terminally Ill Adult

Anticipatory grieving r/t loss of self or significant other

Decisional conflict r/t planning for Advance Directives

Ineffective family coping r/t inability to discuss impending death

Spiritual distress r/t suffering before death

Terminally Ill Child—Infant/Toddler

Ineffective individual coping r/t separation from parents and familiar environment secondary to inability to grasp external meaning of death

Terminally Ill Child—Preschool Child

Fear r/t perceived punishment, bodily harm, feelings of guilt secondary to magical thinking (i.e., believing that thoughts cause events)

Terminally Ill Child—School-Age Child/Preadolescent

Fear r/t perceived punishment, body mutilation, feelings of guilt

Terminally Ill Child/Death of Child—Parent

Altered family processes r/t situational crisis

Altered parenting r/t risk for overprotection of surviving siblings

Anticipatory grieving r/t possible, expected, or imminent death of child

Decisional conflict r/t continuation or discontinuation of treatment, "do not resuscitate" decision, ethical issues regarding organ donation

Family coping: potential for growth r/t impact of crisis on family values, priorities, goals, or relationships; expressed interest or desire to attach meaning to child's life and death

Grieving r/t death of child

Hopelessness r/t overwhelming stresses secondary to terminal illness

Impaired social interaction r/t dysfunctional grieving

Ineffective denial r/t dysfunctional grieving

Ineffective family coping: compromised r/t inability or unwillingness to discuss impending death and feelings with child or to support child through terminal stages of illness

Powerlessness r/t inability to alter course of events

Risk for dysfunctional grieving r/t prolonged, unresolved, or obstructed progression through stages of grief and mourning

Sleep pattern disturbance r/t grieving process

Social isolation: imposed by others r/t feelings of inadequacy in providing support to grieving parents

Social isolation: self-imposed r/t unresolved grief, perceived inadequate parenting skills

Spiritual distress r/t sudden and unexpected death, prolonged suffering before death, questioning the death of youth, questioning meaning of own existence

Tetralogy of Fallot

See Congenital Heart Disease/Cardiac Anomalies

Therapeutic Regimen, Effective Management of: Individual

Effective management of therapeutic regimen: individual r/t adequate ability to manage needed health care

Therapeutic Regimen, Ineffective Management of: Individual

Ineffective management of therapeutic regimen: individual r/t complexity of health care system; complexity of therapeutic regimen; decisional conflicts; economic difficulties; excessive demands made on individual or family; family conflict; family patterns of health care; inadequate number and types of cues to action; knowledge deficits; mistrust of regimen or health care personnel; perceived seriousness, susceptibility, barriers, or benefits; powerlessness; social support deficits

Therapeutic Regimen, Ineffective Management of: Families

Ineffective management of therapeutic regimen: families r/t complexity of health care system, complexity of therapeutic regimen, decisional conflicts, economic difficulties, excessive demands on individual or family, family conflict

Therapeutic Touch

Energy field disturbance r/t low energy levels, disturbance in energy fields, pain, depression, fatigue

Thermoregulation, Ineffective

Ineffective thermoregulation r/t trauma, illness, immaturity, aging, fluctuating environmental temperature

Thoracotomy

Activity intolerance r/t pain, imbalance between oxygen supply and demand, presence of chest tubes

Ineffective airway clearance r/t drowsiness, pain with breathing and coughing

Ineffective breathing pattern r/t decreased energy, fatigue, pain

Knowledge deficit r/t self-care, effective breathing exercises, pain relief

Pain r/t surgical procedure, coughing, deep breathing

Risk for infection r/t invasive procedure

Risk for injury r/t disruption of closed-chest drainage system

Risk for perioperative positioning injury r/t lateral positioning and immobility

Thought Disorders

Altered thought processes r/t disruption in cognitive thinking, processing

Thought Processes, Altered

Altered thought processes r/t head injury, mental disorder, personality disorder, organic mental disorder, substance abuse, severe interpersonal conflict, sleep deprivation, sensory deprivation or overload, impaired cerebral perfusion

Thrombocytopenic Purpura

See ITP

Thrombophlebitis

Altered tissue perfusion: peripheral r/t interruption of venous blood flow

Colonic constipation r/t inactivity, bedrest

Diversional activity deficit r/t bedrest

Impaired physical mobility r/t pain in extremity, forced bedrest

Knowledge deficit r/t pathophysiology of condition, self-care needs, treatment regimen and outcome

Pain r/t vascular inflammation, edema

Risk for injury r/t possible embolus

See Anticoagulant Therapy

Thyroidectomy

Risk for altered verbal communication r/t edema, pain, vocal cord of laryngeal nerve damage

Risk for ineffective airway clearance r/t edema or hematoma formation, airway obstruction

Risk for injury r/t possible parathyroid damage or removal

See Surgery

TIA (Transient Ischemic Attack)

Acute confusion r/t hypoxia

Altered tissue perfusion: cerebral r/t lack of adequate oxygen supply to the brain

Health-seeking behaviors r/t obtaining knowledge regarding treatment and prevention of inadequate oxygenation

Risk for decreased cardiac output r/t dysrhythmia contributing to inadequate oxygen supply to brain

Risk for injury r/t possible syncope

See Syncope

Tinnitus

Altered health maintenance r/t knowledge deficit regarding self-care with tinnitus

Sensory/perceptual alteration: auditory r/t altered sensory reception, transmission, and/or integration

Tissue Damage—Corneal, Integumentary, or Subcutaneous

Impaired tissue integrity r/t altered circulation, nutritional deficit or excess, fluid deficit or excess, knowledge deficit, impaired physical mobility, chemical irritants (including body excretions, secretions, medications), thermal irritants (temperature extremes), mechanical irritants (pressure, shear, friction), radiation irritants (including therapeutic radiation)

Tissue Perfusion, Decreased

Altered tissue perfusion r/t arterial or venous interruption of flow, exchange problems, hypovolemia, hypervolemia

Tocolytic Therapy

Altered health maintenance r/t knowledge deficit regarding management of preterm labor and treatment regimen

Risk for fluid volume excess r/t effects of tocolytic drugs

See Preterm Labor

Toilet Training

Health-seeking behaviors: bladder/bowel training r/t achievement of developmental milestone secondary to enhanced parenting skills

Toileting Problems

Self-care deficit: toileting r/t impaired transfer ability, impaired mobility status, intolerance of activity, neuromuscular impairment, cognitive impairment

Tonsillectomy and Adenoidectomy

See T & A

Total Anomalous Pulmonary Venous Return

See Congenital Heart Disease/Cardiac Anomalies

Total Incontinence

Total incontinence r/t neuropathy, neurological dysfunction, compromised contraction of detrusor reflex, anatomical incontinence (fistula)

Total Joint Replacement—Total Hip/Total Knee

Body image disturbance r/t large scar, presence of prosthesis

Impaired physical mobility r/t musculoskeletal impairment, surgery, prosthesis

Knowledge deficit r/t self-care, treatment regimen, outcomes

Pain r/t possible edema, physical injury, surgery

Risk for infection r/t invasive procedure, anesthesia, immobility

Risk for injury: neurovascular r/t altered peripheral tissue perfusion, altered mobility, prosthesis

Total Parenteral Nutrition

See TPN

Toxemia

See PIH

TPN (Total Parenteral Nutrition)

Altered nutrition: less than body requirements r/t inability to ingest or digest food or absorb nutrients because of biological or psychological factors

Risk for fluid volume excess r/t rapid administration of TPN

Risk for infection r/t concentrated glucose solution, invasive administration of fluids

Tracheoesophageal Fistula

Altered nutrition: less than body requirements r/t difficulties in swallowing

Ineffective airway clearance r/t aspiration of feeding secondary to inability to swallow

Risk for aspiration r/t common passage of air and food

See Respiratory Conditions of the Neonate; Hospitalized Child

Tracheostomy

Anxiety r/t impaired verbal communication, ineffective airway clearance

Body image disturbance r/t abnormal opening in neck

Impaired verbal communication r/t presence of mechanical airway

Knowledge deficit r/t self-care, home maintenance management

Pain r/t edema, surgical procedure

Risk for aspiration r/t presence of tracheostomy

Risk for ineffective airway clearance r/t increased secretions, mucus plugs

Risk for infection r/t invasive procedure, pooling of secretions

Traction and Casts

Constipation r/t immobility

Diversional activity deficit r/t immobility

Impaired physical mobility r/t imposed restrictions on activity secondary to bone or joint disease injury

Pain r/t immobility, injury, or disease

Risk for disuse syndrome r/t mechanical immobilization

Risk for impaired skin integrity r/t contact of traction or cast with skin

Risk for peripheral neurovascular dysfunction r/t mechanical compression

Self-care deficit: feeding, dressing/grooming, bathing/hygiene, toileting r/t degree of impaired physical mobility, body area affected by traction or cast

Transient Ischemic Attack

See TIA

Transposition of the Great Vessels

See Congenital Heart Disease/Cardiac Anomalies

Transurethral Resection of the Prostate

See TURP

Trauma, Risk for

Internal

Risk for trauma r/t weakness, poor vision, balancing difficulties, reduced temperature and/or tactile sensation, reduced large or small muscle coordination, reduced hand-eye coordination, lack of safety education, lack of safety precautions, insufficient finances to purchase safety equipment or effect repairs, cognitive or emotional difficulties, history of previous trauma

External

Risk for trauma r/t slippery floors or walkways, unanchored rugs, bathtub without hand grip or antislip equipment, use of unsteady ladders or chairs, entering of unlighted rooms, unsturdy or absent stair rails, unanchored electrical wires, litter or liquid spills on floors or stairways, high beds, children playing at top of ungated stairs, obstructed passageways, unsafe window protection in home with young children, inappropriate call-for-aid mechanisms for client on bedrest, pot handles facing toward front of stove, bathing in very hot water, unsupervised bathing of young children, potentially ignitable gas leaks, delayed lighting of gas burner or oven, experimenting with chemicals or gasoline, unscreened fires or heaters, wearing of plastic apron or flowing clothes around open flame, children playing with dangerous objects (e.g., matches, candles, cigarettes), inadequately stored combustible items or corrosives, highly flammable children's toys or clothing, overloaded fuse box, contact with rapidly moving objects (e.g., machinery, industrial belts, pulleys), sliding on coarse bed linen or struggling within bed restraints, faulty electrical plugs, frayed wires, defective appliances, contact with acids or alkalis, playing with fireworks or gunpowder, contact with intense cold, overexposure to sun or radiotherapy, misuse of sun lamps, use of cracked dishware or glasses, knives stored uncovered, guns or ammunition stored unlocked, large icicles hanging from the roof, exposure to dangerous machinery, children playing with sharp-edged toys, high-crime neighborhoods and vulnerable clients, driving of a mechanically unsafe vehicle, driving after consuming alcoholic beverages or drugs, driving at excessive speeds, driving without necessary visual aids, children riding in the front seat of car, smoking in bed or near oxygen, overloaded electrical outlets, grease waste collected on stoves, use of thin or worn potholders, misuse of necessary headgear for motorized cyclists, young children carried on adult bicycles, unsafe road or road-crossing conditions, playing or working near vehicle pathways, nonuse or misuse of seat restraints

Trauma in Pregnancy

Anxiety r/t threat to self or fetus, unknown outcome

Impaired skin integrity r/t trauma

Knowledge deficit r/t lack of exposure to situation

Pain r/t trauma

Risk for fetal injury r/t premature separation of placenta

Risk for fluid volume deficit r/t blood loss

Risk for infection r/t traumatized tissue

Traumatic Brain Injury (TBI)

See TBI; Intracranial Pressure, Increased

Traumatic Event

Post-trauma response r/t previously experienced trauma

Trembling of Hands

Anxiety/fear r/t threat to or change in health status, threat of death, situational crisis

Tricuspid Atresia

See Congenital Heart Disease/Cardiac Anomalies

Truncus Arteriosus

See Congenital Heart Disease/Cardiac Anomalies

TSE (Testicular Self-Examination)

Health-seeking behavior r/t procedure for doing self-testicular examinations

Tube Feeding

Risk for altered nutrition: less than body requirements r/t intolerance to tube feeding, inadequate calorie replacement to meet metabolic needs

Risk for aspiration r/t improperly administered feeding, improper placement of tube, improper positioning of client during and after feeding, excessive residual feeding or lack of digestion, altered gag reflex

Risk for fluid volume deficit r/t inadequate water administration with concentrated feeding

TURP (Transurethral Resection of the Prostate)

Knowledge deficit r/t postoperative self-care, home maintenance management

Pain r/t incision, irritation from catheter, bladder spasms, kidney infection

Risk for fluid volume deficit r/t fluid loss and possible bleeding

Risk for infection r/t invasive procedure, route for bacteria entry

Risk for urinary retention r/t obstruction of urethra or catheter with clots

U

Ulcer, Peptic or Duodenal

Altered health maintenance r/t lack of knowledge regarding health practices to prevent ulcer formation

Fatigue r/t loss of blood, chronic illness

Pain r/t irritated mucosa from acid secretion

See GI Bleed

Ulcerative Colitis

See Inflammatory Bowel Disease

Ulcers, Stasis

See Stasis Ulcers

Unilateral Neglect of One Side of Body

Unilateral neglect r/t effects of disturbed perceptual abilities (e.g., hemianopsia), one-sided blindness, neurological illness or trauma

Unsanitary Living Conditions

Impaired home maintenance r/t impaired cognitive or emotional functioning, lack of knowledge, insufficient finances

Urgency to Urinate

Urge incontinence r/t decreased bladder capacity, irritation of bladder stretch receptors causing spasm, alcohol, caffeine, increased fluids, increased urine concentration, overdistention of bladder

Urinary Diversion

See Ileal Conduit

Urinary Elimination, Altered

Altered urinary elimination r/t anatomical obstruction, sensory motor impairment, urinary tract infection

Urinary Incontinence

See Incontinence of Urine

Urinary Retention

Urinary retention r/t high urethral pressure caused by weak detrusor, inhibition of reflex arc, strong sphincter, blockage

Urinary Tract Infection

See UTI

Urolithiasis

See Kidney Stone

Uterine Atony in Labor

See Dystocia

Uterine Atony in Postpartum

See Postpartum Hemorrhage

Uterine Bleeding

See Hemorrhage; Shock; Postparum Hemorrhage

UTI (Urinary Tract Infection)

Altered health maintenance r/t knowledge deficit regarding methods to treat and prevent UTIs

Altered pattern of urinary elimination: frequency r/t urinary tract infection

Pain: dysuria r/t inflammatory process in bladder

V

Vaginal Hysterectomy

Risk for altered urinary elimination r/t edema in area

Risk for infection r/t surgical site

Risk for perioperative positioning injury r/t lithotomy position

Urinary retention r/t edema at surgical site

See Hysterectomy

Vaginitis

Altered health maintenance r/t knowledge deficit regarding self-care with vaginitis

Altered pattern of sexuality r/t abstinence during acute stage, pain

Pain: pruritis r/t inflamed tissues, edema

Risk for infection r/t spread of infection, risk of reinfection

Vagotomy

See Abdominal Surgery

Value System Conflict

Potential for enhanced spiritual well-being r/t desire for harmony with self, others, and higher power/God

Spiritual distress r/t challenged value system

Varicose Veins

Altered health maintenance r/t knowledge deficit regarding health care practices, prevention, and treatment regimen

Altered tissue perfusion: peripheral r/t venous stasis

Chronic pain r/t impaired circulation

Risk for impaired skin integrity r/t altered peripheral tissue perfusion

Vascular Dementia (Formerly called "Multiinfarct Dementia")

See Dementia

Vascular Obstruction—Peripheral

Altered tissue perfusion: peripheral r/t interruption of circulatory flow

Anxiety r/t lack of circulation to body part

Pain r/t vascular obstruction

Risk for peripheral neurovascular dysfunction r/t vascular obstruction

Venereal Disease

See STD

Ventilation, Inability to Sustain Spontaneous

Inability to sustain spontaneous ventilation r/t metabolic factors, respiratory muscle fatigue

Ventilator Client

Dysfunctional ventilatory weaning response r/t inability to sustain respirations without mechanical support

Fear r/t inability to breathe on own, difficulty communicating

Impaired gas exchange r/t ventilation-perfusion imbalance

Impaired verbal communication r/t presence of endotracheal tube, decreased mentation

Inability to sustain spontaneous ventilation r/t metabolic factors, respiratory muscle fatigue

Ineffective airway clearance r/t increased secretions, decreased cough and gag reflex

Ineffective breathing pattern r/t decreased energy and fatigue secondary to possible alteration in nutrition (less than body requirements)

Powerlessness r/t health treatment regimen

Risk for infection r/t presence of endotracheal tube, pooled secretions

Social isolation r/t impaired mobility, ventilator dependence

See Child with Chronic Condition; Hospitalized Child; Respiratory Conditions of the Neonate

Ventilatory, Dysfunctional Weaning Response (DVWR)

Dysfunctional ventilatory weaning response r/t inability to sustain respirations without mechanical support

Vertigo

Altered tissue perfusion: cerebral r/t decreased blood supply to brain

Risk for injury r/t sensory/perceptual alteration

Sensory/perceptual alteration: kinesthetic r/t altered sensory reception, transmission, and/or integration; medications

Violent Behavior

Risk for violence: self-directed or directed at others r/t antisocial character, battered women, catatonic excitement, child abuse, manic excitement, organic brain syndrome, panic states, rage reactions, suicidal behavior, temporal lobe epilepsy, toxic reactions to medication

Vision Impairment

Fear r/t loss of sight

Risk for injury r/t sensory/perceptual alteration

Self-care deficit: specify r/t perceptual impairment

Sensory/perceptual alteration: visual r/t altered sensory reception related to impaired vision

Social isolation r/t altered state of wellness, inability to see

Vomiting

Altered comfort: nausea, retching r/t tension on abdominal muscles

Risk for altered nutrition: less than body requirements r/t inability to ingest food

Risk for fluid volume deficit r/t decreased intake, loss of fluids with vomiting

W

Weakness

Fatigue r/t decreased or increased metabolic energy production

Weight Gain

Altered nutrition: more than body requirements r/t excessive intake in relation to metabolic need

Weight Loss

Altered nutrition: less than body requirements r/t inability to ingest food because of biological, psychological, or economic factors

Wellness-Seeking Behavior

Health-seeking behavior r/t expressed desire for increased control of health practice

Wheezing

Ineffective airway clearance r/t tracheobronchial obstructions or secretions

Withdrawal from Alcohol

See Alcohol Withdrawal

Withdrawal from Drugs

See Drug Withdrawal

Wound Debridement

Impaired tissue integrity r/t debridement, open wound

Pain r/t debridement of wound

Risk for infection r/t open wound, presence of bacteria

Wound Dehiscence, Evisceration

Altered nutrition: less than body requirements r/t inability to digest nutrients, need for increased protein for healing

Fear r/t client fear of body parts falling out, surgical procedure not going as planned

Risk for fluid volume deficit r/t inability to ingest nutrients, obstruction, fluid loss

Risk for injury r/t exposed abdominal contents

Wound Infection

Altered nutrition: less than body requirements r/t biological factors, infection, hyperthermia

Body image disturbance r/t dysfunctional open wound

Hyperthermia r/t increased metabolic rate, illness, infection

Impaired tissue integrity r/t wound, presence of infection

Risk for fluid volume deficit r/t increased metabolic rate

Risk for infection (spread of) r/t altered nutrition: less than body requirements

W

Guide to Planning Care

Activity intolerance

Linda L. Straight

Definition   The state in which an individual has insufficient physiological or psychological energy to endure or complete required or desired daily activities

Defining Characteristics

Verbal report of fatigue or weakness *(critical),* abnormal heart rate or blood pressure in response to activity, exertional discomfort or dyspnea, electrocardiographic changes reflecting dysrhythmias or ischemia, changes in skin color or moisture

Related Factors (r/t)

Bedrest or immobility, generalized weakness, sedentary life-style, imbalance between oxygen supply and demand

Client Outcomes/Goals

- Participates in prescribed physical activity with appropriate increases in heart rate, blood pressure, and breathing rate; maintains monitor patterns (rhythm and ST segment) within normal limits
- States symptoms of adverse effects of exercise and reports onset of symptoms immediately
- Maintains normal skin color that is warm and dry with activity
- Verbalizes an understanding of the need to gradually increase activity based on testing, tolerance, and symptoms
- Expresses an understanding of the need to balance rest and activity
- Demonstrates increased activity tolerance

Suggested NIC Interventions

Activity therapy, energy management

Nursing Interventions and Rationales

- Determine cause of activity intolerance (see Related Factors) and determine whether its cause is physical, psychological, or motivational.
  Determining the cause of a disease can help direct appropriate interventions.
- Assess client daily for appropriateness of activity and bedrest orders.
  Inappropriate prolonged bedrest orders may contribute to activity intolerance.
- If appropriate, ensure clients are getting out of bed. Assist to change position gradually; sit up in bed, dangle, and if tolerated, help to stand and sit.
  Immobilization and enforced bedrest in the supine position have considerable adverse effects on nearly every system in the body (Hoenig, Rubenstein, 1991). The headward body fluid shifts that occur with bedrest may be responsible for many of the untoward effects of bedrest. Getting the patient out of bed is one of the most important countermeasures to fluid shift (Winslow, 1985).
- Ensure that clients change position slowly. Consider using a chair-bed or oscillating bed for clients who cannot get out of bed. Monitor for symptoms of activity intolerance.
  Evidence of orthostatic intolerance begins after as little as 6 hours bedrest (McCally, Pohl, Samson, 1968).
- When getting clients up, observe for symptoms of intolerance such as nausea, pallor, dizziness, visual dimming, and impaired consciousness as well as changes in vital signs.
  There is wide variability in heart rate and blood pressure responses to orthostasis. Vital sign changes by themselves should not define orthostatic intolerance (Winslow, Lane, Woods, 1995).

- Perform range-of-motion exercises if client is unable to tolerate activity.
  Inactivity rapidly contributes to muscle shortening and changes in periarticular and cartilaginous joint structure. These factors contribute to contracture and limitation of motion (Creditor, 1994).
- Refer to physical therapy for help in increasing activity levels.
- Monitor and record client's ability to tolerate activity; note pulse rate, blood pressure, monitor pattern, dyspnea, use of accessory muscles, and skin color before and after activity.
  If the following signs and symptoms of cardiac decompensation develop, activity should be stopped immediately:
  - *Excessive fatigue*
  - *Lightheadedness, confusion, ataxia, pallor, cyanosis, dyspnea, nausea, or any peripheral circulatory insufficiency*
  - *Onset of angina with exercise*
  - *Palpitations*
  - *Dysrhythmia (symptomatic supraventricular tachycardia, ventricular tachycardia, exercise-induced left bundle block, second- or third-degree atrioventricular block, frequent premature ventricular contractions)*
  - *Exercise hypotension (greater than 20 mm Hg drop in systolic blood pressure during exercise)*
  - *Excessive rise in blood pressure (systolic greater than 220 mm Hg or diastolic greater than 110 mm Hg) NOTE: These are upper limits; activity may be stopped before reaching these values.*
  - *Inappropriate bradycardia (drop in heart rate greater than 10 beats/min) with no change or increase in workload*
  - *Increased heart rate above the prescribed limit (Pate et al, 1991)*
- Instruct client to stop activity immediately and report to physician if experiencing the following symptoms: new or worsened intensity or increased frequency of discomfort, tightness, or pressure in chest, back, neck, jaw, shoulders, and/or arms; palpitations; dizziness; weakness; unusual and extreme fatigue; excessive air hunger.
  These are common symptoms of angina and are caused by a temporary insufficiency of coronary blood supply. Symptoms typically last for minutes as opposed to momentary twinges. If symptoms last longer than 5 to 10 minutes, the client should be evaluated by a physician (McGoon, 1993). The client should be evaluated before resuming activity (Thompson, 1988).
- Allow for periods of rest before and after planned exertion periods such as meals, bath, treatments, and physical activity.
  Rest periods decrease oxygen consumption (Prizant-Weston, Castiglia, 1992).
- Refer the cardiac client to cardiac rehabilitation for assistance in developing safe exercise guidelines based on testing and medications.
  Cardiac rehabilitation exercise training improves objective measures of exercise tolerance in both men and women, including elderly patients with coronary heart disease and heart failure. This functional improvement occurs without significant cardiovascular complications or other adverse outcomes (Wenger et al, 1995).
- Ensure that the chronic pulmonary client has had oxygen saturation testing with exercise. Use supplemental oxygen to keep oxygen saturation 90% or above or as prescribed with activity.

Supplemental oxygen increases circulatory oxygen levels and improves activity tolerance (Petty, Finigan, 1968; Casaburi, Petty, 1993).

- Monitor a chronic obstructive pulmonary disease (COPD) client's response to activity by observing for symptoms of respiratory intolerance such as increased dyspnea, loss of ability to control breathing rhythmically, use of accessory muscles, and skin tone changes such as pallor and cyanosis.
- Instruct and assist client in using conscious controlled breathing techniques such as pursing their lips and diaphragmatic breathing.
  Training clients with COPD to slow their respiratory rate with a prolonged exhalation (with or without pursed lips) helps control dyspnea and results in improved ventilation, increased tidal volume, decreased respiratory rate, and a reduced alveolar-arterial oxygen difference. This breathing pattern not only helps relieve dyspnea but can improve the ability to exercise and carry out activities of daily living (ADLs) (Mueller, Petty, Filley, 1970; Casaburi, Petty, 1993).
- Provide emotional support and encouragement to client to gradually increase activity.
  Fear of breathlessness, pain, or falling may decrease willingness to increase activity.
- Refer the COPD client to a pulmonary rehabilitation program.
  Pulmonary rehabilitation has been shown to improve exercise capacity, walking ability, and sense of well-being (Fishman, 1994).
- Observe for pain before activity. If possible treat pain before activity, and ensure client is not heavily sedated.
  Pain restricts the client from achieving a maximal activity level and is often exacerbated by movement.
- Obtain any necessary assistive devices or equipment needed before ambulating client (e.g., walkers, canes, crutches, portable oxygen).
  Assistive devices can increase mobility by helping the client overcome limitations.
- Use a walking belt when ambulating a client who is unsteady.
  With a walking belt the client can walk independently, but the nurse can provide support if the client's knees buckle.
- Refer to physical therapy for help in increasing activity levels.
- Work with client to set mutual goals that increase activity levels.

Geriatric
- Slow the pace of care. Allow client extra time to carry out activities.
- When mobilizing the elderly client, watch for orthostatic hypotension accompanied by dizziness and fainting.
  Orthostatic hypotension is common in the elderly as a result of cardiovascular changes, chronic diseases, and medication effects (Mobily, Kelley, 1991).

Home Care Interventions

- Assess the home environment for factors that precipitate decreased activity tolerance: presence of allergens such as dust, smoke, and those associated with pets; temperature; energy-intensive activity patterns; and furniture placement. Refer to occupational therapy if needed to assist the client in restructuring the home and activity of daily living patterns.
  Clients and families often estimate energy requirements inaccurately during hospitalization because of the availability of support.
- Teach the client/family the importance of and methods for setting priorities for activities, especially those having a high energy demand (e.g., home/family events).
- Discuss the importance of sexual activity as part of daily living. Instruct the client in adaptive techniques to conserve energy during sexual interactions.

Families may make unsafe choices for sexual activity or place added stress on themselves trying to cope with this issue without proper support or teaching.

- Instruct the client and family in the importance of maintaining proper nutrition and rest for energy conservation and rehabilitation.
- Refer to medical social services as necessary to assist the family in adjusting to major changes in patterns of living.
- Assess the need for long-term supports for optimal activity tolerance of priority activities (e.g., assistive devices, oxygen, medication, catheters, massage), especially for hospice patients. Evaluate intermittently.

Assessments ensure the safety and appropriate use of these supports.

- Refer to home health aide services to support the client and family through changing levels of activity tolerance. Introduce aide support early. Instruct the aide to promote independence in activity as tolerated.

Providing unnecessary assistance with transfers and bathing activities may promote dependence and a loss of mobility (Mobily, Kelley, 1991).

- Allow terminally ill clients and their families to guide care.

Control by the client or family promotes effective coping.

- Provide increased attention to comfort and dignity of the terminally ill client in care planning. For example, oxygen may be more valuable as a support to the client's psychological comfort than as a booster of oxygen saturation.

Client/Family Teaching

- Instruct client on rationale and techniques for avoiding activity intolerance.
- Teach client to use controlled breathing techniques with activity.
- Teach client the importance and method of coughing, clearing secretions.
- Instruct client in the use of relaxation techniques during activity.
- Help client with energy conservation and work simplification techniques in ADL.
- Teach client the importance of proper nutrition.
- Describe to client the symptoms of activity intolerance and which to report to the physician.
- Explain to client how to use assistive devices or medications before or during activity.
- Help client set up an activity log to record exercise and exercise tolerance.

REFERENCES   Casaburi R, Petty T: *Principles and practice of pulmonary rehabilitation,* Philadelphia, 1993, WB Saunders.

Creditor M: Hazards of hospitalization of the elderly, *Ann Intern Med* 149:825, 1994.

Fishman AP: Pulmonary rehabilitation research, *Resp Crit Care Med* 149:825, 1994.

Hodgkin JE, Connors GL, Bell CW: *Pulmonary rehabilitation—guidelines to success,* Philadelphia, 1993, JB Lippincott.

Hoenig H, Rubenstein L: Hospital-associated deconditioning and dysfunction, *J Am Geriatr Soc* 39:220, 1991.

Humphrey, Carolyn J: *Home care nursing handbook,* ed 2, Maryland, 1994, Aspen.

McCally M, Pohl SA, Samson PA: Relative effectiveness of selected flight deconditioning countermeasures, *Aerospace Med* 39:722, 1968.

McGoon M: *Mayo Clinic heart book,* New York, 1993, William Morrow.

Mobily PR, Kelley LS: Iatrogenesis in the elderly: factors of immobility, *J Gerontol Nurs* 17:5, 1991.

Mueller RE, Petty TL, Filley GF: Ventilation and arterial blood gas changes induced by pursed lips breathing, *J Appl Physiol* 28:784, 1970.

Pate RR et al: *Guidelines for exercise testing and prescription,* ed 4, Philadelphia, 1991, Lee & Febiger.

Petty TL, Finigan MM: Clinical evaluation of prolonged ambulatory oxygen therapy in chronic airway obstruction, *Am J Med* 45:242, 1968.

Prizant-Weston M, Castiglia K: Hemodynamic regulation. In Bulecheck GM, McCloskey JC, editors: *Nursing interventions: essential nursing treatments,* Philadelphia, 1992, WB Saunders.

Thompson P: The safety of exercise testing and participation. In Blair SN et al, editors: *Resource manual for guidelines for exercise testing and prescriptions,* Philadelphia, 1988, Lea & Febiger.

Wenger NK et al: *Cardiac rehabilitation clinical practice guideline No 17,* ACPHR No 96-0672, Rockville, MD, 1995, US Department of Health and Human Services, Public Health Service, Agency for Health Care and Policy and Research and the National Heart, Lung, and Blood Institute.

Winslow EH: Cardiovascular consequences of bedrest, *Heart & Lung* 14:236, 1985.

Winslow EH, Lane LD, Woods RJ: Dangling: a review of relevant physiology, research, and practice, *Heart & Lung,* 24:263, 1995.

Risk for activity intolerance

Definition   The state in which an individual is at risk of experiencing insufficient physiological or psychological energy to endure or complete required or desired daily activities

Risk Factors

History of intolerance to activity, deconditioned status, presence of circulatory or respiratory problems, inexperience with activity

Related Factors (r/t)

See Risk Factors

Suggested NIC Interventions

Emotional support, energy management

Client Outcomes/Goals, Nursing Interventions and Rationales, Client/Family Teaching

See care plan for **Activity intolerance.**

Impaired adjustment

Gail B. Ladwig

Definition   The state in which an individual is unable to modify life-style or behavior in a manner consistent with a change in health status

Defining Characteristics

Major   Verbalized nonacceptance of health status change, nonexistent or unsuccessful involvement in problem solving or goal setting

Minor   Lack of movement toward independence; extended period of shock, disbelief, or anger regarding change in health status; lack of future-oriented thinking

Related Factors (r/t)

Disability that requires change in life-style, inadequate support systems, impaired cognition, sensory overload, assault to self-esteem, altered locus of control, incomplete grieving

Client Outcomes/Goals

- States acceptance of change in health status
- Lists behaviors needed to adjust to change in health status
- States personal goals for dealing with change in health status
- Experiences a period of grief that is proportional to the actual or perceived effect of the loss

Suggested NIC Interventions

Coping enhancement

Nursing Interventions and Rationales

- Assess client's perception about the illness. Ask client to state feelings related to the change in health status.

  A clinician's ability to understand a client's perceptions of the impact of the illness is crucial to the clinician's ability to be therapeutic. Knowledge of a patient's perceptions about chronic illness will help nurses intervene sensitively and effectively (Yuen-Juen, 1995).

- Assess the individual's feelings about whether change in health status is personally being dealt with effectively.

  Nurses must understand how each individual perceives personal coping with stressful experiences associated with a chronic illness (Downe-Wamboldt, Melanson 1995).

- Allow client adequate time to express feelings about the change in health status.

  Verbalization of feelings leads to acceptance and understanding of changes. The client cannot be pushed into coping with the change in health status (Johnson, 1994).

- Help client work through the stages of grief. Denial is usually the initial response. Acknowledge that grief takes time, and give client permission to grieve; accept crying.

  Acceptance of feelings conveys empathy and promotes movement toward adjustment.

- Discuss resources with client that have worked previously in dealing with changes in life-style or health.

  Past successes can often be repeated, and the client needs to build on existing skills.

- Use open-ended questions to allow the client free expression (e.g., "Tell me about your last hospitalization" or "How does this time compare?").

  Open-ended questions allow the client to be more actively involved in the interaction.

- Discuss client's current goals. If appropriate, have client list goals so they can be referred to and steps taken to accomplish them.

  Self-monitoring serves an important role in the maintenance of internal standards of behavior (Fleury, 1991).

- List client activities that may require assistance and those that can be performed independently.

  This list gives the client permission to ask for help and informs the client that outside resources are available.

- Allow client choices in daily care, particularly choices that result from the change in health status.

  To perceive ownership of change, the client needs to value the proposed change, feel able to carry it out, and accept responsibility for it (Fleury, 1991).

- Allow client time to adjust to new situations. Introduce new material gradually to prevent overload. Ask for frequent feedback.

  The stress of changes in health care can be overwhelming. New material takes longer to learn and absorb, thus clarification of information and frequent repetition may be necessary.

- Give client positive feedback for accomplishments, no matter how small.

  Empathic communication has been shown to be therapeutic and health promoting (Wells-Federman et al, 1995).

- Manipulate environment to decrease stress.

  The change in health status is producing enough stress; thus the environment should be as trouble-free as possible.

- Maintain consistency and continuity in daily schedule.
  Such measures provide some constancy in the client's life.

Geriatric
- Assess for signs of depression resulting from illness-associated changes.
  The elderly are at risk of depression when living with a chronic illness (Badger, 1993).
- Monitor client for agitation.
  The elderly often use agitation to express an inability to accept change.

Home Care Interventions

- Include a spiritual assessment in overall assessment of client and family resources.
- Refer to medical social services to facilitate the listed interventions and support client care goals.
  Support for transition to the home setting can facilitate acceptance of the changes required to maintain the client in the home setting.
- Observe for signs of caregiver stress on an ongoing basis. Refer to necessary support services.
  Caregiver stress may increase as time progresses.

Client/Family Teaching

- Help client maintain a positive outlook by listing current strengths.
  The use of optimistic coping strategies is positively related to psychological well-being (Downe-Wamboldt, Melanson, 1995).
- Teach clients and family relaxation techniques and help them practice.
  Teaching and guiding the client in positive self-care techniques is empowering (Wells-Federman et al, 1995).
- Instruct client to keep a journal documenting positive ways of coping with the current health change.
  By documenting daily experiences, clients are better able to take an active role in treatment (Burham, 1995).
- Allow client to proceed at own pace in learning; provide time for return demonstrations (e.g., self-injection of insulin). Use clear and distinct language free of medical jargon and meaningless values.
  Everyone learns at a different pace, and some clients need frequent repetition. A comfortable teaching atmosphere allows for openness and comfort when delivering disturbing information and facilitates trust (Hopkins, 1994).
- Refer client to counselor or therapist for follow-up care.
  Clients who maintained contacts with counselors or therapists achieved greater levels of success in managing their original problems (Di-Donato, Schaffer, 1994).
- Initiate community referrals as needed (e.g., grief counseling, self-help groups).
  Motivation, sharing of experiences, camaraderie with and support from peers, and the feeling of not being alone have been identified as advantages of group learning (Payne, 1993).
- Involve significant others in planning and teaching.
  The support of significant others facilitates desired changes. Through positive reinforcement and an expression of congruency in behavioral change, significant others often serve as powerful external motivators (Fleury, 1991).
- If long-term deficits are expected, inform the family as soon as possible.
  Early information promotes acceptance and results in decreased anxiety (Hilton, 1994).

- Teach families intervention techniques such as setting limits, communicating acceptable behavior, and having time-outs.
  If there are deficits related to the changed health, there may be anger and agitation; interventions are effective in those situations (Hilton, 1994).

REFERENCES   Badger T: Physical health impairment and depression among older adults, *Image J Nurs Sch* 25:325, 1993.

Burham M: Health diaries in nursing research and practice, *Image J Nurs Sch* 27(2):147, 1995.

Di-Donato BA, Schaffer VL: The importance of outcome data in brain injury rehabilitation, *Rehabil Nurs* 19:219, 1994.

Downe-Wamboldt B, Melanson P: Emotions, coping and psychological well-beings in elderly people with arthritis, *West J Nurs Res* 7:250, 1995.

Fleury D: Empowering potential: a theory of wellness motivation, *Nurs Res* 40:286-291, 1991.

Hilton T: Behavioral and cognitive sequelae of head trauma, *Orthop Nurse* 13:22, 1994.

Hopkins A: The trauma nurse's role with families in crisis, *Crit Care Nurse* 14:35, 1994.

Humphrey C: *Home Care nursing handbook,* ed 2, Maryland, 1994, Aspen.

Yuen-Juen H: The impact of chronic illness on patients, *Rehabil Nurs* 20:221, 1995.

Johnson J: Caring for the woman who's had a mastectomy, *Am J Nurs* 94:25, 1994.

Payne J: The contribution of group learning to the rehabilitation of spinal cord injured adults, *Rehabil Nurs* 18:375, 1993.

Wells-Federman C et al: The mind-body connection: the psychophysiology of many traditional nursing interventions, *Clin Nurse Spec* 9:59, 1995.

Ineffective airway clearance

Betty J. Ackley

Definition   The state in which an individual is unable to clear secretions or obstructions from the respiratory tract

Defining Characteristics

Abnormal breath sounds (e.g., crackles, wheezes), changes in rate or depth of respiration, tachypnea, cough (effective or ineffective and with or without sputum), cyanosis, dyspnea

Related Factors (r/t)

Decreased energy, fatigue, tracheobronchial infection, obstruction, secretions, perceptual or cognitive impairment, trauma

Client Outcomes/Goals

- Demonstrates effective coughing and clear breath sounds, is free of cyanosis and dyspnea
- Maintains a patent airway at all times
- Relates methods to enhance secretion removal
- Relates the significance of changes in sputum to include color, character, amount, and odor
- Identifies and avoids specific factors that inhibit effective airway clearance

Suggested NIC Interventions

Airway management, airway suctioning

Nursing Interventions and Rationales

- Auscultate breath sounds q_____h.

  Breathing sounds are normally clear or scattered fine crackles at bases, which clear with deep breathing. The presence of coarse crackles during late inspiration indicates fluid in the airway; wheezing indicates an airway obstruction.

- Monitor respiratory patterns, including rate, depth, and effort.

  A normal respiratory rate for an adult without dyspnea is 12 to 16. With the secretions in the airway, the respiratory rate will increase.

- Monitor blood gas values.

  Normal blood gas values are a Po_2 of 80 to 100 mmHg and a Pco_2 of 35 to 45 mmHg. Hypoxemia can result from ventilation-perfusion mismatches secondary to respiratory secretions.

- Position client to optimize respiration (e.g., head of bed elevated 45 degrees and repositioned at least every 2 hours).

  An upright position allows for maximal air exchange and lung expansion; lying flat causes abdominal organs to shift toward the chest, which crowds the lungs and makes it more difficult to breathe.

- If the client has unilateral lung disease, alternate a semi-Fowler's position with a lateral position (with a 10 to 15 degree elevation and "good lung down") for 60 to 90 minutes. This method is contraindicated for a client with a pulmonary abscess or hemorrhage or interstitial emphysema.

  Gravity and hydrostatic pressure allow the dependent lung to become better ventilated and perfused, which increases oxygenation (Yeaw, 1992).

- Help client to deep breathe and cough, or use incentive spirometer and cough every ____ hour(s).

  Controlled coughing uses the diaphragmatic muscles, making the cough more forceful and effective. The incentive spirometer is an effective tool that can help prevent atelectasis and retention of bronchial secretions (Peruzzi, Smith, 1995).

- Assist with clearing secretions from pharynx by offering tissues, gentle suction of the oral pharynx if necessary. Do not do nasotracheal suctioning.

  It is preferable for the client to cough up secretions. In the debilitated client, gentle suctioning of the posterior pharynx may stimulate coughing and help remove secretions; nasotracheal suctioning is dangerous because the nurse is unable to hyperoxygenate before, during, and after to maintain adequate oxygenation (Peruzzi, Smith, 1995).

- When suctioning an endotracheal tube or tracheostomy tube for a client on a ventilator, do the following:

  - Hyperoxygenate before, between, and after endotracheal suction sessions.

    Nursing research has demonstrated that the client should be hyperventilated during suctioning if using either the open- or closed-suction system (Winslow, 1993).

  - Use a closed, in-line suction system.

    The closed, in-line suction system is associated with a decrease in noscomial pneumonia (Deppe et al, 1990; Johnson et al, 1994), reduced suction-induced hypoxemia, and fewer physiological disturbances (including decreased development of dysrhythmia) and often saves money.

  - Avoid saline instillation during suctioning.

    Saline instillation before suctioning has an adverse effect on oxygen saturation (Ackerman, 1993; Winslow, 1993b, Raymond, 1995).

- Document results of coughing and suctioning, particularly client tolerance and secretion characteristics such as color, odor, and volume.
- Provide oral care every 4 hours.
  Oral care freshens the mouth after respiratory secretions have been expectorated.
- Encourage activity and ambulation as tolerated. If unable to ambulate client, turn client from side to side at least every 2 hours.
  Body movement helps mobilize secretions. The supine position and immobility have been shown to predispose postoperative clients to pneumonia (Brooks-Brunn, 1995). See interventions for **Impaired gas exchange** *for further information on positioning a respiratory client.*
- Encourage adequate fluid intake of up to 3000 ml/day within cardiac or renal reserve.
  Fluids help minimize mucosal drying and maximize ciliary action to move secretions (Carroll, 1994). Some clients can not tolerate increased fluids because of underlying disease.
- Administer oxygen as ordered.
  Oxygen has been shown to correct hypoxemia, which can be caused by retained respiratory secretions.
- Administer medications such as bronchodilators if ordered. Watch for side effects such as tachycardia or anxiety.
  Bronchodilators decrease airway resistance secondary to bronchoconstriction.
- Assist client with using nebulizers or metered dose inhalers as ordered.
  To use metered dose inhalers, the client must be taught to inspire deeply and coordinate the inspiratory effort with activation of the device (Peruzzi, Smith, 1995).
- Provide postural drainage, percussion, and vibration as ordered.
  Chest physical therapy helps mobilize bronchial secretions, it should be used only when prescribed because it can cause harm if client has underlying conditions such as cardiac disease, increased intracranial pressure (Peruzzi, Smith 1995).
- Refer for physical therapy or respiratory therapy for further treatment.

Geriatric
- Encourage ambulation as tolerated without causing exhaustion.
  Immobility is often harmful to the elderly because it decreases ventilation and increases stasis of secretions, leading to atelectasis or pneumonia (Hoyt, 1992).
- Actively encourage the elderly to deep breathe and cough.
  Cough reflexes are blunted and coughing is decreased in the elderly (Sparrow, Weiss, 1988).
- Ensure adequate hydration within cardiac and renal reserves.
  The elderly are prone to dehydration and therefore more viscous secretions because they frequently use diuretics or laxatives and forget to drink adequate amounts of water (Hoyt, 1992).

Home Care Interventions
- Assess home environment for factors that exacerbate airway clearance problems (e.g., presence of allergens, lack of adequate humidity in the air, stressful family relationships).
- Limit client exposure to upper respiratory infections.
- Provide/teach percussion and postural drainage per physician orders. Teach adaptive breathing techniques.
  Adaptive breathing, percussion, and postural drainage loosen secretions and allow more effective oxygenation.

- Assess client compliance with medical regimen.
- Teach client when and how to use inhalant or nebulizer treatments at home.
- Teach client/family importance of maintaining regimen and having prn drugs easily accessible at all times.
  Success in avoiding emergency or institutional care may rest solely on medication compliance or availability.
- Identify an emergency plan including criteria for usage.
  Ineffective airway clearance can be life threatening.
- Refer for home health aide services for assist with ADL.
  Clients with decreased oxygenation and copious respiratory secretions are often unable to maintain energy for ADL.
- Assess family for role changes and coping skills. Refer to medical social services as necessary.
  Clients with decreased oxygenation are unable to maintain role activities and experience frustration and anger, which may pose a threat to family integrity.
- Provide family with support for care of a client with a chronic or terminal illness.
  Severe compromise to respiratory function creates fear in clients and caregivers. Fear inhibits effective coping.

Client/Family Teaching

- Teach importance of not smoking. Be aggressive in approach, ask to set a date for smoking cessation, and recommend nicotine replacement therapy (nicotine patch or gum). Refer to smoking cessation programs, and encourage clients who relapse to keep trying to quit.
  All health care clinicians should be aggressive in helping smokers quit (AHCPR Guidelines, 1996).
- Teach client how to deep breathe and cough effectively.
  Controlled coughing uses the diaphragmatic muscles, making the cough more forceful and effective.
- Teach client the significance of rest periods between short periods of exertion.
- Teach client/family to identify and avoid specific factors that exacerbate ineffective airway clearance, especially smoking (if relevant) or exposure to second-hand smoke.
- Educate client and family about the significance of changes in sputum characteristics, including color, character, amount, and odor.
  With this knowledge the client and family can identify signs of infection early and seek treatment before acute illness occurs.
- Teach client/family need to take antibiotics until they are gone.
  Taking the entire course of antibiotics until finished helps eradicate bacterial infection, decreasing lingering, chronic infection.

REFERENCES   Ackerman MI: Ask the experts, *Crit Care Nurse* 13(3):103, 1993.
Agency for Health Care Policy and Research: *Smoking cessation,* Clinical Practice Guideline, Washington, DC, 1996, US Government Printing Office.
Brooks-Brunn JA: Postoperative atelectasis and pneumonia: risk factors, *Am J Crit Care* 4:340, 1995.
Carroll P: Safe suctioning prn, *RN* 57(5):32, 1994.
Dam V, Wild MC, Baun MM: Effect of oxygen insufflation during endotracheal suctioning on arterial pressure and oxygenation in coronary artery bypass graft patients, *Am J Crit Care* 3:191, 1994.
Deppe SA et al: Incidence of colonization, nosocomial pneumonia, and mortality in critically ill patients using a Trach Care closed-suction system: prospective, randomized study, *Crit Care Med* 18:1389, 1990.

Hagler DA, Traver GA: Endotracheal sale and suction catheters: sources of lower airway contamination, *Am J Crit Care* 3:444, 1994.

Hoyt MM: Impaired gas exchange in the elderly, *Geriatr Nurs* 13:262, 1992.

Johnson KL et al: Closed versus open endotracheal suctioning: costs and physiologic consequences, *Crit Care Med,* 22:658, 1994.

Marrelli, TM: *Handbook of home health standards and documentation guidelines for reimbursement,* ed 2, St Louis, 1994, Mosby.

Peruzzi WT, Smith B: Bronchial hygiene therapy, *Critic Care Clin* 11:79, 1995.

Raymond SJ: Normal saline instillation before suctioning: helpful or harmful? A review of the literature, *Am J Crit Care* 4:267, 1995.

Redick EL: Closed-system, in-line endotracheal suctioning, *Crit Care Nurse* 13:47, 1993.

Sparrow D, Weiss S: Pulmonary system. In Rose JW, Besdine RS, editors: *Geriatric medicine,* Boston, 1988, Little, Brown.

Winslow EH: Open-and-closed debate on hyperoxygenation: working smart, *Am J Nurs* 13:16, 1993.

Winslow EH: Save the saline, *Am J Nurs* Oct 1993, p. 16.

Yeaw P: Good lung down, *Am J Nurs* 92:27, 1992.

Altered family process: alcoholism

Jane M. Curtis

Definition   The state in which the psychosocial, spiritual, and physiological functions of the family unit are chronically disorganized, leading to conflict, denial of problems, resistance to change, ineffective problem solving, and a series of self-perpetuating crises

Defining Characteristics

Major
Feelings: Decreased self-esteem, worthlessness, anger, suppressed rage, frustration, powerlessness, anxiety, tension, distress, insecurity, repressed emotions, responsibility for alcoholic's behavior, lingering resentment, shame, embarrassment, hurt, unhappiness, guilt, emotional isolation, loneliness, vulnerability, mistrust, hopelessness, rejection
Roles and Relationships: Deterioration in family relationships, disturbed family dynamics, ineffective communication with spouse and other, marital problems, altered role function, disruption of family roles, inconsistent parenting, low perception of parental support, family denial, intimacy dysfunction, chronic family problems, closed communication systems
Behaviors: Inappropriate expression of anger, difficulty with intimate relationships, loss of control of drinking, impaired communication, ineffective problem-solving skills, enabling to maintain drinking, inability to meet emotional needs of family members, manipulation, dependence, criticizing, alcohol abuse, broken promises, rationalization, denial of problems, refusal to get help, inability to appropriately accept and receive help, blaming, inadequate understanding or knowledge of alcoholism

Minor
Feelings: Feeling different from other people, depression, hostility, fear, emotional control by others, confusion, dissatisfaction, loss, misunderstanding, abandonment, confused love and pity, moodiness, failure, feeling unloved, lack of identity
Roles and Relationships: Triangulating family relationships/reduced ability of family members to relate to each other for mutual growth and maturation, lack of necessary skills for relationships, lack of cohesiveness, disrupted family rituals, inability of family to meet security needs of its members, lack of respect for individuality and autonomy of family members, patterns of rejection, economic problems, neglected obligations

Behaviors: Inability to meet spiritual needs of its members, inability to express or accept a wide range of feelings, orientation to tension relief rather than achievement of goals, alcohol-centered family special occasions, escalating conflict, lying, contradictory or paradoxical communication, lack of dealing with conflict, harsh self-judgment, isolation, nicotine addiction, difficulty having fun, self-blaming, unresolved grief, controlled communication, power struggles, inability to adapt to change, immaturity, stress-related physical illnesses, inability to constructively deal with traumatic experiences, seeking of approval and affirmation, lack of reliability, disturbances in academic performance in children, disturbances in concentration, chaos, abuse of substances other than alcohol, failure to accomplish current or past developmental tasks, difficulty with life cycle transitions, verbal abuse of spouse or parent, agitation, diminished physical contact

Related Factors (r/t)

Abuse of alcohol, family history of alcoholism, resistance to treatment, inadequate coping skills, genetic predisposition, addictive personality, lack of problem-solving skills, biochemical influences

Client Outcomes/Goals

Family
- Develops relationship with nurse that demonstrates at least a minimal level of trust
- Demonstrates an understanding of alcoholism as a family illness and the severity of the threat to emotional and physical health of family members
- Develops belief in feasibility and effectiveness of efforts to address alcoholism
- Begins to change dysfunctional patterns by moving from inappropriate to appropriate role relationships, improving cohesion among family members, decreasing conflict and social isolation, and improving coping behaviors
- Maintains improvements

Suggested NIC Interventions

Family process maintenence, substance use treatment

Nursing Interventions and Rationales

- Demonstrate high levels of empathy and expectancy of positive outcomes in interactions with family members.
  Empathy as evidenced by respect, warmth, sympathetic understanding, supportiveness, caring, concern, commitment, and interest has been found to be the most important caregiver trait that affects motivation for treatment among alcoholic clients. The client's perception that the caregiver wants to help and that a positive outcome can be achieved increases commitment and willingness to be influenced (Miller, 1985). Presenting families with realistic facts in a nonjudgmental manner facilitates participation in treatment (American Nurses Association, 1987).
- Educate family members about alcoholism.
- Educate family members about available educational and support programs.
- Encourage participation.
- Stress individual self-focus as a first step in problem resolution.
  Health Beliefs Model Research confirms that client understanding of the severity of the threat to personal and family health and a belief in the feasibility and effectiveness of treatment are important motivating factors in changing health-related behavior (Damrosch, 1991; Giuffra, 1993). Family members can benefit themselves, the family as a whole, and the client through self-focus and participation in education and support activities (Captain, 1989; Williams, 1989). The perception of choice enhances motivation and improves compliance and outcome (Miller, 1985).

- When completing a family assessment, include demographic data, physical and emotional health of individuals, current family structure and roles, communication patterns, relationships among members, current stressors and conflicts, family cohesion, coping behaviors, shared interests and activities, resources and supports, knowledge of the problem, and expectations for recovery.

  NOTE: Assessment factors are included under interventions because it has been noted that assessment questions initiate a family process of self-examination and family problem solving and also provide assessment data (Craft, Willadsen, 1992). Most families are not aware of their adjustment to the addictive behavior, and family structure and function may be altered (e.g., a child assumes a parent's role in absence of parent appropriateness). In addition, individual family members or the family unit itself may be experiencing biological, cognitive, or spiritual responses that require separate interventions (American Nurses Association, 1987; Captain, 1989). The range of possible nursing interventions required for the family members is extremely broad, and the nurse is advised to consult the *Standards of Addictions Nursing* for assistance (American Nurses Association, 1987).

- Help family to restructure family patterns of interaction and function that support the development of consistency, a predictable environment, emotional nurturance, and positive modeling.

  Studies indicate that consistency, a predictable environment, emotional nurturance, and positive social modeling may act as ameliorating factors in the dysfunctional environment (Roberts, 1992; Sielhamer, Jacob, Dunn, 1993). Clinical reports and research also indicate that recovery is partially contingent on the restructuring of family interaction patterns. In assisting the family, the generalist nurse becomes a role model, counselor, educator, and promoter of effective interactions, self-care, and referral sources by using principles of nursing care derived from medical, surgical, psychiatric, and community health nursing. The nurse specialist, who has had specialty training and advanced education, may serve as family therapist (American Nurses Association, 1987).

- Assist with stabilization and maintenance of positive change in the family.

- Focus on the continued use of resources, which may become apparent as family dynamics change.

- To form a basis for realistic and objective evaluation of family changes, continue to provide education pertinent to the appropriate stage of family improvement.

- Support increasing social contacts and family recreational activities, and use contracting or homework assignment techniques to encourage positive behaviors.

- Monitor family closely for return to old patterns of behavior.

  The improvement of family interaction is an important condition for maintaining change. Family cohesion is fostered through the sharing of positive and fun experiences and is a critical factor in lasting recovery (Captain, 1989). A return to previous behavior patterns, termed relapse, *occurs most frequently within the first 3 months. Factors that have been useful in relapse prevention are education, social support, skills training, reinforcement, recreational activities, and the practice of new behaviors (Jones, 1990). Continuation and compliance are behaviors that are influenced by maintaining contact with an empathetic caregiver (Miller, 1985). There is evidence that success is achieved only after several relapses, and the effort to succeed is enhanced by knowledge skills training, support and self-help groups, and other techniques (Damrosch, 1991).*

Home Care Interventions

NOTE: In the community setting, alcoholism as an etiology for altered family process must be considered in two categories. The first is when the client suffers personally from the illness; the second is when a significant other suffers from the illness, that is, the client is not the active alcoholic but may be dependent on the alcoholic for caregiving. The listed considerations apply to both situations with appropriate adaptation for the circumstances.

- Identify client and family expectations of the home care nurse and nurse expectations of the client and family by use of a well-defined contract. Be specific and realistic. Adjust the contract only with clear consent and understanding of the client/family. *A well-defined contract supports success in meeting goals and encourages positive family dynamics. A contract defines conditions under which care can by safely provided and under which care cannot continue. Safety of the staff should never be jeopardized.*
- Establish well-defined contingency and emergency plans for the care of client. *Clinical safety of the client between visits is a primary goal of the home care nurse (Stanhope, Lancaster, 1996).*
- Request concrete, measurable tasks of client and family for caregiving.
- Refer for medical social work services at outset of care. *The social worker can help identify, set the structure for, and guide appropriate client/family and client/family/nurse interactions that will promote the plan of care throughout the length of the stay.*
- Acknowledge without judging when resolution of alcoholism is *not* a goal of care. *It is usually not appropriate for terminally ill or hospice clients or their families to change family life patterns. Recognizing this fact nonjudgmentally helps the client or family use remaining energy to complete other end-of-life work.*

REFERENCES   American Nurses Association, Task Force on Substance Abuse Nursing Practice: *The care of clients with addictions: dimensions of nursing practice,* Kansas City, Mo, 1987, The Association.

Captain C: Family recovery from alcoholism: mediating family factors, *Nurs Clin North Am* 24:55, 1989.

Craft MJ, Willadsen JA: Interventions related to family, *Nurs Clin North Am* 27:517, 1992.

Damrosch S: General strategies for motivating people to change their behavior, *Nurs Clin North Am* 26:833, 1991.

Giuffra MJ: Nursing strategies with alcohol and drug problems in the family. In Naegle MA, editor: *Substance abuse in education in nursing,* Vol III, Pub No 15-2464, New York, 1993, National League for Nursing Press.

Jones J: A proposed model of relapse prevention for adolescents who abuse alcohol, *J Child Adol Psychiatr Ment Health Nurs* 3:139, 1990.

Miller WR: Motivation for treatment: a review with special emphasis on alcoholism, *Psychol Bull* 98:84, 1985.

Roberts BJ: Adult children of alcoholics, *J Am Acad Nurse Pract* 4:22, 1992.

Stanhope M, Lancaster J, editors: *Community health nursing: promoting health of aggregates, families, and individuals,* ed 4, St Louis, 1996, Mosby.

Sielhamer RA, Jacob T, Dunn NJ: The impact of alcohol consumption on parent-child relationships in families of alcoholics, *J Stud Alcohol* 54:189, 1993.

Williams E: Strategies for intervention, *Nurs Clin North Am* 24:95, 1989.

Anxiety

Pam B. Schweitzer

Definition   A vague, uneasy feeling whose source is often nonspecific or unknown to the individual

Defining Characteristics

Subjective   Increased tension; apprehension; painful and persistent feelings; increased helplessness; uncertainty; fear; regret; overexcitement; rattled, distressed, or jittery feelings; feelings of inadequacy; shakiness; fear of unspecific consequences; expressed concerns regarding changes in life events; worry; anxiety

Objective   Sympathetic stimulation evidenced by cardiovascular excitation, superficial vasoconstriction, or pupil dilation; restlessness; insomnia; darting glances; poor eye contact; trembling or hand tremors; extraneous movement (e.g., foot shuffling, hand or arm movements); facial tension; quivering voice; self-focusing; increased wariness; increased perspiration

Related Factors (r/t)

Unconscious conflict regarding essential values or goals of life, threat to self-concept, threat of death, threat to or change in health status, threat to or change in environment, threat to or change in interaction patterns, situational or maturational crises, interpersonal transmission of contagion, unmet needs

Client Outcomes/Goals

- Identifies and verbalizes symptoms of anxiety
- Identifies, verbalizes, and demonstrates techniques to control anxiety
- Verbalizes absence of or decrease in subjective distress
- Has vital signs that reflect baseline or decreased sympathetic stimulation
- Has posture, facial expressions, gestures, and activity levels that reflect decreased distress
- Demonstrates improved concentration and accuracy of thoughts
- Identifies and verbalizes anxiety precipitants, conflicts, and threats
- Demonstrates return of basic problem-solving skills
- Demonstrates increased external focus
- Demonstrates some ability to reassure self

Suggested NIC Interventions

Anxiety reduction

Nursing Interventions and Rationales

- Assess client's level of anxiety and physical reactions to anxiety (e.g., tachycardia, tachypnea, nonverbal expressions of anxiety). Validate observations by asking client, "Are you feeling anxious now?"
  Anxiety is a highly individualized, normal, physical, and psychological response to internal or external life events (Badger, 1994).
- Use presence, touch (with permission), verbalization, or demeanor to remind clients that they are not alone and to encourage expression or clarification of needs, concerns, unknowns, and questions.
  Being supportive and approachable encourages communication (Olson, Sneed, 1995).
- Accept client's defenses; do not confront, argue, or debate.
  If defenses are not threatened, the client may feel safe enough to look at behavior (Rose, Conn, Rodeman, 1994).
- Allow and reinforce client's personal reaction to or expression of pain, discomfort, or threats to well-being (e.g., talking, crying, walking, other physical or nonverbal expressions).
  Talking or otherwise expressing feelings sometimes reduces anxiety (Johnson, 1972).

- Help client identify precipitants of anxiety that may indicate interventions.
  Gaining insight enables the client to reevaluate the threat or identify new ways to deal with the threat (Damrosch, 1991).
- If the situational response is rational, use empathy to encourage client to interpret the anxiety symptoms as normal.
  Anxiety is a normal response to actual or perceived danger (Peplau, 1963).
- If irrational thoughts or fears are present, offer client accurate information.
  Correcting mistaken beliefs reduces anxiety.
- Avoid excessive reassurance; this may reinforce undue worry.
  Reassurance is not helpful for the anxious individual (Garvin, Huston, Baker, 1992).
- Intervene when possible to remove sources of anxiety.
  Anxiety is a normal response to actual or perceived danger; if the threat is removed, the response will stop.
- Explain all activities, procedures, and issues that involve the client; use nonmedical terms and calm, slow speech. Do this in advance of procedures when possible, and validate client's understanding.
  Uncertainty and lack of predictability contribute to anxiety (Garvin, Huston, Baker, 1992).
- Explore coping skills previously used by client to relieve anxiety; reinforce these skills and explore other outlets.
  Methods of coping with anxiety that have been successful in the past are likely to be helpful again.
- Rule out withdrawal from alcohol, sedatives, or smoking as the cause of anxiety.
  Withdrawal from these substances is characterized by anxiety (Badger, 1994).
- Identify and limit, discontinue, or be aware of the use of any stimulants such as caffeine, nicotine, theophylline, terbutaline sulfate, amphetamines, and cocaine.
  Many substances cause or potentiate anxiety symptoms.

Geriatric
- Monitor client for depression. Use appropriate interventions.
  Anxiety often accompanies or masks depression in elderly adults.
- Provide a protective and safe environment. Use consistent caregivers and maintain the accustomed environmental structure.
  Elderly clients tend to have more perceptual impairments and adapt to changes with more difficulty, especially during an illness (Halm, Alpen, 1993).
- Observe for adverse changes if antianxiety drugs are taken.
  Age renders clients more sensitive to both the clinical and toxic effects of many agents.
- Provide a quiet environment with diversion.
  Excessive noise increases anxiety; involvement in a quiet activity can be soothing to the elderly.

Client/Family Teaching
- Teach client and family symptoms of anxiety.
  If client and family can identify anxious responses, they can intervene earlier (Reider, 1994).
- Help client to define anxiety levels (from "easily tolerated" to "intolerable") and select appropriate interventions.
  Mild anxiety enhances learning and adaptation, but moderate to severe anxiety may impede or immobilize progress (Peplau, 1963).
- If antianxiety medications have been prescribed, teach client how to use them appropriately.

- Teach client to identify and use distraction or diversion tactics when possible. *Early interruption of the anxious response prevents escalation.*
- Teach client to allow anxious thoughts and feelings to be present until they dissipate. *Allowing and even devoting time and energy to a thought, purposefully and repetitively, reduces associated anxiety (Beck, Emery, 1985).*
- Teach progressive muscle relaxation techniques.
- Teach relaxation breathing for occasional use—client should breathe in through nose, fill slowly from abdomen upward while thinking "re," and then breathe out through mouth, from chest downward, and think "lax."
- Teach client to visualize or fantasize absence of anxiety or pain, successful experience of the situation, resolution of conflict, or outcome of procedure.
- Teach relationship between a healthy physical and emotional life-style and a realistic mental attitude.
  Health and well-being are influenced by how well defined and met needs are in areas of safety, diet, exercise, sleep, work, pleasure, and social belonging.
- Teach use of appropriate community resources in emergency situations such as hotlines, emergency rooms, law enforcement, and judicial systems.
- Encourage use of appropriate community resources in emergency situations such as family, friends, neighbors, self-help and support groups, volunteer agencies, churches, clubs and centers for recreation, and others with similar interests.

REFERENCES   Badger JM: Calming the anxious patient, *Am J Nurs* 94:46, 1994.

Beck AT, Emery G: *Anxiety disorders and phobias: a cognitive perspective,* New York, 1985, Basic Books.

Damrosch S: General strategies for motivating people to change their behavior, *Nurs Clin North Am* 26:833, 1991.

Garvin BJ, Huston GP, Baker CF: Information used by nurses to prepare patients for a stressful event, *Appl Nurs Res* 5:158, 1992.

Halm MA, Alpen MA: The impact of technology on patients and families, *Nurs Clin North Am* 28:443, 1993.

Johnson J: Effects of structuring patient's expectations on their reactions to threatening events, *Nurs Res* 21:499, 1972.

Olson M, Sneed N: Anxiety and therapeutic touch, *Issues Mental Health Nurs* 16:97, 1995.

Peplau H: A working definition of anxiety. In Burd S, Marshall M, editors: *Some clinical approaches to psychiatric nursing,* New York, 1963, MacMillan.

Reider JA: Anxiety during critical illness of a family member, *Dimen Crit Care Nurs* 13:272, 1994.

Rose SK, Conn VS, Rodeman BJ: Anxiety and self-care following myocardial infarction, *Issues Ment Health Nurs* 15:443, 1994.

Risk for aspiration

Betty J. Ackley

Definition   The state in which an individual is at risk for entry of gastrointestinal secretions, oropharyngeal secretions, or solids or fluids into the tracheobronchial passages

Risk Factors

Reduced level of consciousness; depressed cough and gag reflexes; presence of tracheostomy or endotracheal tube; incomplete lower esophageal sphincter;

gastrointestinal tubes; tube feeding; medication administration; situations hindering elevation of upper body; increased gastrointestinal motility; delayed gastric emptying; impaired swallowing; facial, oral, or neck surgery or trauma; wired jaws

Related Factors (r/t)

See Risk Factors

Client Outcomes/Goals

- Swallows and digests oral, nasogastric, or gastric feeding without aspiration
- Maintains patent airway and clear lung sounds

Suggested NIC Interventions

Aspiration precautions

Nursing Interventions and Rationales

- Monitor respiratory rate, depth, and effort. Note any signs of aspiration such as dyspnea, cough, cyanosis, wheezing, or fever.
  Signs of aspiration should be detected as soon as possible to prevent further aspiration and to initiate treatment that can be lifesaving. Because of laryngeal pooling and residue in clients with dysphagia, silent aspiration (i.e., not manifested by choking or coughing) may occur.
- Auscultate lung sounds q____h and before and after feedings; note any new onset of crackles or wheezing.
- Take vital signs q____h.
- Before initiating oral feeding, check client's gag reflex and ability to swallow by feeling the laryngeal prominence as the client attempts to swallow.
  It is important to check client's ability to swallow before feeding. A client can aspirate even with an intact gag reflex (Baker, 1993).
- When feeding client, watch for signs of impaired swallowing or aspiration, including coughing, choking, spitting food, or excessive drooling. If client is having problems swallowing, see Nursing Interventions for **Impaired swallowing.**
- Have suction machine available for high-risk clients. If aspiration does occur, suction the mouth, pharynx, and trachea immediately.
  A client with aspiration needs immediate suctioning and will need further life-saving interventions such as intubation (Fater, 1995).
- Keep head of bed elevated when feeding and for at least a half four afterwards.
  This position helps keep food in the stomach and decreases aspiration.
- Note presence of any nausea, vomiting, or diarrhea. Treat nausea promptly with antiemetics.
- Listen to bowel sounds q____h, noting if they are decreased, absent, or hyperactive.
  Decreased or absent bowel sounds can indicate an ileus with possible vomiting and aspiration; increased high-pitched bowel sounds can indicate mechanical bowel obstruction with possible vomiting and aspiration.
- Note new onset of abdominal distention or increased rigidity of abdomen.
  Abdominal distention or rigidity can be associated with paralytic or mechanical obstruction and an increased likelihood of vomiting and aspiration.
- If client has a tracheostomy, check for inflation of the tracheostomy cuff before initiating feeding per physician's order; avoid overinflating the cuff. For clients receiving continuous tube feedings, the cuff should be inflated and cuff pressures checked every 8 hours.
  The presence of a tracheostomy tube increases the incidence of aspiration; inflating the

cuff may help decrease aspiration, but overinflating the cuff predisposes the client to aspiration by compression of the esophagus (Elpern, Jacobs, Bone, 1987). If client is receiving continuous tube feedings, cuff pressures should be checked every 8 hours (Eisenberg, 1991; Fater, 1995).

- Feed client only during formal rest periods from restraints.
- If client shows symptoms of nausea and vomiting, position on side.
- If client needs to be fed, feed slowly and allow adequate time for chewing and swallowing.

Enteral feedings

- Check to make sure initial feeding tube placement was confirmed by x-ray, especially if a small-bore feeding tube is used. Keep feeding tube securely taped.
  X-ray verification of placement is the only consistently reliable method to detect inadvertent respiratory placement (Metheny et al, 1990; Rakel et al, 1990). Small-bore feeding tubes have been inadvertently placed in the respiratory tract, and clients did not demonstrate any signs of respiratory distress (Fater, 1995).
- Keep nasogastric tube securely taped. Use pink tape to secure the tube.
  Use of pink tape as opposed to clear tape or butterfly tape increases the length of time a tube stays taped (Bury et al, 1995).
- Determine placement of feeding tube before each feeding or every 4 hours if client on continuous feeding. Check pH of aspirate and note characteristic appearance of aspirate; do not rely on air insufflation method.
  The auscultatory air insufflation method is often not reliable in differentiating between gastric or respiratory placement. Testing the pH can generally predict feeding tube position in the gastrointestinal tract (Metheny et al, 1990b; Metheny et al, 1993), especially if combined with identification of appearance of aspirate (Metheny et al, 1994). Nursing research has suggested use of a manometer to measure pressure in the tube. Positive pressure readings were obtained when the tube was in the stomach, and negative pressure readings were obtained when the tube was in the pulmonary system (Swiech, 1994).
- Check for gastric residual at least every 4 hours during continuous feedings or before feedings; if residual is greater than 100 ml, follow institutional protocol on holding feeding.
  Increased intragastric pressure can result in regurgitation and aspiration.
- If ordered by physician, put several drops of blue or green food coloring in tube feeding to help indicate aspiration.
  Colored secretions suctioned or coughed from the respiratory tract indicate aspiration (Ackerman, 1993; Fater, 1995).
- During feeding, position client with head of bed elevated 30 to 40 degrees; maintain for 30 to 45 minutes after feeding.
  Keeping client's head elevated helps keep food in stomach and decreases incidence of aspiration (Fater, 1995).
- Stop continual feeding temporarily when turning or moving client.
  It is difficult to keep the head elevated to prevent regurgitation and possible aspiration when turning or moving a client.

Geriatric
- Carefully check elderly client's gag reflex and ability to swallow before feeding.
  Laryngeal nerve endings are reduced in the elderly, which diminishes the gag reflex (Close, Woodson, 1989).

- Use central nervous system depressants cautiously; elderly clients may have an increased incidence of aspiration with altered levels of consciousness.
  Elderly clients have altered metabolism, distribution, and excretion of drugs. Some medications can interfere with the swallowing reflex.

Home Care Interventions

- Obtain complete information from the discharging institution regarding institutional management of clients at high risk for aspiration.
  Continuity of care can prevent unnecessary stress for the client and family and can facilitate successful management in the home setting.
- Assess the client and family for willingness and cognitive ability to learn and cope with swallowing, feeding, and related disorders.
  Food and feeding habits may be strongly tied to cultural values of families. Acknowledgment and/or adjustment to cultural values can facilitate compliance and successful family coping.
- Establish emergency and contingency plans for care of client.
  Clinical safety of client between visits is a primary goal of home care nursing (Stanhope, Lancaster, 1996).
- Refer to a speech therapist and occupational therapist for assessment of current status of swallowing or other physiological factors and for strategies to work with the client in the home (e.g., pureeing foods being served at a meal for client; providing adaptive equipment for independence in eating).
  These strategies allow the client to remain part of the family.
- Assess caregiver understanding, and reinforce teaching regarding positioning and assessment of the client for possible aspiration.
- Obtain suction equipment for the home as necessary.
- Teach caregivers safe, effective use of suctioning devices. Teach client and family that only individuals instructed in suctioning should perform the procedure.

Client/Family Teaching

- Teach client and family signs of aspiration and precautions to prevent aspiration.
- Teach client and family how to safely administer tube feeding.

REFERENCES   Ackerman MI: Ask the experts, *Crit Care Nurse,* 13:103, 1993.
Baker DM: Assessment and management of impairments in swallowing, *Nurs Clin North Am* 28:793, 1993.
Burns SM et al: Comparison of nasogastric tube securing methods and tube types in medical intensive care patients, *Am J Crit Care* 4:198, 1995.
Close LG, Woodson GE: Common upper airway disorders in the elderly and their management, *Geriatrics* 44:67, 1989.
Elpern EH, Jacobs ER, Bone RC: Incidence of aspiration in tracheally intubated adults, *Heart Lung* 16:527, 1993.
Fater KH: Determining nasoenteral feeding tube placement, *Medsurg Nurs* 4:27, 1995.
Johnson ER, McKenzie SW, Sievers A: Aspiration pneumonia in stroke, *Arch Phys Med Rehab* 74:973, 1993.
Metheny N et al: Detection of inadvertent respiratory placement of small-bore feeding tubes: a report of 10 cases, *Heart Lung* 19:631, 1990.
Metheny N et al: Effectiveness of the auscultatory method in predicting feeding tube location, *Nurs Res* 39:262, 1990.
Metheny N et al: Effectiveness of pH measurements in predicting feeding tube placement: an update, *Nurs Res* 42:324, 1993.
Metheny N et al: Visual characteristics of aspirates from feeding tubes as a method for predicting tube location, *Nurs Res* 43:282-287, 1994.
Mobarhan S, Trumbore LS: Enteral tube feedings: a clinical perspective on recent advance, *Nutr Rev* 49:129, 1991.

Rakel BA et al: Nasogastric and nasointestinal feeding tube placement: an integrative review of research, *AACN Clin Issues,* 5:194, 1994.

Stanhope M, Lancaster J, editors: *Community health nursing: promoting health of aggregates, families, and individuals,* ed 4, 1996, Mosby.

Swiech K, Lancaster DR, Sheehan R: Use of a pressure gauge to differentiate gastric from pulmonary placement of nasoenteral feeding tubes, *Appl Nurs Res,* 7:183, 1994.

Body image disturbance

Gail B. Ladwig

Definition   Disruption in own body image perception

Defining Characteristics

Objectives   Missing body part, actual change in structure or function, avoidance of looking at or touching body part, intentional or unintentional hiding or overexposure of body part, trauma to nonfunctioning part, change in social involvement, change in ability to estimate spatial relationship of body to environment

Subjective   Change in life-style; fear of rejection or reaction by others; focus on past strength, function, or appearance; negative feelings about body; feelings of helplessness, hopelessness, or powerlessness; preoccupation with change or loss; emphasis on remaining strengths and heightened achievement; extension of body boundary to incorporate environmental objects; personalization of part or loss by name; depersonalization of part or loss by impersonal pronouns; refusal to verify actual change

Related Factors (r/t)

Biophysical, cognitive, perceptual, psychosocial, cultural, or spiritual factors

Client Outcomes/Goals

- States or demonstrates acceptance of change or loss and an ability to adjust to life-style change
- Calls body part or loss by appropriate name
- Looks at and touches changed or missing body part
- Cares for changed or nonfunctioning part without inflicting trauma
- Returns to previous social involvement
- Correctly estimates relationship of body to environment

Suggested NIC Interventions

Body image enhancement

Nursing Interventions and Rationales

- Observe client's usual coping mechanisms during extreme times of stress and reinforce their use in the current crisis.
  Clients are in shock during acute phase, and their own value system must be considered; clients deal better with change over time (Price, 1992).
- Acknowledge denial, anger, or depression as normal feelings in adjusting to changes in body and life-style.
  Changes in body image cause anxiety. People in this situation use a variety of unconscious coping mechanisms to deal with their altered body image (ABI). Defense mechanisms are normal, unless they are used so much that they interfere with rather than improve self-esteem (MacGinley, 1993).

- Clients should not be rushed into sharing their feelings.
  Feelings associated with complicated and emotionally powerful issues involving an altered body image take time to work through and express (Johnson, 1994).
- Do not ask clients to explore feelings unless they have indicated a need to do so.
  Patients reported keeping their feelings to themselves as a frequently used coping strategy (Zacharias et al, 1994).
- Explore strengths and resources with client. Discuss possible changes in weight and hair loss; select a wig before hair loss occurs.
  Emphasizing strengths promotes a positive self-image. Planning for an event such as hair loss helps to decrease the sudden change in appearance.
- Allow client and others gradual exposure to the body change. Begin by having the client touch the affected area; then use a mirror to look at it. Go to a hospital shop with a nurse or support person and discuss feelings associated with the reaction of others to the body change.
  Part of the rehabilitation process is graded exposure—the client moves from a protected to an unprotected environment with the support of the nurse (MacGinley, 1993).
- Encourage client to discuss interpersonal and social conflicts that may arise.
  A good perception of body image is best achieved within a supportive social framework. Clients with an active social support network are likely to make better progress (Price, 1990).
- Encourage client to make own decisions, participate in plan of care, and accept both inadequacies and strengths.
  It is important for clients to be involved in their own care. If they have received information about their altered body image, treatment, and rehabilitation, they will be able to make their own choices. Consequently they will be more likely to come to terms with and adapt to their ABI (Prince, 1986). Healthy adaptation to body image exists when the person is able to maximize ability despite disability (Samonds, Cammermeyer, 1989).
- Help client accept help from others; provide a list of appropriate community resources (e.g., Reach to Recovery, Ostomy Association).
  Motivation, sharing of experiences, camaraderie with and support from peers, and knowledge of not being alone have been identified as advantages of group learning (Payne, 1993).
- Help client describe self-ideal, identify self-criticisms, and be accepting of self.
  The perception of self-image involves knowing the self and what is important and valued. Disability causes individuals to live as changed human beings whether they are willing to or not (Pohl, 1992).
- Avoid looks of distaste when caring for clients who have had disfiguring surgery or injuries. Provide privacy; care should be completed without unnecessary exposure.
  Nurses must be aware of their nonverbal behavior; clients often become acutely aware of nurses' feelings because of their facial expressions, tone of voice, touch, or other behaviors (MacGinley, 1993).
- Encourage client to continue same personal care routine that was followed before the change in body image. It is preferable that this care be completed in the bathroom and not in bed.
  This routine gives the client privacy and also prevents the client from settling into an

"invalid" role. Research has shown that women who resume familiar routines and habits heal better and suffer less depression than those who settle into the role of patient (Johnson, 1994).

Geriatric
- Focus on remaining abilities.
Motivation and self-worth are increased in the elderly by highlighting their capabilities. Even a severely disabled client is usually capable of accomplishing some tasks. Normal changes in body image occur as a result of the aging process (MacGinley, 1993).

Home Care Interventions
- Assess client's stage of grieving or acceptance of body change on return to home setting. Include the future role of sexuality in the psychological assessment of acceptance as appropriate.
- Assess family/caregiver level of acceptance of client's body changes.
- Be accepting of changes in all interactions with client and family/caregivers
Acceptance promotes trusts.
- Help client to see new or changing roles in family. Point out ways in which the community can help support client and family strengths.
- Refer to medical social services for level of acceptance and possible financial impact of changes.
Clients and caregivers may see the nurse's visit as being solely involved with physiological issues such as dressing, especially under managed care systems. Social worker visits can support the client or caregivers with dedicated time and can help the nurse be supportive and adapt interventions to promote acceptance. The nurse or social worker can introduce or reinforce use of community resources.
- Teach all aspects of care. Involve client and caregivers in self-care as soon as possible. Do this in stages if client still has difficulty looking at or touching changed body part.
The quicker the involvement in self-care, the greater the chances for permanent acceptance and positive self-esteem.
- Teach family and client complications of medical condition and when to contact physician.
- Refer to occupational therapy if necessary to evaluate home setting for safety and adaptive equipment and to assist client in returning to normal activities.
The quicker the reinvolvement in daily living activities and self-care, the greater the chances for permanent acceptance and positive self-esteem.
- If appropriate, provide home health aide support to help the client and family through ADL transition.
- Refer to physical therapy if necessary to build range of joint motion (ROJM) flexibility and strength, prevent contractures, assist with transfer/ambulation safety, or obtain use of a prosthetic device in the home setting.
- Assess for and promote good nutrition and sleep patterns. Adapt nutrition to specific physiological situations (e.g., client with ostomy).
Both patterns promote faster healing and better coping.
- Assist family with obtaining needed supplies.
Cost of ostomy supplies and adaptive equipment can be an added stressor for the client. Community resources can assist.

Client/Family Teaching
- Teach appropriate care of surgical site (e.g., mastectomy site, amputation site, ostomy site).

Patient teaching by ET nurses may alleviate problems associated with altered body image in relation to the presence of an ostomy (Tomaselli et al, 1991).

- Inform client of available community support groups; offer to make initial phone call.
  Motivation, sharing of experiences, camaraderie with and support from peers, and knowledge of not being alone have been identified as advantages of group learning (Payne, 1993).
- Refer client to counseling for help adjusting to body change.
  Counseling is important for a client who is trying to create a new body ideal or work through a grief process (Price, 1990).
- Provide printed material and didactic information for significant others.
  Some significant others prefer to receive didactic material rather than vent their feelings as a way of showing support (Northouse, Peters-Golden, 1993).
- Encourage significant others to offer support.
  Social support from significant others enhances both emotional and physical health (Badger, 1990).
- Direct social support as follows: instruct regarding practical care (bandaging), encourage appraisal support (listening), encourage self-esteem support (favorable comparisons between client's and others' appearance), and encourage sense of belonging (assist in socializing).
  The preceding are four categories of support which are recognized in the body-image care model. Clients with an active social support network are likely to make better progress (Price, 1990).

REFERENCES Badger V: Men with cardiovascular disease and their spouses: coping, health and marital adjustment, *Arch Psychiatr Nurs* 4:319, 1990.

Johnson J: Caring for the woman who's had a mastectomy, *Am J Nurs* 94:25, 1994.

MacGinley K: Nursing care of the patient with altered body image, *Br J Nurs* 2:1098, 1993.

Northouse L, Peters-Golden H: Cancer and the family: strategies to assist spouses, *Semin Oncol Nurs* 9:74, 1993.

Payne J: The contribution of group learning to the rehabilitation of spinal cord injured adults, *Rehabil Nurs* 18:375, 1993.

Pohl C, Winland-Brown J: The meaning of disability in a caring environment, *J Nurs Adm* 22:29, 1992.

Price B: Keeping up appearances, *Nurs Times* 82:58, 1986.

Price B: A model for body-image care, *J Adv Nurs* 15:585, 1990.

Price B: Living with altered body image: the classic patient experience, *Br J Nurs* 25:641, 1992.

Samonds R, Cammermeyer M: Perceptions of body image in subjects with mutiple sclerosis: a pilot study, *J Neurosci Nurs* 21:190, 1989.

Tomaselli N, Jenks J, Morin K: Body image in patients with stomas: a critical review of the literature, *J ET Nurs* 18:95, 99, 1991.

Zacharias DR, Gilig CA, Foxall MJ: Quality of life and coping in patients with gynecologic cancer and their spouses, *Oncol Nurs Forum* 21:1699, 1994.

Effective breast-feeding

Vicki E. McClurg and Virginia R. Wall

Definition A state in which a mother-infant dyad exhibits adequate proficiency and satisfaction with the breast-feeding process

Defining Characteristics

Major   Mother able to position infant at breast to promote a successful latch-on response, contented infant after feeding, regular and sustained suckling and swallowing at the breast, age-appropriate infant weight patterns, effective mother-infant communication patterns (e.g., infant cues, maternal interpretation and response)

Minor   Signs or symptoms of oxytocin release (let-down or milk ejection reflex), adequate infant elimination patterns for age, eagerness of infant to nurse, maternal verbalization of satisfaction with breast-feeding process

Related Factors (r/t)

Basic breast-feeding knowledge, normal maternal breast structure, normal infant oral structure, infant gestational age greater than 34 weeks, support sources (e.g., encouraging partner, history of positive breast-feeding experiences among relatives and friends, access to support groups such as La Leche League), maternal confidence, breast-feeding within first hour after birth, exclusive and frequent breast-feeding until milk supply established, maternal determination to breast-feed

Client Outcomes/Goals

- Maintains effective breast-feeding
- Maintains normal growth patterns (infant)
- Verbalizes satisfaction with breast-feeding process (mother)

Suggested NIC Interventions

Breast-feeding assistance

Nursing Interventions and Rationales

- Assess knowledge regarding basic breast-feeding.
  Support and teaching must be individualized to the client's level of understanding. Women prepare to breast-feed by acquiring information. This exposure to a variety of sources of information is an important predictor of breast-feeding duration (Duckett, Henly, Garvis, 1993; Rajan, 1993; Cox, Turnbull, 1994).
- Assess breast and nipple structure.
  Normal nipple and breast structure or early detection and treatment of abnormalities is important for successful breast-feeding (Jensen, Wallace, Kelsay, 1994).
- Assist client with first attachment at breast within first hour after birth.
  During the quiet-alert state in the first hour following birth, the infant is most likely to latch on successfully. Early breast-feeding has a positive effect on lactation performance. A successful first feeding boosts maternal confidence (Crowell, Hill, Humenick, 1994; Lawson, Tulloch, 1995). "Following birth, every effort should be made to put the baby to the breast as soon as possible" (Matthews, 1993).
- Assess client's knowledge of prevention and treatment of common breast-feeding problems.
  Common problems that can lead to early termination of breast-feeding are generally preventable or can be overcome with assistance (Ziemer et al, 1990; Matthews, 1993; Rajan, 1993).
- Monitor the breast-feeding process.
  The nurse's presence and involvement allow for early detection of difficulties and foster success (Rajan, 1993; Quarles et al, 1994).
- Encourage rooming-in and breast-feeding on demand.
  Rooming-in and breast-feeding on demand are positively associated with breast-feeding success (Perez-Escamilla et al, 1994).

- Evaluate adequacy of infant intake.
  Infant intake can be measured by objective criteria such as number and quality of feedings, infant elimination patterns (should have six voidings of light yellow urine per day), and infant weight gain (Hill, 1992).
- Avoid supplemental bottle feedings.
  Supplemental feedings can interfere with the infant's desire to breast-feed, increase the risk of allergies, and convey the subtle message that the mother's breast milk is not adequate. The longer and more exclusively a mother breast-feeds, the greater the health benefits to both her and her infant (Walker, 1993).
- Avoid nipple shields.
  The amount of milk an infant can get through a nipple shield is diminished (Auerbach, 1990).
- Assess support person network.
  Social support is an important factor in the choice of breast-feeding and its success (Gamble, Morse, 1993; Giugliani et al, 1994; Kistin, Abramson, Dublin, 1994; Kessler et al, 1995).
- Give praise for positive mother-infant interactions related to breast-feeding.
  "Strategies that promote not only the initiation, but also the successful continuation of breast-feeding, are particularly important in helping the mother achieve competence and mastery in this important aspect of mothering" (Chute, 1992).
- Do not provide samples of formula at discharge.
  Commercial discharge packs are associated with poor lactation success, especially in vulnerable subgroups such as first-time mothers and low-income women (Perez-Escamilla et al, 1994).
- Provide a nurse-initiated phone call within 2 days of discharge from hospital.
  Outreach of this type is associated with breast-feeding success (Bernard-Bonnin et al, 1989; Quarles et al, 1994).

Client/Family Teaching

- Teach mother importance of maternal nutrition.
  Dieting during lactation can have a negative impact on milk production (Dusdieker, Hemingway, Stumbo, 1994).
- Teach client to be aware of infant's subtle hunger cues (e.g., quiet-alert state, rooting, sucking, hand-to-mouth activity) and to nurse whenever signs are apparent.
  Feedings are initiated more easily when the infant is hungry and in the quiet-alert state (Shrago, 1992). The infant brings certain characteristics to the breast-feeding experience that contribute to breast-feeding success (Lothian, 1995).
- Review guidelines for frequency of feedings (every 2 to 3 hours or at least eight feedings per 24 hours).
  In the first few days, frequent and regular stimulation of the breasts is important to establish an adequate milk supply (Hill, Aldag, 1993; Riordan, Auerbach, 1993).
- Review guidelines for duration of feeding (e.g., until suckling and swallowing slow down).
  The mother should be taught to use infant cues of satiety rather than arbitrary time limits (Hill, Aldag, 1993).
- Provide anticipatory guidance about common breast-feeding problems.
  Lack of knowledge about detection, prevention, and treatment of problems can lead to premature termination of breast-feeding (Rajan, 1993).

- Provide anticipatory guidance about common infant behaviors.
  Lack of knowledge regarding infant growth spurts, temperament, sleep-wake cycles, and introduction of other foods can create parental anxiety and lead to premature termination of breast-feeding (Shrago, 1992; Lothian, 1995).
- Provide information about additional breast-feeding resources.
  Breast-feeding classes, books, materials, and support groups can provide current and accurate information and enhance maternal success and satisfaction with the breast-feeding process (Giugliani et al, 1994).

REFERENCES   Auerbach KG: The effect of nipple shields on maternal milk volume, *J Obstet Gynecol Neonatal Nurs* 19:419, 1990.

Bernard-Bonnin A et al: Hospital practices and breastfeeding duration: a meta-analysis of controlled clinical trials, *Birth* 16:64, 1989.

Chute GE: Promoting breastfeeding success: an overview of basic management, *NAACOG Clin Issues Perinatal Women Health Nurs* 3:570, 1992.

Cox SG, Turnbull CJ: Choosing to breastfeed or bottle-feed: an analysis of factors which influence choice, *Breastfeed Rev* 2:459, 1994.

Crowell MK, Hill PD, Humenick SS: Relationship between obstetric analgesia and time of effective breastfeeding, *J Nurse Midwife* 39:150, 1994.

Duckett L, Henly SJ, Garvis M: Predicting breastfeeding duration during postpartum hospitalization, *West J Nurs Res* 15:177, 1993.

Dusdieker LB, Hemingway DL, Stumbo PJ: Is mild production impaired by dieting during lactation? *Am J Clin Nutr* 59:833, 1994.

Gamble D, Morse JB: Fathers of breastfed infants: postponing and types of involvement, *JOGNN* 22:358, 1993.

Giugliani ERJ et al: Effect of breastfeeding support from different sources on mother's decision to breastfeed, *J Human Lactation* 10:157, 1994.

Hill PD: Insufficient milk supply syndrome, *NAACOG Clin Issues Perinatal Women Health Nurs* 3:605, 1992.

Hill PD, Aldag JC: Insufficient milk supply among black and white breastfeeding mothers, *Res Nurs Hlth* 16:203, 1993.

Jensen D, Wallace S, Kelsay P: LATCH: a breastfeeding charting system and documentation tool, *JOGNN* 23.27, 1994.

Kessler LA, Gielen AC, Diener-west M, Paige DM: The effect of a woman's significant other on her breastfeeding decision, *J Hum Lactation* 11(2):103-9, 1995.

Kistin N, Abramson R, Dublin P: Effect of peer counselors on breastfeeding initiation, exclusivity, and duration among low-income urban women, *J Hum Lactation* 10:11, 1994.

Lawson K, Tulloch MI: Breastfeeding duration: prenatal intentions and postnatal practices, *J Adv Nurs* 22:841, 1995.

Lothian JA: It takes two to breastfeed: the baby's role in successful breastfeeding, *J Nurse Midwife* 40:328, 1995.

Matthews MK: Experiences of primiparous breastfeeding mothers in the first days following birth, *Clin Nurs Res* 2:309, 1993.

North American Nursing Diagnosis Association: *Taxonomy 1,* St Louis, 1990, The Association.

Perez-Escamilla R et al: Infant feeding policies in maternity wards and their effect on breastfeeding success: an analytical overview, *Am J Public Health* 84:89, 1994.

Quarles A et al: Mother's intention, age, education and the duration and management of breastfeeding, *Matern Child Nurs J* 22:102, 1994.

Rajan L: The contribution of professional support, information and consistent correct advice to successful breastfeeding, *Midwifery* 9:127, 1993.

Riordan J, Auerbach KG: *Breastfeeding and human lactation,* Boston, 1993, Jones and Bartlett.

Sears W: The father's role in breastfeeding, *NAACOG's Clin Issues Perinatal Women Health Nurs* 3:713, 1992.

Shrago LC: The breastfeeding dyad: early assessment, documentation, and intervention, *NAACOG Clin Issues Perinatal Women Health Nurs* 3:583, 1992.

Walker M: A fresh look at the risks of artificial infant feeding, *J Hum Lactation,* 9:97, 1993.

Ziemer MM et al: Methods to prevent and manage nipple pain in breastfeeding women, *West J Nurs Res* 12:732, 1990.

Ineffective breast-feeding

Vicki E. McClurg and Virginia R. Wall

Definition   The state in which a mother, infant, or child experiences dissatisfaction or difficulty with the breast-feeding process

Defining Characteristics

Major   Unsatisfactory breast-feeding process

Minor   Actual or perceived inadequate milk supply, infant's inability to latch on to maternal breast correctly, no observable signs of oxytocin release (let-down or milk ejection reflex) either during feeding (uterine cramping, increased lochia flow, dripping from contralateral breast, tingling sensation in breasts, sound of infant swallowing) or after feeding (noticeable softening of breasts), observable signs of inadequate infant intake (e.g., inadequate weight gain, inadequate elimination patterns, dehydration), no sustained suckling or swallowing at the breast, insufficient emptying of each breast at each feeding, persistence of sore nipples beyond the first week of breast-feeding or for the duration of a feed in the first week after birth, insufficient opportunity for suckling at the breast, infant fussiness and crying within the first hour after breast-feeding, infant unresponsiveness to other comfort measures, infant arching and crying at the breast, maternal reluctance to put infant to breast, infant resistance to latch on, sleepiness at the breast

Related Factors (r/t)

Maternal   Breast anomaly (e.g., inverted nipple); drugs; engorgement; fatigue; history of breast-feeding failure; previous breast surgery; sore nipples; anxiety or ambivalence; depression; knowledge deficit; nonsupportive partner, family, or health care provider

Infant   Anomaly (e.g., abnormal oral structure), delayed initiation of breast-feeding, illness, inability to modulate states (sleep-wake cycles), poor sucking reflex, prematurity, receiving supplemental feedings with artificial nipple

Client Outcomes/Goals

- Achieves effective breast-feeding
- Verbalizes or demonstrates techniques to manage breast-feeding problems
- Manifests signs of adequate intake at the breast (infant)
- Manifests positive self-esteem in relation to the infant feeding process
- Explains a safe alternative method of infant feeding if unable to continue exclusive breast-feeding

Suggested NIC Interventions

Lactation counseling

Nursing Interventions and Rationales

- See **Effective breastfeeding.**
- Assess for presence or absence of related factors or conditions that would preclude breast-feeding.
  Some conditions (e.g., maternal drug use, maternal HIV-positive status, infant cleft palate) may preclude breast-feeding so infant needs to be started on a safe alternative method of feeding (Riordan, 1993a; American Academy of Pediatrics, 1994).
- Assess breast and nipple structure.
  Normal nipple and breast structure or early detection and treatment of abnormalities with continuing support are important for successful breast-feeding (The MAIN Trial Collaborative Group, 1994).
- Evaluate and record the mother's ability to position; give cues and help the infant latch on.

Correct positioning and getting the infant to latch on are critical for getting breast-feeding off to a good start and contribute to breast-feeding success (Duckett, Henly Garvis, 1993; Matthews, 1993).

- Evaluate and record the infant's ability to properly grasp and compress the areola with its lips, tongue, and jaw.
  The infant must have a "competent suck" to be successful at breast-feeding. The jaws must compress the milk sinuses beneath the areola—jaws must be well back on the areola, and the tongue should be over the lower gum, forming a trough around the breast; the lips should be flanged and sealed around the breast (Chute, 1992; Lothian, 1995).
- Evaluate and record the infant's suckling and swallowing pattern at the breast.
  When the infant sucks adequately, there is visible muscular movement above the ears. When breast milk is actively flowing, infants suck at a rate of once per second. Swallowing increases as milk supply increases (Shrago, 1992; Lothian, 1995).
- Evaluate and record signs of oxytocin release.
  The let-down reflex (tingling sensation in the breasts, milk dripping from the breasts, uterine cramping) is an indication of oxytocin release and is necessary for transfer of milk to the infant (Newton, 1992; Ueda et al, 1994).
- Evaluate and record infant's state at time of feeding.
  Infants breast-feed best when in the quiet-alert state. Difficulties arise when trying to breast-feed a sleepy, ravenously hungry, or crying infant (Shrago, 1992; Lothian, 1995).
- Assess knowledge regarding psychophysiology of lactation and specific treatment measures for underlying problems.
  Support and teaching must be individualized to the client's level of understanding. The mother must acquire knowledge and become cognitively and emotionally ready (Chute, 1992, Duckett, Henly, Garvis, 1993).
- Assess psychosocial factors that may contribute to ineffective breast-feeding (e.g., anxiety, goals, values, and life-style that contribute to ambivalence about breast-feeding).
  The attitude of the mother toward breast-feeding is critical in achieving successful lactation, influencing milk production, and facilitating the art of breast-feeding (Duckett, Henly, Garvis, 1993; Losch et al, 1995).
- Assess support person network.
  Social support is an important factor in successful breast-feeding (Gamble, Morse, 1993; Giugliani et al, 1994; Kessler et al, 1995; Kistin, Abramson, Dublin, 1994; Losch, et al, 1995).
- Promote comfort and relaxation to reduce pain and anxiety.
  Discomfort associated with breast-feeding can cause some women to discontinue breast-feeding prematurely. Promoting comfort and relaxation can lead to more successful breast-feeding (Chute, 1992; Ziemer, Pigeon, 1993; Buchko et al, 1994).
- Provide support by actively helping mother correctly position baby to attain a good latch on nipple; encourage her to continue trying.
  Many problems that can lead to discontinuing breast-feeding can be prevented by giving a high level of practical and emotional support to the mother (Duckett, Henly, Garvis, 1993; Rajan, 1993).
- Bring infant to quiet-alert state by using alerting techniques (e.g., providing a variety of auditory, visual, and kinesthetic stimuli by unwrapping infant, placing infant upright, or talking to infant) or consoling techniques as needed.

A variety of stimuli can bring the infant to a quiet-alert state. Repetition can soothe a crying baby, thus making it easier to initiate breast-feeding (McCain, 1992; Shrago, 1992).

- Enhance the flow of milk; when infant's swallowing slows down, teach mother to massage breast or burp infant and switch to other breast.

  The mother's perception of inadequate milk supply can lead to early weaning. Infants should breast-feed from both breasts at each feeding. Breast massage can enhance the flow of milk and stimulate production (Hill, 1992; Riordan, Auerbach, 1993).

- Evaluate adequacy of infant intake.

  Infant intake can be measured by objective criteria such as number and quality of feedings, infant elimination patterns (should have six voidings per day of light yellow urine), and infant weight gain (Hill, 1992; Meier et al, 1993).

- Discourage supplemental bottle feedings and encourage exclusive and effective breast-feeding.

  Supplemental feedings can interfere with the infant's desire to breast-feed, increase the risk of allergies, and convey the subtle message that the mother's breast milk is not adequate (Chute, 1992; Duckett, Henly, Garvis, 1993).

- Acknowledge mother's feelings and support her decision to either continue breast-feeding or to choose an alternate plan.

  Mastering infant feeding is an important first step in mothering. The mother needs to be empowered so that she feels competent and capable of making intelligent decisions (Locklin, Naber, 1993; Losch et al, 1995).

- Make appropriate referrals.

  Collaborative practice with neonatal nutritionists, physical or occupational therapists, or lactation specialists helps ensure feeding and parenting success (Meier et al, 1993; Rajan, 1993; Quarles et al, 1994).

- If client is unsuccessful with effective breast-feeding, help her to accept and learn an alternate method of infant feeding.

  Once the decision has been made to provide an alternate method of infant feeding, the mother needs support and education.

Client/Family Teaching

- Provide instruction in correct positioning.

  "Correct positioning is perhaps the most critical single measure for getting breast-feeding off to a good start. Many problems can be attributed to carelessness or inattention to this simple aspect of breast-feeding" (Chute, 1992).

- Reinforce and add to knowledge base regarding underlying problems and specific treatment measures.

  If the mother understands the rationale for recommended treatment, she may be more likely to comply with recommendations and less likely to perceive the problem as insurmountable (Ziemer et al, 1990; Rajan, 1993).

- Provide education to support persons as needed.

  Informational support providers help mother achieve a more positive outcome (McNatt, Freston, 1992; Kessler et al, 1995; Losch et al, 1995).

REFERENCES   American Academy of Pediatrics—Committee on Drugs: Transfer of drugs and other chemicals into human milk, *Pediatrics* 93:137, 1994.

Buchko BL et al: Comfort measures in breastfeeding: primiparous women, *JOGNN* 23:46, 1994.

Chute GE: Promoting breastfeeding success: an overview of basic management, *NAACOG's Clin Issues Perinatal Women Health Nurs* 3:570, 1992.

Duckett L, Henly SJ, Garvis M: Predicting breastfeeding duration during postpartum hospitalization, *West J Nurs Res* 15:177, 1993.

Gamble D, Morse JB: Fathers of breastfed infants: postponing and types of involvement, *JOGNN* 22:358, 1993.

Giugliani ERJ et al: Effect of breastfeeding support from different sources on mother's decisions to breastfeed, *J Hum Lactation* 10:157, 1994.

Hill PD: Insufficient milk supply syndrome, *NAACOG Clin Issues Perinatal Women Health Nurs* 3:650, 1992.

Kessler LA et al: The effect of a woman's significant other on her breastfeeding decision, *J Hum Lactation* 11:103, 1995.

Kistin N, Abramson R, Dublin P: Effect of peer counselors on breastfeeding initiation, exclusivity, and duration among low-income urban women, *J Hum Lactation* 10:11, 1994.

Locklin MP, Naber SJ: Does breastfeeding empower women? Insights from a select group of low-education, low-income minority women, *Birth* 20:30, 1993.

Losch M et al: Impact of attitudes on maternal decisions regarding infant feeding, *J Pediatr* 126:507, 1995.

Lothian JA: It takes two to breastfeed: the baby's role in successful breastfeeding, *J Nurse Midwife* 40:328, 1995.

The MAIN Trial Collaborative Group: Preparing for breast feeding: treatment of inverted and non-protractile nipples in pregnancy, *Midwifery* 10:299, 1994.

Matthews MK: Experiences of primiparous breastfeeding mothers in the first days following birth, *Clin Nurs Res* 2:309, 1993.

McCain GC: Facilitating inactive awake states in preterm infants: a study of three interventions, *Nurs Res* 41:157, 1992,

McNatt MH, Freston MG: Social support and lactation outcomes in postpartum women, *J Hum Lactation* 8:73, 1992.

Meier PP et al: Breastfeeding support services in the neonatal intensive-care unit, *JOGNN* 22:338, 1993.

Newton N: The quantitative effect of oxytocin (Pitocin) on human milk yield, *Ann NY Acad Sci* 652:481, 1992.

Newton N: The relation of milk-ejection reflex to the ability to breastfeed, *Am NY Acad Sci* 652:484, 1992.

North American Nursing Diagnosis Association: *Taxonomy 1,* St. Louis, MO:NANDA 1990, The Association.

Quarles A et al: Mother's intention, age, education and the duration and management of breastfeeding, *Matern Child Nurs J* 22:102, 1994.

Rajan L: The contribution of professional support, information and consistent correct advice to successful breastfeeding, *Midwifery* 9:127, 1993.

Riordan J: AIDS and breastfeeding: the ultimate paradox, *J Hum Lactation* 9:3, 1993.

Riordan J, Auerbach KG: Breastfeeding and human lactation, Boston, 1993, Jones & Bartlett.

Shrago LC: The breastfeeding dyad: early assessment, documentation, and intervention, *NAACOG Clin Issues Perinatal Women Health Nurs* 3:583, 1992.

Ueda T et al: Influence of psychological stress on suckling-induced pulsatile oxytocin release, *Obstet Gynecol* 84:259, 1994.

Ziemer MM et al: Methods to prevent and manage nipple pain in breastfeeding women, *West J Nurs Res* 12:732, 1990.

Ziemer MM, Pigeon JG: Skin changes and pain in the nipple during the first week of lactation, *JOGNN* 22:247, 1993.

Interrupted breast-feeding

Vicki E. McClurg and Virginia R. Wall

Definition

A break in the continuity of the breast-feeding process as a result of inability or inadvisability to put baby to breast for feeding

Defining Characteristics

Major   Insufficient nourishment received by infant at breast for some or all feedings

Minor   Maternal desire to maintain lactation and provide (or eventually provide) her breast milk for her infant's nutritional needs, separation of mother and infant, lack of knowledge regarding expression and storage of breast milk

Related Factors (r/t)

Maternal or infant illness, prematurity, maternal employment, contraindications to breast-feeding (e.g., drugs, true breast milk jaundice), need to abruptly wean infant (with intent to resume at later date)

Client Outcomes/Goals

Infant   • Receives mother's breast milk if not contraindicated by maternal conditions (e.g., certain drugs, infections) or infant conditions (e.g., true breast milk jaundice).

Maternal • Initiates or maintains lactation
          • Achieves effective breast-feeding and satisfaction with the breast-feeding experience
          • Demonstrates effective methods of breast milk collection and storage

Suggested NIC Interventions

Bottle feeding, emotional support, lactation counseling

Nursing Interventions and Rationales

• Evaluate and record mother's desire to begin or continue breast-feeding.
  Maternal commitment to breast-feed is associated with breast-feeding success (Bottorff, 1990; Coates, Riordan, 1992; Quarles, 1994).

• Evaluate advisability of initiating or reinstituting breast-feeding.
  Some conditions (e.g., maternal drug use, HIV-positive status) may be contraindications to breast-feeding. Some conditions (e.g., infant cleft palate, maternal breast surgery) may make it impossible to breast-feed (Riordan, 1993a).

• Evaluate infant's ability to breast-feed and interest in breast-feeding.
  The infant must be able to demonstrate ability to breast-feed and interest in breast-feeding for the mother to resume breast-feeding (Danner, 1992; Lothian, 1995).

• Evaluate whether mother is being supported in her decision to continue breast-feeding.
  Relactating after an interruption is often stressful. The mother will benefit from social support of her efforts (McNatt, Freston, 1992; Giugliani et al, 1994; Kistin, Abramson, Dublin, 1994; Kessler et al, 1995).

• Assess mother's emotional response to events that caused interruption.
  Feelings of grief, guilt, anxiety, and failure are common and may need to be addressed before breast-feeding can be successful (Driscoll, 1992; Matthew, 1993; Meyer et al, 1994).

• Develop a satisfactory feeding plan with mother to allow for continued breast-feeding.
  Involvement of the mother in planning helps her feel able to participate in caretaking (Meyer et al, 1994).

• Assess and record mother's knowledge of breast milk expression techniques.
  During interruption, the mother needs to maintain lactation by expressing milk using either hand expression or a manual or electric breast pump (Zinaman et al, 1992; Auerbach, 1994).

• Assess and record mother's knowledge regarding the way to handle, store, and transport breast milk safely.
  If expressed breast milk is to be fed to an infant, the mother must demonstrate proper storage and handling techniques to ensure that milk remains fresh and uncontaminated (Pittard et al, 1991; Human Milk Banking Association of North America, 1993; Mohandes et al, 1993).

- Assess equipment needs.

"The health care professional needs to base pumping recommendations on many factors and take into account each mother's situation." (Riordan, Auerbach, 1993).

- Provide resource information (e.g., support groups, equipment and supply rental or sales).

The mother needs this information to enable her to follow through with the care plan and receive support as needed (Meyer et al, 1994).

- Promote emotional resolution by encouraging mother to verbalize frustrations and disappointments.

Resolution is important for a satisfactory breast-feeding experience (Driscoll, 1992, Matthews, 1993).

Client/Family Teaching

- Teach mother effective methods for expressing breast milk.

The mother needs to be taught the way to continue lactation during the interruption of breast-feeding.

- Teach mother safe breast milk handling techniques.

The mother needs to be taught the way to handle breast milk to provide a safe product for her infant (Pittard et al, 1991; Mohandes et al, 1993).

- Provide anticipatory guidance for common problems associated with interrupted breast-feeding (e.g., diminishing milk supply, infant difficulty with resuming breast-feeding).

Knowing what to expect helps the mother cope with any difficulties that may arise (Jones, 1995).

- Provide education to support persons as needed.

Informational support providers help the mother achieve a more positive outcome (McNatt, Freston, 1992; Giugliani et al, 1994; Kistin et al, 1994; Kessler et al, 1995).

REFERENCES   Auerbach KG, Walker M: When the mother of a premature infant uses a breast pump: what every NICU nurse needs to know, *Neonatal Network* 13:23, 1994.

Bottorff JL: Persistence in breastfeeding: a phenomenological investigation, *J Adv Nurs* 15: 201, 1990.

Coates M, Riordan J: Breastfeeding during maternal or infant illness, *NAACOG Clin Issues Perinatal Women Health Nurs* 3:683, 1992.

Coreil J, Murphy JE: Maternal commitment, lactation practices, and breastfeeding duration, *JOGNN* 17:273, 1988.

Danner SC: Breastfeeding the neurologically impaired infant, *NAACOG Clin Issues Perinatal Women Health Nurs* 3:640, 1992.

Driscoll JW: Breastfeeding success and failures: implications for nurses, *NAACOG Clin Issues Perinatal Women Health Nurs* 3:565, 1992.

Giugliani ERJ et al: Effect of breastfeeding support from different sources on mother's decisions to breastfeed, *J Hum Lactation* 10:157, 1994.

Hill PD: Insufficient milk supply syndrome, *NAACOG Clin Issues Perinatal Women Health Nurs* 3:605, 1992.

Human Milk Banking Association of North America: *Recommendations for collection, storage, and handling of a mother's milk for her own infant in the hospital setting,* West Hartford, Conn, 1993, The Association.

Jones E: Strategies to promote preterm breastfeeding, *Modern Midwife* 5:8, 1995.

Kessler LA et al: The effect of a woman's significant other on her breastfeeding decision, *J Hum Lactation* 11:103, 1995.

Kistin N, Abramson R, Dublin P: Effect of peer counselors on breastfeeding initiation, exclusivity, and duration among low-income urban women, *J Hum Lactation* 10:11, 1994.

Lothian JA: It takes two to breastfeed: the baby's role in successful breastfeeding, *J Nurse Midwife* 40:328, 1995.

Matthews MK: Experiences of primiparous breastfeeding mothers in the first days following birth, *Clin Nurs Res* 2:309, 1993.

McNatt MH, Freston MG: Social support and lactation outcomes in postpartum women, *J Hum Lactation* 8:73, 1992.

Meyer EC et al: Family-based intervention improves maternal psychological well-being and feeding interaction of preterm infants, *Pediatrics* 93:241, 1994.

Mohandes AE et al: Bacterial contaminants of collected and frozen human milk used in an intensive care nursery, *Am J Infect Control* 21:226, 1993.

Pittard WB et al: Bacterial contamination of human milk: container type and method of expression, *Am J Perinatol* 8:25-7, 1991.

Quarles A et al: Mother's intention, age, education and the duration and management of breastfeeding, *Matern Child Nurs J* 22:102, 1994.

Riordan J: AIDS and breastfeeding: the ultimate paradox, *J Hum Lactation* 9:3, 1993.

Riordan J, Auerbach KG: *Breastfeeding and human lactation,* Boston, 1993, Jones & Bartlett.

Zinaman MJ et al: Acute prolactin and oxytocin responses and milk yield to infant suckling and artificial methods of expression in lactating women, *Pediatrics* 89:437, 1992.

Ineffective breathing pattern

Betty J. Ackley

Definition   The state in which an individual's inhalation and/or exhalation pattern does not enable adequate pulmonary inflation or emptying

Defining Characteristics

Dyspnea, shortness of breath, tachypnea, fremitus, abnormal arterial blood gas, cyanosis, cough, nasal flaring, respiratory depth changes, assumption of three-point position, pursed-lip breathing, prolonged expiratory phase, increased anteroposterior diameter, use of accessory muscles, altered chest excursion

Related Factors (r/t)

Neuromuscular impairment, musculoskeletal impairment, perceptual or cognitive impairment, pain, anxiety, decreased energy, fatigue

Client Outcomes/Goals

- Demonstrates a breathing pattern that supports blood gas results within the client's normal parameters
- Reports ability to breathe comfortably
- Demonstrates ability to perform pursed-lip breathing, controlled breathing, and use relaxation techniques effectively
- Identifies and avoids specific factors that exacerbate episodes of ineffective breathing patterns

Suggested NIC Interventions

Airway management, respiratory monitoring

Nursing Interventions and Rationales

- Monitor respiratory rate, depth, and ease of respiration.
  Normal respiratory rate is 12 to 16 breaths/min in the adult. When the respiratory rate exceeds 24 breaths/min, there is often significant respiratory or cardiovascular disease.
- Note pattern of respiration. If client is dyspneic, note what seems to cause the dyspnea, the way in which the client deals with the condition, and how the dyspnea resolves or gets worse.

A normal respiratory pattern is regular in a healthy adult. To assess dyspnea, it is important to consider all of its dimensions, including antecedents, mediators, reactions, and outcomes (McCord, Cronin-Stubbs, 1992).

- Attempt to determine if client's dyspnea is physiological or psychogenic in cause.
  There are two distinct categories of antecedents to dyspnea: physiological and psychogenic. Psychogenic dyspnea includes dyspnea caused by anxiety, fear, or anger (McCord, Cronin-Stubbs, 1992). Psychogenic dyspnea is commonly known as hyperventilation.

Psychogenic dyspnea—hyperventilation

- Assess cause of hyperventilation by asking client about current emotions and psychological state.
  Hyperventilation can be caused by factors including anxiety, fear, pain, and anger (McCord, Cronin-Stubbs, 1992).
- Ask client to breathe with you to slow down respiratory rate. Maintain eye contact and give reassurance.
  By making the client aware of respirations and giving support, the client may gain control of the breathing rate.
- Consider having client use a paper bag to breathe into and rebreathe expired air.
  Rebreathing air with increased levels of carbon dioxide helps raise the carbon dioxide level in the body and combats the respiratory alkalosis that follows hyperventilation. This will help slow the respiratory rate.
- If pain is the cause of hyperventilation, provide medication routinely to prevent severe pain. Use distraction techniques to help client deal with pain. See interventions for **Pain.**
  An increased respiratory rate is one sign of pain. Providing pain relief will cause the respiratory rate to return to normal.
- If client has chronic problems with hyperventilation, numbness and tingling in extremities, dizziness, and other signs of panic attacks, refer for counseling.

Physiological dyspnea

- Ensure that client in acute dyspneic state has received medications or treatment needed. Coach client to slow respiratory rate and use pursed-lip breathing.
  Anxiety can exacerbate dyspnea, causing the client to enter into a dyspneic panic state. The nurse's presence, reassurance, and help in controlling the client's breathing can be very beneficial.
- Note use of accessory muscles, abdominal breathing, nasal flaring, retractions, irritability, confusion, or lethargy.
  These symptoms signal increasing respiratory difficulty and decreasing Po_2.
- Observe color of tongue, oral mucosa, and skin.
  Cyanosis of the tongue and oral mucosa is central cyanosis and generally represents a medical emergency. Peripheral cyanosis of nailbeds or lips may or may not be serious (Carpenter, 1993).
- Observe sputum, noting color, odor, and volume.
  Normal sputum is clear or gray and minimal; abnormal sputum is green, yellow, or bloody, malodorous, and often copious.
- Auscultate breath sounds, noting decreased or absent sounds, crackles, or wheezes.
  These sounds can indicate a respiratory pathology associated with an altered breathing pattern.

- Monitor client's oxygen saturation and blood gases.
  An oxygen saturation of less than 90% (normal being 95% to 100%) or a Po_2 of less than 80 mmHg (normal being 80 to 100 mmHg) indicates significant oxygenation problems that may result in altered breathing patterns.
- Monitor for presence of pain, and provide pain medication for comfort as needed.
  Pain causes the client to hyperventilate and take shallow breaths that predispose the client to atelectasis.
- Position client in an upright or semi-Fowler's position.
  *An upright position facilitates lung expansion. See nursing interventions for **Impaired gas exchange** for further information on positioning.*
- Increase client's activity up to walking 3 to 4 times daily as tolerated. See nursing interventions for **Activity intolerance.**
  Body movement helps mobilize respiratory secretions.
- Schedule rest periods before and after activity.
  Respiratory clients with dyspnea are easily exhausted and need additional rest.
- Provide small, frequent feedings.
  Small feedings are given to avoid compromising ventilatory effort and to conserve energy. Clients with dyspnea often do not eat sufficient amounts of food because their priority is breathing.
- Encourage client to take deep breaths at prescribed intervals or use incentive spirometry; reinforce client's progress.
- If chronic pulmonary disease is interfering with quality of life, refer client for pulmonary rehabilitation. Pulmonary rehabilitation programs that include desensitization to dyspnea and guided mastery with monitored exercise are preferable.
  Pulmonary rehabilitation has been shown to improve exercise capacity, ability to walk, and sense of well-being (Fishman, 1994). The processes of desensitization and guided mastery for control of dyspnea have helped clients learn to be in control of their condition and has increased the amount of activity they can tolerate (Carrieri-Kohlman, Douglas, Gormley, 1993).

Geriatric
- Encourage ambulation as tolerated.
  Immobility is often harmful to the elderly because it decreases ventilation and increases stasis of secretions (Foyt, 1992).
- Encourage elderly clients to sit upright or stand and to avoid lying down for prolonged periods during the day.
  Thoracic aging results in decreased lung expansion; an erect position fosters maximal lung expansion.

Home Care Interventions

- Assist client and family with identifying other factors that precipitate or exacerbate episodes of ineffective breathing patterns (i.e., stress, allergens, stairs, activities that have high energy requirements).
  Being aware of precipitating factors helps clients avoid them and decrease risk of episodes.
- Assess client knowledge of and compliance with medication regimen.
- Teach client and family importance of maintaining regimen and having prn drugs easily accessible at all times.
  Appropriate and timely use of medications can decrease the risk of exacerbating ineffecting breathing.

- Assess coping skills and refer client for counseling if necessary.
  Many clients with chronic respiratory disease develop depression.
- Identify an emergency plan including when to call the physician or 911.
  Having a ready emergency plan reassures the client and promotes client safety.
- Refer to physical therapy for breathing exercises.
  Breathing exercises can strengthen the respiratory system and give the client increased confidence in personal control of illness.
- Refer to occupational therapy for evaluation and teaching of energy conservation techniques.
- Refer for home health aide services as needed to support energy conservation.
  Energy conservation decreases the risk of exacerbating ineffective breathing.
- Provide family with support for care of client with chronic or terminal illness.
  Severe compromise to respiratory function creates fear in clients and caregivers. Excessive fear inhibits effective coping.

Client/Family Teaching

- Teach pursed-lip and controlled breathing techniques (McConnell, 1992).
  Pursed-lip breathing helps keep alveoli inflated longer to increase oxygenation.
- Using a prerecorded tape, teach client progressive muscle relaxation techniques.
  Relaxation therapy can help reduce dyspnea and anxiety (Gift, Moore, Soeken, 1992).
- Teach about dosage, actions, and side effects of medications.
  Inhaled steroids and bronchodilators can have undesirable side effects, especially when taken in inappropriate doses.
- Teach to monitor sputum for changes in color, amount, or consistency.
  Monitor sputum changes helps the client identify infections earlier.
- Teach client to identify and avoid specific factors that exacerbate ineffective breathing patterns, such as exposure to other sources of air pollution (especially smoking).

REFERENCES   Carpenter, KD: A comprehensive review of cyanosis, *Crit Care Nurse* 13:66, 1993.

Carrieri-Kohlman V et al: Desensitization and guided mastery: treatment approaches for the management of dyspnea, *Heart & Lung,* 22:226, 1993.

Fishman AP: Pulmonary rehabilitation research, *Respir Crit Care Med* 149:825, 1994.

Foyt MM: Impaired gas exchange in the elderly, *Geriatr Nurs* 13:262, 1992.

Gift A, Moore T, Soeken K: Relaxation to reduce dyspnea and anxiety in COPD patients, *Nurs Res* 41:242, 1992.

Kim MJ et al: Inspiratory muscle training in patients with chronic obstructive pulmonary disease, *Nurs Res* 42:356, 1993.

Marrelli TM: *Handbook of home health standards and documentation guidelines for reimbursement,* ed 2, St Louis, 1994, Mosby.

McConnell: Performing pursed-lip breathing, *Nursing* 22:18, 1992.

McCord M, Cronin-Stubbs D: Operationalizing dyspnea: focus on measurement, *Heart & Lung* 21:167, 1992.

Decreased cardiac output

Betty J. Ackley and Linda L. Straight

Definition   The state in which the blood pumped by an individual's heart is sufficiently reduced to the point that it is inadequate to meet the needs of the body's tissues

Defining Characteristics

Variations in blood pressure; dysrhythmia; fatigue; jugular vein distention; color changes of skin and mucous membranes; oliguria; decreased peripheral pulses; cold, clammy skin; crackles; dyspnea; orthopnea; change in mental status; shortness of breath; syncope; vertigo; edema; cough; frothy sputum; gallop rhythm; weakness

Related Factors (r/t)

Myocardial infarction or ischemia, valvular disease, cardiomyopathy, serious dysrhythmia, ventricular damage, altered preload or afterload, pericarditis, sepsis, congenital heart defects, vagal stimulation, stress, anaphylaxis, cardiac tamponade

Client Outcomes/Goals

- Demonstrates adequate cardiac output as evidenced by a blood pressure and pulse rate and rhythm within normal parameters for client, strong peripheral pulses, and an ability to tolerate activity without symptoms of dyspnea, syncope, or chest pain
- Remains free of side effects from the medications used to achieve adequate cardiac output
- Explains actions and precautions to take for cardiac disease

Suggested NIC Interventions

Cardiac care, cardiac care: acute, circulatory care

Nursing Interventions and Rationales

- Monitor for symptoms of heart failure and decreased cardiac output, including diminished quality of peripheral pulses, cool skin and extremities, increased respiratory rate, presence of paroxysmal nocturnal dyspnea or orthopnea, increased heart rate, neck vein distention, decreased level of consciousness, and presence of edema.
  As these symptoms of heart failure progress, cardiac output declines (Murphy, Bennett, 1992; Ahrens, 1995).
- Listen to heart sounds; note rate, rhythm, presence of S_3, S_4, and lung sounds (noting presence of crackles).
  The new onset of a gallop rhythm, tachycardia, and fine crackles in lung bases can indicate onset of heart failure (Janowski, 1996). If client develops pulmonary edema, there will be coarse crackles on inspiration and severe dyspnea.
- Observe for chest pain; note location, radiation, severity, quality, duration, associated manifestations such as nausea, and precipitating and relieving factors.
  Chest pain is generally indicative of an inadequate blood supply to the heart, which can compromise cardiac output. Clients with heart failure can continue to have chest pain with angina or can reinfarct.
- If chest pain is present, have client lie down, monitor cardiac rhythm, give oxygen, run a strip, medicate for pain, and notify the physician.
  These actions can increase oxygen delivery to the coronary arteries and improve client prognosis.
- Place on cardiac monitor; monitor for dysrhythmias, especially atrial fibrillation.
  Atrial fibrillation is common in heart failure (Janowski, 1996).
- Monitor hemodynamic parameters for an increase in pulmonary wedge pressure, an

increase in systemic vascular resistance, or decreases in cardiac output and
Hemodynamic parameters give a good indication of cardiac function.

- Titrate inotropic and vasoactive medications within defined parameters to
contractility, preload, and afterload per physician's order.
*By following parameters, the nurse ensures maintenance of a delicate balance of
medications that stimulate the heart to increase contractility, maintaining adequate
perfusion of the body.*
- Monitor intake and output. If client is acutely ill, measure hourly urine output, and note
decreases in output.
*Decreased cardiac output results in decreased perfusion of the kidneys, with a resulting
decrease in urine output.*
- Note results of thallium scan with ejection fraction, ECG, chest x-ray, complete blood
count, electrolytes, and serum creatinine.
*An ejection fraction in a healthy heart is approximately 50%. Most patients
experiencing heart failure have an ejection fraction of less than 40% (Janowski, 1996).
Clients receiving diuretics are prone to develop hypokalemia. Serum creatinine levels
will elevate in clients with severe heart failure because of decreased perfusion to the
kidneys. Creatinine may also elevate because of ACE inhibitors (Ahren, 1995).*
- Administer oxygen as needed per physician's order.
*"Supplemental oxygen increases oxygen availability to the myocardium" (Prizant-
Weston, Castiglia, 1992).*
- Check blood pressure, pulse, and condition before administering cardiac medications
such as angiotensin converting enzyme (ACE) inhibitors, digoxin, and diuretics. Notify
physician if heart rate or blood pressure is low before holding medications.
*It is important that the nurse evaluate how well the client is tolerating current
medications before administering cardiac medications; do not hold medications
without physician input. The physician may decide to have medications administered
even though the blood pressure or pulse rate has lowered.*
- During acute events, ensure client remains on bedrest or maintains activity level that
does not compromise cardiac output.
Excessive activity will increase myocardial oxygen demands.
- Gradually increase activity when client's condition is stabilized by encouraging slower-
paced activities or shorter periods of activity with frequent rest periods following
exercise prescription; observe for symptoms of intolerance. Take blood pressure and
pulse before and after activity and note changes.
Activity of the cardiac client should be closely monitored. See **Activity intolerance.**
- Serve small low-sodium, low-cholesterol meals. Give small amounts of caffeine-
containing beverages (1 or 2 cups per 24 hours) if no resulting dysrhythmia.
*Low-sodium diets helps decrease fluid volume excess. Low-cholesterol diets helps
decrease atherosclerosis, which causes coronary artery disease. Clients with cardiac
disease tolerate smaller meals better because they require less cardiac output to digest.
One cup of caffeinated coffee has generally not been found to have any significant
effect (Schneider, 1987; Powell, 1993).*
- Monitor bowel function. Provide stool softeners as ordered. Caution client not to strain
when defecating.
*Decreased activity can cause constipation. Straining when defecating that results in the
Valsalva maneuver can lead to dysrhythmia, decreased cardiac function, and sometimes
death.*

- Have clients use a commode or urinal for toileting and avoid use of a bedpan.
  Getting out of bed to use a commode or urinal does not stress the heart any more than staying in bed to toilet. In addition, getting the client out of bed minimizes complications of immobility and is often preferred by the client (Winslow, 1992).
- Provide a restful environment by minimizing controllable stressors and unnecessary disturbances. Schedule rest periods after meals and activities.
  Rest periods decrease oxygen consumption (Prizant-Weston, Castiglia, 1992).
- Weigh client at same time daily (after voiding).
  An accurate daily weight is a good indicator of fluid balance. Increased weight and severity of symptoms can signal decreased cardiac function with retention of fluids.
- Assess for presence of anxiety; see interventions for **Anxiety** to facilitate reduction of anxiety in clients and family.
- Consider using music to decrease anxiety and improve cardiac function.
  Music has been shown to reduce heart rate, blood pressure, anxiety, and cardiac complications (Guzzetta, 1994).
- Closely monitor fluid intake including IV lines. Maintain fluid restriction if ordered.
  In clients with decreased cardiac output, poorly functioning ventricles may not tolerate increased fluid volumes.
- Refer to cardiac rehabilitation program for education, evaluation, and guided support to increase activity and rebuild life.

Geriatric
- Observe for atypical pain; the elderly often have jaw pain instead of chest pain or may have silent myocardial infarctions with symptoms of dyspnea or fatigue.
  The elderly have altered pain pathways and often do not experience the usual chest pain of cardiac patients (Carnevali, Patrick, 1993).
- Observe for syncope, dizziness, palpitations, or feelings of weakness.
  Dysrhythmias are common in the elderly (Carnevali, Patrick, 1993).
- Observe for side effects from cardiac medications.
  The elderly have difficulty with metabolism and excretion of medications; therefore toxic side effects are more common.

Home Care Interventions

- Continue to monitor physiological parameters as described above per physician's order.
  Transition to home can create increased stress and physiological instability related to diagnosis.
- Assess client for understanding and compliance with medical regimen, including medications, activity level, and diet.
- Instruct family and client about complications of disease process, need for weighing daily, and when it is appropriate to call doctor.
  Early recognition of symptoms facilitates early problem solving and prompt treatment (Janowski, 1966).
- Identify emergency plan, including use of CPR.
  Decreased cardiac output can be life threatening.
- Help family adapt daily living patterns to establish life changes that will maintain improved cardiac functioning in the client.
  Transition to the home setting can cause risk factors such as inappropriate diet to reemerge.
- Refer to physical therapy for strengthening exercises if client is not involved in cardiac rehabilitation.

- Refer to medical social services as necessary for counseling about the impact of severe or chronic cardiac disease.
  Social workers can assist the client and family with acceptance of life changes.

Client/Family Teaching

- Teach symptoms of heart failure and appropriate actions to take if client becomes symptomatic.
- Teach importance of smoking cessation and avoidance of alcohol intake.
  Clients who continue to smoke increase their chance of dying by at least 50%, and alcohol depresses heart contractility (Janowski, 1996).
- Teach stress reduction (e.g., imagery, controlled breathing, muscle relaxation techniques).
- Explain necessary restrictions, including consumption of a low-sodium diet, guidelines on fluid intake, and the avoidance of Valsalva's maneuver. Teach the importance of pacing activities, work simplification techniques, and the need to rest between activities to prevent becoming overly fatigued.
- Assist client in understanding the need for and how to incorporate life-style changes. Refer to cardiac rehabilitation for assistance with coping and adjustment.
- Teach client actions, side effects, and importance of consistently taking their cardiovascular medications.
  Medications can prolong the lives of heart failure clients but often are not taken, resulting in hospital readmissions (Agency for Health Care Policy and Research).
- Instruct family regarding cardiopulmonary resuscitation.

REFERENCES Agency for Health Care Policy and Research (AHCPR): *Guidelines for patients with heart failure,* US Department of Health and Human Services, Rockville, Md, AHCPR Publication No 94-0612.

Ahrens SG: Managing heart failure: a blueprint for success, *Nursing,* 25:26, 1995.

Carnevali DL, Patrick M: *Nursing management for the elderly,* ed 3, Philadelphia, 1993, JB Lippincott.

Folta A, Potempa KM: Reduced cardiac output and exercise capacity in patients after MI, *J Cardiovasc Nurs* 6:71, 1992.

Guzzetta CE: Soothing the ischemic heart, *Am J Nurs* 94:24, 1994.

Janowski MJ: Managing heart failure, *RN* 59:34, 1996.

Kern L, Omery A: Decreased cardiac output in the critical care setting, *Nurs Diag* 3:94, 1992.

Murphy T, Bennett EJ: Low-tech, high-touch perfusion assessment, *Am J Nurs* 92:36, 1992.

Powell AH: What's that brewing in the CCU?: Working smart, *Am J Nurs* 93:16, 1993.

Prizant-Weston M, Castiglia K: Hemodynamic regulation. In Bulechek GM, McCloskey JC, editors: *Nursing interventions: essential nursing treatments,* Philadelphia, 1992, WB Saunders.

Schneider JR: Effects of caffeine ingestion on heart rate, blood pressure, myocardial oxygen consumption, and cardiac rhythm in acute myocardial infarction patients, *Heart Lung* 16:167, 1987.

Winslow EH: Panning bedpans, *Am J Nurs* 92:16G, 1992.

Caregiver role strain

Betty J. Ackley

Definition   A caregiver's felt difficulty in performing the family caregiver role

Defining Characteristics

Not enough resources (e.g., time, emotional strength, physical energy, help from others) to provide the care needed; difficulty performing specific caregiving activities such as bathing, cleaning up after incontinence, and managing behavioral problems and pain; worry regarding concerns such as the client's health and emotional state, putting the care receiver in an institution, and caring for the care receiver if something should happen to the caregiver; feelings that caregiving interferes with other important roles such as being a worker, parent, spouse, or friend; feelings of loss because the care receiver is like a different person compared to before caregiving began; in the case of a child, feelings that the care receiver was never the child the caregiver expected; family conflict regarding issues of providing care; other family members not doing their share in providing care to the receiver; feelings that not enough appreciation is shown for what the caregiver does; stress or nervousness in the relationship with the care receiver; depression

Related Factors (r/t)

Pathophysiological

Illness severity of the care receiver, addiction or codependency, premature birth or congenital defect, discharge of family member with significant home care needs, caregiver health impairment, unpredictable illness course or instability in care receiver's health, female caregiver, psychological or cognitive problems of care receiver

Developmental

Caregiver not developmentally ready for caregiver role (e.g., young adult providing care for a middle-aged parent), developmental delay or retardation of the care receiver or caregiver

Psychosocial   Marginal family adaptation or dysfunction before the caregiver situation developed, marginal caregiver coping patterns, past history of poor relationship between caregiver and care receiver, spouse as caregiver, care receiver exhibits deviant or bizarre behavior exhibited by care receiver

Situational   Presence of abuse or violence; presence of situational stressors that normally affect families such as significant loss, disaster, crisis, poverty, economic vulnerability, or major life events (e.g., birth, hospitalization, leaving home, returning home, marriage, divorce, employment, retirement, death); duration of caregiving required; inadequate physical environment for providing care (e.g., housing, transportation, community services, equipment); family or caregiver isolation; lack of respite and recreation for caregiver; inexperience with caregiving; caregiver's competing role commitments; complexity or amount of caregiving tasks

Client Outcomes/Goals

- Maintains physical and psychological health (caregiver)
- Identifies resources available to help in giving care (caregiver)
- Obtains appropriate care (care receiver)

Suggested NIC Interventions

Caregiver support

Nursing Interventions and Rationales

- Monitor quality of care for adequacy and need for improvement.
- Determine physical and psychological health of caregiver and watch for signs of depression; refer to resources as needed.

Caregiving may weaken the immune system and predispose the caregiver to illness in some situations; the incidence of depression in family caregivers is estimated to be 40% to 50% (Stevens, Walsh, Baldwin, 1993).

- Observe for signs of addiction or codependency in caregiver or care receiver.
- Provide for home health services as needed to help with significant home care needs.
- Arrange for intervals of respite care for caregiver; encourage use if available.
  Respite care is beneficial to caregivers, if they can be convinced to use it (Sayles-Cross, DeLorme, 1995).
- Help caregiver to identify supports and decide how to best use them.
  Caregivers sometimes feel abandoned (Given et al, 1990) and sometimes need assistance to activate their support system.
- Encourage caregiver to grieve over loss of care receiver's function. Give caregiver permission to share angry feelings in a safe environment. Refer to nursing interventions for **Grieving.**
  Caregivers grieve the loss of function of their loved one, especially when dementia is involved (Liken, Collins, 1993).
- Identify with caregiver factors that can and cannot be controlled.
- Help caregiver find personal time to meet own needs, and learn stress management techniques.
  Self care is important for the caregiver. Practicing personal wellness measures can increase stamina, energy, and self-esteem and enhance the quality of care given (Ruppert, 1996).
- Encourage caregiver to talk about feelings, concerns, and fears. Acknowledge frustration associated with caregiver responsibilities.
- Arrange for follow-up care following discharge, including the services of a nursing/social work team, to provide medical and social services to caregiver and client.
  A program after discharge that supports the caregiver has been shown to delay nursing home placements, possibly delay some deaths, and save money (Oktay, Volland, 1990). Providing care to a seriously ill family member is a severe financial strain and often depletes most or all of the family savings (Covinsky et al, 1994).
- Give caregiver permission to arrange custodial care in an extended care facility if necessary; support both caregiver and care receiver during this difficult transition.
  Placing a loved one in an extended care facility can relieve the burden of care but does not relieve the stress resulting from financial concerns, guilt, loss of control, or lack of support (Stevens, Walsh, Baldwin, 1993).

Geriatric

- Monitor caregiver for psychological distress and signs of depression, especially if caring for a mentally impaired elder.
  Those caring for mentally impaired elders for an extended time with minimal social support are at high risk for psychological distress or depression (Baille, Norbeck, Barnes, 1988).
- Observe for any evidence of caregiver or care receiver violence; if evidence is present, speak with caregiver and care receiver separately.
  Caregiver violence is possible, especially if the care receiver was violent to the caregiver in the past (Meyer, 1993).
- Recognize that it is hard for the elderly to accept any change in caregivers or in environment.
- Help caregiver identify ways to equitably distribute workload among family or significant others.

Home Care Interventions

- Assess client and caregiver at every visit for quality of care provided and signs of caregiver stress. Document all observations objectively.

  The changing level of support from institutional care to home care and the length of time that care is needed may precipitate cumulative caregiver burden.

- Form a trusting and supportive relationship with caregiver. Allow caregiver to verbalize frustrations.

  Providing attention to the caregiver can decrease caregiver stress and reduce the risk of caregiver violence.

- Provide caregiver with information and education necessary about client's disease and regarding caregiving skills (Hogstel, 1990; Humphrey, 1994).

- Assist caregiver and client with arranging care to be compatible with other household patterns.

  With the right tools the caregiver is better able to plan and have confidence in the caregiver role, thus decreasing potential frustration (Hogstel, 1990; Humphrey, 1994).

- Refer client to home health aide services for activities of daily living (ADLs) assistance and light housekeeping. Allow caregiver to gain confidence in respite provider (Boland, Sims, 1996).

  Home health aide services can provide physical relief and respite for the caregiver.

- Refer to medical social work services as necessary for community resource assistance, financial planning, and supportive counseling for both client and caregiver.

  NOTE: Families of terminally ill clients are especially vulnerable to caregiver role strain because timing of the impending death is unpredictable, and caregiver effort and resources are disproportionately spent early in the caregiving period.

Client/Family Teaching

- Teach caregiver methods for managing behavioral symptoms. Refer to care plan for **Chronic confusion.**

  Caregivers can be taught the way to act when there is problem behavior and an understanding of the behavior (Mastrian, Ritter, Diemling, 1996).

- Teach caregiver how to provide physical care needed.

- Refer to counseling or support groups to assist in adjusting to caregiver role.

REFERENCES   Archbold PG: The PREP system of nursing interventions: a pilot test with families caring for older members, *Res Nurs Health* 18:3, 1995.

Baille V, Norbeck JS, Barnes LE: Stress, social support, and psychological distress of family caregivers of the elderly, *Nurs Res* 37:217, 1988.

Boland D, Sims S: Family caregiving at home as a solitary journey, *Image, Journal of Nursing Scholarship,* 28:55, 1996.

Covinsky KE: The impact of serious illness on patient's families, *JAMA* 272:1839, 1994.

Given B et al: Responses of elder spouse caregivers, *Res Nurs Health* 13:77, 1990.

Hogstel M: *Geropsychiatric nursing,* St Louis, 1990, Mosby.

Humphrey CJ: *Home care nursing handbook,* ed 2, Gaithersburg, Maryland, 1994, Aspen.

Liken MA, Collins CE: Grieving: facilitating the process for dementia caregivers, *J Psychosoc Nurs Ment Health Serv* 31:21, 1993.

Mastrian KG, Ritter C, Diemling GT: Predictors of caregiver health strain, *Home Healthcare Nurse,* 14:209, 1996.

Oktay JS, Volland PT: Post-hospital program for the frail elderly and their caregivers: a quasi-experimental evaluation, *Am J Public Health* 80:39, 1990.

Phillips LR et al: Effects of situational context and interactional process on the quality of family caregiving, *Res Nurs Health* 18:205, 1995.

Robinson KM, Steele D: The relationship between health and social support in caregiving wives as perceived by significant others, *J Adv Nurs* 21:88, 1995.

Ruppert RA: Caring for the lay caregiver, *AJN* 3:40, 1996.

Sayles-Cross S, DeLorme J: Worried, worn out, and angry: providing relief for caregivers: *ABNF J* 6:74, 1995.

Stevens GL, Walsh RA, Baldwin BA: Family caregivers of institutionalized and noninstitutionalized elderly individuals, *Nurs Clin North Am* 28:349, 1993.

What makes caregivers become violent, *Am J Nurs* 93:12, 1993.

Risk for caregiver role strain

Definition   The possibility that a caregiver may experience difficulty in performing the family caregiver role

Related Factors (r/t)

See related factors for **Caregiver role strain.**

Client Outcomes/Goals, Nursing Interventions and Rationales, and Client/Family Teaching

See **Caregiver role strain**

Altered comfort

Betty J. Ackley

Definition   The state in which an individual experiences an uncomfortable sensation in response to a noxious stimulus (Carpenito, 1993)

Defining Characteristics

Major   Verbalization or demonstration of discomfort

Minor   Guarded position, cutaneous irritation, abdominal heaviness, itching, retching

Related Factors (r/t)

Visceral disorders; inflammation; musculoskeletal disorders; treatments; personal situations (e.g., pregnancy, overactivity); chemical irritants (Carpenito, 1993)

Client Outcomes/Goals

- States is comfortable
- Explains methods to decrease itching
- States relief of discomfort of nausea

Suggested NIC Interventions

Pruritis   Skin care: topical treatments

Nausea/vomiting

Medication administration, distraction, progressive muscle relaxation, simple guided imagery, therapeutic touch

Nursing Interventions and Rationales

Pruritis   • Determine cause of pruritis (e.g., dry skin, contact with irritating substance, medication side effect, insect bite, infection, symptom of systemic disease).

The etiology of pruritis helps direct treatment. Pruritis may be caused by serious illnesses such as renal failure, liver failure, malignancy, or diabetes (Eaglestein, 1994), as well as by dry skin and various skin conditions.

- Apply soaks with washcloths wrung out in cool water or ice water as needed.
  The application of cool or cold washcloths can depress the itching sensation.
- Keep client's fingernails short; have client wear mitts if necessary.
  Scratching with fingernails can excoriate the area and increase skin damage.
- Leave pruritic area open to the air if possible.
  Covering the area with a nonventilated dressing can increase itching sensation and warmth in the area.
- Use nonallergenic, mild soap and use it sparingly.
  Many soaps can be irritating to the skin and increase the itching sensation.
- Keep skin well lubricated; apply nonallergenic creams or mineral oil after bathing while the skin is still moist.
  These agents lubricate the skin surface and make the skin feel smoother and less dry (Hardy, 1996). Creams and ointments are more effective than lotions because lotions contain more water (Frantz, 1994).
- If pruritis areas are open and weeping, apply a shake solution such as calamine to the area.
  When they evaporate, these solutions cool the skin and dry weeping lesions (DeWitt, 1990).
- Provide distraction techniques such as music or television.
  These activities help to temporarily distract the client from the itching sensation.
- Consult with physician for medication to relieve itching.
  Medications such as antihistamines can be helpful for pruritis (DeWitt, 1990).

Nausea/vomiting

- Determine cause of nausea and vomiting (e.g., medication effects, viral illness, food poisoning, extreme anxiety, pregnancy).
  The cause of nausea and vomiting often determines the treatment.
- Keep a clean emesis basin and tissues within client's reach.
- Provide oral care after client vomits.
  Oral care helps remove the taste and smell of vomitus, thus reducing the stimulus for further vomiting.
- Stay with client to give support, place hand on shoulder, and hold the emesis basin.
  Human support can be helpful and comforting to an uncomfortable client (Morse, 1994).
- Provide distraction from sensation of nausea using soft music, television, and videos per client preference.
  Distraction can help direct attention away from the sensation of nausea.
- Maintain a quiet, well-ventilated environment.
  Odors from a kitchen or bathroom can trigger nausea (Pervan, 1990).
- Avoid sudden movement of client; allow client to lie still.
  Movement can trigger further nausea and vomiting.
- If client is pregnant, suggest she sit down when experiencing nausea and get more rest.
  Sitting down reduces nausea up to 80% of the time in pregnant women (Dilorio, van Lier, 1989). Fatigue also predisposes to morning sickness (Rhodes, Johnson, McDaniel, 1990).
- Consult with physician regarding need for antiemetic medications, especially if client is receiving chemotherapy. There are antiemetic drugs that can be very effective for clients with nausea from chemotherapy (Goebel, 1996).
- After vomiting is controlled and nausea abates, begin feeding client small amounts of clear fluids such as clear soda or broth and then crackers; progress to a soft diet.

- Remove cover of food tray before bringing it into client's room.
  The sudden, concentrated food odors that come when the cover is removed in front of the client can trigger nausea (Pervan, 1990).

Pruritis
Geriatric
- Limit number of complete baths to every other day. Use a tepid water temperature at 90° to 105° F for bathing.
  Excessive bathing, especially in hot water, depletes aging skin of moisture and increases dryness.
- Use superfatted soap such as Dove, Tone, Basis, or Caress.
  Superfatted soaps help retain moisture in dry, elderly skin (Hardy, 1996).
- Increase fluid intake within cardiac or renal limits to a minimum of 1500 ml/day.
  Dry skin is caused by loss of fluid through the skin; increasing fluid intake rehydrates the skin.
- Use a humidifier or a container of water on heat source to increase humidity in the environment, especially during the winter.
  Increasing moisture in the air helps to keep moisture in the skin (Fenske, Grayson, Newcomer, 1989; Hardy, 1996).

Home Care Interventions
Pruritis
- Assist client and family with identifying and avoiding irritants that exacerbate pruritis (e.g., wool).
  Avoiding irritants decreases discomfort of pruritis.
- Teach family to use mild, nonscented and nonbleach products in laundry.
  Chemical irritants increase discomfort of pruritis.
- Keep temperature of home moderated. Use humidifier as noted previously.
  Overheated home environments increase sweating, which adds salts to the skin and increases irritation.

Nausea
- Assist the client and family with identifying and avoiding irritants in the home setting that exacerbate nausea (e.g., strong odors such as food, plants, perfume, room deodorizers).

Client/Family Teaching
- Teach techniques to use when client is uncomfortable, including relaxation techniques, guided imagery, hypnosis, and music therapy (Jablonski, 1993; Pervan, 1993; Rhodes, Johnson, McDaniel, 1995).
  Guided imagery has been shown to be effective in decreasing nausea associated with chemotherapy (Troesch, 1993). Behavioral interventions for nausea such as hypnosis, progressive muscle relaxation training, systematic desensitization, biofeedback, and distractions have been shown to be effective (Dodd, 1995).
- Teach client with pruritis to substitute rubbing, pressure, or vibration for scratching when itching is severe and irrepressible.

REFERENCES   Abang A, Forrester S: *Practical strategies for nausea and vomiting: the role of oral 5-HT3 antagonists,* 1995, presented to 20th Anniversary Congress of the Oncology Nursing Society.
Carpenito JL: *Nursing diagnosis: application to clinical practice,* ed 5, Philadelphia, 1993, JB Lippincott.
DeWitt S: Nursing assessment of the skin and dermatologic lesions, *Nurs Clin North Am* 25:235, 1990.
Dilorio CK, van Lier DJ: Nausea and vomiting in pregnancy. In Funk SG et al, editors: *Key aspects of comfort: management of pain, fatigue, and nausea,* New York, 1989, Springer.

Dodd MJ: Side effects of cancer chemotherapy, *Res Nurs Prac* 77-101, 1995.

Eaglestein WH, McKay M, Pariser DM: The problems that plague aging skin, *Patient Care* 28:89, 1994.

Fenske NA, Grayson LD, Newcomer VD: Common problems of aging skin, *Patient Care* 23:225, 1989.

Frantz RA, Gardner S: Clinical concerns: management of dry skin, *J Gerontol Nurs* 9:15, 1994.

Frantz RA, Kinney CK: Variables associated with skin dryness in the elderly, *Nurs Res* 35:98, 1986.

Goebel C: Prevention and control of nausea and vomiting for patients with cancer, *Home Health Nurs* 14:15, 1996.

Hardy MA: Dry skin care. In Bulechek GM, McCloskey JC, editors: *Nursing interventions: essential nursing treatments,* ed 2, Philadelphia, 1992, WB Saunders.

Hardy MA: What can you do about your patient's dry skin? *J Gerontol Nurs* 5:11, 1996.

Jablonski RS: Nausea: the forgotten symptom, *Holistic Nurs Pract* 7:64, 1993.

Morse JM, Bottorff JL, Hutchinson S: The phenomenology of comfort, *J Adv Nurs* 20:189, 1994.

Pervan V: Practical aspects of dealing with cancer therapy-induced nausea and vomiting, *Semin Oncol Nurs* 6:3, 1990.

Pervan V: Understanding anti-emetics, *Nurs Times* 89(10):36-37, 1993.

Rhodes VA, Johnson MH, McDaniel RW: Nausea, vomiting, and retching: the management of the symptom experience, *Semin Oncol Nurs* 11:256, 1995.

Troesch LM et al: The influence of guided imagery on chemotherapy-related nausea and vomiting, *Oncol Nurs Forum* 20:1179, 1993.

Impaired verbal communication

Gail B. Ladwig

Definition   The state in which an individual experiences a decreased or an absent ability to use or understand language in human interaction

Defining Characteristics

Inability to speak dominant language *(critical),* difficulties with speech or verbalizations *(critical),* refusal or inability to speak *(critical),* stuttering, slurring, difficulty forming words or sentences, difficulty expressing thoughts verbally, inappropriate verbalizations, dyspnea, disorientation

Related Factors (r/t)

Decrease in circulation to brain, brain tumor, physical barrier (e.g., tracheostomy, intubation), anatomical defect, impaired hearing, cleft palate, psychological barriers (e.g., psychosis, lack of stimuli), cultural difference, developmentally-related or age-related factors

Client Outcomes/Goals

- Uses effective communication techniques
- Uses alternative methods of communication effectively
- Demonstrates congruency of verbal and nonverbal behavior
- Expresses desire for social interactions

Suggested NIC Interventions

Active listening; communication enhancement: hearing deficit; communication enhancement: speech deficit

Nursing Interventions and Rationales

- Determine language spoken; obtain language dictionary or interpreter if possible.
  For clear understanding, the nurse and client must speak the same language or have a means of understanding the other's language.
- Listen carefully. Validate verbal and nonverbal expressions.

Client satisfaction studies have repeatedly shown that what clients want most from their nurses is common courtesy—someone who really listens to their fears and concerns and treats them like a real person, not a disease (Long, Greeneich, 1994).

- Anticipate client's needs until effective communication is possible.
  Anticipation of clients' needs increases client satisfaction (Long, Greeneich, 1994).
- Use simple communication, speak in a well-modulated voice, and smile and show concern for the client.
  Such techniques have been described by clients as demonstrating caring (Clark, 1993).
- Maintain eye contact at client's level, and read client's eyes as able.
  Sitting down is an effective way of listening and helps to build trust (Robinson, 1993).
- Use touch as appropriate. Holding a client's hand or stroking the arm is a simple, nonintrusive way of showing empathy and concern.
  Touch that conveys caring is an appropriate way of communicating, unless the person touched shows discomfort (Wells, 1996).
- Spend time with client, allow time for responses, and make call light readily available.
  Clients consider good care to include listening, helping, and "being there" (Murdaugh et al, 1992).
- Obtain communication equipment such as electronic devices, letterboards, picture boards, and magic slates.
  Alternative methods of communication are necessary when the client is unable to use verbal communication.
- Establish an alternative method of communication such as writing or pointing to letters, word phrases, or picture cards.
  Alternative methods of communication are necessary when the client is unable to use verbal communication.
- Provide pencil and paper for letter writing to facilitate expression of feelings.
  Letter writing has been used with patients who have had amputations to successfully express feelings (Hatipoglu, Temiz, 1995).
- Obtain order for speech therapy. Supplement work of speech therapist with appropriate exercises.
  Consultation and collaboration with a specialist may be necessary to provide the best approach to improving communication.
- Give praise for progress noted. Ignore mistakes and watch for frustration or fatigue.
  Positive reinforcement increases confidence, which can increase communication (Boss, 1991).
- Encourage family to bring in familiar pictures or calendars.
- Establish an understanding of client's symbolic speech (especially with schizophrenic clients). Ask client to clarify particular statements.
  Clarification is a necessary communication skill. Psychoeducation covers the practical problems of living with schizophrenia. Families learn when to ignore problem behaviors and when to intervene (Huddleston, 1992).
- If there is a comprehension deficit, keep environment quiet when communicating and get client's attention before attempting to communicate (e.g., touch client's shoulder, call client's name).
  When the client is confused, a distracting environment interferes with communication; it is necessary to get the client's full attention before any communication can take place (Boss, 1991).

- Use "affection therapy" when the client cannot express thoughts or ideas. Provide frequent and regular reminders that client is wanted and cared about (e.g., physical signs of affection such as a hug or a friendly comment before and after every interaction regardless of client's performance).
  When clients are unable to communicate their thoughts and feelings adequately they may whistle, swear, and make other noises incessantly. "Affection therapy" works when behavior modification techniques do not (Armstrong, 1991).
- Do not raise your voice or shout at the client.
  A loud voice can be frightening and decrease communication.

Geriatric
- Encourage client to wear prescribed eyeglasses and hearing aids.
  Auditory and visual disorders are prevalent among older people. About 40% of adults aged 65 and over have a hearing loss sufficient to interfere with daily conversation (Erber, 1994). About 20% in the same age range experience low vision and reduced visual fields, which can prevent clear perception of a communication partner at a conversational distance (Erber, 1994).
- When communicating with client, face toward client's unaffected side or better ear.
  The position increases the client's awareness of the interaction and enhances the client's ability to interact.
- Provide sufficient light and remove distractions such as glare and background noise.
  Background noise further impairs the elderly client's hearing.
- Use low voice tones and recognize that perception of the sounds *f, s, th, ch, sh, b, t, p, k,* and *d* are impaired with hearing loss that results from aging.
  Presbycusis decreases the ability to hear high-pitched sounds and the consonant sounds listed in the preceding paragraph. Perception of consonants is important to understanding language.
- Allow time for thought comprehension when communicating with client.
  Older clients do not like to be rushed. They fare much better in a calm, consistent environment that functions at a moderately slow pace (Bailey, Bailey, 1993).
- Schedule time to listen to clients' life stories.
  This is a means of finding out what is important to the elderly. The practice of nursing comes alive by listening to individual stories. Each person's story is created out of personal life experiences (Running, 1996).

Home Care Interventions
- Continue with speech therapy services per physician order. Support speech therapy plan of care.
  With appropriate support, clients can continue to make significant progress toward resuming normal or improved communication function.
- Assess family for possible role changes resulting from communication impairment of family member.
  An impairment that prevents a family member from fulfilling the usual role can change the family constellation.
- When possible, encourage family to include client in family activities using enhanced communication techniques with sensitivity.
  Involving the client in family activities promotes earlier return to normal life patterns, but doing so in an awkward or embarrassing way can diminish interest.
- Refer to medical social services as necessary for help in obtaining funds for communication devices and counseling for dealing with long-term impact of communication changes in family.

Client/Family Teaching

- Teach client and family techniques to increase communication.
  Alternative methods of communication are necessary when the client is unable to use verbal communication.
- Encourage touch, such as holding client's hand or stroking the arm.
  Incorporating relatives into this aspect of care provides continuity with the client's real life and fulfills the relatives' need to demonstrate care (MacGinley, 1993).
- Teach client the way to use communication devices.

REFERENCES   Armstrong C: Emotional changes following brain injury: psychological and neurological components of depression, denial and anxiety, *J Rehab* 57:15, 1991.

Bailey DS, Bailey DR: *Therapeutic approaches to the care of the mentally ill,* ed 3, Philadelphia, 1993, FA Davis.

Boss BJ: Managing communication disorders in stroke, *Nurs Clin North Am* 26:985, 1991.

Buckwalter KC et al: Family involvement with communication-impaired residents in long-term care settings, *Appl Nurs Res* 4:77, 1991.

Clark S: Challenges in critical care nursing: helping patients and families cope, *Crit Care Nurs* S2:2, 1993.

Erber N: Conversation as therapy for older adults in residential care: the case for intervention, *Eur J Disord Commun* 29:269, 1994.

Hatipoglu S, Temiz Z: Amputee's diary, *Image* 27:248, 1995.

Huddleston J: Family and group psychoeducational approaches in the management of schizophrenia, *Clin Nurs Spec* 6:118, 1992.

Long C, Greeneich D: Four strategies for keeping patients satisfied, *Am J Nurs* 94:27, 1994.

MacGinley K: Nursing care of the patient with altered body image, *Brit J Nurs* 2:1098, 1993.

Murdaugh C et al: Knowledge about care and caring: state of the art and future developments. In Bulchek G, McCloskey J, editors: *Nursing interventions: essential nursing treatments,* ed 2, Philadelphia, 1992, WB Saunders.

Robinson K: Denial: an adaptive response, *Dimens Crit Care Nurs* 12:102, 1993.

Running A: "The measure of my day" critiqued by the oldest old, *Image* 28:71, 1996.

Wells E: Assisting parents when a child dies in the ICU, *Crit Care Nurs* 16:58, 1996.

Ineffective community coping

Margaret Lunney

Definition   A pattern of community activities for adaptation and problem solving that is unsatisfactory for meeting the demands or needs of the community

Defining Characteristics

Community not meeting its own expectations, deficits of community participation, deficits in communication methods, excessive community conflicts, expressed difficulty in meeting demands for change, expressed vulnerability, high illness rates, stressors perceived as excessive

Related Factors (r/t)

Deficits in social support, inadequate resources for problem solving, powerlessness

Community Outcomes/Goals

- Work in partnership with nurses and other health providers
- Develop improved communication with each other

- Demonstrate cohesiveness in problem solving
- Participate in problem solving
- Develop new strategies for problem solving
- Express power to deal with change and manage problems

Suggested NIC Interventions

- Environmental management: community, health policy monitoring

Nursing Interventions and Rationales

NOTE: The diagnosis of **Ineffective coping** does not apply and should not be used when stress is being imposed by external sources or circumstance. If the community is a victim of circumstances, using the nursing diagnosis **Ineffective coping** would be equivalent to blaming the victim.

- See **Ineffective management of therapeutic regimen: community** and **Potential for enhanced community coping.**
- Establish a collaborative/partnership relationship with the community (see **Ineffective management of therapeutic regimen: community** for references).
- Help community members identify stressors.
  It may be possible to reduce or eliminate some of the stressors.
- Work with community members to increase awareness of ineffective coping behaviors (e.g., conflicts that prevent community members from working together; anger and hate that paralyze the community).
  Problem solving is essential for effective coping. Behaviors that interfere with problem solving can be modified by community members with the assistance of nurses and other health providers (Anderson, McFarlane, 1995).
- Provide support to the community and help identify and mobilize additional supports.
  Social support is associated with positive coping strategies (Pender, 1996).
- Advocate for the community in multiple arenas (e.g., television, newspapers, governmental agencies).
- Write grant proposals to help community members obtain funds for programs that reduce stress or improve coping (Coley, Sheinberg, 1990).
  The programs that are necessary may be expensive, and funds may not be available without the support of the public or privately funded grants.
- Work with members of the community to identify and develop coping strategies that promote a sense of power (e.g., obtaining sources of funding, collaborating with other communities).
  Power is an essential aspect of coping. A first step in attaining a sense of power is for the community to identify and develop its own strategies (Barrett, 1989).

Community Teaching

Teach strategies for stress management.

REFERENCES   Anderson ET, McFarlane J: *Community as partner: theory and practice in nursing,* Philadelphia, 1995, Lippincott-Raven.

Barrett EAM: A nursing theory of power for nursing practice: derivation from Rogers' paradigm. In Riehl-Sisca J, editor: *Conceptual models for nursing practice,* ed 3, Norwalk, Conn, 1989, Appleton & Lange.

Coley SM, Scheinberg CA: *Proposal writing,* Newbury Park, 1990, Sage.

Pender NJ: *Health promotion in nursing practice,* ed 3, Norwalk, Conn, 1996, Appleton & Lange.

Potential for enhanced community coping

Margaret Lunney

Definition   A pattern of community activities for adaptation and problem solving that is satisfactory for meeting the demands or needs of the community but that can also be improved for management of current and future problems and stressors

Defining Characteristics
Major   Deficits in one or a few of the characteristics that indicate effective coping

Minor   Active planning by community for predicted stressors, active problem solving by community when faced with issues, agreement that community is responsible for stress management, positive communication among community members, positive communication between community aggregates and the larger community, programs available for recreation and relaxation, resources sufficient for managing stressors

Community Outcomes/Goals
- Develops enhanced coping strategies
- Maintains effective coping strategies for management of stress

Suggested NIC Interventions
Environmental management: community, health education health policy monitoring

Nursing Interventions and Rationales
NOTE: Interventions depend on the specific aspects of community coping that can be enhanced (e.g., planning for stress management, communication, development of community power, community perceptions of stress, community coping strategies).

- Establish a collaborative partnership with the community (see **Ineffective management of therapeutic regimen: community** for references).
  Collaborative relationships support the community's actions for self-care.
- Describe the role of community/public health nurse in working with healthy communities (Thorpe et al, 1995).
  Members of society are not familiar with nurses' roles in public health.
- Help community obtain funding for additional programs (Coley, Scheinberg, 1990).
  Vulnerable communities often need additional funding sources to strengthen coping resources.
- Encourage positive attitudes toward the community through the media and other sources.
  Negative attitudes or stigmas create additional stress and deficits in social support.
- Help community members collaborate with one another for power enhancement and coping skills.
  Community members may not have sufficient skills to collaborate for enhanced coping. Effective collaboration skills can be promoted by health providers (Higgs, 1995; Courtney et al, 1996).
- Encourage critical thinking.
  Critical thinking supports problem-solving abilities.
- Demonstrate optimal use of resources.
  Optimal use of resources supports community coping; community members benefit from such demonstrations (Miller, 1992). Community members will benefit from observations of nurses' use of resources.
- Collaborate with community members to improve educational levels within the community.

In a study of 18 randomly selected communities and 900 elders living in those communities, higher education levels were associated with less stress pertaining to health and fewer helpers were needed by the elderly (Preston, Bucher, 1996).

Community Teaching
- Review coping skills, power for coping, and the use of power resources.

REFERENCES   Anderson ET, McFarlane J: *Community as partner: theory and practice in nursing,* Philadelphia, 1995, Lippincott-Raven.

Coley SM, Scheinberg CA: *Proposal writing,* Newbury Park, Conn, 1990, Sage.

Courtney R et al: The partnership model: working with individuals, families, and communities toward a new vision of health, *Public Health Nurs* 13:177, 1996.

Higgs ZR: Implementation of a collaborative practice model: an introduction. In Association of Community Health Nursing Educators: *State of the art in community health nursing education, research, and practice, 1993-94 papers,* Skokie, Ill, 1995, The Association.

Miller JF: *Coping with chronic illness: overcoming powerlessness,* ed 2, Philadelphia, 1992, FA Davis.

Pender NJ: *Health promotion in nursing practice,* ed 3, Norwalk, Conn, 1996, Appleton & Lange.

Preston DB, Bucher JA: The effects of community differences on health status, health stress, and helping networks in a sample of 900 elderly, *Public Health Nurs* 13:72, 1996.

Thorpe B et al: Targeting health communities. In Association of Community Health Nursing Educators: *State of the art in community health nursing education, research, and practice, 1993-94 papers,* Skokie, Ill, 1995, The Association.

Ineffective management of therapeutic regimen (community)

Margaret Lunney

Definition   A pattern of regulating and integrating into community processes programs for the treatment of illness and the sequelae of illness that are unsatisfactory for meeting health-related goals

Defining Characteristics
Major   Insufficient number of health care resources for the incidence or prevalence of illnesses

Minor   Expected or unexpected acceleration of illnesses; deficits in advocates for aggregates; deficits in community activities for primary, secondary, and tertiary prevention; deficits in persons and programs to be accountable for illness care of aggregates; illness symptoms above the norm; unavailable resources for illness care

Related Factors (r/t)
Complexity of community and aggregate problems and needs; decreased communication among and between community and society; decreased valuing of community and aggregates by members of society; decreased valuing of health protection; decreased valuing of self by community and aggregates; disorganization of health care system; economic factors (e.g., poor management of available finances); excessive exposure to risk factors (e.g., toxic chemicals); local, state, or national policies

Community Outcomes/Goals
- Obtains for the community persons who are accountable for illness care of specific aggregates

- Remains involved in advocacy for illness care and prevention programs
- Develops health care plans for effective prevention and treatment of illnesses
- Makes resources available for illness care and prevention
- Initiates or improves strategies for prevention of the sequelae of illnesses

Suggested NIC Interventions

Environmental management: community, health policy monitoring

Nursing Interventions and Rationales

NOTE: Nursing interventions are conducted in collaboration with key members of the community, community/public health nurses, and members of other disciplines (Anderson, McFarlane, 1995; Courtney et al, 1996; Higgs, 1995; Lowenberg, 1995; Reuter, Neufeld, Harrison, 1995; Courtney et al, 1996).

- Seek community leaders who are willing to learn about community assessment data and diagnosis and who have the potential to work with interdisciplinary health providers in planning for positive changes.

  Communities need to be involved in obtaining the services and resources they need for illness care and prevention. Only services that are valued and perceived as needed by community members are used effectively. Community health interventions are complex and often require multidisciplinary strategies (Lunney et al [in press]).

- Advocate for and with the community in multiple arenas (e.g., newspapers, television, legislative activities, community boards).

  The community benefits from the advocacy of nurses and other health providers whose opinions are respected (Anderson, McFarlane, 1995).

- Provide information to public and private sources about community assessment and diagnosis and the plan of care.

  The commitment that is needed for improvements in health services can only be obtained when others have adequate information.

- Mobilize support for the community in obtaining the resources necessary for illness care and prevention.

  As with individuals and families, community social supports enable the community to achieve health-related goals (Anderson, McFarlane, 1995).

- Recruit additional health providers as needed.

  If health providers are aware of inadequate community services, they may be able to contribute the necessary services.

- Determine the cultural appropriateness of all programs.

  The cultural appropriateness of a program is an indicator of its potential success (Degazon, 1996).

- Write grants for funding of new programs or expansion of existing programs.

  When they become aware of community problems, public and private sources of funds can often supply the financial bases of health care programs (Coley, Scheinberg, 1990).

- Conduct research needed to convince others of the need for improved services or changes in policy.

  Community assessment and diagnosis may not be sufficient for change. More advanced research findings may be needed to obtain broad support for needed change.

- With other persons and groups, obtain changes in health policy as indicated.

  Health policies set the stage for effective health programs (Milio, 1981; Mason, Talbott, Leavitt, 1993).

REFERENCES   Anderson ET, McFarlane J: *Community as partner: theory and practice in nursing,* Philadelphia, 1995, JB
                 Lippincott-Raven.
             Coley SM, Scheinberg CA: *Proposal writing,* Newbury Park, Conn, 1990, Sage.
             Courtney R et al: The partnership model: working with individuals, families, and communities toward a new
                 vision of health, *Public Health Nurs* 13:177, 1996.
             Degazon C: Cultural diversity and community health nursing practice. In M Stanhope, J Lancaster: *Community
                 health nursing: Process and application for promoting health,* ed 4, St Louis, 1996, Mosby.
             Higgs ZR: Implementation of a collaborative practice model: an introduction. In Association of Community
                 Health Nursing Educators: *State of the art in community health nursing education, research, and practice,
                 1993-94 papers,* Skokie, Ill, 1995, The Association.
             Kang R: Building community capacity for health promotion: a challenge for public health nurse, *Public Health
                 Nurs* 12:312, 1995.
             Lowenberg JS: Health promotion and the "ideology of choice," *Public Health Nurs* 12:319, 1995.
             Lunney et al: (in press).
             Milio N: *Engines and empowerment: using information technology to create health communities and challenge
                 public policy,* Ann Arbor, Mich, 1996, Health Administration Press.
             Reuter L, Neufeld A, Harrison MJ: Using critical feminist principles to analyze programs for low-income urban
                 women, *Public Health Nurs* 12:424, 1995.

Acute confusion

Gail B. Ladwig

Definition   The abrupt onset of a cluster of global, transient changes and disturbances in attention,
cognition, psychomotor activity level of consciousness, or the sleep/wake cycle

Defining Characteristics
Major   Fluctuations in cognition, fluctuations in the sleep-wake cycle, fluctuations in levels of
consciousness, fluctuations in psychomotor activity, increased agitation or restlessness,
misperceptions, lack of motivation to initiate or follow through with goal-directed or
purposeful behavior
Minor   Hallucinations
Related Factors (r/t)
Over 60 years of age, dementia, alcohol abuse, abuse, delirium
Client Outcomes/Goals
- Obtains optimal cognitive functioning
- Obtains adequate amount of sleep
- Maintains an optimal level of consciousness
- Demonstrates normal motor behavior
- Demonstrates decreased agitation and restlessness
- Initiates and follows through with goal-directed or purposeful behavior
- Maintains optimal orientation
Suggested NIC Intervention
Delirium management, delusion management
Nursing Interventions and Rationales
- See care plan for **Chronic confusion.**
- Assess client's behavior at least once daily, preferably at the completion of the day
shift. Also assess client after any episodes of confusion.
Delirious clients have higher fatality rates than demented, depressed, or cognitively

intact persons. Nurses play a vital role in identifying the signs of delirium and can thus affect patient prognosis and outcome through early assessment and intervention (Rabins, Folstein, 1992).

- Obtain a baseline history that includes the recent mental status change (months, years), onset of any symptoms of confusion, time of day of confusional episodes, sleep patterns, medical illnesses, medication use, and education level of client.
  The client's history is the most important aspect of assessing a confused older client (Matzo, 1990).
- Perform an accurate cognitive mental status exam that includes the following:
  1. Overall appearance, manner, and attitude
  2. Behavior observations and level of psychomotor agitation
  3. Mood and affect (presence of suicidal or homicidal ideation as observed by others and reported by client)
  4. Insight and judgment
  5. Cognition as evidenced by level of consciousness, orientation (to time, place, and person), attention, concentration, memory (recent and remote), fund of knowledge, thought process and content (perceptual disturbances such as illusions and hallucinations, paranoia, delusions, abstract thinking)

  Identifying delirium in a hospitalized client depends on the performance of an accurate cognitive mental status examination as part of the routine clinical assessment (Inaba-Roland, Maricle, 1992).

- Assess for physiological alterations (e.g., sepsis, hypoglycemia, hypotension, infection, changes in temperature, fluid and electrolyte imbalances, medications with known cognitive and psychotropic side effects).
  Such alterations may be contributing to confusion and must be corrected (Matthiesen et al, 1994). Medications are considered the most common cause of delirium in the ICU (Harvey, 1996).
- Use orientation techniques—have client identify self and repeat the place and time of day, use wall calendars, have family bring in familiar items for bedside and identify selves—offer reassurance.
  These orientation techniques help the client differentiate between reality and unreality. Confusion associated with delirium is treatable, reversible, and short term (Inaba-Roland, Maricle, 1992).
- Inform, reassure, and orient clients frequently.
  Short-term memory deficits and amnesia are common in ICU patients (Harvey, 1996).
- Offer reassurance to the client and use therapeutic communication at frequent intervals.
  Client reassurance and communication are nursing skills that promote trust and orientation and reduce anxiety (Harvey, 1996).
- Communicate with touch when appropriate.
  Touch is a powerful communication tool that should be used continually unless it is offensive to clients because of their cultural background (Harvey, 1996).
- Encourage family members to stay with clients and find a "safe place" without medical equipment for family members to touch.
  Family members have a calming effect on clients and appreciate the opportunity to stay with clients to calm them (Harvey, 1996).
- Reduce bedside noise as much as possible; eliminate drafts, odors and unnecessary activity.
  These are therapeutic interventions for agitated clients (Harvey, 1996).

- Provide nursing care that enhances sleep (see **Sleep pattern disturbance).**
  Promoting sleep may enhance mental integrity (Richards, 1994).
- Use nursing measures that ensure client comfort—mouth care, eye care, position, tapes and tubes that pull or contort, itching, muscle cramps, thirst.
  Nursing measures that ensure client comfort may be helpful in calming an agitated client (Cooper, 1993).
- Identify, evaluate, and treat pain quickly (see **Pain).**
  Pain is a potential trigger of agitation (Harvey, 1996).
- Use restraints as infrequently as possible.
  Restraints have been shown to increase agitation and have even led to death (Dube, Mitchell, 1986).

Geriatric
- Mobilize client as soon as possible, provide active and passive range of motion.
  Older clients who had a low level of physical activity before injury are at a particular risk for acute confusion (Matthiesen et al, 1994).
- Provide sufficient medication to relieve pain.
  Older clients may give inaccurate pain histories, underreport symptoms, not want to bother the nurse, and exhibit restlessness, agitation, or increased confusion (Matthiesen et al, 1994).
- Nonnarcotic analgesics should be substituted for narcotics.
  Oversedation poses risks for confusion and postoperative complications such as falls (Matthiesen et al, 1994).
- Urinary catheters should be removed as soon as possible.
  Elderly clients are at a high risk for urinary tract infections and urosepsis (Matthiesen et al, 1994).
- Call older clients by the name they prefer.
  Such steps help decrease the unfamiliarity of the health care environment (Campbell, Williams, Mynarczyx, 1986).
- Explain hospital routines and procedures slowly and in simple terms; repeat information as necessary.
  Anxiety and sensory impairment decrease the older client's ability to integrate new information (Matthiesen et al, 1994).
- Give choices regarding hospital routines, but do not give too many options at once. Allow client time to respond.
  Loss of control or independence is difficult for older clients; they need as much control as possible and may need more time to process information (Matthiesen et al, 1994).
- Provide continuity of care when possible (e.g., provide the same caregivers, avoid room changes).
  Continuity of care helps decrease the disorienting effects of hospitalization (Matthiesen et al, 1994).
- If clients know that they are not thinking clearly, acknowledge the concern.
  Confusion is very frightening (Matthiesen et al, 1994).
- Correctly interpret environmental stimuli for the client.
  Acutely confused older clients may misperceive sensory input and experience illusions, delusions, or hallucinations (Campbell, Williams, Mynarczyx, 1986).
- Do not use the intercom to answer a call light.
  The intercom may be frightening to an older confused client (Matthiesen et al, 1994).

- Keep client's sleep-wake cycle as normal as possible (e.g., avoid letting client take daytime naps, avoid waking clients at night, give sedatives but not diuretics at bedtime, provide pain relief and backrubs).
  Acute confusion is accompanied by disruption of the sleep-wake cycle (Matthiesen et al, 1994).

Home Care Interventions

- Using family input and time of home visit, assess client functioning for different times of day. Assess the need for 24-hour or waking hours only supervision of the client.
  A clear profile of the client's usual behavior patterns assists the nurse and family with planning for the client.
- Incorporate cognitive mental status assessments intermittently during client's care to document changes in overall status.
  Client changes may be subtle but progressive. Repeating the assessment allows nurse to benchmark changes and update status.
- Conduct ongoing assessment of physiological parameters and response to medications.
  Determine whether these variables are contributing to changes in client status.
  Changes in medication can result in changes in neurological and cognitive function.
- If the client requires constant supervision to maintain safety, refer to companion or home health aide services to provide respite for family/caregivers. Maintain consistency in staffing. Introduce new staff slowly using an initial joint visit.
  Joint visits reassure the client that the new person is safe and friendly.
- Instruct the family never to leave the confused client at home unattended (caregiver may be in a different room but not out of the house) or restricted by ties to furniture (bed, chair, toilet).
  Leaving the client alone poses unacceptable safety risks. Safety risks and/or restriction by ties may also constitute abuse.
- Teach family and caregivers to keep physical environment constant.
  Constancy in the environment helps maintain spatial orientation.

Client/Family Teaching

- Teach family to recognize signs of early confusion and seek medical help.
  Early intervention prevents long-term complications.
- Have family stay with client in the evening; leave on night light; have call light within reach; turn off television.
  A secure feeling in the evening helps to decrease sundowning phenomenon (Matthiesen et al, 1994).
- Have familiar people or objects present. Encourage family members and friends to visit as often as possible.
  Familiar people help keep an older client oriented (Matthiesen et al, 1994).

REFERENCES   Campbell E, Williams M, Mynarczyx S: After the fall—confusion, *Am J Nurs* 86:151, 1986.
Cooper MC: The intersection of technology and care in ICU, *Adv Nurs Sci* 15:23, 1993.
Dube C, Mitchell E: Accidental strangulation from vest restraints, *JAMA* 256:2725, 1986.
Harvey M: Managing agitation in critically ill patients, *Am J Crit Care* 5:7, 1996.
Inaba-Roland K, Maricle R: Assessing delirium in the acute care setting, *Heart Lung* 21:49, 1992.
Matthiesen V et al: Acute confusion: nursing intervention in older patients, *Orthop Nurs* 13:25, 1994.
Matzo M: Confusion in older adults: assessment and differential diagnosis, *Nurse Pract* 15:32, 1990.
Rabins P, Folstein M: Delirium and dementia: diagnostic criteria and fatality rates, *Br J Psychiatry* 140:149, 1992.
Richards KC: Sleep promotion in the critical care unit, *AACN Clin Issu Crit Care Nurs* 5:152, 1994.

Chronic confusion

Betty J. Ackley and Nancy English

Definition   An irreversible, long-standing, and/or progressive deterioration of intellect and personality that is characterized by a decreased ability to interpret environmental stimuli and a decreased capacity for intellectual thought processes; is manifested by disturbances of memory, orientation, and behavior

Defining Characteristics

Major   Clinical evidence of organic impairment, altered interpretation or response to stimuli, progressive or long-standing cognitive impairment

Minor   No change in level of consciousness, impaired socialization, impaired short-term or long-term memory, altered personality

Related Factors (r/t)

Alzheimer's disease, Korsakoff's psychosis, multi-infarct dementia, cerebral vascular accident, head injury

Client Outcomes/Goals

- Remains content and free from harm
- Functions at maximal of cognitive level
- Participates in activities of daily living at maximal of functional ability

Suggested NIC Interventions

Dementia management, mood management

Nursing Interventions and Rationales

- Determine client's cognitive level using a screening tool such as the Mini Mental State Exam (MMSE).
  Using an evaluation tool such as the MMSE can help determine the client's abilities and assist with planning appropriate nursing interventions (Agostinelli et al, 1994).
- Gather information about client before the onset of confusion including social situation, physical condition, and psychological functioning.
  Knowing the client's background can help the nurse understand clients's behavior if they become delusional and hallucinate. Sharing memories helps soothe clients.
- Assess the client for signs of depression: insomnia, poor appetite, flat affect, withdrawn behavior.
  Between 10% and 40% of people with dementia have depression (Katz, 1996).
- Ensure that client is in a safe environment by removing potential hazards such as sharp objects and harmful liquids.
  Clients with dementia lose the ability to make good judgments and can easily harm self or others.
- Place an identification bracelet on client.
  Clients with dementia wander and can become lost; identification bracelets increase their safety.
- Avoid unfamiliar situations and people as much as possible. Maintain continuity of caregivers. Maintain routines of care through established mealtimes, bathing, and sleeping schedules. Send familiar person with client when client goes for diagnostic testing.
  Situational anxiety associated with environmental, interpersonal, or structural change can escalate into agitated behavior (Gerdner, Buckwalter, 1994).
- Keep environment quiet and nonstimulating; avoid using buzzers and alarms if possible.
  Sensory overload can result in agitated behavior in a client with dementia.

- Begin each interaction with client by identifying self and calling client by name.
- Approach client with a caring, loving, and accepting attitude and speak calmly and slowly.
  Dementia clients can sense feelings of compassion; a calm, slow manner projects a feeling of comfort to the client (Stolley, 1994).
- Touch client gently, stroking hand or arm in a soothing fashion if acceptable in client's culture.
- Give one simple direction at a time and repeat it as necessary. Use verbal and physical prompts, and model the desired action if needed and possible.
  "People with dementia need time to assimilate and interpret your directions, if you rephrase your question, you give them something new to process, increasing their confusion" (Stolley, 1994).
- Break down self-care tasks into simple steps (e.g., instead of saying, "Take a shower," say to client, "Please follow me. Sit down on the bed. Take off your shoes. Now take off your socks. . . .".
  Dementia clients are unable to follow complex commands; breaking down an activity into simple steps makes the activity more feasible (Agostinelli et al, 1994).
- Keep questions simple; yes or no questions are often preferable. Use positive statements and actions and avoid negative communication (e.g., if client is trying to crawl out of bed, help find a method of doing so; lead back to bed later as necessary).
  Negative feedback leads to increased confusion and agitation. It is more effective to go along with the client and then redirect as necessary.
- If eating in the dining room causes increased agitation, let client leave and eat in a quieter environment with smaller numbers of people.
  The noise and confusion in a large dining room can be overwhelming for a dementia client and result in agitated behavior. It is preferable to have dementia clients eat in small groups.
- Provide boundaries by placing red or yellow tape on the floor or by using a stop sign.
  Boundaries help the client identify safe areas; older clients can more easily see red and yellow.
- Write client's name in large block letters in the room and on client's clothing and possessions. Use symbols rather than words to identify areas such as the bathroom or kitchen.
- Limit visitors to two and provide them with guidelines on appropriate topics to discuss with client.
- Set up scheduled quiet periods in a recliner or room for about 40 minutes at 10 AM and 90 minutes at 2 PM. Use afghans and environmental cues to define rest periods.
  Quiet times allow the client's anxiety and building tension levels to decrease (Hall et at, 1995). Fatigue has been associated with the onset of increased confusion and agitation (Stolley, 1994).
- Provide quiet activities such as classical or religious music in the afternoon or early evening.
  An increase in confusion and agitation may occur in the late afternoon and early evening and is referred to as sundowning syndrome. *Quiet activities can provide a calming environment.*
- Provide simple activities for the client to do such as folding washcloths and sorting or

stacking activities. Avoid misleading and frightening stimuli that may include the television, mirrors, and pictures of people or animals.
Dementia clients need activities to keep them busy or may be involved in destructive activities. They see, hear, and perceive a different world; they may not recognize themselves in the mirror and be afraid of the stranger they see so close to them.

- Consider using doll therapy. Ask family members to bring a large, safe doll or stuffed animal such as a teddy bear.
  Doll therapy can be soothing to some dementia clients (Bailey, 1993; Paulanka, Griffin, 1993).

- If client becomes increasingly confused and agitated, perform the following steps:
  - Monitor client for physiological causes, including acute hypoxia, pain, medication effects, infections such as urinary tract infection, fatigue, electrolyte disturbances, and constipation (Gerdner, Buckwalter, 1994).
  - Monitor for psychological causes, including changes in environment, caregiver, and routine; demands to perform beyond capacity; multiple competing stimuli.
  - Avoid confrontations with the client; allow client to dissipate energy by performing repetitive tasks or by pacing.
  - If client is delusional or hallucinating, do not confront him or her with reality. Use validation therapy to verbally reflect back to the emotions that the client appears to be feeling. Use statements such as, "It must be frightening to see a fire at the end of your bed," "I can see you are afraid," "I will stay with you," or "Can you tell me more about what is going on right now?"
    Orienting the client to reality can increase agitation; validation therapy conveys empathy and understanding and can help determine the internal stimulus that is creating the change in behavior (Feil, 1993). Training in validation therapy for staff resulted in decreases doses of psychotherapeutic medications and incidences of behavior problems in one study (Fine, 1995).
  - Decrease stimuli in the environment (e.g., turn off television, take client to a quiet place). Institute activities that are associated with pleasant emotions such as playing soft music the client likes, looking through a photo album, providing favorite food, or using simulated presence therapy.
    Decreasing stimuli can decrease agitation. Reassuring activities can help bring pleasant emotions to help soothe the client, including simulated presence therapy where client listens to a tape of a loved one's phone conversation (Woods, Ashley, 1995).
  - Avoid using restraints if at all possible; obtain physician's order if they become necessary.
    Restrained elderly clients often have increased incidences of falls, possibly because of muscle deconditioning or loss of coordination (Tinetti, Liu, Ginter, 1992).
  - Use prn psychotropic or antianxiety drugs only as a last resort. Start with the lowest possible dose.
    Psychotropic drugs such as Haldol decrease client function and have major side effects including parkinsonian symptoms.

- For predictable difficult times such as during bathing and grooming, try the following:
  - Massage the client's hands lovingly or use therapeutic touch to relax the client.
    Hand massage and therapeutic touch have been shown to induce relaxation that may allow care activities to take place without difficulty (Snyder, Egan, Burns, 1995).

- Use positive behavioral reinforcement for each small step of bathing, such as praising client for walking toward the shower, sitting in the shower chair, and removing items of clothing.
  Positive behavioral reinforcement for desired behavior is effective for clients with dementia (Boehm et al, 1995).
- Treat the client with the utmost respect and give individualized care.
  Treating confused clients with respect and individualizing care can decrease aggression and increase nursing staff satisfaction (Maxfield, Lewis, Cannon, 1996).
- For early dementia clients with mainly symptoms of memory loss, see care plan for **Impaired memory.**
- For clients with self-care deficits, see appropriate care plan **(Self-care deficit: feeding; Self-care deficit: dressing; Self-care deficit: toileting).**

Geriatric   NOTE: Most of the preceding interventions apply to the geriatric client.

- Use reminiscence and life review therapeutic interventions; ask questions about client's work, raising children, or time spent in the service. Ask questions such as "What was really important to you as you look back?"
  Reminiscence and life review can help an older person reframe and accept life events (Burnside, Haight, 1994).

Home Care Interventions

NOTE: In the home setting the goal of maintaining safety for the client takes on primary importance because of the usually less structured nature of community based care and the importance of keeping clients as independent as possible.

- Provide support to family of client with chronic and disabling condition.
- If client will require extensive supervision on an ongoing basis, evaluate client for day care programs. Refer to medical social services to assist with this if necessary.
  Day care programs provide safe, structured care for the client and respite for the family. Respite care for caregivers is an essential part of successful long-term care for a confused client.
- Encourage family to include client in family activities when possible. Reinforce use of therapeutic communication guidelines (Client/Family Teaching) and sensitivity to numbers of people present.
  These steps help the client maintain dignity and lead to familiar socialization of the client.

Client/Family Teaching

- Recommend that the family develop a memory aid wallet or booklet for client, which contains pictures and text that chronicle client's life.
  Using memory aids such as wallets or booklets helps dementia clients make more factual statements and stay on topic and decreases the number of confused, erroneous, and repetitive statements (Bouregois, 1992).
- Teach family how to converse with a memory-impaired person. Guidelines include the following:
  - Ask client to have a conversation with you.
  - Guide conversation to specific, nonthreatening topics, and redirect the conversation back on topic when client begins to ramble.
  - Reassure and help out when the client gets stuck or cannot find the right words.
  - Smile and act interested in what client is saying even if unsure what it means.

- Thank client for talking.
- Avoid quizzing client or asking a lot of specific questions.
- Avoid correcting or contradicting something that was stated even if it is wrong.

  These guidelines can help families interact more effectively with clients and decrease frustration levels (Bouregois, 1992).

• Teach family how to set up environment and use care techniques interventions listed so that client will experience a progressively lowered stress threshold.

  Alzheimer's clients are unable to deal with stress; decreasing stress can decrease confusion and changes in behavior (Hall, 1991; Stolley, 1994).

NOTE: The nursing diagnoses **Impaired environmental interpretation syndrome** and **Chronic confusion** are very similar in definition and interventions. **Impaired environmental interpretation** must be interpreted as a syndrome where other nursing diagnoses would also apply. **Chronic confusion** may be interpreted as the human response to a situation or situations that require a level of cognition no longer available to the individual. Further research is in progress to make this distinction clear to the practicing nurse.

REFERENCES   Agostinelli B et al: Targeted interventions: use of the Mini-Mental State Exam, *J Gerontol Nurs* 20:15, 1994.

Bailey J: To find a soul, *Nursing* 92:63, 1992.

Boehm S et al: Behavioral analysis and nursing interventions for reducing disruptive behaviors of patients with dementia, *Appl Nurs Res* 8:18, 1995.

Bouregois MS: Conversing with memory impaired individuals using memory aids: a memory aid workbook, Gaylord, Mich, 1992, Northern Speech Services.

Burnside I, Haight B: Reminiscence and life review: therapeutic interventions for older people, *Nurse Pract* 55, 1994.

Feil N: *The validation breakthrough: simple techniques for communicating with people with Alzheimer's-type dementia,* Baltimore, 1993, Health Professions.

Fine J, Rouse-Bane S: Using validation techniques to improve communication with cognitively impaired older adults, *J Gerontol Nurs* 21:39, 1995.

Gerdner LA, Buckwalter KC: A nursing challenge: assessment and management of agitation in Alzheimer's patients, *J Gerontol Nurs* 20:11, 1994.

Hall GR: This hospital patient has Alzheimer's, *Am J Nurs* 91:44, 1991.

Hall GR et al: Standardized care plan: managing Alzheimer's patients at home, *J Gerontol Nurs* 21:37, 1995.

Katz IR: On the inseparability of mental and physical health in aged persons, *Am J Geriatr Psych* 4:1, 1996.

Maxfield MC, Lewis RE, Cannon S: Training staff to prevent aggressive behavior of cognitively impaired elderly patients during bathing and grooming, *J Gerontol Nurs* 21:37, 1996.

Paulanka BJ, Griffin LS: Behavioral responses of memory impaired clients to selected nursing interventions, *Phys Occup Ther Geriatr* 12:65, 1993.

Quayhagen MP et al: A dyadic remediation program for care recipients with dementia, *Nursing Res* 44:153, 1995.

Snyder M, Egan EC, Burns KR: Interventions for decreasing agitation behaviors in persons with dementia, *J Gerontol Nurs* 21:34, 1995.

Stolley JM: When your patient has Alzheimer's disease, *Am J Nurs* 94:34, 1994.

Tinetti ME, Liu WL, Ginter SF: Mechanical restraint use and fall-related injuries among residents of skilled nursing facilities, *Ann Intern Med* 116:369, 1992.

Woods P, Ashley J: Simulated presence therapy: using selected memories to manage problem behaviors in Alzheimer's disease patients, *Geriatr Nurs* 16:9, 1995.

Constipation

Kathie D. Hesnan and Betty J. Ackley

Definition   The state in which an individual experiences a change in normal bowel habits characterized by a decrease in frequency of passage of stools and/or passage of hard, dry stools

Defining Characteristics

Decreased frequency of defecation (less than usual pattern or greater than every 3 days); hard, formed stool; straining at stool; feeling of rectal fullness and pressure; abdominal pain; palpable mass; appetite impairment; back pain; headache; interference with daily living; use of laxatives

Related Factors (r/t)

Decreased activity level; decreased fluid intake; inadequate fiber in diet; emotional disturbances; lack of privacy; embarrassment about defecating in hospital environment; decreased peristalsis from hypokalemia or hypothyroidism; side effects from medications such as anticholinergics, antidepressants, antipsychotics, narcotics, antacids, iron, barium, and neuroleptics

Client Outcomes/Goals

- Maintains passage of soft, formed stool every 3 days without straining
- States relief from discomfort of constipation
- Identifies measures that prevent or treat constipation

Suggested NIC Interventions

Constipation/impaction management

Nursing Interventions and Rationales

- Observe usual pattern or have patient keep diary of defection, including time of day; usual stimulus; consistency, amount and frequency of stool; type, amount, and time of food consumed; fluid intake; history of bowel habits or laxative use; diet; exercise patterns; personal remedies for constipation; OB/GYN history; medications; surgeries; alterations in perianal sensation; and present bowel regimen.
  The underlying cause determines the appropriate nursing interventions.
- Review client's current medications.
  Many medications affect normal bowel function, including antidepressants, anticholinergics, diuretics, anticonvulsants, antacids containing aluminum and calcium, muscle relaxants, and narcotics (Cameron, 1992).
- Palpate for abdominal distention and auscultate bowel sounds.
  In clients with constipation the abdomen is often distended with a palpable colon (Held, 1995).
- Check for impaction; perform digital removal per physician's order.
  If impacted, use cleansing regimen until you obtain a very soft stool. A milk and molasses enema is very effective for cleansing. If using an enema, the client must be able to bodily retain the fluid. If the client has poor sphincter tone, use a cone tip irrigating bag to assist the client in retaining in the fluids, which also decreases the amount of fluid necessary for cleansing.
- Assess for anxiety or embarrassment regarding defecation.
- Encourage a fluid intake of 64 oz per day; if oral intake is low, gradually increase fluid intake. Fluid intake must be within the cardiac and renal reserve.
  Adequate fluid intake is necessary to prevent hard, dry stools.

- Encourage ambulation and/or a daily exercise program.
  Activity, even minimal activity such as waist twists, increases peristalsis, which is necessary to prevent constipation (Yakabowich, 1990).
- Encourage adequate fiber intake, about 30 g per day for adults; emphasize foods such as fresh fruits, vegetables, and bran cereals. Add fiber gradually.
  Fiber helps prevent constipation by giving stool bulk. Add fiber gradually because a sudden increase can cause bloating, gas, and diarrhea (Doughty, 1996).
- At each meal, sprinkle bran over client's food as allowed by client and prescribed diet.
  The number of bowel movements is increased and the use of laxatives is decreased in a client who eats wheat bran (Schmelzer, 1990).
- If sprinkling bran over the food is not effective, use the special recipe reported by Behm (1983). Mix 3 cups of sugar-free applesauce, 2 cups of unprocessed coarse wheat bran, and 1½ cups of unsweetened prune juice. Cover and refrigerate. Give client 2 tbsp per day with a glass of water, and titrate the dosage up to 3 tbsp twice a day until adequate bowel function is reached.
  Use of this recipe has been shown to decrease laxative and enema use by 80% and allow clients to experience a regular pattern of bowel function (Smith, Newman, 1989). A number of bran mixtures have been shown to be effective in decreasing constipation (Beverly, Travis, 1992; Gibson et al, 1995), including a mixture called power pudding *(Neal, 1995).*
- Initiate a regular schedule for defecation, using the client's normal evacuation time whenever possible. An optimal time for many individuals is 30 minutes after breakfast because of the gastrocolic reflex.
  A schedule gives the client a sense of control, but more important it promotes evacuation before drying of stool and constipation occur (Doughty, 1992).
- Emphasize to the client the necessary items for a normal bowel regimen (e.g., fluid, fiber, activity, and time).
- Help client onto bedside commode or toilet with client's hips flexed and feet flat. Have client deep breathe through mouth to encourage relaxation of the pelvic floor muscle and use the abdominal muscles to help evacuation.
- Provide laxatives, suppositories, and enemas only as needed and as ordered; establish a client goal of eliminating their use. Avoid soapsud enemas.
  Soapsud enemas can cause damage to the colonic mucosa (Schmelzer, Wright, 1993).
- For the stable neurological client, consider use of a bowel routine of suppositories or a Theravac enema every other day or performing digital stimulation with physician's permission. For persistent constipation, refer to physician for evaluation.
  Constipation can be caused by bowel obstruction, medication effects, irritable bowel syndrome, and psychological problems (Wexner, 1995; Wright, Thomas, 1995).

Geriatric
- Explain the importance of fluid intake and activity for soft, formed stool.
  Activity, fiber, and fluid intake are often decreased in elderly clients. Increasing fiber and fluids can be effective in preventing constipation in the elderly (Rodrigues-Fisher, Bourguignon, Good, 1993).
- Determine client's perception of normal bowel elimination; promote adherence to a regular schedule.
  Misconceptions regarding the frequency of bowel movements can lead to anxiety and overuse of laxatives.

- Explain Valsalva's maneuver and the reason it should be avoided.
  Valsalva maneuver can cause bradycardia and even death in cardiac patients.
- Respond quickly to client's call for help with toileting.
- Avoid regular use of enemas in the elderly.
  Enemas can cause fluid and electrolyte imbalances (Yakabowich, 1990) and damage to the colonic mucosa (Schmelzer, Wright, 1993).
- Use narcotics cautiously. If ordered, use stool softeners and bran mixtures to prevent constipation.
  Narcotics can cause constipation (Cameron, 1992).
- Position client on toilet or commode and place a small footstool under the feet.
  Placing a small footstool under the feet increases intraabdominal pressure and makes defecation easier for an elderly client with weak abdominal muscles.

Home Care Interventions

- Put client in bathroom to toilet when possible.
  Use of purpose-specific surroundings increases psychological stimulus to evacuate and privacy is more easily protected.
- Carefully monitor bowel patterns of clients under pain management with narcotics. Introduce a bowel management program at first sign of constipation.
  Constipation is a major problem for terminally ill or hospice clients who may need very high doses of narcotics for pain management.
- When using a bowel program, establish a pattern that is very regular and allows client to be part of family unit.
  Regularity of program promotes psychological and/or physiological "readiness" to evacuate. Families of home care clients often cannot proceed with normal daily activities until bowel programs are complete.

Client/Family Teaching

- Instruct client on normal bowel function and the necessity of fluid, fiber, and activity in a bowel program.
- Encourage client to heed defecation warning signs and develop a regular schedule of defecation by using a stimulus such as a warm drink or prune juice.
  Most cases of constipation are mechanical and happen from habitual neglect of impulses that signal appropriate for defecation. This results in accumulation of a large, dry fecal mass (Wright, Thomas, 1995).
- Teach client the natural methods of softening stool and increasing peristalsis.
- Encourage client to avoid long-term use of laxatives or enemas and to gradually withdraw their use if they have been used regularly.
- If not contraindicated, teach client how to do bent-leg sit-ups to increase abdominal tone; also encourage client to contract abdominal muscles frequently throughout the day.
- Teach client to increase fluids and roughage.
- Help client develop a daily exercise program to increase peristalsis.

REFERENCES   Beverley L, Travis I: Constipation: proposed natural laxative mixtures, *J Gerontol Nurs* 18:5, 1992.
Cameron T: Constipation related to narcotic therapy, *Cancer Nurs* 15:5, 1992.
Doughty D: A physiologic approach to bowel training, *J WOCN* 23, 1996.
Doughty D: A step-by-step approach to bowel training, *Progressions* 4:12, 1992.
Gibson CJ et al: Effectiveness of bran supplement on the bowel management of elderly rehabilitation patients, *J Gerontol Nurs* 10:21, 1995.

Held JL: Preventing and treating constipation, *Nursing* 3:26, 1995.

Neal LJ: "Power Pudding:" natural laxative therapy for the elderly who are homebound, *Home Healthcare Nurs* 13:66, 1995.

Rodrigues-Fisher L, Bourguignon C, Good BV: Dietary fiber nursing intervention: prevention of constipation in older adults, *Clin Nurs Res* 2:464, 1993.

Schmelzer M: Effectiveness of wheat bran in prevention of constipation in hospitalized orthopaedic surgery patients, *Orthop Nurs* 15:10, 1990.

Schmelzer M, Wright K: Working smart, *Am J Nurs* 93:55, 1993.

Smith D, Newman D: Beating the cycle of constipation, laxative abuse, and fecal incontinence, *THN*, 1989, p. 12.

Wexner SD, Bartolo DC: *Constipation: etiology, evaluation and management,* Jordan Hill, Oxford, 1995, Butterworth & Heineman Linacre House.

Wright PS, Thomas SL: Constipation and diarrhea: the neglected symptoms, *Semin Oncol Nurs* 11:289, 1995.

Yakabowich M: Prescribe with care: the role of laxatives in the treatment of constipation, *J Gerontol Nurs* 16:4, 1990.

Colonic constipation

Definition   The state in which an individual's pattern of elimination is characterized by a hard, dry stool that results from a delay in passage of food residue

Defining Characteristics
Major   Decreased frequency of defecation; hard, dry stool; straining at stool; abdominal distention; painful defecation; palpable mass

Minor   Rectal pressure, headache, appetite impairment, abdominal pain

Related Factors (r/t)
Inadequate fluid intake; inadequate fiber in diet; inadequate dietary intake; decreased activity level; immobility; emotional disturbances; stress; lack of privacy; change in daily routine; decreased peristalsis resulting from hypokalemia, hypocalcemia, or hypothyroidism; deceased gastrointestinal motility resulting from hormonal changes of pregnancy; hesitancy or reluctance to pass stool secondary to previous experience with rectal fissures or bleeding

Client Outcomes/Goals, Nursing Interventions and Rationales, Client/Family Teaching
See care plan for **Constipation**

Perceived constipation

Kathie D. Hesnan

Definition   The state in which an individual makes a self-diagnosis of constipation and ensures a daily bowel movement through the abuse of laxatives, enemas, and suppositories

Defining Characteristics
Expectation of a daily bowel movement that results in an overuse of laxatives, enemas, and suppositories; expectation of a bowel movement at the same time every day

Related Factors (r/t)

Cultural or family beliefs, faulty appraisals, impaired thought processes

Client Outcomes/Goals

- Regularly defecates soft, formed stool without using any aids
- Explains the need to decrease or eliminate the use of laxatives, suppositories, and enemas
- Identifies alternatives to laxatives, enemas, and suppositories for ensuring defecation
- Explains that defecation does not have to occur every day

Nursing Interventions and Rationales

- Observe usual pattern of defecation (e.g., timing, consistency, amount, and frequency of stool passage; diet; fluid intake).
  This bowel record provides both the client and the nurse a way to assess the present bowel program, identify areas of concern, and develop an individualized bowel program.
- Determine client's perception of an appropriate defecation pattern.
  The client may need to be taught that one bowel movement every 1 to 4 days is normal (Yakabowich, 1990).
- Monitor use of laxatives, suppositories, or enemas, and offer alternatives such as natural laxatives.
  Natural laxatives have been shown to be successful in treating constipation (Smith, Newman, 1989; Beverly, Travis, 1992).
- Encourage client to promptly respond to the defecation reflex.
  Not responding to the urge to defecate can be a contributing factor to constipation (Battle, Hanna, 1989).
- Obtain a dietary referral for analysis and input on diet.
- Provide privacy for defecation and encourage client to avoid using a bedpan if possible.
  Many individuals need privacy to defecate. Using a bedpan makes it more difficult to use the abdominal muscles to help evacuate the rectum, and the client may have a feeling of incomplete emptying.
- Observe for potential body image disturbance or the use of laxatives to control or decrease weight; refer for counseling if needed.

Home Care Interventions

- Obtain family and client histories of bowel or other patterned behavior problems.
  Histories may detect psychological etiology to constipation (e.g., withholding).
- Observe family cultural patterns related to eating and bowel habits.
  Cultural patterns may control bowel habits.
- Contract with the client and/or a responsible family member regarding use of laxatives. Have client maintain a bowel pattern diary. Observe for diarrhea or frequent evacuation.
  Intermittent care does not allow for 24-hour supervision. Contracting allows guided control of care by client in partnership with accurate reporting.
- Teach family to carry out bowel program per physician orders.
- Refer for home health aide services to assist with personal care, including bowel program if appropriate.
- Identify contingency plan for bowel care if client is dependent on outside persons for same.

Client/Family Teaching

- Explain normal bowel function and the necessary items for a regular bowel regimen.
- Work with client and family to develop a diet that fits life-style and includes increased roughage and fiber.
- Teach client that it is not necessary to have daily bowel movements and that normal people pass from three stools each day to three stools each week.
- Explain to client the harmful effects of the continual use of defecation aids.
- Encourage client to gradually decrease use of usual laxatives and enemas and to set a date to have eliminated all defecation aids.
- Determine a method of increasing client's fluid intake and fit this practice into client's life-style.
- Explain Valsalva's maneuver and why it should be avoided.
- Work with client and family to design a bowel training routine that is based on previous patterns (before laxative or enema abuse) and incorporates warm fluids, privacy, and a predictable routine.

Additional Nursing Interventions and Rationales, Client/Family Teaching

See care plan for **Constipation.**

REFERENCES   Battle E, Hanna C: Evaluation of a dietary regimen for chronic constipation, *J Gerontol Nurs* 6:527, 1989.

Beverley L, Travis I: Constipation: proposed natural laxative mixtures, *J Gerontol Nurs* 18:5, 1992.

Doughty D: A step by step approach to bowel training, *Progressions* 4:12, 1992.

Doughty D: *Urinary and fecal incontinence: nursing management,* St Louis, 1991, Mosby.

Neal LJ: "Power Pudding": natural laxative therapy for the elderly who are homebound, *Home Healthcare Nurs* 13:66, 1995.

Rodrigues-Fisher L, Bourguignon C, Good BV: Dietary fiber nursing intervention: prevention of constipation in older adults, *Clin Nurs Res* 2:464, 1993.

Schmelzer M: Effectiveness of wheat bran in prevention of constipation in hospitalized orthopaedic surgery patients, *Orthop Nurs* 15:10, 1990.

Smith D, Newman D: Beating the cycle of constipation, laxative abuse, and fecal incontinence, *TNH* 1989.

Yakabowich, M: Prescribe with care: the role of laxatives in the treatment of constipation, *J Gerontol Nurs* 16:4, 1990.

Defensive coping

Gail B. Ladwig

Definition   The state in which an individual repeatedly projects falsely positive self-evaluations based on a self-protective pattern that defends against underlying perceived threats to positive self-regard

Defining Characteristics

Major   Denial of obvious problems or weaknesses, projection of blame or responsibility, rationalization of failures, hypersensitivity to slight criticism, grandiosity

Minor   Superior attitude toward others, difficulty establishing or maintaining relationships, hostile laughter or ridicule of others, difficulties with reality-testing perceptions, lack of follow-through or participation in treatment or therapy

Related Factors (r/t)

Situational crises, psychological impairment, substance abuse

Client Outcomes/Goals

- Accepts responsibility for actions
- Accepts constructive criticism without feeling personally rejected
- Interacts with others
- Participates in therapy and establishes realistic goals

Suggested NIC Interventions

Self awareness enhancement

Nursing Interventions and Rationales

- Ask appropriate questions to assess whether denial is being used in association with alcoholism.
  A short sensitive tool is the CAGE questionaire. (The most widely used tool is the Michigan alcoholism screening test [Mast]. Although it is a very reliable and valid tool, it is not practical for use by a bedside nurse for purposes of assessment.)
- An affirmative answer to two or more of the following questions is considered a basis for suspicion of alcohol abuse:
  C   Have you ever felt you ought to *cut* down on drinking?
  A   Have people *annoyed* you by criticizing your drinking?
  G   Have you ever felt bad or *guilty* about your drinking?
  E   Have you ever had a drink first thing in the morning to steady your nerves or get rid of a hangover *(eye opener)?*
  Because of the denial defense mechanism, asking alcoholics directly about the amount they drink is unlikely to produce an accurate response. Questions must be asked differently to obtain more accurate data. The CAGE questionnaire is a practical tool for a bedside nurse (Kovach, 1991).
- Determine client's perception of the problem, and then provide reality-based examples of the true situation (i.e., witnesses to an accident, blood alcohol levels, problems caused by alcohol).
  Ascribing meaning, altering one's self-perception, and relating the critical event to alcohol is necessary for the alcoholic to transcend denial (Wing, 1995).
- Help client to identify the situations or people that trigger feelings of defensiveness; acknowledge that these are triggers, and emphasize that the client is ultimately responsible for personal behavior.
  Identifying exact situations and feelings helps direct interventions. An emphasis on helping the individual attain a sense of control may facilitate change, ensuring the use constructive rather than obstructive denial (Russell, 1993).
- Encourage client self-worth by using group or individual therapy, role-playing, one-to-one interactions, and role-modeling.
  A positive attitude is the most important characteristic of healing (Criddle, 1993). These traditional interventions promote positive self-esteem.
- Support strengths and normal observations with, "I note that," or "I want you to notice. . ." Tell clients when they do something well.
  By promoting the client's strengths the nurse will be assisting the client to become more secure in the surroundings. As the client's security level increases, the need to use denial decreases (Robinson, 1993).

- Teach client to use positive thinking by blocking negative thoughts with the word *stop* and inserting positive thoughts (e.g., "I'm a good person, friend, or student").
  Once clients learn to recognize negative and distorted thoughts, they can learn to interrupt or stop this self-defeating behavior and replace it with realistic and positive appraisals (Norrus, 1992).
- Provide feedback regarding others' perceptions of the client's behavior through group or milieu therapy or one-to-one interactions.
  Motivation, sharing of experiences, camaraderie with and support from peers and knowledge of not being alone have been identified as advantages of group learning (Payne, 1993).
- Encourage client to use "I" statements and to accept responsibility for and consequences of actions.
  "I" statements encourage personal responsibility and help the client to overcome defensiveness. All clients have the capacity for change (Murray, 1993).

Geriatric
- Assess client for anger and identify previous outlets for anger.
  If appropriate, previously used, familiar outlets for anger can help a client dissipate emotions.
- Explore new outlets for anger, including physical activities within client's capabilities (e.g., hitting a pillow, woodworking, sanding, scrubbing floors).
  Physical activities help the client direct anger outward instead of holding it inside.
- Assess client for dementia or depression.
  Symptoms of dementia or depression may be masked by inappropriate coping techniques. Depression may be overlooked because there is a focus on the physiological problems of aging (Abraham, Neudorfer, Currie, 1992).

Home Care Interventions

- Include in initial assessment client and family histories of mental health problems.
- Observe family dynamics for dysfunctional or supportive communication.
  In the context of some family patterns of communication, defensive coping may be a learned behavior.
- In the absence of primary medical diagnoses, refer to medical social services for assistance with contacting appropriate community services.
- If medical diagnoses coexist with defensive coping, confirm and validate mental health plan for and progress by client. Medical social services may or may not be necessary depending on community support.
- Contract with client for administration of medications. Observe for abuse.
  Successful contracting provides control and improved self-esteem as well as a vehicle for reinforcing clients' responsibility for their actions.

Client/Family Teaching

- Teach client the actions and side effects of medications and the importance of taking them as prescribed, even when the client is feeling "good."
  The client needs to know that feeling "good" may result from the medications and that it is important to continue taking them.
- Refer client to appropriate therapist for grandiose and possibly harmful symptoms such as promiscuity, insomnia, euphoria, overspending, and alcohol or drug abuse.
  Harmful behaviors need appropriate intervention from a qualified professional. Resource personnel should be consulted to assist in identifying and altering patterns of alcohol abuse and addressing the problems that alcoholism creates (Kovach, Weiss, 1991).

- Work with client's support group to identify harmful behaviors and to seek help for client if unable to control behavior.
  The client's support group needs to be involved in the treatment plan to ensure safety and compliance.

REFERENCES   Abraham I, Neudorfer M, Currie L: Effects of group interventions on cognition and depression in nursing home residents, *Nursing Res* 41:196, 1992.
Criddle L: Healing from surgery: a phenomenological study, *Image J Nurs Sch* 25:208, 1993.
Kovach G, Weiss K: Denying alcoholism, *Focus Crit Care AACN* 18:469, 1991.
Murray RB, Bair M: Use of therapeutic milieu in a community setting, *J Psychosoc Nurs Ment Health Serv* 31:11, 1993.
Norris J: Nursing intervention for self-esteem disturbances, *Nurs Diag* 3:48, 1992.
Payne J: The contribution of group learning to the rehabilitation of spinal cord injured adults, *Rehab Nursing* 18:375, 1993.
Robinson K: Denial: an adaptive response, *Dimens Crit Care Nurs* 12:102, 1993.
Russell G: The role of denial in clinical practice, *J Adv Nurs* 18:938, 1993.
Wing D: Transcending alcoholic denial, *Image: J Nurs Sch* 27:121, 1995.

Ineffective individual coping

Gail B. Ladwig

Definition   Impairment of adaptive behaviors and problem-solving abilities in meeting life's demands and roles

Defining Characteristics

Verbalized inability to cope or ask for help (critical), inability to meet role expectations, inability to meet basic needs, inability to problem solve (critical), alteration in social participation, destructive behavior toward self or others, inappropriate use of defense mechanisms, change in usual communication patterns, verbal manipulation, high illness rate, high rate of accidents

Related Factors (r/t)

Situational crises, maturational crises, personal vulnerability

Client Outcomes/Goals

- Verbalizes ability to cope and asks for help when needed
- Demonstrates ability to solve problems and participates at usual level in society
- Remains free of destructive behavior toward self or others
- Communicates needs and negotiates with others to meet needs
- Discusses how recent life stressors have overwhelmed normal coping strategies
- Has illness and accident rates not excessive for age and developmental level

Suggested NIC Interventions

Coping enhancement, decision-making support

Nursing Interventions and Rationales

- Observe for causes of ineffective coping such as poor self-concept, grief, lack of problem-solving skills, lack of support, or recent change in life situations.
  The problem or stressor needs to be identified to plan useful solutions and coping strategies.

- Observe for strengths as the ability to relate facts and recognize source of stressors.
  If a client cannot find something meaningful in life that will give him or her a purpose for living, the client is at risk of focusing on death as an escape route (Buchanan, 1991).
- Monitor risk of harming self or others and intervene appropriately; see **Risk for violence.**
  A client with hopelessness and an inability to problem solve often runs the risk of suicide (Buchanan, 1991). In these cases immediate referral for mental health care is essential (Norris, 1992).
- Help client set realistic goals and identify personal skills and knowledge.
  Involving clients in decision-making helps them move toward independence (Connelly et al, 1993).
- Use empathetic communication, and encourage client to verbalize fears, express emotions, and set goals.
  Clients report increased satisfaction, empowerment, greater compliance with mutually agreed on goals, and less anxiety and depression when communication is empathic (Wells-Federman et al, 1995).
- Encourage client to make choices and participate in planning of care and scheduled activities.
  Participation gives a feeling of control and increases self-esteem.
- Provide mental and physical activities within the client's ability (e.g., reading, television, radio, crafts, outings, movies, dinners out, social gatherings, exercise, sports, games).
  Interventions that enhance body awareness such as exercise, proper nutrition and muscular relaxation may be effective in treating anxiety and depression (Wells-Federman et al, 1995).
- Use touch with permission. Give client a backrub using slow, rhythmic stroking with hands. Use a rate of 60 strokes a minute for 3 minutes on 2-inch wide areas on both sides of the spinous process from the crown to the sacral area.
  Slow stroke back massage decreased heart rate, decreased systolic and diastolic blood pressure, and increased skin temperature at significant levels. The conclusion is that relaxation is induced by slow stroke back massage (Meek, 1993).
- Provide information regarding care before care is given.
  Lack of information is a patient concern that is often reported (Yarcheski, Knapp-Spooner, 1994).
- Discuss changes with client before making them.
  Knowledge about changes gives a feeling of control and increases self-esteem.
- Discuss client's power to change a situation or the need to accept a situation.
  Such a discussion helps the client maintain self-esteem and look at the situation realistically with the aid of a trusted individual (Norris, 1992).
- Use active listening and acceptance to help client express emotions such as crying, guilt, and anger (within appropriate limits).
  Being tuned into the client's feelings and encouraging catharsis are necessary interventions to decrease guilt feelings (Robertson, 1994).
- Avoid false reassurance; give honest answers and provide only the information requested.
  Avoid overload in stressful situations. Honesty promotes trust.

- Encourage client to describe previous stressors and the coping mechanisms used.
  Describing previous experiences strengthens effective coping and helps eliminate ineffective coping mechanisms.
- Be supportive of coping behaviors; allow client time to relax.
  Such support is a positive reinforcement for success.
- Encourage use of cognitive behavioral relaxation (e.g., music therapy, imagery).
  Music is not a cure, but it can lift the human spirit, comfort the heart, and inspire the soul. Imagery is useful for relaxation and distraction (Fontaine, 1994).
- Refer for counseling as needed.
  Follow-up may be needed to reinforce new behaviors.

Geriatric

- Be aware of client's fear of illness. Identify and reinforce patterns the elderly client has previously used to respond to stress.
  The elderly client has had a lifetime of experience dealing with stressful events.
- Observe any physiological imbalance as a contributor to ineffective coping; take appropriate nursing actions to correct imbalances, and notify physician of abnormal laboratory results or medication side effects or interactions.
  Physiological problems may be manifested as emotional problems.
- Increase and mobilize support available to the elderly client. Encourage interaction with family and friends.
  Friends and relatives have shared many of the older person's life experiences. Such mutual interests and overlapping memories can serve to stimulate and focus conversation and contribute effectively to the client's self-esteem (Erber, 1994).
- Maintain continuity of care by keeping the number of caregivers to a minimum.
  The elderly client needs to develop trust before sharing concerns.

Home Care Interventions

- Observe family for coping behavior patterns. Obtain family and client history as able.
  History may dictate current behaviors.
- Assess for suicidal tendencies. Refer for mental health care immediately if indicated. Identify an emergency plan should the client become suicidal.
  A suicidal client is not safe in home environment unless supported by professional help.
- Refer to medical social services for evaluation and counseling, which will promote adequate coping as part of the medical plan of care. If no primary medical diagnosis has been made, request medical social services to assist with community support contacts.
- If the client is involved with the mental health system, actively participate in mental health team planning.
  Home care nurses can often advocate for clients based on knowledge of the home and family. They are often requested to monitor medications and need to know the plan of care.
- If monitoring medications, contract with client or solicit assistance from a responsible caregiver. Prepouring medications may be helpful with some clients.
  Successful contracting provides the client with control of care and promotes self-esteem while establishing responsibility for desired actions.

NOTE: All of the previously mentioned interventions may be applied in the home setting. Home care may offer psychiatric nursing or the services of a licensed clinical social worker under special programs. Traditionally, insurance does not reimburse for counseling that is not related to a medical plan of care unless it is under one of the programs just described. Public health agencies generally do not have the clinical support needed to offer psychiatric nursing services to clients. Clients are usually treated in the ambulatory mental health system.

Client/Family Teaching

- Teach clients to problem solve. Have them define the problem and cause and list the advantages and disadvantages of their options.
- Teach relaxation techniques.
  Problem-solving skills promote the client's sense of control. Relaxation decreases stress and enhances coping (Fontaine, 1994).
- Suggest listening to music.
  Listening to music has been found to decrease total mood disturbances scores (profile of mood states [POMS]). A decrease in POMS scores is indicative of decreased distress and a mood improvement (McNair, Lorr, Droppleman, 1992).
- Teach process imagery (purposely evoking a mental image of a desired effect).
  Using process imagery, a person can look at an old problem in a totally different way, making new connections and freeing the problem from the original memory. Imagery engenders a feeling of control and gives the client an effective tool for self-care (Stephens, 1993).
- Teach client about available community resources (e.g., therapists, ministers, counselors, self-help groups).
  Client and family teaching that promotes the ability to understand and carry out any necessary medical, rehabilitative, or daily living activities contributes to a sense of mastery, competency, and control and is vital to discharge planning and community-based assessments (Norris, 1992).

REFERENCES   Buchanan D: Suicide: a conceptual model for an avoidable death, *Arch Psychiatr Nurs* 5:341, 1991.
Connelly L et al: A place to be yourself: empowerment from the client's perspective, *Image J Nurs Sch* 25:297, 1993.
Erber NP: Conversation as therapy for older adults in residential care: the case for intervention, *Eur J Disord Commun* 29:269, 1994.
Fontaine D: Recognition, assessment, and treatment of anxiety in the critical care setting, *Crit Care Nurse* 3(S):7, 1994.
McNair D, Lorr M, Droppleman L: *Manual for the profile of mood states (POMS),* San Diego, 1992, Educational Testing Service.
Meek S: Effects of slow stroke back massage on relaxation in hospice clients, *Image J Nurs Sch* 25:17, 1993.
Norris J: Nursing interventions for self-esteem disturbances, *Nurs Diag* 3:48, 1992.
Robertson WJ: The concept of guilt, *J Psychosoc Nurs Ment Health Serv* 32:15, 1994.
Stephens R: Imagery: a strategic intervention to empower clients. Review of research literature, *Clin Nurse Spec* 7:170, 1993.
Wells-Federman C et al: The mind-body connection: the psychophysiology of many traditional nursing interventions, *Clin Nurse Spec* 9:59, 1995.
Yarcheski A, Knapp-Spooner C: Stressors associated with coronary bypass surgery, *Clin Nurs Res* 3:57, 1994.

Decisional conflict

Gail B. Ladwig

Definition   The state of uncertainty about the course of action to be taken when choice involves risk, loss, or challenge to personal life values

Defining Characteristics

Major   Verbalization of uncertainty about the choices, verbalization of undesired consequences of alternatives, vacillation between alternative choices, delayed decision-making

Minor   Verbalization of distress while attempting a decision, self-focusing, physical signs of distress or tension (e.g., increased heart rate, increased muscle tension, restlessness), questioning of personal values and beliefs while attempting a decision

Related Factors (r/t)

Unclear personal values or beliefs, perceived threat to value system, lack of experience in or interference with decision making, lack of relevant information, support system deficit, multiple or divergent sources of information, impact of ethical and moral beliefs on choices and health outcomes (e.g., birth of defective child), unplanned life event (e.g., pregnancy)

Client Outcomes/Goals

- States the advantages and disadvantages of choices
- Shares fears and concerns regarding choices and responses of others
- Makes an informed choice

Suggested NIC Interventions

Decision-making support

Nursing Interventions and Rationales

- Observe for factors causing or contributing to conflict (e.g., value conflicts, fears of outcome, poor problem-solving skills).
  Baseline data are important in directing interventions; no single set of values is appropriate for all individuals. Values clarification emphasizes the client's capacity for intelligent, self-directed behavior (Dossey et al, 1988).
- Allow clients to make decisions in a way that is comfortable for them—deferring (allowing others to decide), delaying (choosing an alternative that meets basic requirements), and deliberating (looking at all alternatives).
  Clients confronting health care choices have unique decision-making styles (Pierce, 1993).
- Give client time and permission to express feelings associated with decision-making.
  Decisions become more difficult when feelings are repressed. Once some of this stress is removed by talking through problems or releasing pent-up emotions, the decision process often becomes easier (Burnard, 1992).
- Explore client's perception of the future in relation to different decisions.
  Perceiving the future helps the client focus on what is important. Accurate time orientation (the ability to view the future on the basis of present and past experience) indicates that the client will have better coping skills (Haber et al, 1992).
- Demonstrate reassurance with unconditional respect for and acceptance of client's values, spiritual beliefs, and cultural norms.
  Client reassurance and communication are nursing skills that promote trust and orientation and reduce anxiety (Harvey, 1996).

- Encourage client to list the advantages and disadvantages of each alternative.
  Listing alternatives helps clients learn how to problem solve. Clients might not believe they have alternatives and may need assistance exploring options (Chez, 1994).
- Initiate health teaching and referrals when needed.
  All interventions need to be individualized.
- Facilitate communication between client and family members regarding the final decision; offer support to person actually making the decision.
  Studies suggest that clients' decisions are rarely the same as those of their friends and family members; therefore when possible, clients are best suited to determine their own life support treatment (Beland, Froman, 1995).

Geriatric
- Discuss with client and family the importance of discussing and recording end-of-life decisions.
  These decisions are of extreme importance to an aging client. Discussing these issues gives the client both a sense of control and the opportunity to prepare for the inevitable (Dossey et al, 1988).
- If end-of-life discussions are being avoided, describe the possible consequences.
  The reality of the situation must be confronted.
- Discuss the purpose of a living will and advance directives.
  Elderly clients and their significant others need to know how to legally (laws differ in each state) make end-of-life decisions.
- Discuss choices or changes to be made (e.g., moving in with children, into a nursing home, or into an adult foster care home).
  Exploring options gives the client and family a sense of control. For a change to be effective, it must be accepted and owned by the client (Fleury, 1991).
- Teach family members how to be supportive of final decision or to refrain from being destructive if unable to be supportive.
  It is important to support the decisions that the client makes.

Home Care Interventions

- *Before* providing any home care, assess client plan for advance directives (living will and power of attorney). If no plan exists, offer information on advance directives per agency policy and referral for assistance in completing advance directives. *Do not witness living will.* If plan exists, place copy in client file.
  This is a legal requirement of COBRA legislation.
- Determine relevance of conflict to plan of care.
- Assess client and family for consensus (or lack of) regarding issue in conflict.
- If decision is relevant to plan of care, primary nurse or medical social services may evaluate the need for and call a family conference. If consensus cannot be reached, continue efforts to resolve the conflict. Clients, unless medically incompetent (by legal guidelines) or under authorized power of attorney, may make their own decisions.
  Guided family conferences allow all persons affected by the decision to be heard and have the value system of the client validated. The nurse or social worker serves as the facilitator and client advocate.
- If not relevant to the plan of care, refer to community support appropriate to type of decision and client need.

Client/Family Teaching

- Instruct the client and family members to provide advance directives in the following areas:

- Person to contact in an emergency
- Preference (if any) to die at home or in the hospital
- Desire to sign a living will
- Desire to donate an organ
- Funeral arrangements (i.e., burial, cremation)
- Inform family of treatment options; encourage and defend self-determination.
  The Patient Self-Determination Act, effective since December 1991, has changed the importance of introducing life support options to patients (Beland, Froman, 1995).
- Identify reasons for family decisions regarding care. Explore ways in which family decisions can be respected.
  Family issues need to be identified to provide optimal care (e.g., establish whether the family understands the prognosis or has unresolved issues with the client, whether they are waiting for someone to come from out of town, and whether other issues must be resolved before final decisions can be made [Campbell, 1994]).
- Include families in patient care conferences. As a client's condition changes, it may be necessary to rethink the goal of treatment. It may change from restoration and cure to stabilization of functioning or preparation for comfortable and dignified death.
  Families who are consistently apprised of changes in a client's condition and assisted with exploring what these changes mean are more likely to trust the recommendation of the care team to withdraw or withhold further aggressive treatment (Taylor, 1995).

REFERENCES   Beland K, Froman R: Preliminary validation of a measure of life support preferences, *Image J Nurs Sch* 27:307, 1995.

Burnard PL *Counseling: a guide to practice in nursing,* Oxford, England, 1992, Butterworth-Heinemann.

Campbell M: Making an end-of-life difference, *Crit Care Nurse* 14:111, 1994.

Chez N: Helping the victim of domestic violence, *Am J Nurs* 94:33, 1994.

Dossey B et al: *Holistic nursing: a handbook for practice,* Rockville, Md, 1988, Aspen.

Fleury J: Empowering potential: a theory of wellness motivation, *Nurs Res* 40:268, 1991.

Haber J et al: *Comprehensive psychiatric nursing,* ed 4, St Louis, 1992, Mosby.

Harvey M: Managing agitation in critically ill patients, *Am J Crit Care* 5:7, 1996.

Pierce P: Deciding on breast cancer treatment: a description of decision behavior, *Nurs Res* 42(1), 1993.

Taylor C: Medical futility and nursing, *Image J Nurs Sch* 27:301, 1995.

Ineffective denial

Gail B. Ladwig

Definition   The state of conscious or unconscious attempt to disavow the knowledge or meaning of an event to reduce anxiety and fear to the extent that it is detrimental to health

Defining Characteristics

Major   Delays or refuses health care to the detriment of health, does not perceive personal relevance of symptoms or danger.

Minor   Uses home remedies (self-treatment) to relieve symptoms, does not admit fear of death or invalidism, minimizes symptoms, displaces source of symptoms to other organs, displaces fear of impact of the condition, is unable to admit impact of disease on life pattern, makes dismissive gestures or comments when speaking of distressing events, displays inappropriate affect

Related Factors (r/t)

Fear of consequences, chronic or terminal illness, actual or perceived fear of possible losses (e.g., job, significant other), refusal to acknowledge substance-abuse problem; fear of the social stigma associated with disease

Client Outcomes/Goals

- Seeks out health care attention when needed
- Uses home remedies only when appropriate
- Displays appropriate affect and verbalizes fears
- Acknowledges substance-abuse problem and seeks help

Suggested NIC Interventions

Anxiety reduction, counseling

Nursing Interventions and Rationales

- Assess client's understanding of symptoms and illness.
  Allowing clients to define their own realities shows regard for the client's needs and values and establishes the client as an expert (Ersek, 1992).
- Spend one-to-one time with client.
  The most critical intervention a nurse can make is to offer to spend time with the client (Harrenstein, 1992).
- Allow client to express and use denial.
  At certain stages of an illness, denial may be appropriate. Denial is common and sometimes necessary immediately following the diagnosis of cancer; denial controls the overwhelming information until other coping mechanisms can be mobilized (Weisman, 1992).
- Avoid confrontation.
  Confronting the client too soon may not serve any therapeutic purpose and may do more harm than good (Robinson, 1993).
- Ask appropriate questions to assess whether denial is being used in association with alcoholism. A short sensitive tool is the CAGE questionnaire. (The most widely used tool is the Michigan alcoholism screening test [Mast]. Although it is a very reliable and valid tool, it is not practical for use by a bedside nurse for purposes of assessment.)
- An affirmative answer to two or more of the following questions is considered a basis for suspicion of alcohol abuse:
  C   Have you ever felt you ought to *cut* down on drinking?
  A   Have people *annoyed* you by criticizing your drinking?
  G   Have you ever felt bad or *guilty* about your drinking?
  E   Have you ever had a drink first thing in the morning to steady your nerves or get rid of a hangover *(eye opener)?*
  Because of denial, asking alcoholics directly how much they drink is unlikely to produce an accurate response. Ask questions differently to obtain more accurate data. The CAGE questionnaire is a practical tool for the bedside nurse (Kovach, 1991).
- Sit at eye level.
  Eye-level communication promotes emotional comfort (Ringsven, Bond, 1991).
- Use touch if appropriate and with permission; touch client's hand or arm.
  Touch conveys empathy. Human beings are often hungry for touch (Meek, 1993).

- Explain signs and symptoms of illness; reinforce use of prescribed treatment plan.
  Accurate information and encouragement to follow treatment regimen enhances compliance.
- Have the client make choices regarding treatment and actively involve them in the decision-making process.
  An emphasis on helping the individual attain a sense of control may facilitate change, ensuring the use of constructive rather than obstructive denial (Russell, 1993).
- Help client recognize existing and additional sources of support; allow time for adjustment.
  Involvement of a support system enhances compliance.
- If appropriate, refer family to a skilled mental health counselor for help in planning an intervention to confront client about self-destructive behaviors (e.g., drinking, drugs, eating disorders).
  Specialized treatment may be required for certain potentially harmful behaviors when no productive change is evident (Russell, 1993).
- Allow client to express feelings. Acknowledge client's fear (e.g., say, "I sense that you may be feeling afraid").
  An effective way to build trust is to listen well enough to understand clients' representations or models of the world, thereby perceiving the reason they are using denial (Robinson, 1993).
- Give positive feedback when client follows the appropriate treatment plan.
  By promoting the client's strengths, the nurse will be assisting the client with becoming more secure. As the client's security level increases, the need to use denial decreases (Robinson, 1993).
- Observe whether denial has been or is being used as a coping mechanism in other areas of life.
  Denial can be an adaptive response that helps the client cope (Robinson, 1993).

Geriatric
- Identify recent losses of client, because grieving may prolong denial. Encourage client to take one day at a time.
  An elderly client may have experienced multiple losses and need supportive care and extra time to adapt (Ringsven, Bond, 1991).
- Encourage client to verbalize feelings.
  Verbalization allows the client to release emotions and develop a sense of control.

Home Care Interventions
- Observe family interaction and roles. Assess whether denial is being used to meet the needs of another family member.
  In dysfunctional families, inappropriate or ineffective coping methods may be employed to meet the social needs of the dysfunctional unit.
- Refer client and family to medical social services for evaluation and treatment as indicated per physician order.
  It may be necessary to involve the entire family to effectively treat the client.
- Identify an emergency plan including how to contact hotlines and receive emergency services.
  Denial may be abandoned when the need for emergency care is perceived by the client or the family.

Client/Family Teaching
- Teach signs and symptoms of illness and appropriate responses (e.g., taking

medication, going to the emergency room, calling the physician).
Lack of knowledge about the condition or illness may result in unrealistic goals and hopes. Education is necessary (Robinson, 1993).

- If problem is substance abuse, refer to an appropriate community agency (e.g., Alcoholics Anonymous).
Groups of peer role models confront denial and reinforce that alcohol is a problem (Wing, 1995).

- Teach families of clients with brain injuries that denial has been associated with damage to the right hemisphere. The client may exhibit inappropriate affect and anxiety.
Denial may have an underlying physical cause and may be a necessary coping mechanism to maintain emotional stability and motivation (Armstrong, 1991).

REFERENCES   Armstrong C: Emotional changes following brain injury: psychological and neurological components of depression, denial and anxiety, *J Rehab* 57:15, 1991.

Ersek J: Examining the process and dilemmas of reality negotiation, *Image J Nurs Sch* 24:19, 1992.

Harrenstein E: Young women and depression: origin outcome and nursing care, *Nurs Clin North Am* 26:607, 1992.

Karnes B, Gyulay J: Healing the dying person—theoretical and practical approaches to emotional, mental, and spiritual dimensions, *Am J Hospice Care* 1:28. In Meek S: Effects of slow stroke back massage on relaxation in hospice clients, *Image J Nurs Sch* 25:7, 1993.

Kovach G, Weiss K: Denying alcoholism, *Focus Crit Care AACN* 18:469, 1991.

Ringsven M, Bond D: *Gerontology and leadership skills for nurses,* Albany, NY, 1991, Delmar.

Robinson K: Denial: an adaptive response, *Dimens Crit Care Nurs* 12:102, 1993.

Russell GC: The role of denial in clinical practice, *J Adv Nurs* 18:938, 1993.

Weisman A: Coping with cancer, *Image: J Nurs Sch* 24:19, 1992.

Wing D: Transcending alcoholic denial, *Image: J Nurs Sch* 27:121, 1995.

Diarrhea

Kathie D. Hesnan and Betty J. Ackley

Definition   The state in which an individual experiences a change in normal bowel habits characterized by the frequent passage of loose, fluid, and unformed stools

Defining Characteristics

Abdominal pain and cramping; increased frequency or urgency of defecation; increased frequency of bowel sounds; loose, liquid stool with possible color change

Related Factors (r/t)

Infection (viral, bacterial, protozoan), change in diet or food, gastrointestinal disorders, stress, medication effects, impaction

Client Outcomes/Goals

- Defecates formed, soft stool every day to every third day
- Maintains a rectal area free of irritation
- States relief from cramping and less or no diarrhea
- Explains cause of diarrhea and rationale for treatment
- Maintains good skin turgor and weight at usual level
- Contains stool appropriately (if previously incontinent)

Suggested NIC Intervention
Diarrhea management
Nursing Interventions and Rationales

- Assess pattern of defecation or have client keep a diary that includes the following: time of day defecation occurs; usual stimulus for defecation; consistency, amount, and frequency of stool; type, amount, and time of food consumed; fluid intake; history of bowel habits and laxative use; diet; exercise patterns; OB/GYN, medical, and surgical histories; medications; alterations in perianal sensations; and present bowel regimen.
  Assessment of defecation pattern will help direct treatment (Mertz et al, 1995).
- Identify cause of diarrhea if possible (e.g., viral, including human immunodeficiency virus [HIV]; food; medication effect; radiation therapy; protein malnutrition; laxative abuse). See related factors.
  Identification of the underlying cause is imperative because the treatment and expected outcome depend on it. If the onset of diarrhea is sudden with no obvious cause, a colonoscopy is recommended to rule out colon cancer. When reviewing medication, assess for medications that increase peristalsis, such as metoclopramide (Reglan). HIV infection is also commonly associated with diarrhea (Anastasi, 1993).
- If client has severe diarrhea, a low-grade fever, and a history of antibiotic therapy, consider possibility of *Clostridium difficile* infection.
  C. difficile *infection and pseudomembranous colitis have become increasingly common because of the frequent use of broad-spectrum antibiotics (Vogel, 1995).*
- Use universal precautions when caring for clients with diarrhea to prevent spread of infectious diarrhea.
  C. difficile *has been shown to be contagious and at times epidemic. One study of medical patients demonstrated that more than 30% developed nosocomial diarrhea after admission to a nursing unit, and the majority of cases were caused by* C. difficile *(McFarland, 1995).*
- Obtain stool specimens as ordered to either rule out or diagnose an infectious process (e.g., ova and parasites, *C. difficile* infection, bacterial cultures).
- If client has infectious diarrhea, avoid using medications that slow peristalsis.
  If an infectious process is occurring, such as C. difficile *infection or food poisoning, medication to slow down peristalsis should generally not be given. The increase in gut motility helps eliminate the causative factor.*
- Observe and record number and consistency of stools per day; if desired, use a fecal incontinence collector for accurate measurement of output.
  Documentation of output provides a baseline and helps direct replacement fluid therapy.
- Inspect, palpate, percuss, and auscultate abdomen; note whether bowel sounds are frequent.
- Assess for dehydration by observing skin turgor over sternum and inspecting for longitudinal furrows of the tongue. Watch for hypotension and symptoms of shock.
  Severe diarrhea can cause fluid volume deficit with extreme weakness and cause death in the very young and elderly.
- Observe for symptoms of sodium and potassium loss (e.g., weakness, abdominal or leg cramping, dysrhythmia).
  Stool contains electrolytes; excessive diarrhea causes electrolyte abnormalities that can be especially harmful to clients with existing medical conditions.

- Monitor and record intake and output; note oliguria and dark, concentrated urine. Measure specific gravity of urine if possible.
  Urine amount and specific gravity is an indicator of fluid balance.
- Weigh client daily and note decreased weight.
  An accurate daily weight is the best indicator of fluid balance in the body.
- Give clear fluids as tolerated (e.g., clear soda, Jell-O), serving at lukewarm temperature. For children, give oral replacement therapy liquids as directed by physician.
- Encourage client to eat small, frequent meals and foods that normally cause constipation and are easy to digest (e.g., bananas, crackers, pretzels, rice, potatoes, applesauce). Encourage client to avoid milk products, foods high in fiber, and caffeine (dark sodas, tea, coffee, chocolate).
  Bland, starchy foods are initially recommended when starting to eat food again (Rice, 1994).
- Provide a readily available bedpan, commode, or bathroom.
- Maintain perirectal skin integrity. Apply protective ointment prn after gentle, thorough cleaning. If skin is still excoriated, consider use of perianal pouch or rectal foley catheter with physician's approval.
  Moisture-barrier ointments protect the skin from excoriation. (NOTE: *Rectal Foley catheters can cause rectal necrosis, sphincter damage, or rupture, and the nursing staff may not have the time to properly follow the necessary and very time-consuming steps of their care [Bosley, 1994; Fiers, 1996]).*
- If client is receiving a tube feeding, do not assume it is the cause of diarrhea. Perform a complete assessment to rule out other causes such as medication effects, sorbitol in medications, or an infection.
  Research has shown that tube feedings do not usually cause diarrhea (Campbell, 1994). Sorbitol in medication has been linked to diarrhea (Drug Watch, 1994).
- If client is receiving a tube feeding, suggest formulas that contain a bulking agent. Note rate of infusion, and prevent contamination of feeding by rinsing container every 8 hours and replacing it every 24 hours.
  Rapid administration of tube feeding and contaminated feedings have been associated with diarrhea. Bulking agents are useful in tube feedings to prevent diarrhea (Doughty, 1991; Bockus, 1993).

Geriatric
- Monitor client closely to detect whether an impaction is causing diarrhea; remove impaction as ordered.
  Impactions are more common in the elderly. It is very important that the client be checked for impaction before being given any antidiarrheal medication (Carveveli, Patrick, 1993).
- Seek medical attention if diarrhea is severe, persists for more than 24 hours, or client has symptoms of dehydration or electrolyte disturbances such as lassitude, weakness or prostration.
  Elderly clients can dehydrate rapidly. The greatest concern for elderly clients with severe diarrhea is hypokalemia. Hypokalemia is treatable but when missed can be fatal (Carnaveli, Patrick, 1993).
- Provide emotional support for clients who are having trouble controlling unpredictable episodes of diarrhea.
  Diarrhea can be a great source of embarrassment to the elderly and lead to social isolation and a feeling of powerlessness (Carnaveli, Patrick, 1993).

Home Care Interventions

- Assess the home for general sanitation and methods of food preparation. Reinforce principles of sanitation for food handling.
- Assess for methods of handling soiled laundry if client is bedbound or has been incontinent. Instruct or reinforce universal precautions with family and bloodborne pathogen precautions with agency caregivers.

  The Bloodborne Pathogen Regulations of the Occupational Safety and Health Administration (OSHA) identify legal guidelines for caregivers.
- When assessing medication history, include over-the-counter drugs, both general and currently being used for the diarrhea. Instruct clients not to mix over-the-counter medications when self-treating.

  Mixing over-the-counter medications can further irritate the gastrointestinal system, intensifying the diarrhea or causing nausea and vomiting.
- Instruct adults to avoid electrolyte solutions during first 24 hours of diarrhea.

  Electrolyte solutions can intensify dehydration initially (Humphrey, 1994).

Client/Family Teaching

- Encourage avoidance of coffee, spices, milk products, and foods that irritate or stimulate the gastrointestinal tract.
- Teach appropriate method of taking ordered antidiarrheal medications; explain side effects.
- Explain how to prevent the spread of infectious diarrhea (e.g., careful handwashing, appropriate handling and storage of food).
- Help client to determine stressors and set up an appropriate stress reduction plan.
- Teach signs and symptoms of dehydration and electrolyte imbalance.
- Teach perirectal skin care.

REFERENCES   Anastasi J: Diarrhea in acquired immune deficiency syndrome (AIDS), *Ostomy/ Wound Manag* 39:14-23, 1993.

Bockus S: When your patient needs tube feeding: making the right decision, *Nursing 93* 93:34, 1993.

Bosley C: Three methods of stool management for patients with diarrhea, *Ostomy/Wound Manag* 40:52, 1994.

Campbell C: Research for practice: diarrhea not always linked to tube feedings, *Am J Nurs* 94(4):59, 1994.

Carnaveli DL, Patrick M: *Nursing management for the elderly,* ed 3 Philadelphia, 1993, JB Lippincott.

Doughty D: Maintaining normal bowel function in the patient with cancer, *J ET Nurs* 18:90, 1991.

Drug Watch: Sorbitol: missing link to diarrhea, *Am J Nurs* 10:50, 1994.

Fiers S: Breaking the cycle: the etiology of incontinence dermatitis and evaluating and using skin care products, *Ostomy/Wound Manag* 42:32, 1996.

Forloines-Lynn S: Complications of tube feeding, *Nursing* 3:32, 1996.

Humphrey C: *Home care nursing handbook,* ed 2, Gaithersburg, Md, 1994, Aspen.

McFarland LV: Epidemiology of infectious and iatrogenic nosocomial diarrhea in a cohort of general medicine patients, *Am J Infect Control* 23:295, 1995.

Mertz HR et al: Validation of a new measure of diarrhea, *Digest Dis Sci* 40:1873, 1995.

Rice KH: Oral rehydration therapy: a simple, effective solution, *J Pediatr Nurs* 9:349, 1994.

Vogel LC: Antibiotic-induced diarrhea, *Orthop Nurs* 14:38, 1995.

Risk for disuse syndrome

Betty J. Ackley

Definition   The state in which an individual is at risk for a deterioration of body systems as the result of prescribed or unavoidable musculoskeletal inactivity (NOTE: Complications from immobility can include pressure ulcers, constipation, stasis of pulmonary secretions, thrombosis, urinary tract infection or retention, decreased strength and endurance, orthostatic hypotension, decreased range of joint motion, disorientation, body image disturbance, and powerlessness)

Risk Factors

Paralysis *(critical),* altered level of consciousness, mechanical immobilization, prescribed immobilization, severe pain

Related Factors (r/t)

See Risk Factors

Client Outcomes/Goals

• Maintains full range of motion in joints
• Maintains intact skin, good peripheral blood flow, and normal pulmonary function
• Maintains normal bowel and bladder function
• Expresses feelings about imposed immobility
• Explains methods to prevent complications of immobility

Suggested NIC Interventions

Energy management, exercise therapy: joint mobility, exercise therapy: muscle control

Nursing Interventions and Rationales

• Have client do exercises in bed if not contraindicated (e.g., flexing and extending feet and quadriceps, performing gluteal and abdominal sitting exercises, lifting small weights to maintain muscle strength).
  Unused muscles lose about one eighth of their strength for each week of bedrest; the muscles atrophy, change shape, and shorten, and muscle fatigue occurs more readily (Harper, Lyles, 1988; Corcoran, 1991). In-bed exercises help maintain muscle strength and tone (Metzler, Harr, 1996).
• If not contraindicated by client's condition, obtain referral to physical therapy to use tilt table to provide weight bearing on long bones.
  The upright position helps maintain bone strength, increase circulation, and maintain cardiovascular reflexes. The best way to prevent osteoporosis is to begin weight-bearing exercises as soon as possible (Jiricka, 1994).
• Perform range of motion exercises for all possible joints at least twice daily; perform passive or active range of motion exercises as appropriate.
  If not used, muscles weaken and shorten and are predisposed to contractures; if nonuse continues, the contracture eventually involves the tendons, ligaments, and joint capsules and limits the range of motion (Jiricka, 1994).
• Use high-top sneakers or specialized boots from the occupational therapy department to prevent footdrop; remove shoes twice daily to provide foot care.
  Such shoes help keep the foot in normal anatomical alignment; footdrop can make it difficult or impossible to walk after bedrest.
• Position client so that joints are in normal anatomical alignment at all times.
  Improper positioning can damage peripheral nerves and blood vessels as well as cause joint deformities (Metzlar, Harr, 1996).
• Get client up in chair as soon as appropriate; use a stretcher-chair if necessary.
  Almost all clients can get out of bed now with use of the stretcher-chair, which converts from a stretcher to a chair.
• Consider use of a continuous lateral rotation therapy bed.

Continuous lateral rotation therapy has been shown to be effective in preventing pneumonia in transplant clients (Whiteman, 1995) and deep vein thrombosis in spinal cord injury clients (Von Rueden, Harris, 1995).

- When getting client up after bedrest, do so slowly and watch for signs of postural hypotension, tachycardia, nausea, diaphoresis, or syncope. Take the blood pressure lying, sitting, and standing, waiting 2 minutes in between each reading.
Sitting or standing after 3 or 4 days of bedrest results in postural hypotension because of cardiovascular reflex dysfunction (Jiricka, 1994; Metzlar, Harr, 1996).
- Obtain assistive devices to help client reach and maintain as much mobility as possible.
- Turn client at least every 2 hours and carefully observe skin condition, especially bony prominences.
Turning clients is of paramount importance to prevent all of the complications of bedrest (Metzlar, Harr, 1996). Routine turning has been demonstrated to reduce the length of stay of critical care patients (Von Reudens, Harris, 1995). Systematic inspection can identify impending problems early (Bryant, 1993).
- Provide client with a pressure-relieving mattress.
Pressure-relieving mattresses that reduce pressure below 32 mm Hg prevent pressure ulcers.
- Use antiembolism stockings or a sequential compression system for legs as ordered.
Support hose help decrease edema, and thigh-high compression stockings can be effective in decreasing the incidence of deep vein thrombosis (Brock, 1994).
- Monitor peripheral circulation and especially note color, pulse, and calf or thigh swelling; check Homan's sign.
Bedrest predisposes the client to deep vein thrombosis because of venous stasis, pressure of mattress against veins, and hypercoagulability of blood (Harper, Lyles, 1988). Deep vein thrombosis may result in pulmonary embolism in an immobilized client (Metzlar, Harr, 1996).
- Have client cough and deep breathe or use incentive spirometry every 2 hours while awake.
Bedrest compromises breathing because of decreased chest expansion and decreased size of thoracic compartment; deep breathing helps prevent complications (Jiricka, 1994).
- Monitor respiratory functions, noting breath sounds and respiratory rate. Percuss for new onset of dullness in lungs.
Immobility results in hypoventilation, which predisposes the client to atelectasis, the pooling of respiratory secretions, and thus pneumonia (Corcoran, 1991).
- Note bowel function daily. Provide increased fluids, fiber, and natural laxatives such as prune juice as needed.
Constipation is common in immobilized clients because of decreased activity and food intake (Rubin, 1988).
- Increase fluid intake to 2500 ml per day within the client's cardiac and renal reserve.
Adequate fluids help prevent kidney stones and constipation and help counteract dehydration associated with bedrest (Rubin, 1988).
- Encourage intake of a balanced diet with adequate amounts of fiber and protein.
Reduced muscular activity and lowered metabolism generally reduce the appetite of a client on bedrest (Rubin, 1988).

Geriatric
- Recognize the importance of keeping elderly clients active if possible.
In the elderly, 10% to 15% of muscle strength can be lost for every week that muscles are resting completely (Mobily, Kelley, 1991).

- Keep careful track of bowel function in the elderly; do not allow client to become constipated.
  The elderly can easily develop impactions as a result of immobility.

Home Care Interventions

NOTE: Care for all body systems for the immobilized or otherwise at risk client must continue in the home as stated in the previously mentioned interventions. The primary nurse monitors and adjusts the plan of care accordingly per physician orders.

- Become oriented to all programs of care for client before discharge from institutional care. Confirm the immediate availability of all necessary assistive devices for home.
  Continuity in management of care promotes success in meeting client-centered goals.
- Perform complete physical assessment and recent history at initial visit.
  A complete assessment validates status of client on discharge or defines client problems needing immediate intervention.
- Refer to physical and occupational therapies for immediate evaluations of clients' potential for independence and functioning in the home setting and for follow-up care.
  Early identification of client needs allows for early intervention.
- Allow client to have as much input and control of the plan of care as possible.
  Client perception of control increases self-esteem and motivation to follow medical plan of care.
- Assess knowledge of all care with caregivers. Review as necessary.
  Having the necessary knowledge and skills to perform care decreases caregiver role strain and supports safety of the client.
- Support family of client in assumption of caregiver activities. Refer for home health aide services for assistance and respite as appropriate. Refer to medical social services as appropriate.

Client/Family Teaching

- Teach how to perform range of motion exercises in bed if not contraindicated.
- Teach family how to turn and position client.

NOTE: Nursing diagnoses that are commonly relevant when the client is on bedrest include **Constipation, Risk for impaired skin integrity, Sensory/perceptual alterations, Sleep pattern disturbance,** and **Powerlessness.**

REFERENCES   Bryant R, editor: *Acute and chronic wounds,* St Louis, 1993, Mosby.
Brock JD: Compression stockings: do they prevent DVT?, *Am J Nurs* 94:25, 1994.
Corcoran PJ: Use it or lose it: the hazards of bed rest and inactivity, *West J Med* 154:536, 1991.
Harper CM, Lyles YM: Physiology and complications of bedrest, *J Am Geriatr Soc* 36:1047-1054, 1988.
Jiricka MK: Alterations in activity intolerance. In Porth CM, editor: *Pathophysiology: concepts of altered health states,* Philadelphia, 1994, JB Lippincott.
Metzlar DJ, Harr J: Positioning your patient properly, *Am J Nurs* 96:33, 1996.
Mobily PR, Kelley LS: Iatrogenesis in the elderly: factors of immobility, *J Gerontol Nurs* 17:5, 1991.
Neal LJ: The bedbound home care client, *Home Healthcare Nurse* 13:77, 1995.
Olson EV et al: The hazards of immobility, *Am J Nurs* 67:780, 1967.
Rubin M: The physiology of bed rest, *Am J Nurs* 88:50, 1988.
Von Rueden KT, Harris JR: Pulmonary dysfunction related to immobility in the trauma patient, *AACN Clin Issues* 6:212, 1995.
Vorhies D, Riley BE: Deconditioning, *Geriatr Rehab* 9:745, 1993.
Whiteman K et al: Effects of continuous lateral rotation therapy on pulmonary complications in liver transplant patients, *Am J Crit Care* 4:133, 1995.

Diversional activity deficit

Betty J. Ackley

Definition   The state in which an individual experiences decreased stimulation from or interest or engagement in recreational or leisure activities

Defining Characteristics

Verbalization of boredom (critical), verbalization of desire to do something, inability to undertake usual hobbies in hospital

Related Factors (r/t)

Environmental lack of diversional activity as a result of long-term hospitalization or frequent or lengthy treatments

Client Outcomes/Goals

Engages in personally satisfying diversional activities

Suggested NIC Interventions

Recreation therapy, self-responsibility facilitation

Nursing Interventions and Rationales

- Observe for symptoms of diversional activity deficit: yawning, restlessness, flat facial expression, and statements of boredom (Radziewicz, 1992).
- Observe ability to engage in activities that require good vision and use of hands. *Diversional activities must be tailored to the client's capabilities.*
- Discuss activities with client that are interesting and feasible in the present environment.
- Encourage client to share feelings about situation of inactivity away from usual life activities.
  Work and hobbies provide structure and continuity to life; the client can feel a sense of loss when unable to engage in usual activities.
- Encourage a mix of physical and mental activities (e.g., crafts, videotapes). Provide activities that are entertaining, such as videotapes, joke books, or a "humor room."
  Humor can help clients reduce anxiety and survive in a high technology environment (Radziewicz, 1992).
- Use "bread therapy"—have clients bake bread with a breadmaker two times per day or prn.
  Assembling the ingredients is a group activity that can be therapeutic. The smell of bread baking gives a homelike, loving atmosphere to a health care environment.
- Encourage client to schedule visitors so that they are not all present at once or at inconvenient times.
  A schedule prevents the client from becoming exhausted from frequent company.
- Provide reading material, television, radio, and books on tape.
- If clients are able to write, have them keep journals; if clients are unable to write, have them record thoughts on tape.
  Keeping a journal is diversional and can also help the client deal with the many feelings that result from hospitalization or confinement. A journal can also help the client gain perspective on the situation.
- Request an occupational or art therapist to assist with providing diversional activities.
- Provide a change in scenery; get client out of room as much as possible.
  A lack of sensory stimulation and diversity have significantly adverse effects on clients (Hamilton, 1992).

- Structure the environment as needed to promote optimal comfort and sensory diversity (e.g., by having family bring in posters, banners, or a sound system; changing lighting; changing direction in which bed faces).
  Modification of the environment is sometimes necessary for the well-being of the client (Williams, 1988).
- Recommend activities in which the client can watch movement of animals and develop involvement (e.g., birdwatching, keeping a fishtank).
- Work with family to provide music that is enjoyable to the client.
  Music can help catalyze the client's own self-healing capacity (Guzzeta, 1987).
- Structure client's schedule around personal wishes for time of care, relaxation, and participation in fun activities.
  Increased client control fosters increased self-esteem.
- Spend time with the client when possible or arrange for a friendly visitor.
  Simply being available for the client as a fellow human being is important and helpful (Gardner, 1992).

Geriatric
- Encourage involvement in senior citizen activities (e.g., AARP, YMCA, church groups, Gray Panthers). Arrange transportation to activities as needed.
- Encourage clients to use their ability to help others by volunteering.
  Assisting others can help the client grow as a generative human being.
- Provide an environment that promotes activity (e.g., one that has adequate lighting for crafts, large-print books); allow periods of solitude and privacy.
  Periods of solitude are important for emotional well-being in the elderly.
- Use reminiscence and pet therapy either individually or in groups.
  Reminiscence therapy can increase social interaction, self-esteem, and self-care activities (Hamilton, 1992). Elderly individuals who have or can interact with pets are healthier and live longer.
- Refer client for logo therapy.
  Logo therapy helps the elderly determine the purpose of their lives and can therefore make their lives more meaningful.

Home Care Interventions

NOTE: Many of the previously listed interventions should be administered in the home setting (e.g., modifying the environment to stimulate the client, scheduling visitors to allow for rest and activity). Some adaptations will be necessary.

- Assess the family's ability to respond to client's psychosocial needs regarding stimulation. Assist as able.
  Individuals and caregivers provide care through the context of their own cultural experiences.
- Refer to occupational therapy to assist the client and family with identifying diversional activities within the capability of the client and family.
  Some services require the consultation of specialty prepared professionals.
- Introduce (or continue) friendly volunteer visitors if the client is willing and able to have the company.
  Simply being available for the client as a fellow human being is important and helpful (Gardner, 1992).

Client/Family Teaching

- Work with client and family on learning diversional activities that client desires (e.g., knitting, hooking rugs, writing memoirs).

REFERENCES   Friedland J: Diversional activity: does it deserve its bad name? *Am J Occup Ther* 42:603, 1988.

Gardner DL: Presence. In Bulechek GM, McCloskey JC, editors: *Nursing interventions: essential nursing treatments,* Philadelphia, 1992, WB Saunders.

Guzzetta CE: Effects of relaxation and music therapy on coronary care patients admitted with presumptive acute myocardial infarction, Grant NU-00824, Rockville, Md 1987, Department of Health and Human Services Division of Nursing.

Hamilton DB: Reminiscence therapy. In Bulechek GM, McCloskey JC, editors: *Nursing interventions: essential nursing treatments,* Philadelphia, 1992, WB Saunders.

Radziewicz RM: Using diversional activities to enhance coping, *Cancer Nurs* 15:293, 1992.

Williams MA: The physical environment and patient care, *Am Rev Nurs Res* 6:61, 1988.

Dysreflexia

Betty J. Ackley

Definition

The state in which an individual with a spinal cord injury at thoracic vertebra #7 or above experiences a life-threatening and uninhibited sympathetic nervous system response to a noxious stimulus

Defining Characteristics

Individual with spinal cord injury (T7 or above) with the following symptoms:

Major
Paroxysmal hypertension (sudden, periodic elevated blood pressure greater than 140/90 mm Hg), bradycardia or tachycardia (pulse rate of less than 60 or greater than 100), diaphoresis above the injury, red splotches on skin above the injury, pallor on skin below the injury, headache (diffuse pain in different parts of the head, not confined to any nerve distribution area)

Minor
Chilling, conjunctival congestion, Horner's syndrome (contraction of pupil on one side, partial ptosis of the eyelid, recession of eyeball into the head, occasional loss of sweating over the affected side of the face), paresthesia, pilomotor reflex ("gooseflesh" formation when skin is cooled), blurred vision, chest pain, metallic taste in mouth, nasal congestion

Related Factors (r/t)

Bladder distention, bowel distention, skin irritation, sexual stimulation, lack of client and caregiver knowledge

Client Outcomes/Goals

- Maintains normal vital signs and remains free of dysreflexia symptoms
- Explains symptoms, prevention, and treatment of dysreflexia

Suggested NIC Interventions

Dysreflexia management

Nursing Interventions and Rationales

- Monitor for symptoms of dysreflexia. See Defining Characteristics.
- Observe with physician the cause of dysreflexia (e.g., distended bladder, impaction, pressure sore, urinary calculi, bladder infection, acute abdomen, penile pressure, ingrown toenail, or other source of noxious stimuli).
  Noxious stimuli cause an uncontrolled sympathetic nervous system response (Huston, Boelman, 1995).
- Use the following interventions to prevent dysreflexia:
  - Ensure that drainage from Foley catheter is good and that bladder is not distended.

- Ensure a regular pattern of defecation to prevent fecal impaction.
  Bladder distention and bowel impaction are the most common causes of dysreflexia (Laskowski-Jones, 1993; Huston, Boelman, 1995).
- Frequently change position of client to relieve pressure and prevent the formation of pressure ulcers.
- If ordered, apply an anesthetic agent to any wound below level of injury before performing wound care.

- If symptoms of dysreflexia are present, notify physician, place client in high Fowler's position, remove all support hose or binders, monitor blood pressure every 5 minutes, and determine the identity of the noxious stimuli causing the response immediately.
  These steps promote venous pooling, decrease venous return, and decrease blood pressure. A large number of different stimuli can cause dysreflexia (Adsit, Bishop, 1995). The client should be rapidly evaluated by both the physician and nurse to find the possible cause.
- Initiate antihypertensive therapy as soon as ordered.
  A severely elevated blood pressure needs to be decreased rapidly for client safety.
- Be careful not to increase noxious sensory stimuli. If ordered, use a numbing agent on anus and 1 inch of rectum before attempting to remove a fecal impaction, spray pressure sore with a numbing agent, and also use an agent instilled into bladder.
  Increased noxious sensory stimuli can exacerbate the abnormal response and worsen the client's prognosis.
- Monitor vital signs q____h per day.
- Watch for complications of dysreflexia, including signs of cerebral hemorrhage, seizures, myocardial infarction, or intraocular hemorrhage.
  Extremely high blood pressure can cause rupture of cerebral vessels, myocardial damage, and bleeding within the eye.
- Notify all health care team members of the dysreflexia because episodes can reoccur.
  All health care personnel working with the client should be aware of the dysreflexia because symptoms could begin while the client is away from the nursing unit.
  NOTE: Recognize that dysreflexia happens when spinal shock has worn off and client is in spastic paralysis.

Home Care Interventions

- Instruct client with any known proclivity toward dysreflexia to wear a Medic-Alert bracelet and carry a Medic-Alert wallet card when not in a safe environment (i.e., not with someone who knows client has problem and can respond appropriately).
  Autonomic dysreflexia is life-threatening response.
- Establish an emergency plan: obtain physician orders for medications to be used in situations in which first aid does not work (e.g., nifedipine, nitroglycerin ointment) (Hammond et al, 1989).
  Medication administered immediately can reverse early stage dysreflexia.
- If orders have not been obtained or client does not have medications, use emergency medical services.
- If episode of dysreflexia is resolved, monitor blood pressure every 30 to 60 minutes for next 4 to 5 hours or admit to institution for observation.
  After an episode of autonomic dysreflexia, "it is not uncommon for a second episode or rebound to occur" (Hammond et al, 1989).

Client/Family Teaching

- Teach recognition of the earliest symptoms of dysreflexia, the actions that should be taken when they occur, and the need to summon help immediately.
- Teach steps to take to prevent dysreflexia episodes: bladder, bowel, and skin care and prevention of other forms of noxious stimuli, such as clothing that is too tight. *Dysreflexia can occur anytime after discharge (Spoltore, O'Brien, 1994). Prevention of dysreflexia is the most effective treatment (Nolan, 1994).*

REFERENCES   Adsit PA, Bishop C: Autonomic dysreflexia—don't let it be a surprise, *Orthop Nurs* 14:17, 1995.

Braddom RL, Rocco JF: Autonomic dysreflexia: a survey of current treatment, *Am J Phys Med Rehabil* 70:234, 1991.

Dunn KL: Autonomic dysreflexia: a nursing challenge in the care of the patient with a spinal cord injury, *J Cardiovasc Nurs* 5:57, 1991.

Finocchiaro DN, Herzfeld ST: Understanding autonomic dysreflexia, *Am J Nurs* 90:56, 1990.

Hammond M et al, editors: *Yes you can: a guide to self care for persons with spinal cord injury,* 1989, Paralyzed Veterans of America.

Huston CJ, Boelman R: Autonomic dysreflexia, *Am J Nurs* 93:22, 1995.

Laskowski-Jones L: Acute sci: how to minimize the damage, *Am J Nurs* 93:22, 1993.

Nolan S: Current trends in the management of acute spinal cord injury, *Crit Care Nurs* 17:64, 1994.

Spoltore TA, O'Brien AM: Rehabilitation of the spinal cord injured patient, *Orthop Nurs* 14:7, 1995.

Trop CS, Bennett CJ: Autonomic dysreflexia and its urological implications: a review, *J Urol* 146:1462, 1991.

Energy field disturbance

Helen Kelley and Gail B. Ladwig

Definition   A disruption of the flow of energy surrounding a person's being, which results in a disharmony of mind and spirit

Defining Characteristics

Temperature change (warmth/coolness), visual changes (image/color), disruption of the field (vacant/hold/spike/bulge), movement (wave/spike/tingling/dense/flowing), sounds (tone/words)

Client Outcome/Goals

- States a sense of well-being
- States feeling of relaxation
- Verbalizes decreased pain
- Verbalizes decreased tension
- Demonstrates evidence of physical relaxation (e.g., decreased blood pressure, pulse, respiration rate, muscle tension)

Suggested NIC Interventions

Therapeutic touch

Nursing Interventions and Rationales

- Refer to care plans for **Anxiety** and **Pain**
- Administer therapeutic touch as described in following discussion (may also include healing touch and Reiki practice).

Facilitates energy flow to restore the balance of the recipient's energy field and generalized relaxation (Benson, 1975). Therapeutic touch is the knowledgable and purposeful patterning of the patient environmental energy field process (Meehan, 1992).

Guidelines on therapeutic touch

There are two general guidelines to follow when in training for the use of therapeutic touch. It is recommended by Krieger that nurses who use therapeutic touch should have had at least 6 months of experience in an acute-care setting. Learning should be guided by a nurse who has at least 2 years of experience with therapeutic touch, preferably a Master's degree in nursing, and conforms to the practice guidelines requiring 30 hours of instruction in theory, 30 hours of supervised practice with relatively healthy individuals, and successful completion of written and practice evaluations (Kunz, Krieger, 1975-1990). It is recommended by the Nurse Healers Professional Associates that practitioners should complete a beginning workshop addressing the cognitive and therapeutic aspects of therapeutic touch. A minimum of 12 hours of instruction with a certificate of training is recommended. Family members can be instructed on basic soothing and comforting measures in less time.

- Administer therapeutic touch by performing the following steps:
  1. Centering in the present moment: Shift awareness from the physical environment to an inner focus on the center within self, a center of calm and balance through which nurses perceive themselves and the client as a unitary whole.
     The nurse' attitude becomes clear, and gentle, compassionate attention and focused intent help the client. Although there is awareness of the physical environment, it is not the primary focus (Meehan, 1992).
  2. Assessment: Pass palmar surface of hands 2 to 4 inches over the client's body from head to toe.
     Through the natural sensitivity of the hands, the nurse perceives the state of energy flow as differences in subtle sensations (e.g., congestion, pressure, warmth, coolness, or tingling). During assessment the nurse also obtains information about the client through intuitive and somatic clues (Jurgens, Meehan, Wilson, 1987). Validation study cues include heat, decreased or disrupted energy flow, cold, tingling, pulsating, congestion, heaviness, unbalance, decreased flow, and field symmetry (Mornhinweg, 1996).
  3. Treatment (unruffling): Use hands to brush or smooth out the energy flow. Sweep the hands downward and out of the field from head to toe, and concentrate on the areas of disturbance that were identified during the assessment.
     Areas of static congestion in the energy flow are relieved, and the field is prepared for the reception of healing energy. Clients mobilize their own resources for self-healing, and pain, anxiety, and discomfort are diminished (Jurgens, Meehan, Wilson, 1987).
  4. Direction and modulation of energy: Rest hands on or near the body area where a block of congestion was detected or in other areas of energy imbalance: facilitate transfer of energy to these areas.
     This step corrects energy imbalances (Krieger, 1979).
  5. Stop: Stop procedure when there are no longer any clues or when client indicates it is time to stop. Place hands over the solar plexus (just above the waist), and focus specifically on facilitating the flow of healing energy to the client.
     This final phase allows for rest and evaluation (Jurgens, Meehan, Wilson, 1987).

Home Care Interventions

- See Guidelines on Therapeutic Touch
- Help the client and family accept therapeutic touch as a healing intervention. *Consultation and collaboration with a specialist may be the best approach to nursing care.*
- Assist the family with providing an appropriate space in which therapeutic touch can be administered.

Client/Family Teaching

- Teach the therapeutic touch process to family members. *Family members can use this skill to assist with care and comfort of the client.*
- Teach that when working with the very young, old, or ill or in the head area, therapeutic touch should be gentle and only used for short periods of time. *In these circumstances the client is particularly sensitive to therapeutic touch (Boguslawski, 1980; Borelli, Heidt, 1981). Exercise caution when using therapeutic touch with patients who may exhibit an extreme sensitivity to the process (e.g., premature infants, frail elderly, psychotic clients) (Sayer-Adams, 1994).*
- Teach client how to use guided imagery. *The nurse can facilitate healing by helping the client recontact and reclaim parts of the self (resolve energy disturbance) through guided imagery (Rancour, 1994).*
- Teach the client to relax by deep breathing; ask client to have the disease, affected organ, or symptom assume an image. After the image has been identified, ask the client to speak with the image to address an unresolved issue. *By describing a previously unacknowledged part of the self, liberated energy can transform resistance, defenses, and disease into self-acceptance, peace, and wholeness (Remen, 1994).*

REFERENCES   Benson H: *The relaxation response,* New York, 1975, Avon.

Boguslawski M: Therapeutic touch: a facilitator of pain relief, *Top Clin Nurs* 2:27, 1980.

Borelli M, Heidt P: *Therapeutic touch: a book of readings,* New York, 1981, Springer.

Jurgens A, Meehan T, Wilson H: Therapeutic touch as a nursing intervention, *Holistic Nurs Pract* 2:1, 1987.

Krieger D: *The therapeutic touch: how to use your hands to heal,* Englewood Cliffs, NJ, 1979, Prentice Hall.

Kunz D, Krieger D: *Annual Invitational Workshops on Therapeutic Touch,* 1975-1990, Craysville, NY, Pumpkin Hollow Foundation.

Meehan T: Therapeutic touch. In Bulechek G, McCloskey J, *Nursing interventions: essential nursing treatments,* Philadelphia, 1992, JB Lippincott.

Mornhinweg G: Energy field disturbance—a validation study, *Healing Touch Newsletter* 6:11, 1996.

Rancour P: Interactive guided imagery with oncology patients, *J Holistic Nurs* 12:149, 1994.

Remen N: Psychosynthesis and healing, *J Holistic Nurs* 12:150, 1994.

Sayer-Adams J: Complementary therapies. therapeutic touch—a nursing function, *Nurs Standard* 8:25, 1994.

Impaired environmental interpretation syndrome

Nancy English and Betty J. Ackley

Definition Consistent lack of orientation to person, place, time, or circumstances for longer than 3 to 6 months, necessitating a protective environment

Defining Characteristics

Major Consistent disorientation in known and unknown environments, chronic confusional states

Minor Loss of occupation or social functioning from memory decline, inability to follow simple directions or instructions, inability to reason, inability to concentrate, slow in responding to questions

Related Factors (r/t)

Dementia (e.g., Alzheimer's disease, multiinfarct dementia, Pick's disease, AIDS dementia, Parkinson's disease, Huntington's disease, depression, alcoholism

Client/Outcomes/Goals

- Remains content and free from harm
- Functions at maximal of cognitive level
- Independently participates in activities of daily living at the maximum of functional ability

Suggested NIC Interventions

Dementia management, environmental management surveillance: safety

Nursing Interventions and Rationales

- Determine client's cognitive level using a screening tool such as the Mini Mental State Exam (MMSE).
  An evaluation tool such as the MMSE can help with determining the client's cognitive abilities and planning appropriate nursing interventions (Agostinelli et al, 1994).
- Determine client's background information, including social situation, physical condition, and psychological functioning before the onset of confusion.
  Knowing the client's background can help the nurse understand behavior that includes delusions or hallucinations; sharing memories can help calm the client.
- Determine client's ability to take care of self.
  Assessment of independent self-care activities including hygiene, feeding, and toileting can help the nurse plan care to support and maintain the client's independence.
- Determine the client's daily routine, including sleep-awake cycle, elimination patterns, and morning and evening routines, before the onset of confusion.
  Habitual patterns of behavior are maintained even though the client's cognition is impaired. The knowledge of these usual patterns of daily activity can help the nurse plan individualized care.
- Determine the client's special interests and hobbies before the onset of confusion.
  Knowledge of the client's interests and hobbies can help the nurse distract clients when they become fearful and agitated.
- Ensure that client is in a safe environment by removing potential hazards such as sharp objects and harmful liquids.
  Clients with dementia lose their ability to make good judgments and can easily harm themselves or others.
- Place an identification bracelet on client.
  Clients with dementia wander and may become lost; identification bracelets help increase safety.

- Help client avoid unfamiliar situations and people as much as possible by maintaining continuity of caregivers, maintaining routines of care with established meal times and activities, and having familiar person accompany client during diagnostic testing. *Situational anxiety that is associated with environmental, interpersonal, or structural change can escalate into agitated behavior (Gerdner, Buckwalter, 1994).*
- To keep the environment less stressful, avoid the use of buzzers and alarms around the client if possible. *Sensory overload can result in agitated behavior in a client with dementia.*
- Begin each interaction with client by identifying self and by calling client by name.
- Approach client with a caring, loving, and accepting attitude, and speak calmly and slowly. *Dementia clients can sense compassion; a calm, slow manner promotes a comfortable atmosphere (Stolley, 1994).*
- Touch client gently by stroking hand or arm in a soothing manner.
- Give one simple direction at a time and repeat it exactly as said if necessary. Use verbal and physical prompts, and model the desired actions if needed and possible. *"People with dementia need time to assimilate and interpret your directions. If you rephrase your question, you give them something new to process, increasing their confusion" (Stolley, 1994).*
- Break down self-care tasks into simple steps. Instead of saying, "Take a shower," say "Please follow me. Sit down on the bed. Take off your shoes. Now take off your socks. . . ." *Dementia clients are unable to follow complex commands. Breaking down the activity into simple steps makes the activity more feasible (Agostinelli et al, 1994).*
- Keep questions simple; yes or no questions are often preferable. Use positive statements and actions and avoid negative communication (e.g., if client is trying to crawl out of bed, help client do so and lead back to bed later as necessary). *Negative feedback leads to increased confusion and agitation; it is more effective to be positive and then redirect as necessary.*
- Provide boundaries by placing red or yellow tape on the floor or by using a stop sign. *Boundaries help the client identify safe areas; red and yellow are more easily seen by elderly clients.*
- Write client's name in large block letters in the room and on clothing and possessions.
- Use symbols rather than words to identify areas such as the bathroom, kitchen or bedroom.
- Limit visitors to two and provide them with guidelines on appropriate topics to discuss with client.
- Set up scheduled rest periods in a recliner or room for about 40 minutes at 10 AM and 90 minutes at 2 PM. Use afghans and environmental cues to define rest periods. *Quiet times allow the client's anxiety and building tension levels to decrease (Hall et al, 1995). Fatigue has been associated with the onset of increased confusion and agitation (Stolley, 1994).*
- In the afternoon or early evening, allow client to participate in quiet activities such as listening to classical or religious music. *An increase in confusion and agitation may occur in the late afternoon and early evening, which is referred to as* sundowning syndrome. *Quiet activities can provide a calming environment.*

- Provide open and safe areas for movement.
  Freedom of movement can help relieve the anxiety and agitation that often accompany confusion.
- Recognize that sudden changes of behavior may indicate the need for prompt attention to another underlying condition (e.g., infection, pain, change in cardiac or respiratory status).
  In the Alzheimer's client the new onset of agitated behavior is often associated with a change in physical condition (Gerdner, Buckwalter, 1994).
- Use validation techniques when client experiences an increase in fear and anxiety. For example, say, "I can see you are afraid," "I will stay with you," or "Can you tell me more about what is going on right now?"
  Such statements convey empathy and understanding and can help determine the internal stimulus that is creating the change in behavior (Feil, 1993).
- Consider using doll therapy. Ask family members to bring a large, safe doll or stuffed animal such as teddy bear.
  The use of doll therapy can be soothing to some dementia clients (Bailey, 1992; Paulanka, Griffin, 1993).
- For early dementia clients with memory loss only, see care plan for **Impaired memory.**
- For clients with agitation, see nursing interventions for **Chronic confusion.**
- For guidelines on teaching families to talk with a confused client, see interventions for **Chronic confusion.**
- For clients with self-care deficits, see **Self-care deficit: feeding, Self-care deficit: dressing,** or **Self-care deficit: toileting** as appropriate.

Geriatric   NOTE: Most of the previously mentioned interventions apply to the geriatric client.
- Use reminiscence and life review therapeutic interventions. Ask clients about a favorite Christmas or birthday or a favorite dance or type of music.
  Long-term memory is often preserved even though the client may be unable to remember current events. Reminiscence and life review can help enhance the life of an older person by decreasing depression, resocializing the client, and building relationships (Burnside, Haight, 1994).

Home Care Interventions

Clients with this syndrome are generally not safe at home and medical and psychiatric care should be sought. If the client is in the home, see home care interventions for **Chronic confusion.**

Client/Family Teaching

- Recommend that family members develop a memory aid wallet or booklet for client that has pictures and text chronicling the client's life.
  Memory aids help dementia clients make more factual statements and stay on a certain topic, and they decrease the number of confused, erroneous, and repetitive statements (Bourgeois, 1992).
- Using the previously mentioned interventions, teach family how to set up the environment and use care techniques to progressively lower the stress threshold that client will experience.
  Clients with Alzheimer's disease are unable to deal with stress; decreasing stress can decrease confusion and changes in behavior (Hall, 1991; Stolley, 1994).

NOTE: The nursing diagnoses **Impaired environmental interpretation syndrome** and **Chronic confusion** are very similar in their definitions and nursing interventions.

Impaired environmental interpretation must be interpreted as a syndrome to which other nursing diagnoses would also apply. **Chronic confusion** may be interpreted as the human response to situations that require a level of cognition that is no longer available to the individual. Further research is in progress to make this distinction clear to the practicing nurse.

REFERENCES   Agostinelli B et al: Targeted interventions: use of the Mini-Mental State Exam, *J Gerontol Nurs* 20:15, 1994.
Bailey J: To find a soul, *Nursing* 92:63, 1992.
Bourgeois MS: *Conversing with memory impaired individuals using memory aids: a memory aid workbook,* Gaylord, Mich, 1992, Northern Speech Services.
Burnside I, Haight B: Reminiscence and life review: therapeutic interventions for older people, *Nurse Pract* :55, 1994.
Feil N: *The validation breakthrough: simple techniques for communicating with people with Alzheimer's-type dementia,* Baltimore, Md, 1993, Health Professions Press.
Gerdner LA, Buckwalter KC: A nursing challenge: assessment and management of agitation in Alzheimer's patients, *J Gerontol Nurs* 20:11, 1994.
Hall GR: This hospital patient has Alzheimer's, *Am J Nurs* 91:44, 1991.
Hall GR et al: Standardized care plan: managing Alzheimer's patients at home, *J Gerontol Nurs* 21:37, 1995.
Paulanka BJ, Griffin LS: Behavioral responses of memory impaired clients to selected nursing interventions, *Phys Occup Ther Geriatr* 12:65, 1993.
Stolley JM: When your patient has Alzheimer's disease, *Am J Nurs* 94:34, 1994.

Ineffective family coping, compromised

Beverly Pickett

Definition   A usually supportive primary person (family member or close friend) providing insufficient, ineffective, or compromised support, comfort, assistance, or encouragement, which may be needed by the client to manage or master adaptive tasks related to health challenge

Defining Characteristics
Subjective   Expressed or confirmed concern or complaint by client about significant person's response to client health problem, preoccupation of significant person with personal reaction (e.g., fear, anticipatory grief, guilt, or anxiety about client's illness, disability, other situational or developmental crises), described or confirmed (by significant person) inadequate understanding or knowledge base that interferes with effective assistance or support

Objective   Unsatisfactory attempts by significant person to assist or support client, withdrawal or limited/temporary communication of significant person with the client at time of need, displayed protective behavior on part of significant person that is disproportionate to client's abilities or need for autonomy

Related Factors (r/t)
Lack of adequate or correct information or understanding by a significant person, temporary preoccupation by a significant person who is trying to manage emotional conflicts and personal suffering and cannot perceive or act effectively in regard to client's needs, temporary family disorganization and role changes, situational or developmental

crises or problems the significant person may be facing, lack of support given by client to the significant person, prolonged disease or disability progression that exhausts supportive capacity of significant person

Client Outcomes/Goals

- Verbalizes internal resources to help deal with the situation (family or significant person)
- Verbalizes knowledge and understanding of illness, disability, or disease (family or significant person)
- Provides support and assistance as needed (family or significant person)
- Identifies need for and seeks outside support (family or significant person)

Suggested NIC Interventions

Family involvement, family mobilization, family support

Nursing Interventions and Rationales

- Assess the strengths and deficiencies of the family system.
  Assessments allow for anticipatory care and guidance to help members acquire and maintain supports and coping strategies (Ducharmes, Rowat, 1992).
- Observe for cause of family problems.
  Ongoing assessment provides clues about underlying feelings (Barry, 1989).
- Assist significant person with expanding repertoire of coping skills.
  Coping skills can decrease the family's vulnerability to stress and strengthen and maintain family resources that protect the family.
- Assess how family members interact with each other.
  Understanding how families cope with stress is important. An individual's problems affect the entire family (Mears, 1990).
- Help family identify strengths and make a list that each member can refer to for positive reinforcements.
  Positive feedback from one family member reinforces a particular action or behavior of another member.
- Encourage family members to verbalize feelings; spend time with family members, sit down and make eye contact with them, and offer coffee and other nourishment.
  Acceptance of nourishment indicates a beginning acceptance of the situation.
- Talk with family about the importance of sharing feelings and ways to do so (e.g., role playing, writing a letter to significant other).
  Sharing feelings allows the family an opportunity to communicate in an effective yet nonthreatening manner.
- Involve client and family in planning of care as much as possible.
  Involving the client and family in the planned care or treatment regimen encourages compliance with treatment and enhances the client's feeling of control (Barry, 1989).
- Provide privacy during family visits; if possible, maintain flexible visiting hours to accommodate more frequent family visits.
- If possible, arrange staff assignments so the same staff members have contact with the family. Familiarize other staff members with the situation in the absence of the usual staff spokesperson.
- Determine whether family is suffering from additional stressors (e.g., child care, financial problems).
- Refer family to appropriate resources for assistance as indicated (e.g., counseling, psychotherapy, financial or spiritual support).

If family members do not know who to contact, many useful services may be underused (Mears, 1990).

- Encourage family-centered care of clients during and after discharge.
  Family-centered care supports families by building on their strengths and respecting their different coping methods (Ahmann, 1994).

Geriatric
- Assess needs of significant person and meet needs while visiting (e.g., ensure a person with diabetes eats meals).
- Assist in finding transportation to enable family members to visit.
- If family member is homebound and unable to visit, encourage phone contact to provide ongoing scheduled progress reports.

Home Care Interventions

- During time of compromised coping, increase visits to ensure safety of client, support of family, and assistance with coping strategies.
  Increased time for expressions of support and empathy can nurture the client and family and move them toward more effective coping.
- Assess the needs of the caregiver in the home. Intervene to meet needs as appropriate to total case management (e.g., add home health aide services to relieve caregiver's fatigue, give more specific information about client needs and ways to meet them).
  Meeting the need of caregivers supports their ability to meet the needs of the client.
- Refer family to medical social services for evaluation and supportive counseling.
  Dedicating time for nurturing the caregivers and reassuring the client allows them to express feelings and feel hope.
- Serve as a role model for caregiving. Write or contract for the care needed by the client.
  Concrete task definition and assignment reinforces positive coping strategies and allows caregivers to feel less guilty when tasks are delegated to multiple caregivers.
- When a terminal illness is the precipitating factor for ineffective coping, offer hospice volunteers and support groups as possible resources.
  Nonjudgmental support from helpers with no agenda allows verbalization of feelings.
- Support positive individual and family coping efforts.
  Positive feedback reinforces desired behaviors and supports the family unit.

Client/Family Teaching

- Provide information for family and significant people regarding client's specific illness or condition.
- Involve client and family in planning of care as often as possible.
- Refer to appropriate resources for assistance as indicated (e.g., counseling, psychotherapy, financial support, spiritual support).

REFERENCES   Ahmann E: Family centered care: the time has come, *Pediatr Nurs* vol 20, 1994.

Barry P: *Psychosocial nursing assessment and intervention,* Philadelphia, 1989, JB Lippincott.

Ducharmes F, Rowat K: Conjugal support, family coping behaviors and the well being of elderly couples, *Can J Nurs Res* 24:5, 1992.

Marsden A, Dracup K: Different perspectives: the effect of heart disease on patients and spouses, *AACN Clin Issues Crit Care Nurs* 2:285, 1991.

Mears D: Enhancing family coping skills, *Nurs Homes* 39:32, 1990.

Perry A, Potter P: *Fundamentals of nursing: concepts, process, and practice,* St Louis, 1993, Mosby.

Watson P: Family issues in rehabilitation, *Holistic Nurs Pract* 6:51, 1992.

Ineffective family coping, disabling

Beverly Pickett

Definition   The state in which behavior of a significant person (family member or other primary person) disables own capacities and client's capacities to effectively address tasks essential for adaptation to the health challenge

Defining Characteristics

Neglectful care of the client in regard to basic human needs or illness; distortion of reality regarding client's health problem, including extreme denial about its existence or severity; intolerance; rejection; abandonment; desertion; continuation of usual routines and disregard for client's needs; psychosomaticism; adoption of client's symptoms; family decisions and actions that are detrimental to economic or social well-being; agitation; depression; aggression; hostility; impaired restructuring of a meaningful life for self; impaired individualization; prolonged overconcern for client; neglectful relationships with other family members; client's development of helpless, inactive dependence

Related Factors (r/t)

Chronically unexpressed feelings of guilt, anxiety, hostility, or despair by the significant person; discrepancy between the significant person and client or among significant people regarding ways to cope with adaptive tasks; highly ambivalent family relationships; arbitrary handling of family's resistance to treatment, which tends to solidify defensiveness by dealing inadequately with underlying anxiety

Client Outcomes/Goals

- Expresses realistic understanding and expectations of the client (family or significant person)
- Participates positively in client's care within the limits of their abilities (family)
- Expresses feelings openly, honestly, and appropriately (significant person)

Suggested NIC Interventions

Family support, family therapy

Nursing Interventions and Rationales

- Observe for causative and contributing factors.
  Ongoing assessments provide clues about underlying feelings (Barry, 1989).
- Review the client's background.
  The client's background is largely responsible for reactions (Lipkin, Cohen, 1992).
- Identify patterns of family behaviors and interactions before the illness occurred.
  Most family members have certain roles that are disrupted by illnesses and hospitalizations; this disruption results in shifts in family functioning.
- Identify current behaviors of family members, such as withdrawal (e.g., not visiting, briefly visiting, ignoring client when visiting), anger and hostility toward client and others, or expression of guilt.
  Many of these behaviors are defense mechanisms used by the ego to protect itself until it can fully accept the implications of the illness.
- Note other stressors in family (e.g., financial, job related).
  These facts allow the nurse to develop an appropriate plan of care.
- Encourage family to verbalize feelings.
  Many families find it difficult to maintain open and empathic communication during times of acute stress.

- Provide a role model for interpersonal skills that will help the family improve their verbal interactions.
  Interpersonal skills such as warmth, friendliness, empathy, consideration, and competence are essential in promoting a therapeutic relationship.
- Provide information regarding illness and recovery of client to family.
  Families need a framework that can serve as a measure against which they can monitor progress (Northouse, Peters-Golden, 1993).
- Provide structure for family interactions (e.g., length of visiting time, number of visitors, content of interactions).
  Structure provides stability during times of stress and crisis.
- Help family identify its personal strengths.
  Individual coping skills assist in adjusting to life crises.
- Encourage family members to participate in appropriate support programs (e.g., chronic obstructive pulmonary disease [COPD], Arthritis, I Can Cope, Alzheimer's support groups).
  Direct contact establishes more open communication and facilitates an easier exchange of information (Northouse, Peters-Golden, 1993).
- Provide continuity of care by maintaining effective communication between staff members. Initiate a multidisciplinary client-care conference that involves the client and family in problem-solving.
- Explore available hospital and community resources with the family.
  Resources will provide the family with information and assistance if necessary and appropriate.
- Observe for any symptoms of elder or child abuse or neglect.
  Abuse can take several forms such as physical assaults that may or may not result in injury, verbal attacks, isolation, and social and emotional neglect.
- Prompt reporting of abuse according to local state laws is necessary.

Geriatric
- Refer family to appropriate community resources (e.g., senior centers, Medicare assistance, meal programs).
- If abuse or neglect is an issue, report it to social services.
  The purpose of protective services is to preserve the family.
- Encourage family member to participate in appropriate support groups (e.g., COPD, Arthritis, I Can Cope, Alzheimer's support groups).
  Support groups provide people with a setting in which they can discuss their illness-related problems with other people who have the same illness.
- Teach family ways to manage common problems related to normal aging.

Home Care Interventions

NOTE: This diagnosis presents the complex and difficult problem of securing an appropriate response by the family to a client's illness and caregiving needs. The same problem in the home setting creates an unusually high risk for abuse of the client. The nurse is cautioned that the margin of time for planning and effectively supporting the family unit to avoid abuse may be minimal or even negligible.
- If the client has been in an institution, establish empathetic contact with the client and family before discharge.
  Contact with the family in a nonthreatening manner helps establish a trusting relationship.
- Assess completely client's health care needs and family response at each visit.
  Assessment of the client's health status promotes early detection and treatment of

problems. Changes in the client's health status (especially any deterioration in status) can precipitate more problems with the family or caregiver and place the client at greater risk.

- Identify any changes in skills needed for client care and support caregiving efforts.
  Support from the nurse by teaching and positive feedback assists the caregivers with having a realistic perception of client expectations and shows them they are valued for efforts made.
- Refer for home health aide services when possible.
  Home health aides may be used as role models for caregiving and can observe the status of the client and family. Caution the home health aide to document objectively.
- Refer for medical social services for evaluation, supportive counseling, and assistance with community referrals.
  Dedicating time for nurturing the family and reassuring the client allows them to express feelings and develop a feeling of hope.
- When terminal illness is the precipitating factor for ineffective coping, offer hospice volunteers and hospice support groups as possible resources.
  Nonjudgmental support from helpers with no agenda and no judgment allows verbalization of feelings.

Client/Family Teaching

- Discuss with family appropriate ways to demonstrate feelings.
- Teach family the skills required for client care.
- Help family identify the health care needs of the client and family.

REFERENCES   Barry P: *Psychosocial nursing assessment and intervention,* Philadelphia, 1989, JB Lippincott.

Ducharme F, Rowat K: Conjugal support, family coping behaviors and the well being of elderly couples, *Can J Nurs Res* 24:5, 1992.

Kupferschmid B et al: Families: a link or a liability, *Families* 2:252, 1991.

Lipkin G, Cohen R: *Effective approaches to patient's behavior,* New York, 1992, Springer.

Northouse L, Peters-Golden H: Cancer and the family: strategies to assist spouses, *Semin Oncol Nurs* 9:74, 1993.

Perry A, Potter P: *Fundamentals of nursing: concepts, process and practice,* St Louis, 1993, Mosby.

Watson P: Family issues in rehabilitation, *Holistic Nurs Pract* 6:51, 1992.

Family coping: potential for growth

Beverly Pickett

Definition   Effective managing of adaptive tasks by family member who is involved with the client's health challenge and is now exhibiting desire and readiness for enhanced health and growth in relation to self and the client

Defining Characteristics

Family members attempting to describe growth aspect of crisis according to own values, priorities, goals, or relationships; family members moving in direction of a health-promoting and enriching life-style that supports and monitors maturational processes, audits and negotiates treatment programs, and generally chooses experiences that optimize wellness; individual expressing interest in making contact either with another person who has experienced a similar situation either on a one-to-one basis or in a group setting

Related Factors (r/t)

Needs sufficiently gratified and adaptive tasks effectively addressed to allow achievement of self-actualization goals

Client Outcomes/Goals

- States a plan for growth (family)
- Performs tasks needed for change (family)
- States positive effects of changes made (family)

Suggested NIC Interventions

Developmental enhancement, family support, normalization promotion, pass facilitation

Nursing Interventions and Rationales

- Observe traits family possesses that will help initiate change, such as having a positive attitude or a stating that change is possible.
  The nurse can then identify strengths on which the family may rely and weaknesses from which the family needs protection.
- Allow family time to verbalize their concerns; provide one-to-one interaction with the family.
  Interactions allow family to gather and impart information, decrease anxiety, and provide input for plan of care.
- Provide information and constructive advice about the client's illness and treatment.
  Knowledge about the illness helps assist family members with developing their coping strategies (Van Hammond, Deans, 1995).
- Have family share responsibility for change and encourage all members to have input.
  It is important to view the entire family as a system when trying to promote positive change.
- Encourage family members to write down their goals.
  The more involved the family is in goal development, the greater the probability that their goals will be achieved.
- Explore with family ways to attain their goals (e.g., adult education classes; enrichment courses; family activities such as sports, cooking, or reading; sharing time together).
- Educate client and family regarding illness and take time to answer questions.
  Empowering of family members through education increases the family's knowledge and understanding and ability to deal with the illness (Van Hammond, Deans, 1995).
- Encourage "fun-time"—a time with no tasks—to enjoy each other's company; family members might need to set up a schedule to do this because everyone is busy.
- Help family members communicate with each other using techniques they are comfortable with, such as role-playing, letter writing, or tape recording messages.
  These techniques give the family an opportunity to communicate in an effective yet nonthreatening manner.

Geriatric
- Encourage family members to reminisce with the older family member.
- Start and maintain a log of anecdotal stories about the older family member.
- Encourage children in family to spend time with and share activities with the older family member.
  These activities allow for knowledge of and respect for one another.

Home Care Interventions

The nursing interventions described previously should be used in the home environment with slight adaptations as necessary.

Client/Family Teaching

- Teach that it is normal for changes in family relationships to occur.
- Refer to parenting classes and classes for coping with older parents.
- Identify groups that discuss similar problems and concerns (e.g., Al-Anon, I Can Cope).

REFERENCES   Kupferschmid B et al: Families: a link or a liability, *Families* 2:252, 1991.

Mears D: Enhancing family coping skills, *Nurs Homes* 39:32, 1990.

Perry A, Potter P: *Fundamentals of nursing: concepts, process and practice,* St Louis, 1993, Mosby.

Van Hammond T, Deans C: A phenomenological study of families and psychoeducation support groups, *J Psychosoc Nurs* 33: 1995.

Van Watson P: Family issues in rehabilitation, *Holistic Nurs Pract* 6:51, 1992.

Altered family processes

Beverly Pickett

Definition

The state in which a normally functional family is dysfunctional

Defining Characteristics

Family system unable to meet physical, emotional, or spiritual needs of its members; parents not demonstrating respect for each other's views on child-rearing practices; family unable to express or accept a wide range of feelings; family unable to express or accept feelings of its members; family unable to meet security needs of its members; family members unable to relate to each other for mutual growth and maturation; family uninvolved in community activities; family unable to appropriately accept or receive help; family maintaining rigidity in function and roles; family not demonstrating respect for individuality and autonomy of its members; family unable to adapt to change or deal constructively with traumatic experiences; family unable to accomplish current or past developmental tasks; family using unhealthy decision-making process; family unable to send and receive clear messages; family maintaining boundaries inappropriately; family inappropriately or poorly communicating rules, rituals, and symbols; family holding on to unexamined myths; family maintaining inappropriate level and direction of energy

Related Factors (r/t)

Situational transition or crisis, developmental transition or crisis

Client Outcomes/Goals

- Expresses feelings (family)
- Identifies ways to cope effectively and use appropriate support systems (family)
- Treats impaired family member as normally as possible to avoid overdependence (family)
- Meets physical needs of members or seeks appropriate assistance (family)
- Demonstrates knowledge of illness or injury, treatment modalities, and prognosis (family)
- Participates in the development of the plan of care to the best of ability (impaired family member)

Suggested NIC Interventions

Family integrity promotion, family process maintenance, normalization promotion

Nursing Interventions and Rationales

- Observe for cause of change in family's normal pattern of functioning.
  Ongoing assessment of family members can provide important clues about a possible family disruption.
- Assess the strengths and deficiencies of the family system.
  The nurse can then help client and family with acquiring and maintaining support and coping strategies (Ducharme, Rowat, 1992).
- Discuss with the family how they have handled previous crises.
  Such a discussion gives the nurse clues and information that can help in plan of care. Families that have a broad and diverse array of coping behaviors are more likely to meet needs and have a good outcome (Coleman, Taylor, 1995).
- Spend time with family members; allow them to verbalize their feelings.
  Interactions help the client and family feel relieved and allow anxiety levels to decrease.
- Acknowledge the stages of grief when there is a change of health status in a family member; tell family members it is "normal" to be angry, afraid, etc.
  It is important to understand the wide range of feelings experienced during normal grief and to reassure those experiencing such feelings.
- Encourage family members to list their personal strengths.
  A list of strengths provides information that family members can refer to for positive feedback.
- Involve family members in the care and information/patient teaching sessions with the client.
  Family focused activities can help families cope better with the hospital experience (Worthington, 1995).
- Encourage family to visit client; adjust visiting hours to accommodate family's schedule (e.g., schedule around work, school, babysitting needs).
- Assist with sleeping arrangements if family is spending the night; provide a place to lie down, pillows, and blankets.
- Allow and encourage family to assist in the client's care.
  Assisting with client's care helps maintain family's connectedness.
- Have family participate in client conferences that involve all members of the health care team.
  Conferences allow for distribution of information, input by all members at one time, and a decrease in anxiety of family members.
- Refer to appropriate support groups if needed (e.g., counseling, social services, self-help groups, pastoral care).

Geriatric
- Teach family members about impact of developmental events (e.g., retirement, death, change in health status and household composition).
- Support group problem solving among family members and include the older or ill member.
- Refer family to counseling with a psychotherapist who is knowledgeable about gerontology.

Home Care Interventions

- Refer for or support already existing community-based family counseling.
  Family disruptions precipitating greatly altered family process may require the assistance of a specialist in family dynamics and personal thought processes.
- When terminal illness is the precipitating factor for altered family process, offer hospice volunteers and support groups as possible resources.
  Nonjudgmental support from helpers with no agenda allows verbalization of feelings and respite from caregiving.
- Provide concrete direction for caregiving while family processes disruption. Teach skills required for client care. Keep expectations of family simple and clear.
  Keeping care tasks simple or spread among multiple caregivers allows family members to dedicate energy necessary to psychological healing.

Client/Family Teaching

- Identify community agencies that might be helpful such as Meals on Wheels, Respite Care (agency that provides care for the caregiver), and I Can Cope (group for clients diagnosed with cancer).
- Teach family how to care for client and give medications and treatments.

REFERENCES   Barry P: *Psychosocial nursing assessment and intervention,* Philadelphia, 1984, JB Lippincott.

Coleman W, Taylor E: Family-focused pediatrics: issues, challenges, and clinical methods, *Pediatr Clin North Am* 42, 1995.

Ducharme F, Rowat K: Conjugal support, family coping behaviors and the well-being of elderly couples, *Can J Nurs Res* 24:5, 1992.

Kupferschmid B et al: Families: a link or a liability, *Families* 2:252, 1991.

Lipkin GB, Cohen RG: *Effective approaches to patients' behavior,* New York, 1992, Springer.

Marsden A, Drapcup K: Different perspectives: the effect of heart disease on patients and spouses, *AACN Clin Issues Crit Care Nurs* 2:285, 1991.

Mears D: Enhancing family coping skills, *Nurs Homes* July 1990, pp. 32-33.

Watson P: Family issues in rehabilitation, *Holistic Nurs Pract* 6:51, 1992.

Worthington R: Effective transitions for families: life beyond the hospital, *Pediatr Nurs* 21:8, 1995.

Fatigue

Betty J. Ackley

Definition   An overwhelming, sustained sense of exhaustion and decreased capacity for physical and mental work

Defining Characteristics

Major   Verbalization of an unremitting and overwhelming lack of energy, inability to maintain usual routines

Minor   Perceived need for additional energy to accomplish routine tasks, increase in physical complaints, emotional lability or irritability, impaired ability to concentrate, decreased performance, lethargy or listlessness, disinterest in surroundings, introspection, decreased libido, accident prone

Related Factors (r/t)

Decreased or increased metabolic energy production, overwhelming psychological or emotional demands, increased energy requirements to perform activities of daily living, excessive social or role demands, discomfort, altered body chemistry (e.g., medications, drug withdrawal, chemotherapy)

Client Outcomes/Goals

- Verbalizes increased energy and improved well-being
- Explains energy conservation plan to offset fatigue

Suggested NIC Interventions

Energy management

Nursing Interventions and Rationales

- Assess severity of fatigue on a scale of 0 to 10; assess frequency of fatigue, activities associated with increased fatigue, ability to perform activities of daily living (ADLs), times of increased energy, and usual pattern of activity.
  Such assessments establish a baseline for symptoms of fatigue (Tiesinga, Dassen, Halfens, 1996).
- Evaluate adequacy of nutrition and sleep. Encourage the client to get adequate rest. Refer to **Altered nutrition: less than body requirements** or **Sleep pattern disturbance** if appropriate.
  The most commonly suggested treatment for fatigue is rest (Nail, Winningham, 1995). Inadequate nutrition or poor sleep can contribute to fatigue.
- Determine whether there is a physiological/psychological cause of fatigue that could be treated such as anemia, electrolyte imbalance, hypothryroidism, depression, or medication effect.
  Fatigue should not be tolerated if it can be readily reversed with treatment.
- Schedule rest periods of at least 30 minutes after strenuous activity.
  Clients with fatigue need rest to recover for the next activity.
- Encourage client to express feelings about fatigue—use active listening techniques and help identify sources of hope.
  Fatigue has been associated with depression, anxiety, anger, and mood disturbances (Potempa, 1993).
- Encourage client to keep a journal of activities, symptoms of fatigue, and feelings.
  The journal helps the client monitor progress toward resolving or coping with fatigue and express feelings, which helps with adjustment (Jones, 1992).
- Assist client with ADLs as necessary; encourage independence without causing exhaustion.
- Help client set small, easily achieved short-term goals such as writing two sentences in a journal daily or walking to the end of the hallway twice daily.
- With physician's approval, refer to physical therapy for carefully monitored aerobic exercise program.
  Aerobic exercise and physical therapy can reduce fatigue in some oncology clients (MacVicar, 1989).
- Refer client to diagnosis-appropriate support groups such as National Chronic Fatigue Syndrome Association or Multiple Sclerosis Association.
  Support groups can help clients deal with bodily changes and cope with the frequent depression that accompanies fatigue (Jones, 1992).
- Help client identify essential and nonessential tasks and determine what can be delegated. Give client permission to limit social and role demands if needed (e.g., switch to part-time employment, hire cleaning service).

The nurse can help the client look at life realistically to balance available energy and energy demands.

- For cardiac client, refer to cardiac rehabilitation for carefully prescribed and monitored exercise program.
  Carefully monitored exercise is thought to decrease symptoms of fatigue in heart patients (Friedman, 1995).
- For attentional fatigue, suggest restorative activities such as sitting outside, birdwatching, and gardening (Erickson, 1996).
  Being outside and enjoying nature can help people recover their strength and think more clearly.
- Refer to occupational therapy to learn new energy-conserving ways to perform tasks.
  Occupational therapy can help clients learn how to perform ADLs without exhaustion.
- If very weak, refer to physical therapy for prescription and use of a mobility aid such as a walker.

Geriatric
- Identify recent losses; monitor for depression as a possible contributing factor to fatigue.
  Depression and fatigue are closely correlated; the elderly are more prone to depression because they frequently experience significant losses as they age.
- Review medications for side effects.
  Medications may cause fatigue in the elderly (e.g., beta blockers, antihistamines, pain medications).

Home Care Interventions

- Assess client's history and current patterns of fatigue as they relate to the home environment.
  Fatigue may be more pronounced in specific settings for physical or psychological reasons (e.g., rooms associated with loss of loved ones).
- Assess home for environment and behavioral triggers of increased fatigue (e.g., stairs required to reach bathroom, patterns of movement around home, cleaning activities that require high energy).
- When assisting client with adapting to home and daily patterns, avoid activities of high energy output. Refer to occupational therapy to accomplish this if necessary.
- Assist client with identifying or creating a safe, restful place within the home that can be used routinely (e.g., a room with familiar, nonthreatening or nonfrightening belongings).

Client/Family Teaching

- Share information about fatigue and how to live with it.
  Client education legitimizes fatigue and enhances client's control through self-care (Skalla, Lacasse, 1992).
- Teach strategies for energy conservation (e.g., sitting instead of standing during showering, storing items at waist level).
- Teach client to carry a pocket calendar, make lists of required activities, and post reminders around the house.
  Chronic fatigue is often associated with memory loss and sometimes mild confusion (Jones, 1992).
- Teach the importance of following a healthy life-style—adequate nutrition and rest, pain relief, and appropriate exercise—to decrease fatigue.
- Teach stress reduction techniques such as controlled breathing, imagery, and use of music. See **Anxiety** care plan if appropriate; anxiety is correlated with increased fatigue.

REFERENCES   Belza BL et al: Correlrates of fatigue in older adults with rheumatoid arthritis, *Nurs Res* 42:93, 1993.

Erickson JM: Anemia, *Semin Oncol Nurs* 12:2, 1996.

Friedman MM, King KK: Correlates of fatigue in older women with heart failure, *Heart Lung* 24:512, 1995.

Gift AG, Pugh LC: Dyspnea and fatigue, *Nurs Clin North Am* 28:373, 1993.

Jones CA: These patients truly need our help, *RN* 55:46, 1992.

MacVicar M: Effects of aerobic interval training on cancer patient's functional capacity, *Nurs Res* 38:348, 1989.

Milligan RA, Pugh LC: Fatigue during the childbearing period, *Res Nurs Prac* vol 33.

Nail LM, Winningham ML: Fatigue and weakness in cancer patients: the symptom experience, *Semin Oncol Nurs* 11:272, 1995.

Potempa KM: Chronic fatigue, *Annu Rev Nurs Res* 11:57, 1993.

Reeves N et al: Fatigue in early pregnancy: an exploratory study, *J Nurse Midwife* 36:303, 1991.

Skalla KA, Lacasse C: Patient education for fatigue, *Oncol Nurs Forum* 19:1537, 1992.

Tiesinga LJ, Dassen TW, Halfens RJ: Fatigue: a summary of the definitions, dimensions, and indicators, *Nurs Diagnosis* 7:51, 1996.

Fear

Pam B. Schweitzer

Definition   Feeling of dread related to an identifiable source that the person validates

Defining Characteristics

Subjective   Ability to identify source of fear, scared, rattled, wired, jittery, shaky, nervous, worried, anxious, experiencing acute feelings of helplessness or fear of specific consequences

Objective   Sympathetic stimulation (e.g., cardiovascular excitation, superficial vasoconstriction, pupil dilation, increased perspiration), hyperventilation, muscular tension, vocal and hand tremors, wide-eyed appearance, darting glances, tearfulness, insomnia, restlessness, excessive reassurance seeking, excessive self-focus, avoidance behavior

Related Factors (r/t)

Environmental stressors, hospitalization, treatments, pain, powerlessness, separation from support system, language barrier, sensory impairment, real or imagined threat to own well-being, knowledge deficit, vicarious learning, conditioned response

Client Outcomes/Goals

- Verbalizes known fears
- States accurate information about the situation
- Identifies, verbalizes, and demonstrates those coping behaviors that reduce own fear
- Reports and demonstrates reduced fear

Suggested NIC Interventions

Anxiety reduction, coping enhancement, security enhancement

Nursing Interventions and Rationales

- Assess source of fear with client.
  Fear is a normal response to actual or perceived danger and helps mobilize protective defenses.
- Discuss situation with client and help distinguish between real and imagined threats to well-being.
  The first step in helping the client deal with fear is to collect information about the situation and its effect on the client and significant others (Bailey, Bailey, 1993).

- If irrational fears based on incorrect information are present, provide accurate information.
  Correcting mistaken beliefs reduces anxiety (Beck, Emery, 1985).
- If client's fear is a reasonable response, empathize with client. Avoid false reassurances and be truthful.
  Reassure clients that seeking help is both a sign of strength and a step toward resolution of the problem (Bailey, Bailey, 1993).
- If possible, remove the source of the client's fear.
  Fear is a normal response to actual or perceived danger; if the threat is removed, the response will stop.
- If possible, help the client confront the fear.
  Self-discovery enhances feelings of control.
- Stay with clients when they express fear; provide verbal and nonverbal (touch and hug with permission) reassurances of safety if it is within control.
  The nurse's presence and touch demonstrate caring and diminish the intensity of feelings such as fear (Olson, Sneed, 1995).
- Explain all activities, procedures (in advance when possible), and issues that involve the client; use nonmedical terms and calm, slow speech, and verify client's understanding.
  Knowledge deficit or unfamiliarity is one factor associated with fear (Johnson, 1972; Garvin, Huston, Baker 1992; Whitney, 1992).
- Explore coping skills used previously by client to deal with fear; reinforce these skills and explore other outlets.
  Methods of coping with anxiety that have previously been successful are likely to be helpful again (Clunn, Payne, 1982).

Geriatric
- Establish a trusting relationship so that all fears can be identified.
  An elderly client's response to a real fear may be immobilizing.
- Monitor for dementia and use appropriate interventions.
  Fear may be an early indicator of disorientation or impaired reality testing in elderly clients.
- Provide a protective and safe environment, use consistent caregivers, and maintain the accustomed environmental structure.
  Elderly clients tend to have more perceptual impairments and adapt to changes with more difficulty, especially during an illness.
- Observe for untoward changes if antianxiety drugs are taken.
  Age renders clients more sensitive to both the clinical and toxic effects of many agents.

Home Care Interventions
- During initial assessment, determine whether current or previous episodes of fear relate to the home environment (e.g., perception of danger in home or neighborhood or of relationships that have a history in the home).
  Investigating the source of the fear allows the client to verbalize feelings and determination of appropriate interventions.
- Identify with client what steps may be taken to make the home a "safe" place to be.
  Identifying a given area as a safe place reduces fear and anxiety when the client is in that area.
- Encourage the client to seek or continue appropriate counseling to reduce fear associated with stress or to resolve alterations in thought processes.
  Correcting mistaken beliefs reduces anxiety.

- Encourage the client to have a trusted companion, family member, or caregiver present in the home for periods of time when fear is most prominent. Pending other medical diagnoses, a referral to homemaker/home health aide services may meet this need. *Creating periods of time when fear and anxiety can be reduced allows the client periods of rest and supports positive coping.*
- Offer to sit with a terminally ill client quietly as needed by the client or family, or provide hospice volunteers to do the same. *Terminally ill clients and their families often fear the dying process. The presence of a nurse or volunteer lets clients know they are not alone. Fears are reduced and the dying process becomes more easily tolerated.*

Client/Family Teaching

- Teach client the difference between warranted and excessive fear. *Different interventions are indicted for rational and irrational fears.*
- Teach client that fear itself is not dangerous and that avoidance increases fear.
- Teach client to visualize or fantasize absence of the fear or threat and successful resolution of the conflict or outcome of the procedure.
- Teach client to identify and use distraction or diversion tactics when possible. *Early interruption of the anxious response prevents escalation (Pope, 1995).*
- Teach client to allow fearful thoughts and feelings to be present until they dissipate. *Purposefully and repetitively allowing and even devoting time and energy to a thought reduces associated anxiety (Beck, Emery, 1985).*
- Teach use of appropriate community resources in emergency situations (e.g., hotlines, emergency rooms, law enforcement, judicial systems). *Serious emergencies need immediate assistance to ensure the client's safety.*
- Encourage use of appropriate community resources in nonemergency situations (e.g., family, friends, neighbors, self-help and support groups, volunteer agencies, churches, recreation clubs and centers, seniors, youths, others with similar interests).
- Teach client appropriate use of ordered medications.

REFERENCES   Bailey DS, Bailey DR: *Therapeutic approaches to the care of the mentally ill,* ed 3, Philadelphia, 1993, FA Davis.

Beck AT, Emery G: *Anxiety disorder and phobias: a cognitive perspective,* New York, 1985, Basic Books.

Bulechek G, McCloskey J: *Nursing interventions: essential nursing treatments,* ed 2, Philadelphia, 1992, WB Saunders.

Clunn PA, Payne DB: *Psychiatric mental health nursing,* Garden City, NJ, 1982, Medical Examination.

Garvin BJ, Huston GP, Baker CF: Information used by nurses to prepare patients for a stressful event, *Appl Nurs Res* 5:158, 1992.

Johnson J: Effects of structuring patient's expectations on their reactions to threatening events, *Nurs Res* 21:499, 1972.

Olson M, Sneed N: Anxiety and therapeutic touch, *Issues Mental Health Nurs* 16(2):97, 1995.

Pierce LL: Fear held by caregivers of people with stroke: a concept analysis, *Rehab Nurs Res* 3(2):69, 1994.

Pope DS: Music noise and the human voice in the nurse-patient environment, *Image J Nurs Sch* 27:291, 1995.

Rose SK, Conn VS, Rodeman BJ: Anxiety and self-care following myocardial infarction, *Issues Ment Health Nurs* 15:433, 1994.

Whitney G: Concept analysis of fear, *Nurs Diag* 3:159, 1992.

Fluid volume deficit

Martha A. Spies

Definition   The state in which an individual experiences vascular, cellular, or intracellular dehydration related to failure of regulatory mechanisms or active loss

Defining Characteristics

Change in urine output and dilution (increase in volume of dilute urine in relationship to intake if deficient antidiuretic hormone; decrease in volume of concentrated urine in relationship to intake as a response to active loss from the intravascular space; may be less intake than total output with severe active loss of fluids); increased serum osmolality (will increase with loss of fluid in excess of loss of solutes); increased serum sodium, blood urea nitrogen (BUN), hematocrit; sudden weight loss; decreased venous filling; hypotension; increased pulse rate, body temperature; decreased skin turgor, pulse volume/pressure; change in mental state (confusion); speech difficulty; thirst; dry tongue and mucous membranes; longitudinal tongue furrows; dry skin; sunken eyeballs; weakness, especially of upper body; possible weight gain, edema (with third space loss)

Related Factors (r/t)

Failure of regulatory mechanisms (e.g., diabetes insipidus or any condition resulting in polyuria), hyperosmolar imbalance, active loss (e.g., gastrointestinal losses through vomiting, diarrhea, suction, or fistulas; bleeding; third space loss; diaphoresis), insufficient fluid intake

Client Outcomes/Goals

- Maintains urine output greater than 1300 ml per day (or at least 30 ml per hour) and within 500 ml of intake *PH 7.35-7.45 PaCO$_2$ 35-45 mmHg HCO$_3$ 22-26 mEq/L PaO$_2$ 80-100 K - 3.5-5.1 mEq/L Ca 4.0-5.5 (8.9-10.1) Na 135-145*
- Maintains normal blood pressure, pulse, central venous pressure, pulmonary capillary wedge pressure, and body temperature *Hemoglobin 95-98%*
- Maintains elastic skin turgor, moist tongue, and mucous membranes; absence of longitudinal tongue furrows; capillary filling within 3 to 5 seconds, absence of thirst; normal upper body muscle strength; orientation to person, place, time; clear speech; normal eyeball turgor *Chloride 95-105 Mg 1.5-2.5 Phosphate 1.8-2.6 (all mEq/L)*
- Maintains body weight, gains 2 lbs per week until ideal body weight attained *500-800*
- Maintains serum osmolality less than 295 *280-300* mOsm/kg, urine osmolality between 100 and 800 mOsm/kg, serum sodium less than 145 mEq/L, blood urea nitrogen (BUN) less than 20 mg/dl, hematocrit less than 52% (males) or 47% (females) *Urine PH 4.6-8.0*
- Explains measures that can be taken to treat or prevent fluid volume loss; describes symptoms that indicate the need to consult with health care provider

Suggested NIC Interventions

Electrolyte management, fluid management, fluid monitoring, hypovolemia management, intravenous therapy, shock management: volume

Nursing Interventions and Rationales

- Monitor for the existence of or development of risk factors for fluid volume deficit (e.g., gastrointestinal losses, difficulty maintaining oral intake, uncontrolled type II diabetes, diuretic therapy).

  Early identification of risk factors and early intervention can decrease the occurrence and severity of complications from fluid volume deficit. The gastrointestinal system is the most common site of abnormal fluid loss (Horne, Heitz, Swearingen, 1991). Respiratory failure and coagulopathy were risk factors for gastrointestinal bleeding in a population of critically ill clients; these clients require stress ulcer prophylaxis (Cook et al, 1994).

- Monitor total fluid intake and output every 8 hours (or every hour for the unstable client) for clients with output less than 30 ml/hour or less than 1300 ml/24 hours. Watch trends in output over 3 days, include all routes of intake and output, and note color and specific gravity of urine.

  A urine output of less than 30 ml/hour is insufficient for normal renal function. Monitoring for trends will allow timely identification of serious changes that reflect kidneys' attempt to compensate for decreased intravascular volume. Dark-colored urine with increasing specific gravity reflects increased urine concentration.

- Monitor daily weight for sudden decreases, especially in the presence of decreasing urine output or active fluid loss. Weigh client on same scale with same type of clothing at same time of day, preferably before breakfast.

  Body weight changes reflect changes in body fluid volume. Clinically it is extremely important to get an accurate body weight of a client with fluid imbalance (Metheny, 1996).

- Monitor vital signs of clients at risk for fluid volume deficit every 4 hours or every 15 minutes to 1 hour for the unstable client. Observe for hypotension, postural hypotension, decreased pulse pressure, tachycardia, decreased pulse volume, and increased or decreased body temperature. When client's fluid status is unstable, monitor central venous pressure, right atrial pressure, and pulmonary capillary wedge pressure for decreases.

  Decreased intravascular volume results in hypotension and decreased tissue oxygenation. Increased body temperature is related to hypernatremia (Metheny, 1992). Hemodynamic parameters are sensitive indicators of intravascular fluid volume.

- Monitor serum and urine osmolality, serum sodium, blood urea nitrogen (BUN)/creatinine (Cr) ratio, and hematocrit for elevations.

  These are all measures of concentration and will be elevated with decreased intravascular volume.

- Monitor for decreased venous filling by observing for flat jugular veins when the client is supine and capillary refill time of greater than 3 seconds.

  Decreased intravascular volume results in increased capillary refill time; capillary refill time reflects the degree of fluid volume deficit, especially in young children (Meyers, 1995).

- Monitor for inelastic skin turgor, thirst, dry tongue and mucous membranes, longitudinal tongue furrows, speech difficulty, dry skin, sunken eyeballs, weakness (especially of upper body), and confusion.

  Tongue dryness, longitudinal tongue furrows, dryness of the mucous membranes of the mouth, upper body muscle weakness, confusion, speech difficulty, and sunkenness of eyes have the highest correlation with fluid volume deficit in the elderly (Gross et al, 1992).

- Document fluid volume status at least every 8 hours or more frequently when client's condition is unstable.

  Documentation facilitates the identification of trends in fluid balance by indicating status of condition and response to therapy.

- Use blood-conserving arterial line system for clients who require frequent blood sampling.

  The mean total volume of blood sent to the laboratory for testing in a sample of clients was 257 ml/7-day period. Using the blood-conserving arterial line system resulted in a lower mean blood discard volume of 156/7-day period when compared to the use of a conventional arterial line (Silver et al, 1993).

- Promote oral intake by providing frequent oral hygiene, oral fluids preferred by patient, (with a straw within easy reach), and fresh water (distribute over 24 hours [e.g., 1200 on days, 800 on evenings, and 200 on nights, etc.]); provide prescribed diet; offer snacks (frequent drinks, fresh fruits, fruit juice, etc.); instruct significant other to assist patient with feedings as appropriate.
  The enteral route for maintaining fluid balance is preferred (Metheny, 1996). Oral hygiene decreases unpleasant tastes in the mouth and allows the client to respond to the sensation of thirst. Distributing the intake over the entire 24 hours and providing snacks and preferred beverages increases the likelihood that the client will maintain the prescribed oral intake.
- Provide free water with tube feedings as appropriate (50 to 100 ml every 4 hours).
  This provides water for replacement of intravascular or intracellular volume as necessary.
- Institute measures to rest the bowel when client is vomiting or has diarrhea (e.g., restrict food of fluid intake when appropriate, decrease intake of milk products).
  The most common cause of fluid volume deficit is gastrointestinal loss of fluid.
- Provide oral replacement therapy as ordered with a glucose-electrolyte solution or rice syrup, solids-based solution when the client has acute diarrhea or is nauseous or vomiting. Provide small, frequent quantities of slightly chilled solutions. Administer antidiarrheals and antiemetics as appropriate. Teach proper hygiene.
  Maintenance of oral intake stabilizes the ability of the intestines to digest and absorb nutrients; glucose-electrolyte solutions increase net fluid absorption while correcting fluid volume deficit (Harig, Ramaswamy, 1989; Cohen et al, 1995).
- If client requires intravenous (IV) fluid replacement, maintain patent IV access, set an appropriate IV infusion flow rate, administer hypotonic solutions (e.g., $D_5/\frac{1}{2}NS$) or isotonic solutions (normal saline, lactated Ringer's) at constant flow rate as ordered.
  Hypotonic solutions allow intracellular rehydration (Cullen, 1992); isotonic fluids allow replacement of intravascular volume.
- When ordered, initiate a fluid challenge of crystalloids or combine crystalloid (normal saline, lactated Ringer's) and colloid (Hespan albumin) solutions for replacement of intravascular volume. If the client is hypotensive, administer volume replacement first and then vasoconstrictive medications; monitor client's response to prescribed fluid therapy and fluid challenge.
  Administration of a colloid solution facilitates the movement of fluid from the interstitial space into the intravascular space (Kaminski, Haase, 1992). Vasoconstrictive medications work poorly in clients in shock if there is systemic fluid volume deficit.
- If client requires the administration of blood or blood products, arrange for availability of blood products, prepare for administration (check blood with client identification, prepare infusion set-up, administer with normal saline), set an appropriate blood infusion flow rate, and observe for complications.
  Blood or blood products may be given to a client who is actively bleeding or has a deficit of one or more components (e.g., platelets). The product administered must be compatible with the client's blood to prevent transfusion reactions. The administration of blood products at a rate faster than the client can tolerate may result in fluid volume excess. The administration of blood or blood products can result in complications such as hemolysis and febrile and allergic reactions.

- Correct preoperative dehydration.
  Fluid volume deficit is more difficult to correct intraoperatively (Metheny, 1996).
  Thirst, drowsiness, and dizziness were significantly lower in postoperative clients when isotonic electrolyte solutions were given preoperatively before general anesthesia at a rate of 20 ml/kg over 30 minutes for short ambulatory surgery (Yogendran et al, 1995).
- Assist with ambulation if client has postural hypotension.
  Postural hypotension can cause dizziness, which places the client at higher risk for injury.
- Position client flat with legs elevated when hypotensive.
  This position enhances venous return thus contributing to the maintenance of cardiac output. ① If PH is ↓7.35 -Acidosis Above 7.45 Alkalosis
  Alkalosis - kicks PH up Acidosis kicks PH down
- Promote skin integrity (e.g., monitor areas for breakdown, note frequent weight shifts, prevent shearing, promote adequate nutrition). Position for peripheral perfusion.
  Fluid volume deficit decreases tissue oxygenation which makes the skin cells more vulnerable to breakdown. ② If PaCO₂ is ↓ 35mmHg -Resp. Alkalosis AT 45 ↑2 esp Acidosis
- Consult physician if signs and symptoms of fluid volume deficit persist or worsen.
  Prolonged fluid volume deficit increases the risk for the development of complications.

Geriatric
- Encourage fluid intake by offering fluid regularly to cognitively impaired clients.
  The elderly have a decreased thirst sensation (Metheny, 1996), and short-term memory loss may impede the client's memory of fluid intake.
- Incorporate regular hydration into daily routines (e.g., extra glass of fluid with medication or social activities). ③ If HCO₃ ↓22 - met. acidosis ↑ 26 met. acid.
  Integration of hydration into regular routines increases the chance that the client will meet the daily fluid requirements. ④ If PaCO₂, HCO₃ & BE are abnormal, with one indicating acidosis & one alkalosis, body is compen.
- Monitor elderly clients for fluid volume excess during the treatment of fluid volume deficit. ⑤ PaO₂ is 60-80 - mild hypoxemia   below 40mmHg severe Hypox.
  PaO₂ 40-60 moderate hypoxemia
  The elderly client has a decreased ability to adapt to rapid increases in intravascular volume and can quickly develop heart failure.

Home Care Interventions Hyponatremia - Na deficit in plasma (water moves from vascular space to
(Hypovolemia)   interstitial then to intracellular (signs - confusion)
- Determine the importance of fluid volume deficit to the home care client's plan of care.
  Fluid volume deficit may be a symptom of impending death in terminally ill clients, therefore treating the symptoms may not be desirable. Respiratory ① opposite Some PH↑ PCO₂↓ Alkal.
  PH↓ PCO₂↑ acids.
- Teach family how to monitor output in the home (use of commode, "hat" in the toilet, urinal or bedpan, or catheter and closed drainage). Instruct them to monitor both intake and output.
  An accurate measure of fluid intake and output is an indicator of client status. m-metab. PH↑ HCO₃↑ Alkalosis
  E-equal PH↓ HCO₃↓ Acid.
- When weighing client, use same scale each day as previously noted. Be sure scale is on a flat, not cushioned, surface. Do not weigh with scale on any kind of rug. Use bed or chair scales for clients who are unable to stand.
  An accurate daily weight is an excellent reflection of fluid balance.
- Teach family complications of fluid volume deficit and when to call physician.
- If the client is on intravenous fluids, there must be a responsible caregiver in the home. Teach caregiver administration of fluids, complications of IV administration (e.g., fluid volume overload, speed of medication reactions) and when to call for assistance. Assist caregiver with administration for as long as necessary to maintain client safety.
  Administration of IV fluids in the home is a high-technology procedure and needs sufficient professional support to ensure safety of the client.

- Identify an emergency plan, including when to call 911.
  Some complications of fluid volume deficit cannot be reversed in the home and are life threatening. Clients progressing toward hypovolemic shock should seek emergency care.

Client/Family Teaching

- Instruct client to avoid rapid position changes, especially from supine to sitting or standing.
- Teach client and family about appropriate diet and fluid intake.
- Teach client and family how to accurately measure and record intake and output.
- Teach client and family about measures instituted to treat hypovolemia and prevent or treat fluid volume loss.
- Instruct client and family about signs indicating they should contact health care provider: tongue dryness, dryness of the mucous membranes of the mouth, capillary refill longer than 3 to 5 seconds, upper body muscle weakness, confusion, speech difficulty, sunken eyes, decreased volume of urine output.

REFERENCES   Cohen M et al: Use of a single solution for oral rehydration and maintenance therapy of infants with diarrhea and mild to moderate dehydration, *Pediatrics* 95:639, 1995.

Cook D et al: Risk factors for gastrointestinal bleeding in critically ill patients, *N Eng J Med* 330:377, 1994.

Cullen L: Interventions related to fluid and electrolyte imbalance, *Nurs Clin North Am* 27:569, 1992.

Gross C, Lindquist R, Wooley A et al: Clinical indicators of dehydration severity in elderly patients, *J Emerg Med* 10:267, 1992.

Harig J, Ramaswamy K: Acute diarrhea in adults: management with emphasis on oral rehydration therapy, *Postgrad Med* 89:131, 1989.

Horne M, Heitz U, Swearingen P: *Fluid, electrolyte, and acid-base balance: a case study approach,* St Louis, 1991, Mosby.

Kaminski M, Haase T: Albumin and colloid osmotic pressure implications for fluid resuscitation, *Crit Care Clin* 8:311, 1992.

Metheny N: *Fluid and electrolyte balance: nursing considerations,* ed 3, Philadelphia, 1996, JB Lippincott.

Meyers A: Modern management of acute diarrhea and dehydration in children, *Am Fam Phys* 51:1103, 1995.

Silver et al: Reduction of blood loss from diagnostic sampling in critically ill patients in using a blood-conserving arterial line system, *Chest* 104:1711, 1993.

Yogendran S et al: A prospective randomized double-blinded study of the effect of intravenous fluid therapy on adverse outcomes on outpatient surgery, *Anesth Analg* 80:682, 1995.

Risk for fluid volume deficit

Martha A. Spies

Definition   The state in which an individual is at risk for experiencing vascular, cellular, or intracellular dehydration

Risk Factors

Extremes of age, extremes of weight, excessive losses through normal routes (e.g., diarrhea), loss of fluids through abnormal routes (e.g., indwelling tubes), deviations affecting access to or intake or absorption of fluids (e.g., physical immobility), factors influencing fluid needs (e.g., hypermetabolic state), knowledge deficit regarding fluid volume, medication effect (e.g., diuretics)

Related Factors (r/t)

> See Risk Factors

Suggested NIC Interventions

> Autotransfusion, electrolyte management, fluid management, fluid monitoring, hypovolemia management, intravenous therapy, shock management: volume

Client Outcomes/Goals, Nursing Interventions and Rationales, Client/Family Teaching

> See **Fluid volume deficit**

Fluid volume excess

Martha A. Spies

Definition   The state in which an individual experiences increased fluid retention and edema

Defining Characteristics

> Edema; effusion; anasarca; weight gain; dyspnea; orthopnea; crackles in lungs; pulmonary congestion on chest x-ray; S_3 heart sound; increased central venous pressure (CVP) and pulmonary capillary wedge pressure (PCWP); jugular vein distention; positive hepatojugular reflex; decreased serum osmolality, sodium, hematocrit, blood urea nitrogen (BUN) (except with renal failure); intake greater than output; decreased urine osmolality and specific gravity; oliguria; restlessness; anxiety; confusion

Related Factors (r/t)

> Compromised regulatory mechanism (e.g., decreased glomerular filtration rate associated with renal, heart, and liver failure), excess fluid intake, excess sodium intake

Client Outcomes/Goals

- Remains free of edema, effusion, anasarca; weight appropriate for client
- Maintains clear lung sounds, no evidence of dyspnea or orthopnea
- Remains free of jugular vein distention and hepatojugular reflex
- Maintains normal CVP and PCWP, cardiac output, and vital signs
- Absent S_3
- Maintains serum osmolality greater than 175 mOsm/kg, serum sodium greater than 135 mEq/L, hematocrit greater than 42% (males) or 37% (females), and BUN greater than 10 mg/L
- Maintains urine output within 500 ml of intake and normal urine osmolality and specific gravity
- Demonstrates no restlessness, anxiety, or confusion
- Explains measures that can be taken to treat or prevent fluid volume excess, especially fluid and dietary restrictions and medications
- Describes symptoms that indicate the need to consult with health care provider

Suggested NIC Interventions

> Fluid management, fluid monitoring

Nursing Interventions and Rationales

- Monitor location and extent of edema; use a millimeter tape in the same area each day to measure edema in extremities. Monitor for ascites by measuring abdominal girth, noting presence of shifting dullness on percussion or fluid wave with palpation. *Heart failure and renal failure are usually associated with dependent edema because of increased hydrostatic pressure; dependent edema will cause swelling in the legs and feet of ambulatory clients and the presacral region of clients on bedrest. Dependent edema was found to demonstrate the greatest sensitivity as a defining characteristic for fluid volume excess (Rios et al, 1991). Generalized edema (e.g., in the upper extremities and eyelids) is associated with decreased oncotic pressure as a result of nephrotic syndrome. Ascites is associated with portal hypertension. Measuring the extremity or abdominal girth with a millimeter tape is more accurate than using the +1 to +4 scale (Metheny, 1996).*

- Monitor daily weight for sudden increases using same scale and type of clothing at same time each day, preferably before breakfast.

  Body weight changes reflect changes in body fluid volume. Clinically it is extremely important to get an accurate body weight of a client with fluid imbalance (Metheny, 1996).

- Monitor lung sounds for crackles, monitor respirations for effort, and determine the presence and severity of orthopnea.

  Pulmonary edema results from excessive shifting of fluid from the vascular space into the pulmonary interstitial space and alveoli. Pulmonary edema can interfere with the oxygen-carbon dioxide exchange at the alveolar-capillary membrane (Metheny, 1996).

- With head of bed elevated 30° to 45°, monitor jugular veins for distention in the upright position; monitor for positive hepatojugular reflex.

  Increased intravascular volume results in jugular vein distention, even in a client in the upright position and with positive hepatojugular reflex.

- Monitor central venous pressure (CVP), mean arterial pressure (MAP), pulmonary artery pressure (PAP), pulmonary capillary wedge pressure (PCWP), and cardiac output; note and report trends indicating increasing pressures over time. Monitor vital signs; note decreasing blood pressure, tachycardia, and tachypnea. Monitor for gallop rhythms. If signs of heart failure are present, see **Decreased cardiac output.**

  Increased vascular volume with decreased cardiac contractility increases intravascular pressure. Hemodynamic monitoring had one of the highest intervention content validity scores for the hypervolemia management intervention label (Cullen, 1992). Over time, this increased pressure can result in uncompensated heart failure. Heart failure results in decreased cardiac output and decreased blood pressure. Tissue hypoxia stimulates increased heart and respiratory rates.

- Monitor serum osmolality, serum sodium, BUN/creatinine ratio, and hematocrit for decreases.

  These are all measures of concentration and will decrease (except in the presence of renal failure) with increased intravascular volume. In clients with renal failure the BUN will increase because of decreased renal excretion.

- Monitor intake and output; note trends reflecting decreasing urine output in relation to fluid intake.

  The monitoring of intake and output had one of the highest intervention content validity scores for the hypervolemia management intervention label (Cullen, 1992). Any mechanism that results in decreased glomerular filtration rate will decrease the volume of urine output in relationship to the client's intake.

- Monitor client's behavior for restlessness, anxiety, or confusion; use safety precautions if symptoms are present.

  When fluid volume excess compromises cardiac output, the client will experience tissue hypoxia; cerebral tissue is extremely sensitive to hypoxia and the client may demonstrate restlessness and anxiety before any physiological alterations occur. When the fluid volume excess results in hyponatremia, the cerebral function will also be altered because of cerebral edema (Metheny, 1992).

- Monitor for the development of conditions that increase the client's risk for fluid volume excess.

  Common causes are heart failure, renal failure, and liver failure, which all result in decreased glomerular filtration rate and fluid retention. Other causes are increased intake of oral or intravenous fluids in excess of the client's cardiac and renal reserve levels, increased levels of antidiuretic hormone (ADH), or movement of fluid from the interstitial space to the intravascular space (Horne, Heitz, Swearingen, 1991). Early detection allows the institution of specific treatment measures before the client develops pulmonary edema.

- Provide a low-sodium diet as appropriate.

  Restricting the sodium in the diet will favor the renal excretion of excess fluid. Take care to avoid hyponatremia.

- Monitor serum albumin level and provide protein intake as appropriate.

  Serum albumin is the main contributor to serum oncotic pressure, which favors the movement of fluid from the interstitial space into the intravascular space. When serum albumin is low, peripheral edema may be severe.

- Administer prescribed loop, thiazide, and/or potassium-sparing diuretics as appropriate; these may be given intravenously or orally.

  Therapeutic responses to diuretic therapy include natriuresis, diuresis, elimination of edema, vasodilation, reduction of cardiac filling pressures, decreased renal vasculature resistance, and increased renal blood flow. Additional responses to sodium depletion and diuretic therapy include increased renin and aldosterone levels and increased sympathetic nervous system activity, which can counteract the diuretic effort (Cody, Kubo, Pickworth, 1994).

- Monitor for side effects of diuretic therapy—orthostatic hypotension (especially if also receiving angiotensin-converting enzyme [ACE] inhibitors) and electrolyte and metabolic imbalances (hyponatremia, hypocalcemia, hypomagnesemia, hyperuricemia, and metabolic alkalosis)—in clients receiving loop or thiazide diuretics observe for hypokalemia. Observe for hyperkalemia in clients receiving a potassium-sparing diuretic, especially with the concurrent administration of an ACE inhibitor.

  The blood pressure reduction in response to ACE inhibitors is greater in the presence of sodium depletion and diuretic therapy. The incidence of electrolyte and metabolic imbalances ranges from 14% to 60%; the most common is hypokalemia (Cody, Kubo, Pickworth, 1994).

- Implement fluid restriction as ordered, especially when serum sodium is low; include all routes of intake. Schedule fluids around the clock, and include the type of fluids preferred by the client. Maintain the rate of all intravenous infusions carefully.

  A fluid restriction may decrease intravascular volume and myocardial workload. Overzealous fluid restriction should not be used because hypovolemia can worsen heart failure. Instituting a fluid restriction, distributing fluids over 24 hours, and using the fluid restriction when the client had hyponatremia all had high intervention content validity scores for the fluid management intervention label (Cullen, 1992). Client involvement in planning will enhance participation in the necessary fluid restriction.

- Turn clients with dependent edema frequently (i.e., at least every 2 hours).

  Edematous tissue is vulnerable to ischemia and pressure ulcers (Cullen, 1992).

- Provide for scheduled rest periods.
  Bedrest can induce diuresis related to diminished peripheral venous pooling resulting in increased intravascular volume and glomerular filtration rate (Metheny, 1996).
- Promote a positive body image and self-esteem.
  Visible edema may alter the client's body image (Cullen, 1992).
- Consult with physician if signs and symptoms of fluid volume excess persist or worsen.
  Because fluid volume excess can result in pulmonary edema, it must be treated promptly and aggressively (Cullen, 1992).

Geriatric
- Recognize that the presence of risk factors for fluid volume excess is particularly serious in the elderly.
  Decreased cardiac output and stroke volume are normal aging changes that increase the risk for fluid volume excess (Metheny, 1996).

Home Care Interventions

- Assess client and family knowledge of disease process causing fluid volume excess. Teach disease process and complications of fluid volume excess including when to contact physician.
  Knowledge of disease and complications promotes early detection of and intervention for pending problems.
- Assess client and family knowledge and compliance with medical regimen including medications, diet, rest, and exercise. Assist family with integrating restrictions into daily living.
  Knowledge promotes compliance. Assistance with integration of cultural values, especially those related to foods, with medical regimen, promotes compliance and decreased risk of complications.
- If client is on bedrest or has difficulty reclining, follow previously mentioned positioning recommendations.
- Teach and reinforce knowledge of relationships between medications. Instruct client not to use over the counter medications (e.g., diet medications) without first consulting the physician. Instruct client to make primary physician aware of medications ordered by other physicians.
  There is potential for undesirable interaction among multiple medications, especially when over the counter and other prescribed medications are not monitored.
- Identify emergency plan for rapidly developing or critical levels of fluid volume excess when diuresing is not safe at home.
  When out of control, fluid volume excess can be life threatening.
- Teach signs and symptoms of fluid volume deficit and when to call physician.
  Fluid volume balance can change rapidly with aggressive treatment.

Client/Family Teaching

- Describe signs and symptoms of fluid volume excess and actions to take if they occur.
- Teach the importance of fluid and sodium restrictions. Help client and family to devise a schedule for intake of fluids over entire day. Refer to dietitian concerning implementation of low-sodium diet.
- Teach how to take diuretics correctly: take one dose in the morning and second dose (if taken) no later than 4:00 pm. Adjust potassium intake as appropriate for potassium-losing or potassium-sparing diuretics. Note the appearance of side effects such as weakness, dizziness, muscle cramps, numbness and tingling, confusion, hearing impairment, palpitations or irregular heartbeat, and postural hypotension. Consult with health care provider before taking over the counter medications (Byers, Goshorn, 1995).

REFERENCES   Byery J, Goshorn J: How to manage diuretic therapy, *Am J Nurs* 95:38, 1995.

Cody R, Kubo S, Pickworth K: Diuretic treatment for the sodium retention of congestive heart failure, *Arch Int Med* 154:1905, 1994.

Cullen L: Interventions related to fluid and electrolyte imbalance, *Nurs Clin North Am* 27:569, 1992.

Horne M, Heitz U, Swearingen P: *Fluid, electrolyte, and acid-base balance: a case study approach,* St Louis, 1991, Mosby.

Metheny N: *Fluid and electrolyte balance: nursing considerations,* ed 3, Philadelphia, 1996, JB Lippincott.

Rios H et al: Validation of defining characteristics of four nursing diagnoses using a computerized data base, *J Prof Nurs* 7:293.

Impaired gas exchange

Betty J. Ackley

Definition

The state in which an individual experiences a decreased passage of oxygen and/or carbon dioxide between the alveoli of the lungs and the vascular system

Defining Characteristics

Confusion, somnolence, restlessness, irritability, inability to move secretions, hypercapnea, hypoxia

Related Factors (r/t)

Ventilation-perfusion imbalance

Client Outcomes/Goals

- Maintains a patent airway at all times
- Demonstrates improved ventilation and adequate oxygenation as evidenced by blood gases within client's normal parameters
- Maintains clear lung fields and remains free of signs of respiratory distress
- Verbalizes understanding of oxygen and other therapeutic interventions

Suggested NIC Interventions

Acid-base management, airway management

Nursing Interventions and Rationales

- Monitor respiratory rate, depth, and effort, including use of accessory muscles, nasal flaring, and abnormal breathing patterns.
  Increased respiratory rate, use of accessory muscles, nasal flaring, abdominal breathing, and a look of panic in the client's eyes may be seen with hypoxia.
- Auscultate breath sounds q_____h.
  Presence of crackles and wheezes may alert the nurse to an airway obstruction that may lead to or exacerbate existing hypoxia.
- Monitor client's behavior and mental status for onset of restlessness, agitation, confusion, and in the late stages, extreme lethargy.
  Changes in behavior and mental status can be early signs of impaired gas exchange (Misasi, Keyes, 1994).
- Monitor oxygen saturation continuously, using pulse oximeter. Note blood gas results as available.
  An oxygen saturation of less than 90% (normal—95% to 100%) or a Po_2 of less than 80 (normal—80 to 100) indicates significant oxygenation problems.

- Observe for cyanosis in skin; especially note color of tongue and oral mucous membranes. *Central cyanosis in tongue and oral mucosa is indicative of serious hypoxia and is a medical emergency. Peripheral cyanosis in extremities may or may not be serious (Carpenter, 1993).*
- If client has unilateral lung disease, alternate semi-Fowler's position with lateral position (with a 10° to 15° elevation and "good lung down") for 60 to 90 minutes. This method is contraindicated for clients with a pulmonary abscess or hemorrhage or interstitial emphysema. *Gravity and hydrostatic pressure cause the dependent lung to become better ventilated and perfused, which increases oxygenation (Yeaw, 1992; Lasater-Erhard, 1995).*
- If client has a bilateral lung disease, position client in either semi-Fowler's or side-lying positions that increase oxygenation as indicated by pulse oximetry. Turn client every 2 hours. Monitor mixed venous oxygen saturation closely after turning critically ill client. If saturation drops more than 9% or fails to return to baseline promptly, turn the client back into supine position and evaluate oxygen status. *Turning is important to prevent complications of immobility, but in critically ill clients with low hemoglobins or decreased cardiac output turning on either side can result in desaturation (Winslow, 1992). Critically ill clients should be turned carefully and watched closely.*
- If client is obese or has ascites, consider positioning in reverse Trendelenberg at 45° for periods of time as tolerated. *A study demonstrated that use of the reverse Trendelenberg position at 45° resulted in increased tidal volumes and decreased respiratory rates in a group of intubated patients with obesity, abdominal distention, and ascites (Burns et al, 1994; Winslow, 1996).*
- Consider positioning the client prone with upper thorax and pelvis supported, allowing the abdomen to protrude. *Pao_2 has been shown to increase in the prone position, possibly because of greater contraction of the diaphragm and increased function of ventral lung regions (Douglas, 1977; Lasater-Erhard, 1995).*
- Encourage deep breathing and coughing or use of incentive spirometry every q_____h. *Controlled coughing uses the diaphragmatic muscles, which makes the cough more forceful and effective. The incentive spirometer is an effective tool that can help prevent atelectasis and retention of bronchial secretions (Peruzzi, Smith, 1995).*
- Monitor the effects of sedation and analgesics on client's respiratory pattern. *Both analgesics and medications that cause sedation can depress respiration at times. However, these medications can be very helpful with decreasing the sympathetic nervous system discharge that accompanies hypoxia.*
- Schedule nursing care to provide rest and minimize fatigue. *The hypoxic client has limited reserves; inappropriate activity can increase hypoxia.*
- Administer humidified oxygen through appropriate device (e.g., nasal cannula or face mask per physician's order); watch for onset of hypoventilation as evidenced by increased somnolence after initiating or increasing oxygen therapy. *A chronic lung client may need a hypoxic drive to breathe and may hypoventilate during oxygen therapy.*
- Provide adequate fluids to liquefy secretions within the client's cardiac and renal reserve.
- If client is severely debilitated from chronic respiratory disease, consider use of a wheeled walker to help ambulate.

Use of a wheeled walker has been shown to result in significant decrease in disability, hypoxemia, and breathlessness during a 6-minute walk test (Honeyman, Barr, Stubbing, 1996).

- Refer to pulmonary rehabilitation team if client has chronic respiratory disease.
  This team is multidisciplinary, and working together can help make the client's life more livable (Tiep, 1993).
  NOTE: If client becomes ventilator dependent, see **Inability to maintain spontaneous ventilation.**

Geriatric
- Use central nervous system depressants carefully to avoid decreasing respiration rate.
  An elderly client is more prone to respiratory depression.
- Maintain low-flow oxygen therapy.
  An elderly client is more susceptible to oxygen-induced respiratory depression.
- Encourage client to stop smoking.
  There are substantial health benefits for elderly clients who stop smoking (Foyt, 1992).
- To maximize oxygen exchange, encourage client to sit or stand in the most upright position possible.
  The size of the chest cavity is decreased with aging.

Home Care Interventions

- Assess the home environment for irritants that impair gas exchange. Assist the client to adjust home environment as necessary (e.g., installing air filter to decrease presence of dust).
- Refer to occupational therapy as necessary to assist client with adapting to home and environment and with energy conservation.
- Assist client with identifying and avoiding situations that exacerbate impairment of gas exchange (e.g., stress related situations, proximity to noxious gas fumes such as chlorine bleach).
  Irritants in the environment decrease the effectiveness with which the client can access oxygen during breathing.
- Instruct client to keep home temperature above 68° and to avoid cold weather.
  Cold air temperatures cause constriction of the blood vessels and increased moisture, impairing the client's ability to absorb oxygen.
- Instruct client to limit exposure to persons with respiratory infections.
- Instruct family in complications of disease and importance of maintaining medical regimen, including when to call physician.
- Assess nutritional status. Instruct client to eat several small meals and use dietary supplements as necessary.
  Clients with decreased oxygenation have little energy to use for eating and will avoid meals. Malnutrition significantly affects muscle aerobic capacity and exercise tolerance in the chronic obstructive pulmonary disease (COPD) clients (Palange et al, 1995).
- Refer for home health aide services as necessary to assist with activities of daily living (ADLs).
  Clients with decreased oxygenation have decreased energy to carry out personal and role activities.
- Assess family role changes and coping ability. Refer to medical social services as appropriate for assistance in adjusting to chronic illness.
  Inability to maintain level of social involvement before illness leads to frustration and anger in the client and may create a threat to the family unit. Clients with chronic lung

problems were described as negative, helpless, confused, and socially obstreperous by their family members in one study (Leidy, Traver, 1996).
- Support family of client with chronic illness.
  Severely compromised respiratory functioning causes fear and anxiety in clients and their families. Reassurance from the nurse can be helpful.

Client/Family Teaching
- Teach client how to perform pursed-lip breathing and controlled diaphragmatic breathing. Have client watch pulse oximetry to note improvement in oxygenation with breathing techniques.
  Use of breathing techniques can help the client increase oxygenation in times of acute dyspnea.
- Teach client energy conservation techniques and the importance of alternating rest periods with activity. See nursing interventions for **Fatigue.**
- Teach importance of not smoking; be aggressive in approach and ask client to set a date for smoking cessation. Recommend nicotine replacement therapy (nicotine patch or gum). Refer client to smoking cessation programs. Encourage clients who relapse to keep trying to quit.
  All health care clinicians should be aggressive in helping smokers quit (AHCPR, 1996).
- Instruct client and family on home care regimen. Refer to social services for special home therapy if necessary.
- Instruct family regarding home oxygen therapy (e.g., delivery system, liter flow, safety precautions).
- Teach client relaxation therapy techniques to help reduce stress responses and panic attacks resulting from dyspnea.
  Relaxation therapy includes progressive muscle relaxation, autogenic techniques, visualization, and diaphragmatic breathing. This therapy can help modify the symptoms of dyspnea and help the client deal with feelings associated with the chronic disease (Jerman, Haggerty, 1993).

REFERENCES   AHCPR Guidelines, *Smoking cessation: clinical practice guideline,* 1996, US Government.

Ahrens R: Changing perspectives in the assessment of oxygenation, *Crit Care Nurse* 13:78, 1993.

Burns SM et al: Effect of body position on spontaneous respiratory rate and tidal volume in patients with obesity, abdominal distention and ascites, *Am J Crit Care* 3:102, 1994.

Carpenter KD: A comprehensive review of cyanosis, *Crit Care Nurse* 13:66, 1993.

Douglas W et al: Improved oxygenation in patients with acute respiratory failure: the prone position, *Am Rev Respir Dis* 115:559, 1977.

Epstein CD, Henning RJ: Oxygen transport variables in the identification and treatment of tissue hypoxia, *Heart Lung* 22:328, 1993.

Foyt MM: Impaired gas exchange in the elderly, *Geriatr Nurs* 13:262, 1992.

Honeyman P, Barr P, Stubbing DG: Effect of a walking aid on disability, oxygenation, and breathlessness in patients with chronic airflow limitation, *J Cardiopulm Rehab* 16:63, 1996.

Jerman A, Haggerty MC: Relaxation and biofeedback: coping skills training. In Casaburi R, Petty L, editors: *Principles and practice of pulmonary rehabilitation,* Philadelphia, 1993, WB Saunders.

Lasater-Erhard M: The effect of patient position on arterial oxygen saturation, *Crit Care Nurse* Oct:31, 1995.

Leidy NK, Traver GA: Adjustment and social behavior in older adults with chronic obstructive pulmonary disease: the family's perspective, *J Adv Nurs* 23:252, 1996.

Misasi RS, Keyes JL: The pathophysiology of hypoxia, *Crit Care Nurse* 14:55, 1994.

Palange P et al: Nutritional state and exercise tolerance in patients with COPD, *Chest* 107:1206, 1995.

Peruzzi W, Smith B: Bronchial hygiene therapy, *Crit Care Clonics* 11:79, 1995.

Winslow EH: High Fowler's won't always ease breathing, *Am J Nurs* 96:59, 1996.

Winslow EH: Turn for the worse, *Am J Nurs* 92:16C, 1992.

Yeaw P: Good lung down, *Am J Nurs* 92:27, 1992.

Grieving

Betty J. Ackley

Definition   The state in which an individual or group of individuals reacts to an actual or perceived loss, which may be a person, object, function, status, relationship, or body part

Defining Characteristics

Verbal expression of distress at loss; anger; sadness; crying; difficulty in expressing loss; alterations in eating habits, sleep patterns, dream patterns, activity levels, or libido; reliving of past experiences; interference with life function; alterations in concentration or pursuit of tasks

Related Factors (r/t)

Actual or perceived object loss that may include people, possessions, job, status, home, ideals, or parts and processes of the body

Client Outcomes/Goals

- Expresses feelings of guilt, fear, anger, or sadness
- Identifies problems associated with grief (e.g., changes in appetite, insomnia, loss of libido, decreased energy, alteration in activity level)
- Plans for future one day at a time
- Functions at normal developmental level and performs activities of daily living

Suggested NIC Interventions

Grief work facilitation, grief work facilitation: perinatal death

Nursing Interventions and Rationales

- Allow family members to participate in care of the body if desired. Help survivors say good-bye in the most loving and caring way possible.
  These experiences can help facilitate positive outcomes to grieving.
- Allow family "holding" behaviors, including taking photographs of the deceased or clipping a piece of hair.
  Holding behaviors can help the family preserve the fact and meaning of the loved one's existence (Carter, 1989).
- Help bereaved client survive during times of acute grief—ensure that client maintains proper nutrition, and help client determine a routine to make it through each day.
  A newly bereaved person can be stunned and helpless (Gifford, Cleary, 1990).
- Encourage client to share memories of the person or loss by saying, "Tell me about your wife (husband, parent)." Do an in-depth personal interview to learn about client and loved one or loss.
  A personal history can help a nurse understand the unique loss the person has experienced, the meaning of the loss to the individual, and the strengths the person brings to the situation (Solari-Twadell et al, 1995). Bereaved clients need someone to listen while they sort out the complex emotional reactions to the new reality of the situation.
- Actively listen to the client's expression of grief; do not interrupt, do not tell own story, and do not offer meaningless platitudes such as, "It will be better this way."
  These behaviors do not help and can often hurt (Gifford, Cleary, 1990).
- Encourage client to "cry out" their grief and express feelings including sadness and anger.
  Grief work is work and is best treated as an active process in which the grieving client expresses and feels the grief (Grainger, 1990).
- Help client identify previous personal coping strategies.
  Coping strategies used previously are helpful in dealing with loss.

- Refer client to spiritual counseling if desired.
  Spiritual counseling can help the client gain perspective about the loss and give comfort.
- Provide information about the grief process, including the stages of grieving (denial, anger, bargaining, and acceptance). Help client realize that the grieving process takes time and is painful.
  This information helps normalize the grief experience and provides clients with hope that they can survive (Gifford, Cleary, 1990).
- Help client determine the best way and where to find social support.
  Social support has been identified as an important predictor of positive bereavement (Cooley, 1992; Herth, 1990).
- Assess for causes of dysfunctional grieving (e.g., sudden death, highly dependent or ambivalent relationship with deceased, lack of coping skills, lack of social support, previous physical or mental health problems, death of a child).
  Life circumstances can interfere with normal grieving (Cooley, 1992; Stewart, 1995).
- Encourage family members to set aside time to talk with each other about the loss without criticizing each other or belittling others' feelings.
  Once these feelings are shared, family members can begin to accept the unacceptable (Gifford, Cleary, 1990).
- Identify available community resources, including bereavement groups from local hospitals and hospice.
  Support groups can have positive effects on bereavement outcomes (Cooley, 1992; Heiney, Dunaway, Webster, 1995; Stewart, 1995).
- Recognize times when you as a nurse are affected by loss and need grief resolution. Attend a grief resolution group, ask for help from pastoral care, speak with a kind friend who is supportive, or seek counseling.
  Nursing staff can experience unresolved grief from the death of a client or suffer other losses that require grief resolution to function effectively and be able to give to others (Hittle, 1995).

Home Care Interventions

- If the agency has served the deceased as a client, allow primary caregivers to attend services.
  Families experiencing the loss of a loved one perceive staff attendance at services as a significant statement of caring and support.
- Plan first home visit within 10 days following loss by client, guided by type of loss and schedule of family following loss.
  Support is a contributing factor to completion of grief work. The nurse can provide support and guidance.
- If the loss is a loved one, allow client to express feelings about loss through interaction with the home environment (e.g., looking at pictures, keeping special chairs or clothing).
  Symbols of the lost loved one can be comforting and allow the bereaved to accept the loss in stages.
- Refer the bereaved to hospice bereavement programs.
  Support can be provided by groups of people sharing similar pain. Bereavement programs can support the bereaved through the first full year following the loss using personal contact, telephone calls, and cards.

- Refer the client to medical social services as necessary for losses not related to deaths. *Support is helpful to grief work from all types of losses. Social workers can assist the client with planning for financial changes as a result of job losses and assist with community referrals as appropriate.*

NOTE: Grieving is not an official NANDA nursing diagnosis but is included because the authors believe that grieving is part of the normal human response to loss and that nurses can use interventions to help the client grieve. Grieving is a wellness-oriented nursing diagnosis.

REFERENCES   Carter SL: Themes of grief, *Nurs Res* 38:354, 1989.
Cooley ME: Bereavement care: a role for nurse, *Cancer Nurs* 15:125, 1992.
Gifford BJ, Cleary BB: Supporting the bereaved, *Am J Nurs* 90:49, 1990.
Grainger RD: Successful grieving, *Am J Nurs* 90:12, 1990.
Heiney SP, Dunaway C, Webster J: Good grieving—an intervention program for grieving children, *ONF* 22:649-655, 1995.
Herth K: Relationship of hope, coping styles, concurrent losses, and setting to grief resolution in the elderly widow(er), *Res Nurs Health* 13:109, 1990.
Hittle JM: Grieving together, *Am J Nurs* July 1995, pp. 55-57.
Jaffe MS, Skidmore-Roth L: *Home Health Care Plans,* ed 2, St Louis, 1993, Mosby.
Solari-Twadell PA, Bunkers SS, Wange EC et al: The pinwheel model of bereavement, *Image* 27:323, 1995.
Stewart ES: Family-centered care for the bereaved, *Pediatr Nurs* 21:181, 1995.

Anticipatory grieving

Betty J. Ackley

Definition   Intellectual and emotional responses and behaviors used by an individual to modifying the self-concept based on the perception of potential loss

Defining Characteristics

Potential significant loss, expression of distress at potential loss, denial of potential loss, guilt, anger, sorrow, choked feelings, changes in eating habits, alterations in sleep patterns, alterations in activity level, altered libido, altered communication patterns

Related Factors (r/t)

Perceived or actual impending loss of people, objects, possessions, job, status, home, ideals, or parts and processes of body (Carpenito, 1993)

Client Outcomes/Goals

- Expresses feelings of guilt, anger or sorrow
- Identifies problems associated with anticipatory grief (e.g., changes in activity, eating, or libido)
- Seeks help in dealing with anticipated problems
- Plans for the future one day at a time

Suggested NIC Interventions

Grief work facilitation, grief work facilitation: perinatal death

Nursing Interventions and Rationales

- If grief results from impending death of a loved one, allow family members to say with

loved one during the dying process if desired, and help them determine appropriate times to take breaks.
Families often feel disorganized and helpless; they need support from nurses to be with the dying person (Walters, 1995).

- Encourage family to touch dying client if they are comfortable with doing so.
Sharing personal space with touch can help establish connectedness and help with grieving (Walters, 1995).

- Encourage family members to listen carefully to messages given by the dying loved one; they may hear symbolic or obscure language referring to the dying process.
As people approach death, they develop an understanding of how their death will unfold, and they communicate this awareness in symbolic language (Callanan, 1994).

- If dying client is denying seriousness of their condition, do not negate the denial.
Denial protects clients from hopelessness and may be their coping mechanism to deal with reality. Not everyone needs to go through the stages of dying (McClement, Degner, 1995).

- Help dying client maintain hope by focusing on the moment, reviewing their assets, and maintaining important relationships.
Hope is not a cure for the dying; hope maintains a connection to the world (McClement, Degner, 1995).

- Help family members let the loved one go if appropriate; give the loved one permission to die.
Sometimes dying people wait until they know their family members are strong enough to accept the loss before they allow themselves to die (Callanan, 1994).

- Use therapeutic communication with open-ended questions such as, "What are your thoughts and fears?".
Nurses need to give a grieving client permission and opportunity to talk about the anticipated loss.

- Actively listen to client's expression of grief; do not interrupt, do not tell own story, and do not offer meaningless platitudes such as, "It will be better this way."
These behaviors do not help and can often hurt (Gifford, Cleary, 1990).

- Encourage client to "cry out" grief and express feelings including sadness or anger.
Grief work is work and is best treated as an active process in which the grieving client expresses and feels the grief.

- Encourage client to take care of any unfinished business if appropriate. Client can talk to dying person or use simulated conversations to resolve issues.
Unfinished business must be resolved before the grieving client can heal and move on (Grainger, 1990).

- Refer to spiritual counseling if desired and appropriate.
Spiritual counseling can help the client gain perspective about the loss and give comfort.

- Help client determine how to best obtain social support.
Social support has been identified as the most important predictor of positive bereavement (Cooley, 1992).

- Be honest; do not give false reassurances.

- Identify problems with eating or sleeping and intervene with suggestions as appropriate.
A grieving client can be stunned and helpless (Gifford, Cleary, 1990).

- Encourage caregiver of a dying person to live one day at a time and recognize that mourning is occurring while caring for the loved one. Help caregiver express feelings

of loss, and encourage the caregiver to practice self-care.

Caregivers grieve as they give care to the dying person and can develop an increased intimacy and involvement in the relationship, which can help them obtain a positive bereavement outcome (Brown, Powell-Cope, 1993).

Home Care Interventions

NOTE: Hospice care encourages individuals and families to experience final days in the setting of choice. All of the above interventions can and should be applied in the home setting when that is the setting of choice.

- When potential loss is of a loved one, refer grieving client to hospice volunteer services for support.

Social support has been identified as the most important predictor of positive bereavement (Cooley, 1992). Hospice volunteers are available to the grieving person and support is their only agenda.

REFERENCES   Brown MA, Powell-Cope G: Themes of loss and dying in caring for a family member with AIDS, *Res Nurs Health* 16:179, 1993.

Callanan M: Farewell messages: dealing with death, *Am J Nurs* 94:19, 1994.

Carpenito JL: *Nursing diagnosis: applications to clinical practice,* ed 5, Philadelphia, 1993, JB Lippincott.

Cooley ME: Bereavement care: a role for nurses, *Cancer Nurs* 15:125, 1992.

Gifford BJ, Cleary BB: Supporting the bereaved, *Am J Nurs* 90:49, 1990.

Grainger RD: Successful grieving, *Am J Nurs* 90:12, 1990.

McClement SE, Degner LF: Expert nursing behaviors in care of the dying adult in the intensive care unit, *Heart Lung* 24:408, 1995.

Walters AJ: A hermeneutic study of the experiences of relatives of critically ill patients, *J Adv Nurs* 22:998, 1995.

Dysfunctional grieving

Betty J. Ackley

Definition   Extended, unsuccessful use of intellectual and emotional responses used by individuals to work through modifying self-concepts on the basis of the perception of loss

Defining Characteristics

Verbal expression of distress at loss; denial of loss; excessive expression of guilt or unresolved issues; excessive anger, sadness, or crying; difficulty in expressing loss; alterations in eating habits, sleep or dream patterns, activity levels, or libido; idealization of lost object; reliving of past experiences; interference with life functions; developmental regression; labile affect; alterations in concentration or pursuit of tasks

Client Outcomes/Goals

- Expresses appropriate feelings of guilt, fear, anger, or sadness
- Identifies problems associated with grief (e.g., changes in appetite, insomnia, nightmares, loss of libido, decreased energy, alteration in activity levels)
- Seeks help in dealing with grief-associated problems
- Plans for future one day at a time; identifies personal strengths
- Functions at a normal developmental level and performs activities of daily living after an appropriate length of time

Suggested NIC Interventions

Grief work facilitation, grief work facilitation: perinatal death

Nursing Interventions and Rationales

- Assess client's grieving stage. Educate client regarding stages and emotions that accompany them.
  This information helps normalize the grief experience and provides clients with hope that they can survive (Gifford, Cleary, 1990).
- Assess for causes of dysfunctional grieving (e.g., sudden bereavement [less than 2 weeks to prepare for the oncoming loss], highly dependent or ambivalent relationship with the deceased, inadequate coping skills, lack of social support, previous physical or mental health problems, death of a child).
  Life circumstances can interfere with normal grieving and be risk factors for dysfunctional grieving (Cooley, 1992; Steele, 1992; Stewart, 1995).
- Observe for the following reactions to loss, which predispose a client to dysfunctional grieving:
  - Delayed grieving: the bereaved exhibits little emotion and continues with a busy life.
  - Inhibited grieving: the bereaved exhibits various physical conditions and does not feel grief.
  - Chronic grieving: the behaviors of the normal grief periods continue beyond a reasonable time.
  These maladaptive grief reactions indicate that the client needs help with grief work (Gifford, Cleary, 1990).
- Identify problems of eating and sleeping; ensure that basic human needs are being met.
- *Losses often interrupt appetite and sleep (Gifford, Cleary, 1990; Bateman et al, 1992).*
- Develop a trusting relationship with client by using therapeutic communication techniques.
  An accepting, trusting relationship facilitates communication and serves as a foundation for healing.
- Establish a defined time to meet and discuss feelings about the loss and to perform grief work.
- Encourage client to "cry out" grief and to talk about feelings of anger, sadness and guilt.
  Grief work is work and is best treated as an active process in which the bereaved expresses and feels the grief. Expression of guilt or anger is necessary for progressing through the grieving process and feeling better (Bateman et al, 1992).
- Help clients recognize that although sadness will occur at intervals for the rest of their lives, it will become bearable.
  The sadness associated with chronic sorrow is permanent, but as the grief resolves there can be times of satisfaction and even happiness (Grainger, 1990; Teel, 1991). Grief has a lasting nature; it changes and softens but never ends (Carter, 1989).
- Help the client complete the following "guilt work" exercises:
  - Identifying "if onlys" and putting them into perspective
  - Dealing with "I didn't do" by looking at what was accomplished
  - Forgiving self; say to client, "You are being awfully hard on yourself; try not to hurt yourself over something you could not have controlled."
  The client may need to resolve guilt before successfully grieving and moving on in life.
- Review past experiences, role changes, and coping skills.
- Help client to identify own strengths for use in dealing with loss; reinforce these strengths.

- Expect client to meet responsibilities; give positive reinforcement.
- Help client identify areas of hope in life and determine their purposes if possible.
  A significant positive relationship has been found between the level of grief resolution and the level of hope (Herth, 1990). Grieving people with little purpose in life often experience more anger than individuals with more purpose.
- Encourage client to make time to talk to family members about the loss with the help of professional support as needed and without criticizing or belittling each others' feelings about the loss.
  Once these feelings are shared, family members can begin to accept the unacceptable (Gifford, Cleary, 1990).
- Identify available community resources, including bereavement groups from local hospitals and hospice.
  Support groups can have positive effects on bereavement for both children and adults (Cooley, 1992; Heiney et al, 1995; Stewart, 1995).
- Identify whether client is experiencing depression, suicidal tendencies, or other emotional disorders. Refer for counseling as appropriate.
  Counseling, including use of relaxation therapy, desensitization, and biofeedback, in addition to traditional psychotherapy has been shown to be helpful (Arnette, 1996).
- Depression and the risk of suicide can accompany dysfunctional grieving.

Geriatric
- Use reminiscent therapy in conjunction with the expression of emotions.
- Identify previous losses and assess client for depression.
  Losses and changes in older age often occur in rapid succession without adequate recovery time. More than two concurrent losses increases the incidence of unresolved grief (Herth, 1990).
- Evaluate the social support system of elderly client. If support system is minimal, help client determine how to increase available support.
  The elderly who have poor grieving outcomes often do not live with family members and have a minimal support system.

Home Care Interventions

- Encourage the client to make choices about daily living and the home environment that acknowledge the loss.
  Helping with grief work allows client to accept reality of loss and realize that grieving is a healthy response.
- Evaluate the long-term support system of bereaved client. Encourage client to interact with the support system at defined intervals.
  Regular contact with support systems allows for regular expression of feelings and grief resolution.
- Refer to or encourage continued interaction with hospice volunteers and bereavement programs as continuing forms of support.
- Refer to medical social services, especially the hospice program social worker, for assistance with grief work.
  Consulting with or referring to specialty services is sometimes the best way to provide care.

REFERENCES   Arnette JD: Physiological effects of chronic grief: a biofeedback treatment approach, *Death Stud* 20:59, 1996.
Bateman A et al: Dysfunctional grieving, *J Psychosoc Nurs* 30:5, 1992.
Cooley ME: Bereavement care: a role for nurses, *Cancer Nurs* 15:125, 1992.

Gifford BJ, Cleary BB: Supporting the bereaved, *Am J Nurs* 90:49, 1990.

Grainger RD: Successful grieving, *Am J Nurs* 90:12, 1990.

Hainsworth MA, Eakes GG, Burke ML: Coping with chronic sorrow, *Issues Ment Health Nurs* 15:59, 1994.

Heiney SP, Dunaway NC, Webster J: Good grieving—an intervention program for grieving children, *Oncol Nurs Forum* 22:649, 1995.

Herth K: Relationship of hope, coping styles, concurrent losses, and setting to grief resolution in the elderly widow(er), *Res Nurs Health* 13:109, 1990.

Steele L: Risk factor profile for bereaved spouses, *Death Stud* 16:387, 1992.

Stewart ES: Family-centered care for the bereaved, *Pediatr Nurs* 21:181, 1995.

Teel CS: Chronic sorrow: analysis of the concept, *J Adv Nurs* 16:1311, 1991.

Altered growth and development

Peggy Wetsch

Definition   The state in which an individual demonstrates deviations from the norms of own age group

Defining Characteristics

Major   Delay or difficulty in performing skills (motor, social, or expressive) typical of age group, altered physical growth, inability to perform age-appropriate self-care or self-control activities

Minor   Flat affect, listlessness, decreased responses

Related Factors (r/t)

Inadequate caretaking; indifferent, inconsistently responsive, or multiple caretakers; separation from significant others; environmental and stimulative deficiencies; physical disability; prescribed dependence

Client Outcomes/Goals

- Describe realistic, age-appropriate patterns of growth and development (parents/primary caregiver)
- Promote activities and interactions that support age-related developmental tasks (parents/primary caregiver)
- Displays consistent, sustained achievement of age-appropriate behaviors (social, interpersonal and/or cognitive) and/or motor skills (child)
- Achieves realistic developmental and/or growth milestones based on existing abilities, extent of disability, and functional age (mentally and/or physically challenged)
- Exhibits limited temporary behavioral regression that reverses shortly after episode of illness/hospitalization (child)
- Attains steady gains in growth patterns (child)

Suggested NIC Interventions

- Developmental enhancement
- Nutritional monitoring, nutrition therapy, self-responsibility facilitation

Nursing Interventions and Rationales

NOTE: Determination of the etiology for altered growth and development is critical because it will direct the selection of interventions for treating the diagnosis. Parenting skill deficits, lack of consistency between caregivers, and hospitalization versus a chronic medical condition/developmental disability will necessitate different strategies. A hospitalization experience with regressive behaviors can be a transient occurrence as opposed to a chronic situation, which may have more severe and longer delays requiring more in-depth intervention. Parenting skills and consistent expectations between multiple caregivers can be addressed by more intensive education efforts (Stutts, 1994; Seideman, Kleine, 1995).

- Identify child at risk for or with actual developmental delays using standard developmental screening surveillance tests.
  Developmental surveillance is a flexible, ongoing process that uses both skilled observation of the child and concerns of parents, health professionals, teachers, and others to identify children at risk for variation in normal growth and development (Curry, Duby, 1994).
- Interview parents to determine risk for or actual deviations in normal development. Note and emphasize positive attributes of parents/family.
  Early intervention into developmental issues is beneficial to both parents and children and leads to improved outcomes (Curry, Duby, 1994). Accepting the family's value system with respect will support and encourage parents/family to increase their involvement (Reis, 1993).
- Compare height and weight measurements for child or adolescent to established age-appropriate norms and previous measurements over time (if available).
  This process identifies altered growth patterns and deviations from the norm (United States Department of Health and Human Services, 1995).
- Initiate referrals for a more comprehensive growth and/or development evaluation if indicated.
  Presence of a risk factor alone does not always obviate the need for referrals. The number and weight of risk factors and normal differences of each child must be considered (Curry, Duby, 1994).
- Identify coexisting health or medical conditions that may be contributing to the alteration in growth and/or development and refer to appropriate health care discipline for management.
  Treatment of underlying or coexisting conditions such as metabolic disorders, obstructive sleep apnea, parasitic infestations, or brain injury may facilitate return to previous developmental levels or growth patterns (Spahis, 1994).
- Examine parental/caregiver expectations of future learning, ability, and developmental achievements of children with developmental disabilities.
  Initiation of measures to support or enhance family/child motivation and ability increases achievement (Edwards-Beckett, 1994).
- Assist family with discerning child's regressive responses to illness, hospitalization, or chronic health conditions. Explain manifestations of regression, magical thinking, separation anxiety, and fears.
  A child may regress to prior developmental levels. Children's responses differ from adults' depending on their stage of cognitive development and prior encounters. When parents are able to attribute their child's usual reactions to stress and illness, they are better able to support the child (Ziegler, Prior, 1994).
- Provide meaningful stimulation for hospitalized infants and children.
  Stimulation is essential to the development of gross and fine-motor adaptive skills, language, and personal-social functioning in infants and children. Disruption of this process for infants, even those without preexisting developmental delays, can occur without intervention. Hospitalized infants are often subjected to understimulation or an overabundance of meaningless stimulation (Slusher, McClure, 1995).
- Engage child in appropriate play activities. Refer to play/recreational therapist (if available) for supplemental strategies.
  Play is the work of childhood. It supports the development of expanding gross and fine motor skills, social, and interactional behaviors (LeVieux-Anglin, Sawyer, 1993).
- Enlist and encourage parents and/or family involvement as participants in care, particularly for the hospitalized infants, toddlers, preschoolers or school-age children,

whenever possible without exceeding the parent/family's emotional and physical limits. *Frequent and consistent parent/family contact and care diminishes normal separation anxiety. Most infants and toddlers find this presence comforting and are better able to cope with the situation and stress (Craft, Willadsen, 1992).*

- Model age and cognitively appropriate caregiver skills by doing the following:
  - Communicating with child at an appropriate cognitive level of development
  - Giving the child tasks and responsibilities appropriate to age or functional age level
  - Instituting safety devices such as assistive equipment
  - Encouraging child to perform activities of daily living (ADLs) as appropriate

  These actions illustrate parenting and child-rearing skills and behaviors for parents and family members (McCloskey, Bulecheck, 1992).
- Furnish an environment that promotes additional sleep and rest opportunities.
  A balance of sleep, rest, and activity is essential for sustained progression of growth and development (White, 1990).

Client/Family Teaching

- Provide anticipatory guidance for parents/caregivers regarding expectations for realistic attainment of growth and development milestones. Clarify expectations and correct misconceptions.
  Parents/caregivers who understand both what is normal and realistic for their child are better equipped to provide a nurturing, supportive environment (Denehy, 1990).
- Have parents/caregivers rehearse coping strategies with approaching developmental milestones and acknowledge positive actions/behaviors.
  As children progress to another developmental stage such as adolescence, families are challenged to master developmental tasks that seem enigmatic. Anticipating and preparing can strengthen their ability to mediate situations and enhance achievement (Reisch, Forsyth, 1992).
- Teach methods of providing meaningful stimulation for infants and children.
  Stimulation is essential to the development of gross and fine-motor adaptive skills, language, and personal-social functioning in infants and children (Slusher, McClure, 1995).
- Advise client regarding activities and play, nutrition, discipline, and safety that are age appropriate and support growth and development.
  Parents are better equipped to promote the growth and development of the child (McCloskey, Bulecheck, 1992).
- Elicit involvement of parents/caregivers in social support groups and parenting classes. Furnish information about community resources.
  Support groups and other opportunities to obtain guidance serve to empower parents and clarify and reinforce knowledge and parenting skills (Kinney, Mannetter, Carpenter, 1992; McCloskey, Bulecheck, 1992).

REFERENCES   Craft MJ, Willadsen JA: Interventions related to family. In Bulecheck GM, McCloskey JC, editors: Symposium on nursing interventions, *Nurs Clin North Am* vol 27, 1992.

Curry DM, Duby JC: Developmental surveillance by pediatric nurses, *Pediatr Nurs* 20:40-44, 1994.

Denehy JA: Anticipatory guidance. In Craft MJ, Denehy JA, editors: *Nursing interventions for infants and children,* Philadelphia, 1990, WB Saunders.

Edwards-Beckett, J: Caregivers' expectations of future learning of dependents with a developmental disability, *J Pediatr Nurs* 9:27, 1994.

Kinney CK, Mannetter R, Carpenter MA: Support groups. In Bulecheck GM, McCloskey JC, editors: *Nursing interventions: essential nursing treatment,* Philadelphia, 1992, WB Saunders.

LeVieux-Anglin L, Sawyer EH: Incorporating play interventions into nursing care, *Pediatr Nurs* 19:459, 1993.

McCloskey JC, Bulecheck GM, editors: *Nursing interventions classification (NIC),* St Louis, 1992, Mosby.

Reis M: The neglected preschooler, *Can Nurse* 89:42, 1993.

Reisch SK, Forsyth DM: Preparing to parent the adolescent: a theoretical overview, *J Child Adolese Psych Ment Hlth Nurs* 5:31, 1992.

Seideman RJ, Kleine PF: A theory of transformed parenting: parenting a child with developmental delay/mental retardation *Nurs Res* 44:38, 1995.

Slusher IL, McClure MJ: Infant stimulation during hospitalization, *J Pediatr Nurs* 7:276, 1995.

Spahis J: Sleepless nights: obstructive sleep apnea in pediatric patient, *Pediatr Nurs* 20:469, 1994.

Stutts AL: Selected outcomes of technology dependent children receiving home care and prescribed child care services, *Pediatr Nurs* 20:501, 1994.

US Public Health Service: Body measurement, *J Am Acad Nurs Pediatr* 7:339, 1995.

White MA et al: Sleep onset latency and distress in hospitalized children, *Nurs Res* 39:134, 1990.

Ziegler DB, Prior MM: Preparation for surgery and adjustment to hospitalization, *Nurs Clin North Am,* 29:655, 1994.

Altered health maintenance

Suzanne Skowronski

Definition   The inability to identify, manage, or seek out help to maintain health

Defining Characteristics

Lack of knowledge regarding basic health practices; lack of adaptive behaviors to internal and external environmental changes; inability to take responsibility for meeting basic health practices in any or all functional pattern areas; history of lack of health-seeking behavior; expressed interest in improving health behaviors; lack of equipment, finances, and other resources; impaired personal support systems

Related Factors (r/t)

Lack of or significant alteration in communication skills (written, verbal, or gestural), inability to make deliberate and thoughtful judgments, perceptual-cognitive impairment (complete or partial lack of gross or fine motor skills), ineffective individual coping, dysfunctional grieving, unachieved developmental tasks, ineffective family coping, disabling spiritual distress, lack of material resources

Client Outcomes/Goals

- Discusses fear of or blocks to implementing a health regimen
- Follows mutually agreed on health care maintenance plan
- Meets goals for health care maintenance

Suggested NIC Interventions

Health system guidance, support system enhancement

Nursing Interventions and Rationales

- Assess client's feelings, values, and reasons for not following prescribed plan of care; see related factors.
  "When individual rights for autonomy and control of one's own life are recognized, strengths can be developed, even in limited cases" (Jones, Meleis, 1993).
- Encourage client to share feelings about change in health status and its effects on life.
  "Perceived benefits of a specific behavior are positively correlated with implementation of that behavior" (Gillis, 1993).

- Help client determine how to arrange a daily schedule that incorporates the new health care regimen (e.g., taking pills before meals).
- Determine what the client believes to be the most important aspect of the health care plan; start education and reinforcement in that area.
  "Self efficacy is the strongest determinant of participating in a health-promoting life style" (Gillis, 1992). Clients engage in health behaviors that they find relevant and acceptable (Pender, 1987).
- Refer to social services for financial assistance if needed.
- Identify support groups related to the disease process (e.g., Reach to Recovery for a mastectomy client).
- Have client identify at least two significant support people and have them attend teaching sessions if possible.
- Refer client to community agencies for appropriate follow-up care (e.g., day treatment or adult day health program).
  Social support affects health by fostering meaning in life, facilitating health-promoting behaviors, and regulating thoughts toward health. Increased social support has been related to a reduction in mortality rates and incidences of physical and mental illness (Callaghan, Morrissey, 1993).
- Obtain or design educational material that is appropriate for the client, using pictures if possible.
  An inadequate reading level may be significant barrier to patients' understanding of their diagnosis and treatments. Medical information on a fourth-grade reading level may even be a barrier (Williams, 1995). The three major learning styles are visual (seeing), aural (listening), and psychomotor (experiencing).
- Make sure follow-up appointments are scheduled before client is discharged; discuss a way to ensure that appointments are kept.
  Many people do not complete organized programs and many others do not maintain newly adopted health behaviors. Direct attention toward preventing relapse tendencies (Redland, Stuifbergen, 1993).

Geriatric
- Assess sensory deficits and psychomotor skills in terms of client's ability to comply with a health program.
  "Reactions to common danger signals such as smoke or rotten food are impaired because there has not been appropriate intensity of stimuli due to loss of receptors in aging" (Edelman, Mandle, 1990).
- Recognize any resistance to change in lifelong patterns of personal health care.
  "Problem solving, managing identical prescriptions from different physicians, communicating effectively with health care providers about medications, managing medications during lifestyle changes all contribute to compliance issues" (Conn, 1991). Change in one aspect of life can precipitate adjustment in all other aspects.
- Provide aids to assist with compliance (e.g., prepare medication schedules and put week's medications in daily containers).
- Discuss with client realistic goals for changes in health maintenance.
  The focus of a chronic illness may be care rather than cure.

Home Care Interventions
- If the client is returning home from institutional care, reaffirm client priorities for health maintenance.
  Clients will pursue desired health actions based on perceptions of susceptibility and severity if the cost is not greater than the benefit (Rosenstock, 1974).

- Provide sufficient outside supports (e.g., written notices, calendars, planned ride shares) to assist with follow-through of the agreed-on actions.
  Cues play a significant role in stimulating completion of desired health actions.
- Refer to medical social services to resolve conflicts about illness or condition.
  Medical social services can provide structured support for conflict resolution.
- Meet with client following the proposed actions to review the contract and determine the next course of action. Do this until the client is able to initiate and follow through independently.
  Successful completion of contracts promotes improved self-esteem and positive coping.

Client/Family Teaching

- Teach client and family prescribed health care treatments (e.g., medications, treatments, diet, activities of daily living, methods of coping, seeking help when necessary).
  "Social support has been related to reduction in mortality rates and the incidence of both mental and physical illness" (Callaghan, Morrissey, 1993).
- Have client and family demonstrate at least twice any procedures to be done at home.
  Practice of a procedure exposes problems, enhances skill levels, and promotes confidence in new behaviors.
- Explain nonthreatening material before introducing more anxiety producing.
  Anxiety focuses attention, so anxious clients may perceive details as more important than the overall health-maintenance program.
- Establish a written contract with client to follow the agreed-on health care regimen.
  "Individuals fall into old behavior patterns when confronted with situations promoting the former patterns" (Redland, Stuifbergen, 1993). Written agreements reinforce the verbal agreement and serve as a reference.

REFERENCES Callaghan P, Morrissey G: Social support and health: a review, *J Adv Nurs* 203:18, 1993.
Conn V et al: Medication regimen complexity and adherence among older adults, *Image* 23:231, 1991.
Edelman C, Mandle C. *Health promotion throughout the lifespan*, St Louis, 1990, Mosby.
Gillis A: Determinants of a health-promoting lifestyle: an integrative review, *J Adv Nurs* 18:345, 1993.
Jones P, Meleis A: Health is empowerment, *Adv Nurs Sci* 1:1-14, 1993.
Pender N: *Health promotion in nursing practice*, ed 2, Norwalk, Conn, 1987, Appleton & Lange.
Redland A, Stuifbergen A: Strategies for maintenance of health promoting behaviors, *Nurs Clin North Am* 28:427, 1993.
Rosenstock I: Health belief model and preventive behavior. In Becker M, editor: *The health belief model and personal health behavior*, Thorofare, NJ, 1974, CB Slack.
Williams M, et al: Inadequate functional health literacy among patients at two public hospitals, *JAMA* 274:1677, 1995.

Health-seeking behaviors

Suzanne Skowronski

Definition The state in which an individual in stable health actively seeks ways to alter personal health habits or the environment to move toward a higher level of health
NOTE: *Stable health status* is defined as the achievement of age-appropriate illness prevention measures, a client's report of good or excellent health, and the control of any signs and symptoms of disease.

Defining Characteristics
Major Expressed or observed desire to seek a higher level of wellness for self or family

Minor   Expressed or observed desire for increased control of health practice, expressed concern about the effect of current environmental conditions on health status, stated or observed unfamiliarity with wellness community resources, demonstrated or observed lack of knowledge regarding health-promoting behaviors

Related Factors (r/t)

Role change; change in developmental level (e.g., marriage, parenthood, "empty-nest" syndrome, retirement); lack of knowledge regarding the need for preventive health behaviors, appropriate health screenings, optimal nutrition, weight control, regular exercise programs, stress management, supportive social networks, and responsible role participation

Client Outcomes/Goals

- Maintains ideal weight and is knowledgeable about nutritious diet
- Explains ways to fit newly prescribed change in health habits into life-style
- Lists community resources available for assistance in achieving wellness ✓
- Explains ways to include wellness behaviors in current life-style ✓

Suggested NIC Interventions

Health education, self-modification assistance

Nursing Interventions and Rationales

- Determine health habits of client and family (e.g., diet, exercise, sleep, smoking, alcohol intake, stress levels).
  "Holistic health integrates body-mind-spirit lived within a supportive environmental system" (Edelman, Mandle, 1990).
- Determine with client the most important wellness behavior on which to work. ✓
  The client is individually responsible for coping and maintaining health (Jones, Meleis, 1990). "Facilitating empowerment begins with helping individuals develop a critical awareness of their situation and enabling them to master their environment to achieve self-determination" (Jones, Meleis, 1990).
- Identify environmental and social factors that the client perceives as health promoting. ✓
  "Exposure to a health-promoting environment had statistically significant direct and indirect effects" (Conrad et al, 1996).

Nutrition
- Determine client's height and weight; compare with recommended weight for age or height.
- Encourage a diet low in salt, fat, sugar, and preservatives; encourage an appropriate intake of complex carbohydrates, fruits, vegetables, protein, and fat.
  Dietary intake provides nutrients that promote wellness, prevent illness, and enhance the social quality of life (Edelman, Mandle, 1990).
- Refer client to dietician or weight-loss program for further assessment of diet and help with compliance.

Exercise
- Determine amount of exercise client needs per week and ability to tolerate exercise; refer client to physician for testing to determine ability to tolerate exercise.
- Explore weightlifting options with client to increase muscle strength and stamina.
- Help client to focus on the enjoyment of exercise; set up a support and reward system.
  "Older men whose health is not good are less likely to engage in exercise and nutrition health promotion despite high income or high self-esteem" (Duffy, 1993). "Men evaluated exercise less positively than women, yet participate at considerably higher levels. Social

influences to exercise increase with age in men, but not in women. As women age, the receive less social influence to motivate them to exercise" (Hawkes, 1993).

- Encourage aerobic exercise that increase heart rate within the prescribed limit; encourage ✓ client to exercise at least 3 times per week for 20 or more minutes using exercises that the client prefers (e.g., walking, jogging, aerobics, swimming, bicycling, yoga, Tai Chi). *Exercise should involve large-muscle groups, last for about 20 minutes 3 times a week, and use 60% of a client's cardiorespiratory capacity (Emmunds, 1991).*

Stress management

- Ask client to define stress in terms of life-style events, and assign the events a value on a scale from one to five.
  This exercise helps distinguish between anxiety as a personality trait and anxiety as a coping response toward threatening events.
- Determine usual ways in which the client relieves stress, and evaluate their effectiveness.
  "A combination of stress management techniques was found more effective than one technique (muscle relaxation) with medication management in the care of patients with essential hypertension" (Bok Han, 1993).
- Determine client's social support network.
- Determine amount of personal time client has; if necessary, decide how this time can be increased.
- Teach stress-relieving techniques (e.g., deep and slow breathing, progressive muscle relaxation, exercise, meditation, power strategies, problem solving, imagery, verbalization of feelings, spiritual practices [prayer]).
  Stress management addresses the sources of tension in physical performance, emotional expression, transcendent spiritual experiences, social relationships, and the surrounding environment.

Smoking, drinking, self-medication

- Determine the frequency of risk-taking habits.
- Refer smokers to Smoke Enders or a similar community-based program; discuss ways in which client can deal with loss of the behavioral habit or addiction.
  "Although complete cessation of smoking is preferred, sustained reduction is likely to reduce the risk of disease and is a valuable public health outcome" (Wakefield et al, 1992).
- Refer clients who drink excessively to Alcoholics Anonymous. Identify a support person to help client into the organization.
  "Post treatment from alcohol use is a major life transition that requires extensive coping efforts, social support, and environmental control" (Murphy, 1993).
- Discuss whether a significant other's excessive alcohol consumption is a family- or work-related problem. Refer client to Alcoholics Anonymous.
  "Attention needs to be directed to family adjustment factors. Women recovering from alcohol abuse are at risk for relapse if their spouse continues to drink alcohol" (Murphy, 1993).
- Identify patterns of self-medication (e.g., antibiotics, mood-altering drugs).
  Excessive alcohol intake, cigarette smoking, and self-administered use of mood-altering drugs affects major body organs and predisposes the client to a chronic or life-threatening illness.

Health-seeking behaviors

- Teach stress-relieving techniques (e.g., deep and slow breathing, progressive muscle relaxation, exercise, medication, power strategies, problem solving, imagery, verbalization of feelings, spiritual practice [prayer]).

Stress management addresses the sources of tension in physical performance, emotional expression, transcendent spiritual experiences, social relationships, and the surrounding environment.

Health screening, appropriate health care

- Assess frequency of illness-preventing practices such as yearly physical examinations, dental examinations, flu shots, monthly breast self-examinations (and mammograms as recommended) for women, testicular self-examinations and prostate examinations for men, screening for familial diseases such as glaucoma and elevated cholesterol. See **Altered health maintenance.**

  "CDC recommends yearly flu vaccination for adults with chronic disease, those over 65 years, and children age 2 and older with chronic illness" (Morbidity & Mortality Weekly Report, 1984).

Geriatric
- Assess client's awareness of deficits that may result from normal aging (e.g., changes in sleep patterns or in frequency of urination, loss of visual acuity in night driving, loss of hearing, dietary changes, memory changes, loss of significant others).

- Identify coping mechanisms that promote wellness and place control of life choices back with the client. Stress early retirement planning.

  "An active sense of accountability for one's own well-being provides the necessary motivation to pursue a health-enhancing life style" (Walker, 1993).

- Find suitable housing that provides support, safety, protection, meals, and social events.

  "Only 5% of older adults live in an institution at one time. The risk of institutionalization increases with age" (Walker, 1993).

- Give client information about community resources for the elderly (e.g., transportation to appointments, Meals-on-Wheels, home visitors, pets, American Association of Retired Persons).

  The aging process occurs throughout the lifespan. The elderly client hopes to remain independent and useful as long as possible without being a burden to others.

- Provide information about pneumococcal vaccinations for those over 65.

  "Pneumococcal vaccines are given only once and recommended for those over 65."

- Teach health-protecting behaviors to the elderly.

  "The Surgeon General recommends flu vaccines yearly, and pneumonia vaccines once in a lifetime, wearing auto seat belts, installing smoke detectors, preventing falls, not smoking, decreasing alcohol consumption and using medications safely" (US Department of Health and Human Services, 1991).

Home Care Interventions

NOTE: All of the previously listed nursing interventions are applicable to the home care setting. For more information, see home care interventions for **Altered health maintenance.**

Client/Family Teaching

- Discuss the role of environmental and social factors in supporting a healthy family life.
- Provide and review pamphlets about health-seeking opportunities and wellness resources in the community.

  Community nurses implement health promotion in a variety of settings including schools, industry, and ambulatory care settings. Through evaluation techniques they heighten awareness of such factors as billboards advertising tobacco and alcohol and this influence on the health of a community (Edelman, Mandle, 1990).

- Identify physical and emotional threats to family security (e.g., domestic violence, child abuse, school violence).
  Wellness and health-promoting behaviors can only be met when personal and social safety and security issues are solved.

REFERENCES   Bok Han Y et al: The effect of thermal biofeedback and progressive muscle relaxation training in reducing the blood pressure of patients with essential hypertension, *Image* 25:204, 1993.

Conrad K et al: The work site environment as a cue to smoking reduction, *Res Nurs Health* 19:21, 1996.

Duffy M: Determinants of health promoting lifestyles in older persons, *Image* 25:53, 1993.

Edelman C, Mandle C: *Health promotion throughout the lifespan,* St Louis, 1990, Mosby.

Emmunds M: Strategies for promoting physical fitness, *Nurs Clin North Am* 26:4, 1991.

Hawkes J, Holm K: Gender differences in exercise determinants, *Nurs Res* 42:166, 1993.

Jones P, Meleis A: Health is empowerment, *Adv Nurs Sci* 1:15, 1990.

Morbidity & Mortality Weekly Report, *New Engl J Med* 33:275, 1984.

Murphy S: Coping strategies of abstainers from alcohol up to 3 years post treatment, *Image* 25:32, 1993.

US Department of Health and Human Services: *Healthy people 2000 national health promotion and disease prevention objectives.* DHHS Publication No (PHS) 91-50212, Washington DC, 1991, US Government Printing Office.

Wakefield M et al: Workplace smoking restrictions, occupational status and reduced cigarette consumption, *J Occup Med* 34, 1992.

Walker S: Wellness for elders, *Holistic Nurs Pract* 38:7, 1993.

Impaired home maintenance management

Suzanne Skowronski

Definition   The inability to independently maintain a safe and growth-promoting immediate environment

Defining Characteristics

Subjective   Household members express difficulty in maintaining their home in a comfortable fashion *(critical),* household members request assistance with home maintenance *(critical),* household members describe outstanding debts or financial crises *(critical)*

Objective   Disorderly environment, unwashed or unavailable cooking equipment, clothes, or linens (critical); accumulation of dirt, food wastes, or hygienic wastes (critical); offensive odors, inappropriate household temperature, overtaxed family members (e.g., exhausted, anxious) *(critical);* lack of necessary equipment or aids, presence of vermin or rodents; repeated hygienic disorders, infestations, or infections *(critical)*

Related Factors (r/t)

Client or family member disease or injury, insufficient family organization or planning, insufficient finances, unfamiliarity with neighborhood resources, impaired cognitive or emotional functioning, lack of knowledge, lack of role models, inadequate support systems

Client Outcome/Goals

- Wears clean clothing, eats nutritious meals, and has a sanitary and safe home
- Has the resources to cope physically and emotionally with the chronic illness process
- Uses community resources to assist with treatment needs

Suggested NIC Interventions

Home maintenance assistance

Nursing Interventions and Rationales

- Help client and family with identifying what they need to provide care in a home environment.
  Continuity of care from hospital to home may require adjustment of equipment and supplies and rearrangement of the environment to promote safety.
- Assess family members' concerns, especially those of the primary caregiver, about long-term home-care issues.
  "The stress of caregiving may be so intense that the burden of caring is not automatically reduced when the elder is institutionalized" (Sayles-Cross, 1993).
- Set up a system of relief for the main caregiver in the home and a plan for sharing household duties.
  The caregiving career does not have a specific endpoint; it lasts as long as the chronically ill person is cared for at home (Lindgren, 1993).
- Encourage social relationships with family and friends, even if only by phone.
  "Social distance and high cost of caring were associated with tension and potential for conflict between caregivers and family members" (Sayles-Cross, 1993).
- Assess the characteristics of the current caregiving stage.
  "The encounter stage calls for rapid adjustment, the enduring stage is the heavy-duty caring phase, the exit stage requires the care giver to relinquish most duties" (Lindgren, 1993).
- Initiate a referral to community agencies as needed, including housekeeping aides, Meals-on-Wheel, wheelchair-compatible transportation, and oxygen therapy.
  Community-based agencies provide financial help, education, and emotional support for in-home care, which reduces the burden of care for families coping with chronic sickness.
- Obtain adaptive equipment as appropriate to help family members continue to maintain the home environment.
- Refer client to social services to help with debt consolidation or financial concerns.
  Financial help ranges from Medicaid and private insurance to specific foundations such as Shriner's Burn Center for Children. Hospital discharge planners are an important resource for coordinating agencies.
- Community health agencies can evaluate whether the home is safe enough to provide health care to a chronically ill person, can provide direct care, and can assist with resource coordination.

Geriatric
- Explore community resources to assist with home care (e.g., senior centers, Department of Aging, hospital discharge planners, churches).
  People who are more than 65 years of age have difficulty paying for goods and services on a fixed retirement income. Persons who are age 85 or older are most likely to have incomes at or below the poverty level (Edelman, Mandle, 1990).
- Visit client's home to assess safety features (e.g., no throw rugs, safety bars in the bathroom, stair borders that distinguish each step, adequate nonglare light).
  "In aging there is decreased accommodation ability in the eyes which causes difficulty distinguishing objects in a bright light and decreased ability to distinguish intensities of light" (Edelman, Mandle, 1990).
- Be alert to signs of elder abuse during the home visit such as unattended medical problems, poor hygiene, dehydration, substandard housing, and verbal abuse from family, neighbors, or professional caregivers.
  About 3% to 4% of the nation's elderly are victims of elder mistreatment (Edelman, Mandle, 1990).

- Assess client's nutritional status and ability to meet daily self-care needs.
  "Energy and energy expenditure decline with age; it is important that the nutrient density of the diet be high. Lactose intolerance may decrease dairy intake. Loneliness and untreated depression may alter eating patterns" (Walker, 1992).
- See care plan for **Risk for injury.**

Home Care Interventions

NOTE: By definition this nursing diagnosis consists of primarily community-based interventions. Home care and public health nursing are two community resources that can assist the family to restore or improve home management. The previous interventions incorporate these resources.

Client/Family Teaching

- Teach caregiver the need to sct aside some personal time every day to meet own needs.
  "Constant vigilance was found to be one of the primary caregiver burdens for parents of technologically dependent children at home (gastrostomy, tracheostomy, peritoneal dialysis)" (Burke, 1991).
- Teach family members how to perform home-maintenance activities (e.g., cooking, cleaning, fire prevention).
  When one family member becomes ill and requires home care, the role of other family members may change.
- Identify support groups within the community to assist families in the caregiver career.
  "New caregivers could benefit from support groups that address adjustments at this stage. Support groups may not be the answer if caregivers are 'veterans' and discuss extensive care giving tasks and frustrations" (Lindgren, 1993).
- Ask family to identify support people who can help with home maintenance.
  Churches, nursing home health agencies, and hospice organizations are sources for reliable in-home support.

REFERENCES   Burke S et al: Hazardous secrets and reluctantly taking charge: parenting a child with repeated hospitalizations, *Image* 23:39, 1991.

Edelman C, Mandle C: *Health promotion throughout the lifespan,* ed 3, St Louis, 1990, Mosby.

Lindgren C: The caregiver career, *Image* 214:25, 1993.

Sayles-Cross S: Perceptions of familial caregivers of elder adults, *Image* 25:88, 1993.

Walker S: Wellness for elders, *Holi Nurs Pract* 7:38, 1992.

Hopelessness

Gail B. Ladwig

Definition

The subjective state in which an individual sees limited or unavailable alternatives or personal choices and is unable to mobilize energy on own behalf

Defining Characteristics

Major   Passivity, decreased verbalization, decreased affect, verbal cues (e.g., saying "I can't," sighing)

Minor   Lack of initiative, decreased response to stimuli, decreased affect turning away from speaker, closing of eyes, shrugging responses, decreased appetite, increased or decreased sleep, lack of involvement in care, passively allowing care

Related Factors (r/t)

Prolonged activity restriction that creates isolation, failing or deteriorating physiological condition, long-term stress, abandonment, lost beliefs in transcendent value or in God

Client Outcomes/Goals

- Verbalizes feelings, participates in care
- Makes positive statements (e.g., "I can," or "I will try")
- Makes eye contact, focuses on speaker
- Maintains appropriate appetite for age and physical health
- Sleeps appropriate amount of time for age and physical health

Suggested NIC Interventions

Hope instillation

Nursing Interventions and Rationales

- Monitor and document potential for suicide. See **Risk for violence: self-directed** for specific interventions.
  Hopelessness is correlated with an increased risk of suicide (Buchanan, 1991).
- Evaluate the client by realistically assessing the predicament or threat.
  Unless there is a threat that is acknowledged and assessed, hope does not exist (Morse, Doberneck, 1995).
- Determine appropriate approaches based on the underlying condition or situation that is contributing to feelings of hopelessness—either encourage a positive mental attitude (discourage negative thoughts) or brace client for negative outcomes (i.e., they may have to accept some long-term limitations).
  A person awaiting a transplant may need to only express hope or optimism whereas a person with an injury with long-term effects such as a spinal-cord injury may need to prepare for possible negative outcomes and slow progress (Morse, Doberneck, 1995).
- Assist clients with looking at alternatives and setting goals that are important to them.
  Clients who do not know what to hope for are without hope. Thus an integral part of developing of hope is determining and setting goals. The significance of the goal to the individual is complex and critical to sustaining hope (Morse, Doberneck, 1995).
- When dealing with possible long-term deficits, work with the client to set small, attainable goals.
  Spinal-cord injured clients focused hope only on small gains, one step at a time. "Every little step I took was more important to me than what I had in the end" (Morse, Doberneck, 1995).
- Spend one-to-one time with client. Use empathy; try to understand what a client is saying and communicate this understanding to the client.
  There is a demonstrated connection between nurse-expressed empathy and positive patient outcomes (Olson, 1995).
- Encourage expression of feelings and acknowledge acceptance of them.
  A client's ability to express a negative emotion can be a very healthy sign; strong emotions are potentially dangerous if not expressed (Barry, 1994).
- Give client time to initiate interactions. After an appropriate amount of time is allowed, approach client in an accepting and nonjudgmental manner.
  Clients who have feelings of hopelessness need extra time to initiate relationships but sometimes are not able. Approaching the client in an unhurried, nonjudgmental manner allows the client to feel secure and provides an atmosphere conducive to venting fears and asking questions (Anderson, 1992).

- Encourage client to participate in group activities.
  Group activities provide social support and help identify alternative ways to problem solve.
- Encourage exercise of the mind to alleviate boredom. Watching or listening to the news, listening to music, and letter writing help to relieve the monotomy of hospitalization.
  Boredom may become a serious problem, leading to apathy, loss of hope, and depression (Anderson, 1992).
- Review client's strengths with client. Have client list strengths on a note card and carry it for future reference.
  Listing strengths provides reinforcement of positive self-regard.
- Use humor as appropriate.
  Humor is an effective intervention for hopelessness (Hunt, 1993).
- Involve family and significant others in plan of care.
  Frequent meetings with the staff and family can provide a safe, positive atmosphere for discussing feelings (Anderson, 1992).
- Encourage family and significant others to express care, hope, and love for client.
  Clients awaiting transplants had only one alternative and that was hoping to receive a transplant. These clients solicited mutually supportive relationships. They sought social and emotional support from staff, family, clergy, and friends, and it was the intensity of these social relationships that enabled them to survive the precarious nature of their physical conditions (Morse, Dobernect, 1995).
- Use touch if appropriate and with permission to demonstrate caring, and encourage the family to do the same.
  Touch is a basic human need and it lets clients know that they are valued (MacGinley, 1993).
- For additional interventions see **Spiritual distress (distress of the human spirit), Potential for enhanced spiritual well-being,** and **Sleep pattern disturbance.**

Geriatric
- Assess for clinical signs and symptoms of depression; differentiate depression from functional or organic dementia.
  It can be difficult to distinguish depression from dementia in people older than age 65 because some symptoms (e.g., disorientation, memory loss, and distractibility) may suggest dementia. Concurrent medical illnesses, prescription medications, and concealed alcohol or substance abuse can also appear to be dementia (Agency for Health Care Policy and Research, 1993).
- Take threats of self-harm or suicide seriously.
  Elderly people who are depressed or have experienced recent losses and live alone are at the highest risk.
- Identify significant losses that might be leading to feelings of hopelessness.
- Discuss stages of emotional responses to multiple losses.
- Use reminiscence and life review therapies to identify past coping skills.
  The memory and reminiscence have been used successfully with elderly persons to evoke pleasure and achieve therapeutic goals (Woods, Ashley, 1995).
- Express hope to client and give positive feedback whenever appropriate.
- Identify client's past sources of spirituality. Help client explore life and identify those experiences that are noteworthy. Clients may want to read the Bible or have it read to them.
  Older adults frequently identified spirituality as a source of hope (Gaskins, Forte, 1995).
- Use simulated presence therapy (SPT): SPT is a personalized audiotape composed of a family member's or caregiver's portion of a telephone conversation and soundless

spaces that correspond to the client's side of the conversation. On the SPT audiotape, a caregiver "converses" about cherished memories, loved ones, family antidotes, and other cherished experiences of the patient's life. The SPT audiotape is played using headphones and lightweight, automatic reverse cassette player that is inserted into a hip pack. (SPT is a patented product of SIM-PRES Incorporated, Boston, Mass.)

SPT builds on strengths of cognitively impaired elderly people because it relies on their remote memory, which is more likely to be retained than their recent memory. SPT produces an positive environment for cognitively impaired elderly people; the selected memories of SPT seem to provide enough stimulation to evoke the elder's interest, involvement, and pleasure (Woods, Ashley, 1995).

- Encourage visits from children.
  Children stimulate a sense of hope in many older adults (Gaskins, Forte, 1995).
- Position clients by window, take them outside, or encourage activities such as gardening if they are able.
  Enjoyment of nature fosters hope (Gasking, Forte, 1995).

Home Care Interventions

- Assess for isolation within the family unit.
- Encourage clients to participate in family activities. If clients cannot participate, encourage them to be in the same area and watch family activities. If possible, move client's bed or primary sitting are to active household area.
  Participation in events increases energy and the sense of belonging.
- Reminisce with clients about their lives.
  Reminiscing gives meaning to life and helps maintain the individual's self-esteem and identity.
- Identify areas in which client can have control. Allow client to set achievable goals in these areas.
  Having control enhances self-esteem.
- If illness precipitated the hopelessness, discuss knowledge of and previous experience with the disease. Help client with identifying strengths.
  Uncertainty is a danger when it results in pessimism. Knowledge of and previous experience with the disease decreases uncertainty.
- Provide plant or pet therapy if possible.
  Caring for pets or plants helps redefine the client's identity and helps them feel needed and loved.
- Provide a safe environment so clients cannot harm themselves. (See also "no suicide" contract in following section). Provide one-to-one contact when necessary. Refer for immediate mental health treatment if needed.
  Hopelessness is a accurate indicator of suicidal risk. A safe environment reassures the client.

Client/Family Teaching

- Teach stress reduction, relaxation, and imagery. Many cassette tapes are available on relaxation and meditation. Assist the client with relaxation based on the client's preference from the initial assessment.
  Such techniques are useful in combating depression, hopelessness, powerlessness, and a poor self-image (Anderson, 1992).
- Encourage families to express love, concern, and encouragement and allow the client to vent.
  Hope was partially sustained through relationships with the social networks—families. The availability of significant sources of support can perpetuate hopefulness with cardiac transplant recipients (Hirth, Stewart, 1994).

- Refer client to self-help groups such as I Can Cope and Make Today Count.
  These groups allow the client to recognize the love and care of others, and they promote a sense of belonging (Bulechek, McCloskey, 1992).
- Supply a crisis phone number and secure a "no suicide" contract from the client stating the crisis number will be used if thoughts of self-harm occur.
  A no suicide contract is one type of intervention used with clients who have suicidal thoughts (Valente, 1989).

REFERENCES   Abraham I, Neundorfer M, Currie L: Effect of group interventions on cognition and depression in nursing home residents, *Nurs Res* 41:196, 1992.

Agency for Health Care Policy and Research Clinical Practice Guideline, Publication 93-0550, *Depression in primary care. Volume 1: Detection and diagnosis,* Rockville, Md, 1993, US Department of Health and Human Services.

Anderson SB: Guillain-Barre syndrome: giving the patient control, *J Neurosci Nurs* 24:158, 1992.

Barry P: *Mental health and mental illness,* ed 5, Philadelphia, 1994, JB Lippincott.

Buchanan DM: Suicide: a conceptual model for an avoidable death, *Arch Psychiatr Nurs* 5:341, 1991.

Bulechek G, McCloskey J: *Nursing interventions: essential nursing treatments,* ed 2, Philadelphia, 1992, JB Lippincott.

Clemons S, Cummings S: Helplessness and powerlessness: caring for clients in pain, *Hol Nurs Pract* 6:76, 1991.

Gaskins S, Forte L: The meaning of hope: implications for nursing practice and research, *J Gerontol Nurs* 21:17, 1995.

Hirth A, Stewart M: Hope and social support as coping resources for adults waiting for cardiac transplantation, *Canad J Nursing Res* 26;31, 1994.

Hunt AH: Humor as a nursing intervention, *Cancer Nurs* 16:34, 1993.

Jaffe, Marie S, Skidmore-Roth, Linda: *Home health nursing care plans,* ed 2, St Louis, 1993, Mosby.

MacGinley K: Nursing care of the patient with altered body image, *Brit J Nurs* 2:1098, 1993.

Molenbeach EE, Sarit SH: Current research issues in caregiving to the elderly, *Int J Aging Hum Dev* 31:103, 1991. In Morse J, Doberneck B: Delineating the concept of hope, *Image* 27:277, 1995.

Olson J:Relationships between nurse-expressed empathy, patient perceived empathy and patient distress, *Image* 27:317, 1995.

Rawlins R. Heacock P: *Clinical manual of psychiatric nursing,* ed 2, St Louis, 1993, Mosby.

Valente SM: Adolescent suicide: assessment and intervention, *J Child Adol Psychiatr Ment Health Nurs* 2:34, 1989.

Woods P, Ashley: Simulated presence therapy: using selected memories to manage problem behaviors in Alzheimer's disease patients, *Geriatr Nurs* 16:9, 1995.

Hyperthermia

Marcia LaHaie and Terry VandenBosch

Definition   The state in which an individual's body temperature is elevated above normal range
NOTE: Body temperature is controlled by the hypothalamus and increases in response to internal and external factors such as infection, tissue injury, and hypothalamus dysfunction. Fever is present whenever a person's temperature elevates above his or her normal daily range or above 100° F. Normally there is a proportional increase in immune system enhancement for every degree of temperature rise up to 104° F. Fever is believed to be adaptive at levels below 104° F (Kluger, 1991). Hyperthermia is a significant elevation in body temperature, usually above 104° F, and it occurs in the presence of hypothalamic dysfunction. Hyperthermia is not considered adaptive (Holtzclaw, 1992).

Defining Characteristics

Major   Increase in body temperature above normal range (NOTE: Temperature greater than 104° F)

Minor   Flushed or hot skin, increased respiratory rate, tachycardia, seizures, convulsions

Related Factors (r/t)

Exposure to hot environment, vigorous activity, medications or anesthetics, inappropriate clothing, increased metabolic rate, illness or trauma, dehydration, inability or decreased ability to perspire

Client Outcomes/Goals

- Maintains oral temperature within adaptive levels (below 104° F) (NOTE: A lower temperature may be necessary, depending on the presence of cardiopulmonary disease or on the client's neurological status)
- Remains free of dehydration problems
- Remains free of seizure activity (febrile seizure activity rare in adults)

Suggested NIC Interventions

Fever treatment, malignant hyperthermia precautions, temperature regulation, temperature regulation: inoperative, vital signs monitoring

Nursing Interventions and Rationales

- Take client's temperature at least once a day between 3 PM and 7 PM or according to institutional standards.
  Temperature screening for afebrile patients can be based on daily circadian rhythm patterns. Take client's temperature at the peak of the circadian rhythm (Beaudry, VandenBosch, Anderson, 1995).
- Once a temperature elevation has been detected, retake temperature if clients experience chills or state that they feel warmer and after instituting interventions.
  Shivering indicates a rising body temperature.
- Notify physician of temperature according to institutional standards or written orders.
- Administer antipyretic medications on the basis of physician's order, client comfort level, and/or a temperature greater than 102.5° F. (NOTE: This method represents conservative management of fever.)
  Fever is a symptom used to diagnose, monitor a disease process, and determine the effectiveness of a treatment. Fever is adaptive; for every degree of temperature increase up to 104° F, there is a proportional increase in immune system enhancement (Kluger, 1991).
- Assess client for a history of febrile seizures; give antipyretics more aggressively only in clients with a positive history.
  In adults, there is very little evidence of an association between fever and seizures and neurological damage (Styrt, Sugarman, 1990). Children who have a high fever (more than 104° F) at the time of an initial febrile seizure are less likely to have a recurrence of such seizures than children who have more moderate fevers at the time of an initial seizure (El-Radhi et al, 1986).
- Assess fluid loss and administer intravenous fluids or facilitate oral intake to promote fluid replacement.
  Increased metabolic rate and diaphoresis cause a loss of body fluids.
- Notify physician of changes in client's mental status.
  A change in mental status may indicate the onset of septic shock.
- When diaphoresis is present, maintain client's comfort by assisting with clothing changes and bathing.
  Clothing changes and bathing increase comfort and decrease the possibility of continued shivering resulting from water evaporation from the skin.

- Do not use external cooling measures such as ice packs, tepid water baths, or the removal of blankets and clothing for fever management unless temperature is greater than 104° F; these measures cause shivering.

  Shivering results in significantly increased oxygen consumption (Holtzclaw, 1993). If the client's temperature drops as a result of external cooling measures, the hypothalamus resets the body temperature at a higher level, which results in more shivering (Enright, Hill, 1989).

- Use a cooling blanket if client's fever is higher than 105° F or if a high body temperature is related to hypothalamus dysfunction.

  Cooling blankets are used when the client's oral temperature exceeds 105° F and cannot be controlled by antipyretics (Styrt, Sugarman, 1990) or when the fever is caused by a heat-related illness or is neurologically related (Morgan, 1990).

Geriatric
- In hot weather, encourage clients to drink 8 to 10 glasses of fluid per day regardless of whether they are thirsty (within the cardiac and renal reserve). Encourage the use of fans or air conditioning.

  The elderly are more susceptible to heat because of a decreased sensitivity to heat, decreased sweat gland function, and decreased thirst (Brody, 1994).

Home Care Interventions

- Prior to the condition of hyperthermia, confirm that the client or family has a thermometer and knows how to read it. Instruct as needed.

  An accurate temperature is one indicator of the client's condition.

- Employ nursing interventions listed previously with physician's orders. Keep physician informed if temperature does not stabilize below 104° F.

- Use emergency plan under physician's direction or when temperature indicators approach hyperthermia.

  Hyperthermia is an acute and possibly life-threatening symptom. The client cannot stay at home safely.

- If the client is in hospice or is terminally ill, follow advance directives and the client's wishes and physician's orders. Keep the client comfortable and free of pain.

  The goal of terminal care is to provide comfort and dignity during the dying process.

Client/Family Teaching

- Teach that fever enhances the immune system response in the presence of infection; the peak of beneficial effects occurs at an oral temperature of 104° F.

  Fevers of less than 104° F enhance immune system functioning (Roberts, 1991).

- Recommend a liberal intake of nonalcoholic and noncaffeinated fluids.

  Liberal fluid intake replaces fluid lost through perspiration and respiration. The presence of alcohol and caffeine in fluids can promote diuresis.

- Teach client the detrimental effects of shivering and to avoid activities that can cause shivering (e.g., blanket removal, lower room temperature, tepid water bath, ice packs).

  External cooling measures result in shivering and discomfort (Styrt, Sugarman, 1990).

- Teach that the use of antipyretics is the most effective way to reduce an infection-related fever below 104° F if the client is uncomfortable.

  Antipyretics effectively reduce infection-related fevers (Clark, 1991).

- Teach client to avoid vigorous physical activity, wear light clothing, and wear a hat to minimize sun exposure during periods of excessive outdoor heat.

  Such methods reduce exposure to high environmental temperatures, which can cause heat stroke.

REFERENCES   Beaudry M, VandenBosch T, Anderson J: Research utilization: once a day temperatures for afebrile patients, *Clin Nurs Spec* 10:21, 1995.

Brody GM: Hyperthermia and hypothermia in the elderly, *Clin Geriatr Med* 10:213, 1994.

Bruce J, Grove SK: Fever: pathology and treatment, *Crit Care Nurse* 12:40-48, 1992.

Clark WG: Antipyretics. In Mackowiak P, editor: *Fever: basic mechanisms and management,* New York, 1991, Raven Press.

El-Radhi AS et al: Recurrence rate of febrile convulsions related to the degree of pyrexia during the first attack, *Clin Pediatr* 25:311, 1986.

Enright T, Hill MG: Treatment of fever, *Focus Crit Care* 16:96, 1989.

Holtzclaw BJ: *Clinical predictors and metabolic consequences of postoperative shivering after cardiac surgery,* Paper presented at the meeting of the Fifth National Conference on Research for Clinical Practice, Chapel Hill, NC, April 23, 1993.

Holtzclaw BJ: The febrile response in critical care: state of the science, *Heart Lung* 21:482, 1992.

Kluger MJ: The adaptive value of fever. In Mackowiak PA, editor: *Fever: basic mechanisms and management,* New York, 1991, Raven Press.

Mackowiak PA: A critical appraisal of 98.6° F, the upper limit of the normal body temperature and other legacies of Carl Reinhold August Wunderlich, *JAMA* 268:1578, 1992.

May A, Bauchner H: Fever phobia: the pediatrician's contribution, *Pediatrics* 90:851, 1992.

Morgan, SP: A comparison of three methods of managing fever in the neurologic patient, *J Neurosci Nurs* 22:19, 1990.

Roberts NJ: The immunological consequences of fever. In Mackowiak PA, editor: *Fever: basic mechanisms and management,* New York, 1991, Raven Press.

Samples JF et al: Circadian rhythms: basis for screening for fever, *Nurs Res* 34:377, 1985.

Styrt B, Sugarman B: Antipyresis and fever, *Arch Intern Med* 150:1589, 1990.

Hypothermia

Sandra K. Cunningham

Definition   The state in which an individual's body temperature is reduced below normal range

Defining Characteristics

Major   Reduction in body temperature below normal range, mild shivering, cool skin, moderate pallor

Minor   Slow capillary refill, piloerection, cyanotic nail beds, bradycardia, bradypnea, decreased mentation, drowsiness, confusion (Carpenito, 1993), hypotension, positive deflection in the RT segment on electrocardiogram (ECG) with temperature of less than 82.4° F.

Related Factors (r/t)

- Exposure to cool or cold environment, illness, trauma, damage to hypothalamus, inability or decreased ability to shiver, malnutrition, inadequate clothing, alcohol consumption, medications that cause vasodilation, evaporation of perspiration from skin in cool environment, decreased metabolic rate, inactivity, aging, extremes of age (elderly or newborn)

Client Outcomes/Goals

- Maintains body temperature within normal range
- Identifies risk factors of hypothermia
- States measures to prevent hypothermia
- Identifies symptoms of hypothermia and the actions to take when hypothermia is present

Suggested NIC Interventions

Hypothermia treatment, temperature regulation, temperature regulation: inoperative, vital signs monitoring

Nursing Interventions and Rationales

- Determine factors leading to hypothermic episode; see related factors.
  It is important to assess risk factors and precipitating events.
- Remove client from cause(s) of hypothermic episode (e.g., cold environment, cold or wet clothing).
  This eliminates causative or contributing factors.
- Institute a low-reading, continuous core-temperature monitoring device as appropriate.
  Monitor client's response to interventions. The normal range is 96.8° F to 100.4° F (Black, Matassarin-Jacobs, 1993).
- Monitor client's vital signs every hour and as appropriate. Note changes associated with hypothermia such as decreased pulse, irregular pulse rhythm, decreased respiratory rate, or initially increased then decreased blood pressure.
  Decreased circulating volume during hypothermia results in decreased cardiac output and depressed oxygen delivery. Hypoxia, metabolic acidosis, and intrinsic irritability of a cold myocardium result in various dysrhythmias (Larach, 1995).
- Monitor for signs of hypothermia (e.g., shivering, cool skin, piloerection, pallor, slow capillary refill, cyanotic nail beds, decreased mentation, coma).
  This monitors the client's response to interventions and provides evidence of persistent hypothermia.
- Rewarm client passively (e.g., set room temperature at 70° F to 75° F, layer clothing and blankets, cover client's head, offer warm fluid with physician's order); allow client to rewarm at own pace. Passive rewarming is not encouraged for clients with temperatures below 82.4° F (28° C).
  Passive rewarming prevents heat loss via radiation and evaporation. Clients' responses rely on their ability to generate heat (Dexter, 1990). Gradual rewarming limits complications associated with hypothermia. Passive rewarming is a slow process and may increase risk of cardiac arrest in severe hypothermia (Larach, 1995).
- Rewarm client actively (e.g., with warmed cotton blankets or a forced warm air blanket, radiant heat lights as available). Following a physician's order, use hydrothermic blankets, administer heated and humidified oxygen (40° C [104° F]), and carefully administer heated intravenous fluids at prescribed temperature.
  Increases heat gain via the four major mechanisms of heat transfer—radiation, conduction, convection, and evaporation (Stevens, 1993; Giuffre, Heidenreich, Pruitt, 1994).
- Rewarm client using active core rewarming techniques (e.g., colonic lavage, hemodialysis, peritoneal lavage, extracorporeal blood rewarming, bladder irrigations) following physician's order.
  This type of rewarming increases heat gain via conduction. Heat transfer depends on the difference between the inlet and outlet water temperatures and the water flow rate (Gentilello, 1995).
- Request a social service referral to help client obtain the heat, shelter, and food needed to maintain body temperature.
  A preventive approach that includes adequate food and fluid intake, shelter, heat, and clothing decreases the risk of hypothermia.

Geriatric

- Encourage proper nutrition and hydration. Request a dietician referral to identify minimum dietary needs.
  Insufficient calorie and fluid intake predispose the client to hypothermia.
- Assess neurological signs frequently.
  Older adults are less likely to shiver or complain of feeling cold. Early signs of hypothermia are subtle (Miller, 1990).
- Warm a hypothermic elderly client slowly—a rate of 1° F per hour.
  Slow warming avoids overheating and allows body to accommodate decreasing risk of complications (Miller, 1995).

Home Care Interventions

NOTE: Hypothermia is not a symptom that presents in the normal course of home care. When it presents, it is a clinical emergency and the client/family should access emergency medical services immediately.

- Prior to medical crisis, confirm that client or family has a thermometer and can read it. Instruct as needed.
  An accurate temperature is one indicator of the client's condition.
- Instruct client or family to take temperature when client displays cyanosis, pallor, or shivering. Monitor every hour as noted previously.
- If temperature of client begins dropping below normal range, apply layers of clothing or blankets or adjust environmental heat to comfort level. Do not overheat. Contact physician.
  Active rewarming is the only method of rewarming appropriate to home care under normal circumstances.
- If temperature continues dropping, activate emergency system and notify physician.
  Hypothermia is a clinically acute condition that may not be managed safely in the home.
- If client is a hospice client or is terminally ill, follow advance directives, client wishes, and physician's orders. Keep client free of pain.
  The goal of terminal care is to provide dignity and comfort during the dying process.

Client/Family Teaching

- Teach client/family signs of hypothermia and method for taking a temperature (age appropriate).
- Teach client methods to prevent hypothermia—wearing adequate clothing, heating environment to a minimum of 68° F, and ingesting adequate food and fluid.
  Simple measures such as layering clothes, wearing a hat, and avoiding extremes in temperature prevent significant heat loss.
- Teach client and family about medications such as antidepressants and barbiturates that predispose client to hypothermia (as appropriate).
  If client has had hypothermia in the past, using alternative medications (such as a monoamine oxidase (MAO) inhibitor instead of a tricyclic antidepressant) is an option if there is no contradiction (Miller, 1990).

REFERENCES   Black JM, Matassarin-Jacobs E: *Luckmann and Sorenson's medical-surgical nursing: a psychophysiologic approach,* Philadelphia, 1993, WB Saunders.
Carpenito JL: *Nursing diagnosis: application to clinical practice,* ed 5, Philadelphia, 1993, JB Lippincott.
Danzl DF, Ghezzi KT: Hot tips on handling hypothermia, *Patient Care* 25:89, 1991.
Dexter WW: Hypothermia: safe and efficient methods of rewarming, *Postgrad Med* 88:55, 1990.
Gentilello LM: Advances in the management of hypothermia, *Surg Clin North Am* 75:243, 1995.

Giuffre M, Heidenreich T, Pruitt L: Rewarming cardiac surgery patients: radiant heat versus forced warm air, *Nurs Res* 43:174, 1994.

Giuffre M et al: Rewarming postoperative patients: lights, blankets, or forced warm air, *J Post Anesth Nurs* 6:387, 1991.

Hortzclaw BJ: Monitoring body temperature, *AACN Clin Issues Crit Care Nurs* 4:44, 1993.

Larach MG: Accidental hypothermia, *Lancet* 354:493, 1995.

Miller CA: *Nursing care of older adults,* ed 2, Glenview, Ill, 1995, Scott Foresman/Little, Brown.

Miller CA: *Nursing care of older adults: theory and practice,* Glenview, Ill, 1990, Scott Foresman/Little, Brown.

Stevens T: Managing postoperative hypothermia, rewarming, and its complications, *Crit Care Nurse* 16:60, 1993.

Summers S: Inadvertent hypothermia: clinical validation in postanesthesia patients, *Nurs Diag* 3:54, 1992.

Bowel incontinence

Mikel Gray

Definition

The state in which an individual experiences a change in bowel elimination habits characterized by involuntary passage of stool

Defining Characteristics

Involuntary passage of stool *(critical),* change in frequency of stool elimination

Related Factors (r/t)

Change in stool consistency (e.g., diarrhea, constipation, fecal impaction), defects in gastrointestinal motility (e.g., metabolic disorders, inflammatory bowel disease, infectious diseases, drug-induced motility disorders, food intolerance), defects in rectal vault function (e.g., low rectal compliance from ischemia, fibrosis, radiation, infectious proctitis, Hirschprung's disease, local or infiltrating neoplasm, severe rectocele), sphincter dysfunction (e.g., obstetric or traumatic induced incompetence, fistula or abscess, prolapse, third-degree hemorrhoids, pseudodyssynergia of the pelvic muscles), neurological disorders impacting gastrointestinal motility, rectal vault function and sphincter function (e.g., cerebrovascular accident, spinal injury, traumatic brain injury, central nervous system tumor, advanced stage dementia, encephalopathy, profound mental retardation, multiple sclerosis, myelodysplasia and related neural tube defects, gastroparesis of diabetes mellitus, heavy metal poisoning, chronic alcoholism, infectious or autoimmune neurological disorders, myasthenia gravis)

Client Outcomes/Goals

- Maintains regular, complete evacuation of fecal contents from the rectal vault (pattern may vary from every day to every 3 to 5 days) (Roig et al, 1993)
- Regulates stool consistency (soft, formed stools)
- Reduces or eliminates frequency of incontinent episodes
- Maintains intact skin in the perianal/perineal area
- Demonstrates the ability to isolate, contract, and relax pelvic muscles (when incontinence related to sphincter incompetence or pseudodyssynergia)
- Increases pelvic muscle strength (when incontinence related to sphincter incompetence)

Suggested NIC Interventions

Bowel incontinence care, bowel incontinence care: encopresis, bowel training

Nursing Interventions

- Complete a focused nursing history including previous and present bowel elimination routines, dietary history, frequency and volume of uncontrolled stool loss, and aggravating and alleviating factors.

A nursing history is needed to determine the patterns of stool elimination, characterize involuntary stool loss, and determine the likely etiology of the incontinence.

- Complete a focused physical assessment including inspection of perineal skin, pelvic muscle strength assessment, digital examination of the rectum for presence of impaction and anal sphincter strength, and evaluation of functional status (mobility, dexterity, visual acuity).

  A focused physical examination assists in determining the severity of fecal leakage and its likely etiology. A functional assessment provides information concerning the impact of functional status on stool elimination patterns and incontinence (Gray, Burns, 1996).

- Complete an assessment of cognitive functioning.

  Include dementia, acute confusion, and mental retardation and risk factors for fecal incontinence (Doughty, 1991; O'Donnell et al, 1992).

- Document patterns of stool elimination and incontinent episodes via a bowel record including frequency of bowel movements, stool consistency, frequency and severity of incontinent episodes, precipitating factors, and dietary and fluid intake.

  This document is used to confirm the verbal history (Resnick et al, 1994), to assist in determining the likely etiology of stool incontinence, and to serve as a baseline to evaluate treatment efficacy.

- Identify the probable causes of fecal incontinence.

  Fecal incontinence is frequently multifactorial (Doughty, 1991); identification of the probable etiology of fecal incontinence is necessary to select a treatment plan likely to control or eliminate the condition.

- Improve access to toileting by doing the following:
  - Identify usual toileting patterns among persons in the acute care or long-term care facility and plan opportunities for toileting accordingly.
  - Provide assistance with toileting for patients with limited access or impaired functional status (e.g., mobility, dexterity, access).
  - Institute a prompted toileting program for persons with impaired cognitive status (e.g., retardation, dementia).
  - Provide adequate privacy for toileting.
  - Respond promptly to requests for assistance with toileting.

  Acute or transient fecal incontinence frequently occurs in the acute care or long-term care facility because of inadequate access to toileting facilities, insufficient assistance with toileting, or inadequate privacy when attempting to toilet (Ouslander, Schnelle, 1995; Wong, 1995; Gray, Burns, 1996).

- For clients with intermittent episodes of fecal incontinence related to acute changes in stool consistency, begin a bowel reeducation program consisting of the following:
  - Cleansing impacted stool from the bowel if indicated
  - Normalizing stool consistency by adequate intake of fluids (30 ml/kg of body weight per day) and dietary or supplemental fiber
  - Establishing a regular routine of fecal elimination based on established patterns of bowel elimination (patterns established prior to onset of incontinence)

  Bowel reeducation is designed to reestablish normal defecation patterns and normalize stool consistency to reduce or eliminate the risk of recurring fecal incontinence associated with changes in stool consistency (Doughty, 1996).

- Begin a prompted defecation program for adults with dementia, mental retardation, or related learning disabilities.
  Prompted urine and fecal elimination programs have been shown to reduce or eliminate incontinence in long-term care facilities and community settings (Ouslander, Snelle, 1995; Smith et al, 1994; Doughty, 1996).
- Begin a scheduled stimulation-defecation program for clients with neurological conditions causing fecal incontinence. Include the following steps:
  - Cleanse the bowel of impacted fecal material before beginning the program.
  - Implement strategies to normalize stool consistency including adequate intake of fluid and fiber and avoidance of foods associated with diarrhea.
  - Determine a regular schedule for bowel elimination (typically every day or every other day) based on prior patterns of bowel elimination whenever feasible.
  - Provide a stimulus prior to assisting the patient to a position on the toilet—digital stimulation, a stimulating suppository, or a "mini-enema" or pulsed-evacuation enema may be used for stimulation.
  The scheduled, stimulated program relies on consistency of stool and a mechanical or chemical stimulus to produce a bolus contraction of the rectum with evacuation of fecal material (Munchiando, Kendall, 1993; Dunn, Galka, 1994; King, Currie, Wright, 1994; Doughty, 1996).
- Begin a pelvic floor reeducation or muscle exercise program for clients with sphincter incompetence or pseudodyssynergia of the pelvic muscles, or refer clients with fecal incontinence related to sphincter dysfunction to a nurse specialist or other therapist with clinical expertise in these techniques of care.
  Pelvic muscle reeducation, including biofeedback, pelvic muscle exercise, and/or pelvic muscle relaxation techniques, are safe and effective treatments for selected clients with fecal incontinence related to sphincter or pelvic floor muscle dysfunction (McIntosh et al, 1993; Arhan et al, 1994; Enck et al, 1994; Keck et al, 1994).
- Begin a pelvic muscle biofeedback program among patients with urgency to defecate and fecal incontinence related to recurrent diarrhea.
  Pelvic muscle reeducation, including biofeedback, can reduce uncontrolled loss of stool in clients who experience urgency and diarrhea as provocative factors for fecal incontinence (Chiarioni et al, 1993).
- Cleanse skin following each episode of fecal incontinence. When incontinence occurs frequently, use an incontinence cleansing product specifically designed for this purpose.
  Frequent cleaning with soap and water may compromise perianal skin integrity and enhance the irritation produced by fecal leakage (Lyder et al, 1992; Byers et al, 1995).
- Apply mineral oil or a petroleum-based ointment to the perianal skin when frequent episodes of fecal incontinence occur.
  These products form a moisture and chemical barrier to the perianal skin that may prevent or reduce the severity of comprised skin integrity with severe fecal incontinence (Doughty, 1991).
- Assist the client with selecting and applying a containment device for occasional episodes of fecal incontinence.
  A fecal containment device will prevent soiling of clothing and reduce odors in clients with uncontrolled stool loss.
- Teach clients with more frequent stool loss to apply an anal continence plug in consultation with the physician.

The anal continence plug is a device that can reduce or eliminate persistent liquid or solid stool incontinence in selected patients (Blair et al, 1992).

- Apply a fecal pouch to the patient with frequent stool loss, particularly when fecal incontinence produces altered perianal skin integrity.
Fecal pouches keep stool loss contained, reduce odor, and protect the perianal skin from chemical irritation related to contact with stool (Doughty, 1991).
- Consult the physician concerning the use of a rectal tube for the patient with severe fecal incontinence.
A large French-sized indwelling catheter has been used for fecal containment when incontinence is severe and perianal skin integrity significantly compromised (Birdsall, 1986). The safety of this technique remains unknown (Doughty, 1991; Doughty, Broadwell-Jackson, 1993).

Geriatric
- Evaluate all elderly clients for established or acute fecal incontinence when they enter the acute or long-term care facility and intervene as indicated.
The rate of fecal incontinence in acute-care facilities is as high as 3% and in long-term care facilities is as high as 50% (Leigh, Turnburg, 1982; Egan, Plymad, Thomas, 1983).
- Evaluate cognitive status of elderly clients with a NEECHAM confusion scale (Neelan et al, 1992); for acute cognitive changes, use a Folstein Mini-Mental Status Examination (Folstein, Folstein, 1975) or other tool as indicated.
Acute or established dementia increase the risk of fecal incontinence among elderly persons.

Home Care Interventions
- Assess and teach medication regimens and bowel programs to support continence.
- Provide clothing that is nonrestrictive, can be manipulated easily for toileting, and can be changed with ease.
Avoidance of complicated maneuvers increases the chance of success in toileting programs and decreases the client's embarrassment.
- Assist the family with arranging care in a way that allows the client to participate in family or favorite activities without embarrassment.
Careful planning can maintain the dignity of the client and integrity of family patterns.
- If client is limited to bed or bed and chair, provide a commode or bedpan that can be easily accessed. If necessary, refer client to physical therapy services for teaching safe transfers and building strength for transfers.
- If client is frequently incontinent, refer for home health aide services to assist with client hygiene and skin care.
Support services provide continuity of skin care and valuable respite for caregivers.

Client/Family Teaching
- Teach client and family to perform a bowel reeducation; program a scheduled, stimulated program; or to use other strategies to manage fecal incontinence.
- Teach client and family of common dietary sources of fiber as well as providing supplemental fiber or bulking agents as indicated.
- Refer the family to support services for assistance with home management of fecal incontinence as indicated.
- Teach nursing colleagues and nonprofessional care providers importance of providing toileting opportunities and adequate privacy for clients in acute- or long-term care facilities.
NOTE: See **Diarrhea** and **Constipation** for detailed management of these related conditions.

REFERENCES   Arhan P et al: Biofeedback reeducation of fecal incontinence in children, *Int J Colorectal Dis* 9:128, 1994.

Birdsall C: Would you put a Foley in the rectum? *Am J Nurs* 9:1050, 1986.

Blair et al: The bowel management tube: an effective means for controlling fecal incontinence, *J Pediatr Surg* 27:1269, 1992.

Byers PH et al: Effects of incontinence care cleansing regimens on skin integrity, *J Wound Ostomy Cont Nurs* 22:187, 1995.

Chiarinoni G et al: Liquid stool incontinence with severe urgency: anorectal function and effective biofeedback treatment, *Gut* 34:1576, 1993.

Doughty DB: A physiological approach to bowel training, *J Wound Ostomy Cont Nurs* 23:46, 1996.

Doughty DB, editor: *Urinary and fecal incontinence: nursing management,* St Louis, 1991, Mosby.

Doughty DB, Broadwell-Jackson D: *Gastrointestinal disorders,* St Louis, 1993, Mosby.

Dunn KL, Galka ML: A comparison of the effectiveness of Therevac SB and bisacodyl suppositories in SCI patients' bowel programs, *Rehab Nurs* 19:334, 1994.

Egan M, Plymad K, Thomas T: Incontinence in patients in two district general hospitals, *Nurs Times* 79:22, 1983.

Enck P et al: Long term efficacy of biofeedback for fecal incontinence, *Dis Colon Rectum* 37:997, 1994.

Folstein MF, Folstein EF, McHugh P: Mini mental state: a practical method of grading the cognitive status of the patient for the clinician, *J Psychiatr Rev* 12:189-98, 1975.

Gray ML, Burns SM: Continence management. *Crit Care Nurs Clin North Am* 8:29, 1996.

Keck JO et al: Biofeedback training is useful in fecal incontinence but disappointing in constipation, *Dis Colon Rectum* 37:1271, 1994.

King JC, Currie DM, Wright E: Bowel training in spina bifida: importance of education, patient compliance, age, and anal reflexes, *Arch Phys Med Rehab* 75:243, 1994.

Leigh, RJ, Turnberg LA: Fecal incontinence: the unvoiced symptom, *Lancet* 1:1349, 1982.

Lyder CH et al: Structured skin care regimen to prevent perineal dermatitis in the elderly, *J ET Nurs* 19:12, 1992.

McIntosh LJ et al: Pelvic floor rehabilitation in the treatment of incontinence, *J Reprod Med* 38:662-666, 1993.

Munchiando JF, Kendall K: Comparison of the effectiveness of two bowel programs for CVA patients, *Rehab Nurs* 18:168, 1993.

Neelan VJ et al: Use of the NEECHAM confusion scale to assess acute confusional states of hospitalized older patients. In Funk SG et al, editors: *Key aspects of elder care: managing falls, incontinence and cognitive impairment,* New York, 1992, Springer.

O'Donnell BF et al: Incontinence and troublesome behaviors predict institutionalization in dementia, *J Geriatr Psych Neurol* 5:45, 1992.

Ouslander JG, Schnelle JF: Predictors of successful prompted voiding among incontinent nursing home residents, *JAMA* 273:1366, 1995.

Resnick NM et al: Short term viability of self report of incontinence in older persons, *J Am Geriatr Soc* 42:202, 1994.

Roig Vila JV et al: The defecation habits in a normal working population, *Rev Esp Enferm Dig* 84:224, 1993.

Smith LJ et al: A behavioral approach to retraining bowel function after long-standing constipation and fecal impaction in people with learning disabilities, *Dev Med Child Neurol* 36:41, 1994.

Functional incontinence

Mikel Gray

Definition   The state in which an individual finds it difficult or is unable to reach the toilet because of impaired functional status including impaired mobility, dexterity, cognitive defects including dementia or mental retardation, or environmental barriers

Defining Characteristics

Urination occurs prior to locating the toilet, removing clothing, or sitting on the toilet

Client Outcomes/Goals

- Eliminates or reduces incontinent episodes
- Eliminates or overcomes environmental barriers to toileting

- Uses adaptive equipment to reduce or eliminate incontinence related to impaired mobility or dexterity
- Uses portable urinary collection devices or urine containment devices when access to the toilet is not feasible

Suggested NIC Interventions

Urinary habit training, urinary incontinence care

Nursing Interventions and Rationales

- Perform a focused history of the incontinence including duration, frequency, and severity of leakage episodes and alleviating and aggravating factors.
  The history provides clues to the etiology and severity of the condition and its management.
- Complete a bladder log of diurnal and nocturnal urine elimination patterns and patterns of urinary leakage.
  The bladder log provides a more objective verification of urine elimination patterns than the history (Resnick et al, 1994) and a baseline against which the results of management can be evaluated.
- Assess client for potentially reversible causes of acute/transient urinary incontinence (e.g., urinary tract infection, atrophic urethritis, constipation or impaction, sedatives or narcotics interfering with the ability to reach the toilet in a timely fashion, antidepressants or psychotropic medications interfering with efficient detrusor contractions, parasympatholytics, alpha adrenergic antagonists, polyuria caused by uncontrolled diabetes mellitus or insipidus).
  Transient or acute incontinence can be eliminated by reversing the underlying cause (Urinary Incontinence Guideline Panel, 1996).
- Assess client for established/chronic incontinence (stress incontinence, urge incontinence, reflex or extraurethral ["total"] incontinence). If present, begin treatment for these forms of urine loss.
  Functional incontinence often coexists with another form of urinary leakage, particularly among the elderly (Gray, 1992).
- Assess the home, acute-care or long-term care environment for accessibility to toileting facilities. Pay particular attention to the following:
  - Distance of toilet from bed, chair, and general living quarters
  - Characteristics of the bed, including presence of side rails and distance of bed from the floor
  - Characteristics of the pathway to the toilet, including barriers such as stairs, loose rugs on the floor, and inadequate lighting
  - Characteristics of the bathroom, including patterns of use, lighting, height of toilet from floor, presence of hand rails to assist transfers to toilet, breadth of door and its accessibility for wheelchair, and presence of walker or other assistive device
  Functional continence requires access to the toilet; environmental barriers blocking this access can produce functional incontinence (Wells, 1992).
- Assess client for mobility, including ability to rise from chair and bed, ability to transfer to toilet, ability to ambulate, and need for physical assistive devices such as a cane, walker, or wheelchair.
  Functional continence requires the ability to gain access to a toilet facility, either independently or with the assistance of devices to increase mobility (Jirovec, Wells, 1990; Wells, 1992).
- Assess client for dexterity, including the ability to manipulate buttons, hooks, snaps, Velcro, and zippers needed to remove clothing.
  Functional continence requires the ability to remove clothing to urinate (Wells, 1992).

- Evaluate cognitive status with a NEECHAM confusion scale (Neelan et al, 1992) for acute cognitive changes, a Folstein Mini Mental Status Examination (Folstein, Folstein, McHugh, 1975), or other tool as indicated.

  Functional continence requires sufficient mental acuity to respond to sensory input from a filling urinary bladder by locating the toilet, moving to it, and emptying the bladder (Jirovec, Wells, 1990; Colling et al, 1992).

- Remove environmental barriers to toileting in the acute care, long-term care or home setting. Assist the client with removing loose rugs from the floor and improving lighting in hallways and bathrooms.

- Provide an appropriate, safe urinary receptacle such as a 3-in-1 commode or a female or male hand-held or no-spill urinal when toileting access is limited by immobility or environmental barriers.

  These receptacles provide access to a substitute toilet and enhance the potential for functional continence (Wells, 1992).

- Assist clients with limited mobility with obtaining an evaluation from a physical therapist and obtaining assistive devices as indicated. Help clients select shoes with nonskid soles to maximize traction when getting out of a chair or transferring to the toilet.

- Assist clients with altering their wardrobe to maximize toileting access. Select loose-fitting clothing with stretch waist bands rather than buttoned or zipper waists, minimize buttons, snaps, and multilayered clothing, and substitute Velcro or other easily loosened fasteners for buttons, hooks, and zippers in existing clothing.

- Begin a prompted voiding program or patterned urge response toileting program with functional incontinence and dementia for elderly clients in the home or a long-term care facility.

  - Determine the frequency of current urination using an alarm system or check and change device.
  - Record urinary elimination and incontinent patterns on a bladder log to use as a baseline for assessment and evaluation of treatment efficacy.
  - Begin a prompted toileting program based on the results of this program; toileting frequency may vary from every 1.5 to 2 hours to every 4 hours.
  - Praise the client when toileting occurs with prompting.
  - Refrain from any socialization when incontinent episodes occur. Change clients' clothes and make them comfortable.

  Prompted voiding and patterned urge response toileting have been shown to markedly reduce or eliminate functional incontinence in selected clients in long-term care facilities and the community setting (Colling et al, 1992; Jilek, 1993; McDowell et al, 1994).

Geriatric

- Institute aggressive continence management programs for clients living in the community by having a consultation with the patient and family.

  Uncontrolled incontinence can lead to institutionalization in elderly clients who prefer to remain in a home care setting (O'Donnell et al, 1992).

- Monitor elderly clients in long-term care facilities, acute care facilities, or home for dehydration.

  Dehydration can exacerbate urine loss, produce acute confusion, and increase the risk of morbidity and mortality, particularly in frail elderly clients (Colling, Owen, McCreedy, 1994).

Home Care Interventions

- Assist the family with arranging care in a way that allows the client to participate in family or favorite activities without embarrassment.

Careful planning can retain the dignity of the client and integrity of family patterns.

- Refer client for home health aide services for hygiene and skin care.

Maintaining cleanliness helps the client retain dignity.

- Refer to occupational therapy for help in obtaining assistive devices and adapting the home for accessibility.
- Consider the use of an indwelling catheter to perform continuous drainage for a client who is terminal, homebound, and bedbound (requires physician order).

The primary goal may be caregiver support and client comfort, not correction of the incontinence.

- If using an indwelling catheter, follow prescribed maintenance protocols for skin care, catheter care, and changing. Maintain universal precautions for protection of the client and staff. Teach infection control measures.

Proper care decreases the risk of infection or other catheter-related problems.

- Instruct client to notify nurse or physician if urine is cloudy or blood streaked and if drainage is associated with abdominal pain or distention.

Early detection and reporting of problems allows immediate treatment.

Client/Family Teaching

- Work with client, family, and their extended support systems to assist with needed changes in the environment and wardrobe and other alterations needed to maximize toileting access.
- Work with client and family to establish a reasonable, manageable prompted voiding program using environmental and verbal cues, such as television programs, meals, and bedtime, to remind caregivers of voiding intervals.
- Teach family to use alarms as toileting cues or to perform a check and change program and maintain an accurate log of voiding and incontinent episodes.

REFERENCES   Colling JC, Owen TR, McCreedy MR: Urine volumes and voiding patterns among incontinent nursing home residents, *Geriatr Nurs* 15:188, 1994.

Colling JR et al: The effects of patterned urge response toileting (PURT) on urinary incontinence among nursing home residents, *J Am Geriatr Soc* 40:135, 1992.

Doughty DB, editor: *Urinary and fecal incontinence: nursing management,* St Louis, 1991, Mosby.

Folstein MR, Folstein EF, McHugh P: Mini mental state: a practical method of grading the cognitive status of the patient for the clinician, *J Psychiatr Rev* 12:189, 1975.

Gray ML: *Genitourinary disorders,* St Louis, 1992, Mosby.

Jeter K, Faller N, Norton C editors: *Nursing for continence,* Philadelphia, 1990, WB Saunders.

Jilek R: Elderly toileting: is two hours too often? *Nurs Standard* 47:25, 1993.

Jirovec MM, Wells TJ: Urinary incontinence in nursing home residents with dementia: the mobility-cognition paradigm, *Applied Nurs Res* 3:112, 1990.

McCormick K et al: Nursing management of urinary incontinence in geriatric inpatients, *Nurs Clin North Am* 23:231, 1988.

McDowell BJ et al: Successful treatment using behavioral interventions of urinary incontinence in homebound elder adults, *Geriatr Nurs* 15:303, 1994.

Neelan VJ et al: Use of the NEECHAM confusion scale to assess acute confusional states of hospitalized older patients. In Funk SG, Tornquist EM et al, editors: *Key aspects of elder care: managing falls, incontinence and cognitive impairment,* New York, 1992, Springer.

O'Donnell BF et al: Incontinence and troublesome behaviors predict institutionalization in dementia, *J Geriatr Psychiatr Neurol* 5:45, 1992.

Pinkowski PS: Prompted voiding in the long term care facility, *J Wound Ostomy Cont Nurs* 23:110, 1996.

Resnick NM et al: Short term variability of self report of incontinence in older persons, *J Am Geriatr Soc* 42:202, 1994.

Urinary Incontinence Guidelines Panel: *Urinary incontinence in adults: clinical practice guidelines,* ed 2, Rockville, Md, 1996, Agency for Health Care Policy and Research.

Wells TJ: Managing incontinence through managing the environment, *Urol Nurs* 12:48, 1992.

Reflex incontinence

Mikel Gray

Definition   The state in which an individual experiences an involuntary loss of urine caused by a defect in the spinal cord between the nerve roots at or below the first cervical segment and above the second sacral segment

Defining Characteristics

Absent or diminished awareness of bladder filling, absent urge to urinate; hyperreflexic detrusor contractions or other factors (e.g., positional changes, exposure of the perineum to the air, dipping hands in water) producing unpredictable urine loss with bladder filling; hyperreflexic detrusor contractions frequently accompanied by dyssynergia of the striated sphincter mechanism, producing functional outlet obstruction of the bladder

Related Factors (r/t)

Paralyzing spinal disorder affecting spinal segments C1 to S2.

Client Outcomes/Goals

- Follows prescribed schedule for bladder evacuation
- Demonstrates successful use of triggering techniques to stimulate voiding
- Maintains intact perineal skin
- Remains free of symptomatic urinary infection
- Demonstrates ability to use containment device or indwelling catheter or provides caregiver with instructions to perform these procedures
- Demonstrates awareness of risk of autonomic dysreflexia and its prevention and management

Suggested NIC Interventions

Urinary bladder training: urinary catheterization, intermittent

Nursing Interventions and Rationales

- Assess client's neurological status, including type of neurological disorder, functional level of neurological impairment and its completeness (affect on motor and sensory function), and ability to perform bladder management (e.g., intermittent catheterization, application of a condom catheter).

  The type of the neurological disorder as its associated functional level, completeness, and underlying disorder affect the severity of the urinary leakage, risk of striated sphincter dyssynergia, and subsequent management (Gray, 1992).

- Perform a focused assessment of the urinary system including a perineal skin assessment, evaluation of the vaginal vault, and reproduction of the sign of stress incontinence (see **Stress incontinence**). Perform a neurological examination including reproduction of the bulbocavernosus reflex and testing of perineal sensation.

  The focused physical examination will provide objective evidence of coexisting stress incontinence and indirect evidence of bladder and urethral sensation.

- Complete a bladder log to determine the pattern of urine elimination, incontinent episodes, and current bladder management program.

The bladder log provides an objective record of urine elimination confirming the accuracy of the historical report and providing a baseline for assessment and evaluation of treatment efficacy.

- Consult with the physician concerning current bladder function and the potential of the bladder to produce upper urinary tract distress (hydronephrosis, vesicoureteral reflux, febrile urinary tract infection, or compromised renal function).

  Reflex incontinence is typically accompanied by detrusor striated sphincter dyssynergia, which increases the risk of upper urinary tract distress (Gray et al, 1991; Killorin, 1992).

- Determine a bladder management program in consultation with the patient, family, and rehabilitation team.

  The bladder management program impacts the client and significant others. The program is determined by a holistic assessment that addresses potential of the bladder to create upper urinary tract distress, potential for continence and related complications, patient and family preference, and perceived impact of the bladder management program on the patient's life-style (Anson, Gray, 1993; Gray, Rayome, Anson, 1995).

- In a consultation with the rehabilitation team, counsel client and family concerning merits and potential risks associated with each bladder management program including spontaneous voiding, intermittent self-catheterization, reflex voiding program with condom catheter containment, and indwelling catheterization.

  All bladder management programs carry some risk of urinary incontinence or serious urinary system complications. Spontaneous voiding and intermittent catheterization carry greater risk of urine loss as compared to condom catheter containment or indwelling catheters, but these strategies carry higher risk for serious urinary system complications including upper urinary tract distress when evaluated over a period of years (Anson, Gray, 1993; Gray, Rayome, Anson, 1995).

- Teach all clients with reflex incontinence to consume an adequate amount of fluids on a daily basis (30 ml/kg of body weight).

  Dehydration exacerbates urine loss and increases the risk of related complications, including constipation and urine infection (Pearson, 1993; Gray, Rayome, Anson, 1995).

- Teach client using spontaneous voiding to self-administer an alpha adrenergic blocking medication as directed and to recognize and manage potential side effects.

  Clients who spontaneously urinate often take alpha adrenergic blocking drugs to reduce urethral resistance to voiding (Gray, 1996).

- Teach male clients (and their families) who have reflex incontinence and choose not to perform intermittent catheterization or cannot perform catheterization to obtain, select, and apply a condom catheter with drainage bag. Assist them with choosing a product that adheres to the penile shaft without allowing seepage of urine onto surrounding skin or clothing, a material and adhesive that do not produce hypersensitive reactions on the skin, and a leg bag that is easily concealed under clothing and does not cause irritation to thigh skin.

  Multiple components of the condom catheter affect the product's ability to contain urinary leakage, protect underlying skin, and preserve the client's dignity (Watson, 1989; Watson, Kuhn, 1990).

- Teach clients using intermittent catheterization to self-administer antispasmodic (parasympatholytic) medications as directed and to recognize and manage potential side effects.

  Clients who manage reflex incontinence by intermittent catheterization frequently require antispasmodic medications to manage the hyperreflexic detrusor contractions that produce urine loss (Gray, 1996).

- Teach the client using a condom catheter to routinely inspect the skin with each catheter change for evidence of lesions caused by pressure from the containment device or by exposure to urine.
  Skin breakdown is a common complication associated with routine use of the condom catheter (Anson, Gray, 1993).
- Teach clients using intermittent or indwelling catheters to recognize signs of significant urinary tract infections and promptly seek care when these signs appear. The signs of significant infection are the following (National Institute on Disability and Rehabilitation Research, 1992):
  - Discomfort over the bladder area or during urination
  - Acute onset of urinary incontinence
  - Fever
  - Markedly increased spasticity of muscles below the level of the spinal lesion
  - Malaise, lethargy
  - Hematuria
  - Autonomic dysreflexia (hyperreflexia)
  Intermittent catheterization is typically associated with asymptomatic bacteriuria, and the indwelling catheter is routinely associated with asymptomatic colonization. Antibiotic treatment of asymptomatic bacteriuria has not proven helpful, but prompt management of significant infection is necessary to prevent urosepsis or related complications (Waites, Cannupp, DeVivo, 1991; Stover, 1993).

Geriatric
- If having difficulties teaching elderly clients, refer them to a nurse who specializes in care of aging clients with urinary incontinence.

Home Care Interventions
- Instruct client in complications of reflex incontinence and when to report to physician or primary nurse.
  Early detection allows for early diagnosis and treatment of potential problems.
- If client is taught intermittent self-catheterization, arrange for contingency care in the event client is unable to perform self-catheterization.
  Self-catheterization supports client independence.
- Assess and instruct client and family in care of catheter and supplies in the home.
  Proper care of supplies decreases risk of infection.
- Assist the family with arranging care in a way that allows the client to participate in family or favorite activities without embarrassment.
  Careful planning can help client retain dignity and maintain the integrity of family patterns.
- If medications are ordered, instruct family or caregivers and client in medication administration, use, and side effects.
  Adherence to a medication regimen increases its chances of success and decreases the risk of losing the regimen as an option for care when other options are unacceptable.

Client/Family Teaching
- Teach signs of autonomic dysreflexia to all clients with a spinal injury, its relationship to bladder fullness, and management of the condition (see **Dysreflexia**).
- Teach client and several significant others techniques of intermittent catheterization, indwelling catheter care and removal, and condom catheter management as appropriate.
- Teach client and family techniques to clean intermittent catheters including washing with soap and water and allowing to air dry and using the microwave.

REFERENCES   Anson C, Gray ML: Secondary complications after spinal cord injury, *Urol Nurs* 13:107, 1993.

Gray ML: *Genitourinary disorders,* St Louis, 1992, Mosby.

Gray ML: *Urology nursing drug reference,* St Louis, 1996, Mosby.

Gray ML, Rayome RG, Anson C: Incontinence and clean intermittent catheterization following spinal cord injury, *Clin Nurs Res* 4:6, 1995.

Gray ML et al: Urethral pressure gradient in the prediction of upper urinary tract distress following spinal cord injury, *J Am Paraplegia Soc* 14:105, 1991.

Jeter K, Faller N, Norton C: *Nursing for continence,* Philadelphia, 1990, WB Saunders.

Killorin WK et al: Evaluative urodynamics and bladder management in the prediction of upper urinary infection in male spinal cord injury, *Paraplegia* 30:437, 1992.

National Institute on Disability and Rehabilitation Research: Prevention and management of urinary tract infections among people with spinal cord injuries, *J Am Paraplegia Soc* 15:194, 1992.

Pearson BD: Liquidate a myth: reducing liquid intake is not advisable for elderly with urine control problems, *Urol Nurs* 13:80, 1993.

Stover SL: Management of bacteriuria and infection in neurogenic bladder, *Rehab Clin North Am* 4:343, 1993.

Waites KB, Cannupp KC, DeVivo MJ: Efficacy and tolerance of norfloxacin in treatment of complicated urinary tract infection in outpatients with neurogenic bladder secondary to spinal cord injury, *Urology* 38:589, 1991.

Watson R: A nursing trial of urinary sheath systems on male hospitalized patients, *J Adv Nurs* 14:467, 1989.

Watson R, Kuhn M: The influence of component parts on the performance of urinary sheath systems, *J Adv Nurs* 15:417, 1990.

Stress incontinence

Mikel Gray

Definition   The state in which an individual experiences a urine loss of less than 50 ml accompanied by increased intraabdominal pressure (NOTE: The restriction of the volume of urine loss to less than 50 ml may be exceeded by women and men with severe stress incontinence caused by intrinsic sphincter deficiency. This is sometimes classified as "total incontinence." However, in this book, "total incontinence" will be used to refer exclusively to extraurethral incontinence; all forms of stress incontinence are reviewed under this diagnosis regardless of severity.)

Defining Characteristics

Observed urine loss with physical exertion (sign of stress incontinence), reported loss of urine associated with physical exertion or activity (symptom of stress incontinence), urine loss associated with increased abdominal pressure (urodynamic confirmation of stress incontinence)

Related Factors (r/t)

Urethral hypermobility (familial predisposition, multiple vaginal deliveries, delivery of large for gestational age baby, forceps assisted or breech delivery, obesity, changes in estrogen levels at climacteric, extensive abdominopelvic or pelvic surgery), intrinsic sphincter deficiency (multiple urethral suspensions in women, radical prostatectomy in men, uncommon complication of transurethral prostatectomy or cryosurgery of prostate, spinal lesion affecting sacral segments 2 through 4 or cauda equina, pelvic fracture)

Client Outcome/Goals

- Reports relief from stress incontinence or a decrease in the incidence or severity of incontinent episodes
- Achieves a reduction in grams of urine loss measured objectively by a pad test
- Identifies containment devices that assist in the management of stress incontinence

Suggested NIC Interventions

Pelvic floor exercise, urinary incontinence care

Nursing Interventions and Rationales

- Complete a history of urine loss including duration, severity and frequency of symptoms, precipitating factors, and current management of symptoms of urge incontinence.

  A history of stress incontinence helps determine the likely cause of leakage and best treatment options.

- Perform a focused physical assessment including perineal skin assessment, evaluation of the vaginal mucosa, reproduction of the sign of stress incontinence, and observation or urethral hypermobility and related pelvic descent (prolapse).

  The physical evaluation provides information about the severity of urine loss and objective evidence of the condition and determines the presence of urethral hypermobility (Gray, Rayome, Moore, 1995).

- Determine the client's current use of containment devices; evaluate selections for ability to adequately contain urine loss, protect clothing, and control odor. Assist client with identifying containment devices designed to contain urinary leakage.

  Clients, particularly women, may select feminine hygiene pads for urine containment. These items are designed to contain menstrual flow and are not well suited for urine loss (Jeter, Faller, Norton, 1990).

- Review treatment options with client (in close consultation with physician) including behavioral management, drug therapy, pessary use, and surgery. Outline potential benefits, efficacy, and side effects.

  Multiple treatments have been used to manage stress incontinence; behavioral management options should be offered initially (Urinary Incontinence Guideline Panel, 1996).

- Assess client for signs of urge incontinence (see **Urge incontinence**), and discuss the impact of this coexisting condition with clients suspected of having mixed urge and stress urinary leakage.

  Many options offered for stress incontinence also have a beneficial effect on the frequency and severity of urge incontinence (Urinary Incontinence Guideline Panel, 1996).

- Begin pelvic muscle reeducation for clients who choose this treatment option. Assess the client's pelvic muscle strength using pressure manometry, a digital evaluation technique, or urine stop test.

  A baseline of pelvic muscle strength is needed for initial assessment and evaluation of treatment efficacy (Worth, Dougherty, McKey, 1986; Dougherty et al, 1991; Sampselle, DeLancey, 1992; Brink et al, 1992).

- Teach the patient undergoing pelvic muscle reeducation to identify, contract, and relax the periurethral muscles without contracting distant muscle groups (such as the abdominal muscles) using biofeedback techniques.

  Pelvic muscle strengthening and reeducation are enhanced by the use of biofeedback (Burns et al, 1985; Berghmann et al, 1996).

- Incorporate principles of physiotherapy to a pelvic muscle exercise program including the following:
  - Graded program beginning with 5 to 10 repetitions and advancing gradually to 35 to 50 repetitions every day or every other day
  - Sustained exercise sessions over a period of 3-6 months
  - Integration of the exercise program into activities of daily living

- ▪ Repeated evaluations (no more than weekly) to encourage continued compliance with the muscle reeducation program, evaluate increases in pelvic muscle strength, and assess alleviation of stress incontinence

Pelvic reeducation alleviates or cures stress incontinence by a combination of factors including biofeedback and strength training. Application of principles of physiotherapy maximize the value of the exercise program (Dougherty et al, 1991; Dougherty et al, 1992; Brink et al, 1992; Nygaard et al, 1996).

- Teach client to reeducate pelvic muscles using weighted vaginal cones.

  Weighted vaginal cones have been shown to correct or alleviate stress urinary incontinence (Kondo, Yamada, Niijima, 1995; Fischer, Baessler, Linde, 1996).

- Begin transvaginal or transrectal electrical stimulation therapy among selected persons with stress incontinence in consultation with client and physician.

  Electrical stimulation alleviates stress incontinence, probably by strengthening the pelvic muscles and possibly via a biofeedback effect (Sand et al, 1995).

- Teach the patient to self-administer alpha adrenergic medications, imipramine, and topical or oral estrogens as directed.

  Pharmacotherapeutic agents alleviate or temporarily cure stress incontinence in selected women (Gray, 1996).

- Refer female clients who wish to employ a pessary to manage stress incontinence to a nurse specialist or gynecologist with expertise in the placement and maintenance of these devices.

  Pessary devices may alleviate or correct stress incontinence; however, they may cause serious complications unless applied correctly and monitored closely (Gray, 1992).

- Place a bladder neck support prosthesis in female clients who wish to use this device to manage stress incontinence.

  The bladder neck support prosthesis has been shown to reduce or correct stress incontinence among selected women (Bernier, Harris, 1995).

- Discuss potentially reversible or controllable risk factors with clients who have stress incontinence and assist them with formulating a strategy to alleviate or eliminate these conditions.

  Although research supports a strong familial predisposition to stress incontinence among women, other risk factors associated with the condition, including obesity and chronic coughing from smoking, are reversible (Skoner, Thompson, Caron, 1994; Mushkat, Bukovsky, Langer, 1996).

- Provide information about support groups such as the SIMON foundation or National Foundation for Continence.

- Refer clients with persistent stress incontinence to a continence service or physician or nurse who specializes in management of this condition.

  Complex stress incontinence is best managed with a multidisciplinary approach (McDowell, 1992).

Geriatric
- Evaluate the elderly client's functional and cognitive status to determine the impact functional limitations exert on the frequency and severity of urine loss, and plans for management.

Home Care Interventions

- Consider the use of an indwelling catheter to perform continuous drainage for a client who is terminal, homebound, and bedbound (Requires physician order).

  The primary goal may be caregiver support and client comfort, not correction of the incontinence.

- If using an indwelling catheter, follow prescribed maintenance protocols for skin care, catheter care, and changing. Use universal precautions for protection of client and staff. Teach infection control measures.
  Proper care decreases the risk of infection or other catheter-related problems.
- Instruct client to notify nurse or physician if urine is cloudy or blood streaked or drainage is associated with abdominal pain or distention.
  Early detection and reporting of problems support immediate treatment.

Client/Family Teaching

- Teach client to perform pelvic muscle exercises using an audiotape or a videotape if indicated.
- Teach client the importance of avoiding dehydration and to consume 30 ml/kg of body weight daily of fluids.
- Teach client the importance of avoiding constipation by a combination of adequate fluid and dietary fiber intakes and exercise.
- Teach client to apply and remove support devices such as the bladder neck support prosthesis.
- Teach the client to select and apply urine containment devices.

REFERENCES   Berghmann LCM et al: Efficacy of biofeedback when included with pelvic muscle exercise treatment for stress incontinence, *Neurourol Urodynamics* 15:37, 1996.

Bernier F, Harris L: Treating stress incontinence with the bladder neck support prosthesis, *Urol Nurs* 15:5, 1995.

Brink CA et al: A digital test for pelvic muscle strength in older women with urinary incontinence, *Nurs Res* 38:196, 1989.

Brink CA et al: Pelvic muscle exercise for elderly incontinent women. In Funk SG et al: *Key aspects of elder care: managing falls, incontinence and cognitive impairment,* New York, 1992, Springer.

Burns PA et al: Kegel's exercises with biofeedback therapy for treatment of stress incontinence, *Nurse Pract* 10:32, 1985.

Dougherty MC et al: Graded exercise: effect of pressures developed by the pelvic muscles. In Funk SG et al: *Key aspects of elder care: managing falls, incontinence and cognitive impairment,* New York, 1992, Springer.

Dougherty MC et al: Variations in intravaginal pressure measurements, *Nurs Res* 40:282, 1991.

Fischer W, Baessler K, Linde A: Pelvic floor conditioning with vaginal weights—post partum and in urinary incontinence, *Zentralbl Gynakol* 118:18, 1996.

Gray ML: *Genitourinary disorders,* St Louis, 1992, Mosby.

Gray ML: *Urology nursing drug reference,* St Louis, 1996, Mosby.

Gray ML, Rayome RG, Moore KN: The urethral sphincter: an update, *Urol Nurs* 15:40-53, 1995.

Jeter K, Faller N, Norton C, editors: *Nursing for continence,* Philadelphia, 1990, WB Saunders.

Kondo A, Yamada Y, Niijima R: Treatment of stress incontinence by vaginal cones: short- and long-term results and predictive parameters, *Brit J Urol* 76:464, 1995.

McDowell B et al: An interdisciplinary approach to the assessment and behavioral treatment of urinary incontinence in geriatric outpatients, *J Am Geriatr Soc* 40:370, 1992.

Mushkat Y, Bukovsky I, Langer R: Female urinary stress incontinence—does it have familial prevalence? *Am J Obstet Gynecol* 174:617, 1996.

Nygaard IE et al: Efficacy of pelvic floor muscle exercise in women with stress, urge and mixed urinary incontinence, *Am J Obstet Gynecol* 174:120, 1996.

Sampselle CM, DeLancey JOL: The urine stream interruption test and pelvic muscle function, *Nurs Res* 41:73, 1992.

Sand PK et al: Pelvic floor electrical stimulation in the treatment of genuine stress incontinence: a multicenter placebo controlled trial, *Am J Obstet Gynecol* 173:72, 1995.

Skoner MM, Thompson WD, Caron VA: Factors associated with risk of stress urinary incontinence in women, *Nurs Res* 43:301, 1994.

Urinary Incontinence Guideline Panel: *Urinary incontinence in adults: clinical practice guideline,* ed 2, Rockville, Md, 1996, Agency for Health Care Policy and Research.

Worth AM, Dougherty MC, McKey PL: Development and testing of the circumvaginal muscle (CVM) rating scale, *Nurs Res* 35:166, 1986.

Total incontinence

Mikel Gray

Definition   The state in which an individual experiences a continuous and unpredictable loss of urine (NOTE: In this book, the diagnosis of total incontinence will be used to refer to continuous urine loss from an extraurethral loss, and stress incontinence will be used to refer to leakage from sphincter incompetence, regardless of severity.)

Defining Characteristics

Continuous urine flow varying from dribbling incontinence superimposed on an otherwise identifiable pattern of voiding to severe urine loss without identifiable micturition episodes

Related Factors (r/t)

Ectopia (ectopic ureter opens into the vaginal vault or cutaneously, bladder ectopia with exstrophy/epispadias complex), fistula (opening from bladder or urethra to vagina or skin that bypasses urethral sphincter mechanism, allowing continuous urine loss)

Client Outcomes/Goals

- Adequately contains urine loss, keeps clothing unsoiled, controls odor
- Maintains intact perineal skin
- Maintains dignity—hides urine containment devices in clothing, minimizes bulk and noise related to the device

Suggested NIC Interventions

Urinary incontinence care

Nursing Interventions and Rationales

- Obtain a history of duration and severity of urine loss, prior management, and aggravating or alleviating features.
  The symptom of "continuous incontinence" may be caused by extraurethral leakage or other types of incontinence that have been inadequately evaluated and/or managed. The patient history will provide clues to the etiology of the urinary leakage (Doughty, 1991).
- Perform a focused physical assessment including inspection of the perineal skin, examination of the vaginal vault, reproduction of the sign of stress incontinence (see **Stress incontinence**), and testing of bulbocavernosus reflex and perineal sensations.
  The physical examination will provide evidence supporting the diagnosis of extraurethral or another type of incontinence (stress, urge, or reflex) and provide the basis for further evaluation and/or treatment (Doughty, 1991).
- Complete a bladder log of urine elimination patterns, frequency, and severity of urine loss.
  The bladder log provides further information allowing the nurse to differentiate extraurethral from other forms of urine loss, providing the basis for further evaluation and treatment (Doughty, 1991).
- Assist client with selecting and applying urine containment device(s). Review types of containment products with client, including advantages and potential complications associated with each type of product.
  Urine containment products include a variety of absorptive pads, incontinent briefs, underpads for bedding, absorptive inserts that fit into specially designed undergarments, and condom catheters. Careful selection of an absorptive device and education concerning its use maximizes its effectiveness in controlling urine loss in a particular individual (Gray, 1992; McKibben, 1995).

- Evaluate disposable versus reusable products for urine containment, considering factors such as setting (home care versus acute care versus long-term care), preferences of the patient and caregiver(s), and immediate versus long-term costs.
  The economic and related impacts of routine use of urine containment devices are significant, regardless of the setting. Economic factors, as well as patient and caregiver preferences, affect the success and ultimate cost of a reusable versus disposable urine containment device (Hu, Kaltreider, Igou, 1990; Ledger, 1993; Cummings et al, 1995).
- Cleanse skin with an incontinence cleansing product system or plain water when changing urinary containment devices or pads. Use soap and water on the perineum no more than once daily or every other day as necessary.
  Excessive cleansing of the perineal skin may exacerbate alterations in skin integrity, particularly in the elderly (Lindell, Olsson, 1990; Byers et al, 1995).
- Apply a skin moisturizer following cleansing.
  Moisturizers promote comfort and may reduce the risk of skin breakdown (Kemp, 1994).
- Apply a protective barrier or ointment to the perineal skin when incontinence is severe, double fecal and urinary incontinence exist, or the risk of a pressure ulcer is significant.
  A moisture barrier is indicated when the risk of altered skin integrity is complicated by coexisting factors of shear, fecal incontinence, or exposure to prolonged pressure (Doughty, 1991; Kemp, 1994).
- Consult physician concerning use of an antifungal powder or ointment when perineal dermatitis is complicated by monilial infection. Teach client to use product sparingly when applying to affected areas.
  Antifungal powders or ointments provide effective relief from monilial rash; however, application of excessive amounts of the product retains moisture and diminishes its effectiveness (Doughty, 1991).
- Consult physician concerning placement of an indwelling catheter when severe urine loss is complicated by urinary retention, when careful fluid monitoring is indicated, when perineal dryness is required to promote healing a stage three or four pressure ulcer, during periods of critical illness, or in a terminally ill client when use of absorbent products produces pain or distress.
  Although not routinely indicated, the indwelling catheter provides an effective, transient management technique for carefully selected patients (Treatment of Pressure Ulcers Guideline Panel, 1994; Urinary Incontinence Guideline Panel, 1996).
- Refer clients with intractable or extraurethral incontinence to a continence service or specialist for further evaluation and management of urine loss.
  The successful management of complex, severe urinary incontinence requires specialized evaluation and treatment from a health care provider with special expertise (Doughty, 1991; Gray, 1992).

Geriatric
- Provide privacy and support when changing incontinent devices of elderly clients.
  Elderly, hospitalized clients frequently express feelings of shame, guilt, and dependency when undergoing urinary containment device changes (Biggersson et al, 1993).
- Employ meticulous infection control procedures when using an indwelling catheter.

Home Care Interventions
The interventions identified are all applicable in the home setting. Please review the interventions for appropriateness to individual clients.

Client/Family Teaching
- Teach family to obtain, apply, and dispose or clean and reuse urine containment devices.

- Teach family a routine perineal skin care regimen, including daily or every other day hygiene and cleansing with containment product changes.
- Teach client and family to recognize and manage perineal dermatitis, ammonia contact dermatitis, and monilial rash.
- Teach client to maintain adequate fluid intake (30 ml/kg of body weight per day).
- Teach client and family to recognize and manage urinary infection.

REFERENCES   Bierwirth W: Which pad is for you? *Urol Nurs* 12:75, 1992.

Biggersson AB: Elderly women's feelings about being incontinent, using napkins and being helped by nurses to change napkins, *J Clin Nurs* 2:165, 1993.

Byers PH et al: Effects of continence care cleansing regimens on skin integrity, *Wound Ostomy Cont Nurs* 22:187, 1995.

Cummings V et al: Costs and management of urinary incontinence in long term care, *J Wound Ostomy Cont Nurs* 22:193, 1995.

Doughty DB, editor: *Urinary and fecal incontinence: nursing management,* St Louis, 1991, Mosby.

Gray ML: *Genitourinary disorders,* St Louis, 1992, Mosby.

Hu T, Kaltreider DL, Igou J: The cost-effectiveness of disposable versus reusable diapers: a controlled experiment in a nursing home. *J Gerontol Nurs* 16:19, 1990.

Jeter K, Faller N, Notron C, editors: *Nursing for continence,* Philadelphia, 1990, WB Saunders.

Kemp MG: Protecting the skin from moisture and associated irritants, *J Gerontol Nurs* 20:8, 1994.

Lindell ME, Olsson HM: Personal hygiene in external genitalia of health and hospitalized elderly women, *Health Care Women Int* 11:151, 1990.

McKibben, E: Pad use in perspective, *Nurs Times* 91:60,62, 1995.

Philp J, Cottenden A, Ledger D: Well disposed? Comparison between reusable and disposable incontinence products, *Nurs Times* 89:65, 1993.

Treatment of Pressure Ulcers Guideline Panel: *Treatment of pressure ulcer: clinical practice guideline,* Rockville, MD, 1994, Agency for Health Care Policy and Research.

Urinary Incontinence Guideline Panel: *Urinary incontinence in adults: clinical practice guideline,* ed 2, Rockville, MD, 1996, Agency for Health Care Policy and Research.

Verdell L, editor: *Resource guide of continence products and services,* ed 6, Union, SC, 1994, Help for Incontinent People/National Association for Continence.

Urge incontinence

Mikel Gray

Definition   The state in which an individual experiences involuntary passage of urine occurring with a precipitous desire to urinate

Defining Characteristics

Diurnal urinary frequency (void more frequently than every 2 hours), urgency (subjective report of the immediate desire to urinate with bladder filling or provocation), urge incontinence (involuntary passage of urine unless a toilet is located very soon after the symptom of urgency is perceived), nocturia or enuresis (awakened more than once per night by the desire to urinate or uncontrolled loss of urine during sleep)

Related Factors (r/t)

Neurological disorders (disorders of the brain including cerebrovascular accident [CVA], brain tumor), stress urinary incontinence (often coexisting with stress incontinence—with relationship between stress and urge incontinence unclear), irritative voiding disorders (urinary tract infection in susceptible individuals, bladder calculi, bladder tumors including papillary transitional cell carcinoma tumors and carcinoma in situ; inflammatory lesions of the bladder), bladder outlet obstruction (see **Urinary retention**)

Suggested NIC Interventions

Urinary habit training, urinary incontinence care

Nursing Interventions and Rationales

- Perform a nursing history focusing on duration of urinary incontinence, frequency and severity of symptoms, and alleviating and aggravating factors.

  A focused history helps determine the cause of urge incontinence and its management.

- Perform a urinalysis to evaluate client for causes of acute urinary incontinence including urinary tract infection and diabetes mellitus.

  These disorders may cause acute or transient urinary incontinence that is reversible with treatment of the underlying condition (Urinary Incontinence Guideline Panel, 1996).

- Perform a focused physical assessment including perineal skin inspection evaluation of the vaginal vault for atrophic changes or hypermobility and a neurological examination including testing of the bulbocavernosus and perineal skin sensation.

  The physical examination provides clues to the cause of urge incontinence, including the presence of atrophic vaginal and urethral changes that can produce transient urge leakage that is reversible with treatment of this underlying condition (Urinary Incontinence Guideline Panel, 1996).

- Complete a bladder log including frequency of diurnal micturition and nocturia, patterns of incontinence, symptoms accompanying urine loss, and the type and volume of fluids consumed.

  The bladder log provides a more objective record of diurnal urinary frequency, nocturia, and symptoms of urgency and urge incontinence as compared to the history (Resnick et al, 1994). Recording fluid consumption allows assessment of the intake of bladder irritants and assessment of the volume of fluid consumption over a 24-hour period.

- Review medications client is receiving, paying particular attention to sedatives, narcotics, diuretics, antidepressants, psychotropic drugs, cholinergics, and alpha adrenergic agonists or antagonists. Consult physician concerning altering or eliminating these medications if they are suspected of affecting continence.

  The side effects of multiple medications may produce or exacerbate urge incontinence (Urinary Incontinence Guideline Panel, 1996).

- Assess the client for urinary retention (see **Urinary retention**).

  Urinary retention associated with bladder outlet obstruction may be a contributing cause of urge incontinence (Rozier et al, 1995) and urinary retention, regardless of its cause, significantly impacts the management of this condition (Doughty, 1991; Gray, 1992).

- Assess the client for functional limitations (environmental factors, limited mobility or dexterity, impaired cognitive function) that produce or exacerbate urge incontinence (see **Functional incontinence**).

  Functional limitations impact the severity and management of urge incontinence (Gray, 1992).

- Consult the physician concerning diabetic management, pharmacotherapy for a urinary infection, or hormonal therapy for atrophic vaginitis/urethritis when indicated.

  Urge incontinence may be corrected or significantly alleviated by managing these underlying disorders (Urinary Incontinence Guideline Panel, 1996).

- Establish a habit retraining program based on data gathered from the bladder log, physical assessment, and functional assessment.
  Bladder retraining has been shown to reduce or correct urge incontinence among selected patients (Fantl et al, 1991).
- Review fluid consumption with the client; identify, reduce, or eliminate bladder irritants including alcohol, caffeinated beverages, aspartame, and carbonated beverages.
  Bladder irritants may increase urinary urgency and exacerbate urge incontinence. The precise effect of these irritants on the bladder remains unclear (Doughty, 1991; Gray, 1992).
- Evaluate the volume of fluids consumed and gradually increase fluid intake to the Recommended Daily Allowance (RDA) of 30 ml/kg of body weight (National Academy of Sciences, Food and Nutrition Board, 1980).
  Dehydration exacerbates rather than alleviates the risk of urine loss (Pearson, Larsen, 1992; Pearson, 1993).
- Use biofeedback techniques to teach client to contract pelvic muscles in response to a precipitous urge to urinate.
  Biofeedback is effective in the management of urge incontinence in selected patients (Burgio, Engel, 1990).
- Begin transvaginal or transrectal electrical stimulation using a low Hertz frequency (5 to 20 Hz) in consultation with the physician.
  Transvaginal, transrectal, or transcutaneous electrical stimulation is effective in controlling urge incontinence in selected patients (Moore, Gray, Rayome, 1995).
- Teach client to self-administer antispasmodic (parasympatholytic) drugs as directed. Assist client with determining and implementing a timed schedule while on these medications.
  The effectiveness of antispasmodic medications is enhanced when the patient voids on a timed schedule (prior to occurrence of hyperactive unstable detrusor contractions) (Gray, 1992; Gray, 1996).
- Assist client with selecting, obtaining, and applying a urine containment device for urge incontinence as indicated (see **Total incontinence**).
- Assist client with establishing a skin care cleansing regimen for urge incontinence when indicated (see **Total incontinence**).
- Provide client with information about incontinence support groups such as the National Association for Continence (NAFC) and the SIMON Foundation.

Geriatric
- Assess functional and cognitive status of all elderly clients with urge incontinence.
- Plan care in long-term or acute care facilities based on knowledge of the elderly client's established voiding patterns, paying particular attention to patterns of nocturia.

Home Care Interventions

- If the family is under financial stress, assist in identifying alternatives to incontinence products or other financial resources.
  Continence supplies are considered cosmetic. They are expensive—they are used frequently and on a long-term basis by nature of the problem, and insurance does not cover them as supplies.

Client/Family Teaching

- Teach client and family to recognize foods and beverages that are likely to irritate the bladder.
- Teach client and family the significance of avoiding dehydration and the paradoxical relationship between reduction of fluid intake and urge incontinence.

- Teach client and family to recognize and manage side effects of anticholinergic, antispasmodic medications sometimes used to manage urge incontinence.
- Teach family and client to identify and correct environmental barriers to toileting within the home.

REFERENCES   Burgio KL, Engel BT: Biofeedback behavioral therapy for elderly men and women, *J Am Geriatr Soc* 38:338, 1990.

Doughty DB, editor: *Urinary and fecal incontinence: nursing management,* St Louis, 1991, Mosby.

Fantl JA et al: Efficacy of bladder training in older women with urinary incontinence, *JAMA* 265:609, 1991.

Gray ML: *Genitourinary disorders,* St Louis, 1992, Mosby.

Gray ML: *Urology nursing drug reference,* St Louis, 1996, Mosby.

Jeter K, Faller N, Notron C, editors: *Nursing for continence,* Philadelphia, 1990, WB Saunders.

Moore KN, Gray ML, Rayome R: Electric stimulation and urinary incontinence: research and alternatives, *Urol Nurs* 15:94, 1995.

National Academy of Sciences, Food and Nutrition Board: *Recommended daily allowances,* ed 9, Washington, DC, 1980, The Academy.

Pearson BD: Liquidate a myth: reducing liquids is not advisable for elderly with urine control problems, *Urol Nurs* 13:86, 1993.

Pearson BD, Larsen JM: Urine control by elders: noninvasive strategies. In Funk SG et al: *Key aspects of elder care: managing falls, incontinence, and cognitive impairment,* New York, 1992, Springer.

Resnick NM et al: Short term variability of self report of incontinence in older persons, *J Am Geriatr Soc* 42:202, 1994.

Rozier PFWM et al: Is detrusor instability in males related to the grade of obstruction? *Neurourol Urodynamics* 14:625, 1995.

Urinary Incontinence Guideline Panel: *Urinary incontinence in adults: clinical practice guideline,* ed 2, Rockville, Md, 1996, Agency for Health Care Policy and Research.

Disorganized infant behavior

Mary A. Fuerst-DeWys

Definition   Altered regulation and balanced functioning of the neurobehavioral subsystems (i.e., physiological/autonomic, motor, state, attention-interaction, and self-regulatory systems) that is manifested in disorganized behavior patterns (modified from NANDA)

Defining Characteristics

Major   **Physiological/autonomic cues:** *Cardiorespiratory changes beyond normal limits:* tachycardia, bradycardia, tachypnea, apnea
Color changes: pale, mottled, red, dusky, cyanotic
Visceral: gagging, regurgitation, digestive intolerance, hiccoughs
Neurological: seizures, twitches, tremors/tremorlike movements of head, hands, lips, and feet
Motor cues: *Posture/tone:* fluctuating muscle tone and hyperextended, hyperflexed, hyperflaccidity of the neck, face, trunk, arms, legs, fingers, toes
Movement: excessive startles, body squirms, jerky and/or frantic movements, cycles of uncontrolled high activity, disorganized motor behaviors interfering with purposeful activities
State cues: Lack of full range of states from deep sleep to robust crying, display of unclear diffuse states

States of infant alertness

State I	Deep Sleep: irregular respirations, occasional startles, twitches
State II	Light Sleep: twitches, grimaces, whimpers
State III	Drowsy: transitional sleep, diffuse movements, fusses, whimpers
State IV	Quiet Awake: dull appearance, diffuse non-alert wakefulness, non-interactive
State V	Active Awake: distressed appearance, hyperaroused, increased body activity, fussing
State VI	Crying: diffuse, strained or weak crying

Modified from Als H: A synactive model of neonatal organization: framework for the assessment and support of the neurobehavioral development of the premature infant and his parents in the environment of the neonatal intensive care unit, Phys Occup Ther Pediatr 6:3, 1986.

Ineffective state modulation: problems maintaining a clear state for a period of time (e.g., client is hyperaroused, irritable); problems transitioning smoothly from one state of sleep and wakefulness to another (e.g., abrupt state changes)

Sleep problems: initiating sleep and maintaining sleep, irregular sleep-wake patterns

Ineffective habituation: problems "shutting out" noxious stimuli (hyperresponsive to stimuli)

Attentional-interaction cues: *Altered attentional and interaction capabilities:* problems initiating attention, maintaining attention, and shifting attention easily from one stimulus to another; poor impulse control; easily distracted with several, new, or changing stimuli; problems engaging in mutual and reciprocal interactions without significant display of avoidance/stress behaviors; difficulty being consoled or inconsolable

Self-regulatory cues: *Ineffective self-regulation and control:* imbalance of disorganized behaviors versus organized behaviors that interferes with adaptive functioning (e.g., physiological regulation, sleep problems, hyperarousal, irritability, attentional and interaction problems), inability to console self

Minor   Yawning, sighing, coughing, straining and stooling with stress

Related Factors (r/t)

Internal   Pain; colic; hunger; fatigue; discomfort; respiratory, visceral, or neurological compromise; altered sensory threshold (hypersensitive, hyposensitive, sensory defensiveness); infection; malnutrition; anxiety; poor adaptability; low energy level and/or energy depletion; pathological condition resulting from prematurity, neurological sequelae; prenatal exposure to alcohol, cocaine, and/or other substances; maternal infection; congenital anomalies

External   Cognitive and emotional stimulation and care that are noncontingent to infant-child's state, cues, level of sensory and energy thresholds, health status, and level of recovery and maturity; environmental stresses such as bright lights, temperature changes, visual clutter, sudden loud noises, prolonged sound levels above 50 to 55 decibels; disorganized and/or chaotic environment lacking structure and predictability; inappropriate handling and positioning; invasive or painful procedures

Client Outcomes/Goals

Infant-child   • Displays organized and balanced neurobehavioral functioning in all systems
• Displays minimal or no maladaptive or abnormal compensatory behavior patterns

Parent/significant other

- Recognizes infant-child behaviors as a unique way of communicating needs and goals
- Recognizes infant behavior used to communicate stress/avoidance and approach/ regulatory
- Recognizes and supports infant-child's drive and behaviors used to self-regulate
- Demonstrates ways of being more responsive to infant-child cues and needs
- Recognizes the way their interactions affect the infant's responses and that allowing the infant-child to take lead in the interaction fosters adaptive communication patterns
- Structures and modifies the environment in response to infant-child behaviors
- Identifies appropriate positioning and handling techniques to enhance comfort and normal development and prevent abnormalities

Suggested NIC Interventions

Environmental management: positioning

Nursing Interventions and Rationales

- Identify infant-child's level of neurobehavioral organization as a unique way of communicating.
  The infant's principal method of communicating goals, needs, and limits for stress and stability is by behavior; therefore the infant's own behaviors provide a guide for individualizing care and interactions and promoting development (Als, 1982).
- Recognize behavior used to communicate stress/avoidance and approach/regulatory.
  The ability to read and interpret infant behavior provides a framework for responding to infants in a way that communicates the infant-child's importance and that they are able to affect their environment (Als, 1982; Blackburn, Vandenberg,1991).
- Identify and support the infant-child's self-regulatory coping behaviors used for mastery of the environment.
  A continuous interaction takes place between the infant and the environment; behaviors such as hand-to-mouth/face, hand grasping, foot and leg bracing, sucking on fingers/fists, auditory and visual fixation, and postural changes are used to maintain or regain a balanced adaptation between the self and the environment. Supporting infant behaviors enhances the coregulatory fit between the infant and the environment (Als, 1986).
- Correlate the evidence of stress/disorganization to internal factors (e.g., pain, hunger, discomfort) or external factors (e.g., lights, noise, handling).
  Noise is one of the common stresses in hospital ICUs resulting in sensory overload with the potential for alteration in development (DePaul, Chambers, 1995; Elander, 1995). Infant colic characterized by increased irritability, diminished soothability, and excessive restlessness reflects immature sleep-wake regulation (an internal factor) (Keefe et al, 1996). Intrauterine cocaine exposure can result in disorganized behavior patterns of infants (DeWys, 1994).
- Structure and modify care and environment.
  A developmental care approach designed to reduce environmental and procedural stress and facilitate motor and sleep-wake organization results in improved behavioral organization during the preterm period (Newman, 1986; Becker et al, 1991). Patterns of sound and light and caretaking task should minimize stress, conserve energy, and protect the developing neonate from inappropriate environmental stimuli (Blackburn, Vandenberg, 1991).
- Facilitate the use of developmentally supportive positioning and handling.
  Developmentally correct positioning can prevent position-induced deformities (e.g., neck hyperextension, retracted shoulders, wide and abducted hips, and lack of midline

orientation), provide comfort, and enhance interactions and long-term sensorimotor development (Fay, 1988; Semmler, 1986). Normal sensorimotor development provides the foundation for normal movement patterns that are directed toward adaptive and purposeful activities (Gilfoyle, Grady, Moore, 1982).

- Identify techniques to assist development of state modulation and organization.
Providing care and stimulation contingent to the state of the infant are critical to state organization (Fajardo et al, 1990). Assisting parents to recognize infant states and state modulation and self-consoling strategies provides caregivers with greater sense of competence (Nursing Child Assessment Satellite Training, 1994).

- Identify and support infant-child's attentional capabilities.
In organized attentive states, infants are able to focus attention and interact with their environments purposefully (Burns et al, 1994).

- Facilitate and enhance mutual and reciprocal social interactions.
Reciprocal interactions are essential in establishing positive patterns with partners who are mutually adapting their behaviors to each other (Brazelton, Koslowski, Main, 1974). Authors suggested a developmental perspective for assessing mutual engagement and reciprocal interactions, which assesses the ability to attend and remain calm for a period of time (e.g., 5+ seconds by 3 to 4 months of age, 30+ seconds by 8 to 10 months of age, 2+ minutes by 2 years of age, and 15 minutes by 4 years of age) (National Center for Clinical Infant Programs, 1994).

- Enhance normal developmental patterns through appropriate sensorimotor stimulation.
Healthy 33 to 34 week postconceptual-age infants who received 15 minutes of auditory, visual, tactile, and vestibular stimulation each day were found to be better at state modulation. Their ability to maintain quiet-alertness enhances parent-infant interactions and feedings (White-Traut et al, 1993). Enhancing normal experiences through appropriate sensory stimulation, handling, and social interactions appropriate to infant's developmental level can minimize secondary problems (Anderson, Auster-Liebhaber, 1984).

REFERENCES   Als H: A synactive model of neonatal behavioral organization: framework for the assessment and support of the neurobehavioral development of the premature infant and his parents in the environment of the neonatal intensive care unit, *Phys Occup Ther Pediatr* 6:3, 1986.

Als H: Toward a synactive theory of development: promise for the assessment and support of infant individuality, *Infant Ment Health J* 3:229, 1982.

Anderson J, Auster-Liebhaber J: Developmental therapy in the neonatal intensive care unit, *Phys Occup Ther Pediatr* 4:89, 1984, Haworth Press.

Becker et al: Outcomes of developmentally supportive nursing care for very low birth weight infants, *Nurs Res* 40:150, 1991.

Blackburn S: Fostering behavioral development of high-risk infants, *J Obstet Gynecol Neonat Nurs* 3 (suppl):76, 1983.

Blackburn S, Vandenberg K: Assessment and management of neonatal development. In Kenner C et al: *Comprehensive neonatal nursing: a physiologic approach,* Toronto, 1991, WB Saunders.

Brazelton TB, Koslowski B, Main M: The origins of reciprocity: the early mother-infant interaction. In Lewis M, Rosenblum I, editors: *The effect of infant on its caregiver,* New York, 1974, John Wiley.

Burns M et al: Infant stimulation: modification of an intervention based on physiologic and behavioral cues, *JOGNN* 23:581, 1994.

D'Apolito K: What is an organized infant? *Neonatal Network* 10:23, 1991.

DePaul D, Chambers SE: Environmental noise in the neonatal intensive care unit: implications for nursing practice, *J Perinatol Neonat Nurs* 8:71, 1995, Aspen.

DeWys M, McComish-Fry J: Infants states and cues: facilitating effective parent-infant interactions. In *Caring for infants: a resource manual for caring for infant trainers,* 1992, East Lansing, Mich, Michigan State University Board of Trustees.

Elander G, Hellstrom G: Reduction of noise levels in intensive care units for infants: evaluation of an intervention program, *Heart Lung* 24:376, 1995.

Fay M: The positive effects of positioning, *Neonatal Network* 7:23, 1988.

Fajardo B et al: Effect of nursery environment on state regulation in very-low-birth-weight premature infants, *Infant Beh Dev* 13:287, 1990.

Gilfoyle E, Grady A, Moore J: *Children adapt,* 1982, Thorofare, NJ, Slack.

Keefe M et al: A longitudinal comparison of irritable and nonirritable infants, *Nurs Res* 45:4, 1996.

National Center for Clinical Infant Programs: *Diagnostic classification: zero to three diagnostic classification of mental health and developmental disorders in infancy and early childhood,* Virginia, 1994, The Center.

Newman L: Social and sensory environment of low birth weight infants in a special care nursery, *J Nerv Ment Dis* 169:448, 1986.

Semmler C: Positioning and position-inducing deformities: In Semmler C, editor: *A guide to care and management of low birth weight infants: a team approach,* Tucson, 1986, Therapy Skill Builders.

University of Washington, School of Nursing: *NCAST caregiver/parent-child interaction feeding manual,* Seattle, 1994, Nursing Child Assessment Satellite Training.

White-Traut R et al: Patterns of physiological and behavioral response of intermediate care preterm infants to intervention, *Pediatr Nurs* 19:625, 1993.

Potential for enhanced organized infant behavior

Mary A. Fuerst-DeWys

Definition   A pattern of balanced regulation and integration of an infant-child's neurobehavioral subsystems of functioning (i.e., physiological/autonomic, motor, state, attentional-interaction systems, self-regulatory) that is satisfactory but can be improved and results in higher levels of modulation, what is manifested in organized behavior patterns

Defining Characteristics

Physiological/autonomic cues: cardiorespiratory within normal limits, minimal color changes, smooth digestive functioning with minimal regurgitation, minimal tremors and twitches, no seizures

Motor cues: progressive development toward well-controlled posture; consistent well-balanced flexor or extensor tone; smooth, well-differentiated movements pertinent for purposeful activities; midline orientation and control; minimal startles

State cues: display of full range of states from deep sleep to robust crying

States of infant alertness	
State I	Deep sleep: non-REM, regular respirations, no spontaneous activity
State II	Light sleep: REM, low level activity, mild sucking or few mouthing movements
State III	Drowsy: semidozing, glassy-eyed look, mild startles
State IV	Quiet-awake: alert, bright-eyed, minimal activity, focused attention
State V	Active-awake: aroused but not hyperaroused, increased activity, less focused attention
State VI	Crying: robust, rhythmical crying, more than 15 seconds; nonattentive

Modified from Als H: A synactive model of neonatal behavioral organization: framework for the assessment and support of the premature infant and his parents in the environment of the neonatal intensive care unit, Phys Occup Ther Pediatr *6:3, 1986.*

Effective state modulation: maintenance of a clear, well-defined state for a period of time, display of smooth transition from one state of sleep and wakefulness to another, display of regular sleep-wake patterns

Effective habituation: ability to "shut out" noxious stimuli without excessive underresponsiveness

Attention-interaction cues: initiation, maintenance, and shift of attention smoothly from one stimulus to another; inhibition of distractions and engagement in reciprocal social interactions with minimal avoidance/stress behaviors; consoled easily

Self-regulation cues: effective regulation of subsystems (e.g., balance of approach and avoidance behaviors and effectively consoles self)

Related Factors (r/t)

Internal   Pain; colic; hunger; fatigue; discomfort; respiratory, visceral, or neurological compromise; altered sensory threshold (hypersensitive, hyposensitive, sensory defensiveness); infection; malnutrition; anxiety; poor adaptability; low energy level and/or energy depletion; pathological condition resulting from prematurity; neurological sequelae; prenatal exposure to alcohol, cocaine, and/or other substances; maternal infection; congenital anomalies

External   Cognitive and emotional stimulation and care that are noncontingent to infant-child's state, cues, level of sensory and energy thresholds, health status, level of recovery, and maturity; environmental stressors such as bright lights, temperature changes, visual clutter, sudden loud noises, prolonged sound levels above 50 to 55 decibels; disorganized environment lacking in structure and predictability; inappropriate handling and positioning; invasive or painful procedures

Client Outcomes/Goals

Infant-child   • Displays organized and balanced neurobehavioral functioning in all systems

                • Displays minimal or no maladaptive or abnormal compensatory behaviors patterns

Parent/significant other

                • Recognizes infant-child behaviors as a unique way of communicating needs and goals

                • Recognizes infant behaviors that communicate approach or avoidance/stress

                • Recognizes and supports infant-child's drive and behaviors used to self-regulate (Als, 1982)

                • Demonstrates ways of being more responsive to infant-child cues and needs

                • Recognizes the way their interactions affect the infant's responses and that allowing the infant-child to take the lead in interactions fosters adaptative communication patterns

                • Structures and modifies the environment in response to infant-child behaviors

                • Identifies appropriate positioning and handling techniques to enhance comfort and normal development and prevent abnormalities

Suggested NIC Interventions

Environmental management: attachment process, sleep enhancement

Nursing Interventions and Rationales

                • Identify infant-child's level of neurobehavioral organization as a unique way of communicating.
                The infant's principal method of communicating goals, needs, and limits for stress and stability is by behavior; therefore the infant's own behaviors provide a guide for individualizing care and interactions and promoting development (Als, 1982).

                • Recognize behavior used to communicate stress/avoidance and approach/regulatory.
                The ability to read and interpret infant behavior provides a framework for responding to infants in a way that communicates their importance and that they are able to affect their environment (Als, 1982; Blackburn, Vandenberg, 1991).

- Identify and support the infant-child's self-regulatory coping behaviors used for mastery of the environment.

  A continuous interaction takes place between the infant and the environment; behaviors such as hand-to-mouth/face, hand grasping, foot and leg bracing, sucking on fingers/fists, auditory and visual fixation, and postural changes are used to maintain or regain a balance between the self and the environment. Supporting infants' behaviors enhances the coregulatory fit between the infant and the environment (Als, 1986).

- Correlate the evidence of stress/disorganization to internal factors (e.g., pain hunger, discomfort) or external factors (e.g., lights, noise, handling).

  Noise is one of the common stressors in hospital ICUs, resulting in sensory overload with the potential for alteration in development (DePaul, Chambers, 1995; Elander, Hellstrom, 1995). Infant colic characterized by increased irritability, diminished ability to be soothed, and excessive restlessness reflects immature sleep-wake regulation (an internal factor) (Keefe et al, 1996). Intrauterine cocaine exposure can result in disorganized infant behavior patterns (DeWys, 1992).

- Structure and modify the care and environment.

  A developmental care approach designed to reduce environmental and procedural stress and facilitate motor and sleep-wake organization results in improved behavioral organization during the preterm period (Becker et al, 1991; Newman, 1986). Patterns of sound and light and caretaking tasks should minimize stress, conserve energy, and protect the developing neonate from inappropriate environmental stimuli (Blackburn, 1991).

- Facilitate the use of developmentally supportive positioning and handling.

  Developmentally correct positioning can prevent position-induced deformities (e.g., neck hyperextension, retracted shoulders, wide and abducted hips, and lack of midline orientation), provide comfort, and enhance interactions and long-term sensorimotor development (Fay, 1988; Semmler, 1989). Normal sensorimotor development provides the foundation for normal movement patterns that are directed toward adaptative and purposeful activities (Gilfoyle, Grady, Moore, 1982).

- Identify techniques to assist development of state modulation and organization.

  Providing care and stimulation contingent to the state of the infant are critical to state organization (Fajardo, 1990). Assisting parents with recognizing infant states and state modulation and self-consoling strategies provides caregivers with greater sense of competence (Nursing Child Assessment Satellite Training, 1994).

- Identify and support the infant-child's attentional capabilities.

  In organized, attentive states infants are able to focus attention and interact with their environment in a purposeful way (Burns et al, 1994).

- Facilitate and enhance mutual and reciprocal social interactions.

  Reciprocal interactions are essential for establishing positive patterns of interactions with partners who mutually adapt their behaviors to each other (Brazelton, Koslowski, Main, 1974). Authors suggested a developmental perspective for assessing mutual engagement and reciprocal interactions, which assess the ability to attend and remain calm for a period of time (e.g., 5+ seconds by 3 to 4 months of age, 30+ seconds by 8 to 10 months of age, 2+ minutes by 2 years of age, and 15 minutes by 4 years of age). (National Center for Infant Clinical Programs, 1994).

- Enhance normal developmental patterns through appropriate sensorimotor stimulation.

  Healthy 33- to 34-week postconceptional age infants who received 15 minutes of auditory, visual, tactile, and vestibular stimulation each day were found to be better at state modulation. Their ability to maintain quiet-alertness enhances parent-infant interactions and feedings (White-Traut et al, 1993). Enhancing normal experiences through appropriate sensory stimulation, handling, and social interactions appropriate to infant's developmental level can minimize secondary problems (Anderson, 1984).

REFERENCES   Als H: A synactive model of neonatal behavioral organization: framework for the assessment and support of the neurobehavioral development of the premature infant and his parents in the environment of the neonatal intensive care unit, *Phys Occup Ther Pediatr* 6:3, 1986.

Als H: Toward a synactive theory of development: promise for the assessment and support of infant individuality, *Infant Ment Health J* 3:229, 1982.

Anderson J, Auster-Liebhaber J: Developmental therapy in the neonatal intensive care unit, *Phys Occup Ther Pediatr* 4:89, 1984.

Becker et al: Outcomes of developmentally supportive nursing care for very low birth weight infants, *Nurs Res* 40:150, 1991.

Blackburn S: Fostering behavioral development of high-risk infants, *J Obstet Gynecol Neonatal Nurs* 3 (suppl):76, 1983.

Blackburn S, Vandenberg K: Assessment and management of neonatal development. In Kenner C et al: *Comprehensive neonatal nursing: a physiologic approach,* Toronto, 1991, WB Saunders.

Brazelton TB, Koslowski B, Main M: The origins of reciprocity: the early mother-infant interaction. In Lewis M, Rosenblum I, editors: The effect of infant on its caregiver, New York, 1974, John Wiley.

Burns M et al: *JOGNN* 23:581, 1994.

D'Apolito K: What is an organized infant? *Neonatal Network* 10:23, 1991.

DePaul D, Chambers SE: Environmental noise in the neonatal intensive care unit: implications for nursing practice, *J Perinat Neonatal Nurs* 8:71, 1995.

DeWys M, McComish-Fry J: Infants states and cues: facilitating effective parent-infant interactions. In *Caring for infants: a resource manual for caring for infant trainers,* 1992, East Lansing, Mich, Michigan State University Board of Trustees.

Elander G, Hellstrom G: Reduction of noise levels in intensive care units for infants: evaluation of an intervention program, *Heart Lung* 24:376, 1995.

Fajardo B et al: Effect of nursery environment on state regulation in very-low-birth-weight premature infants, *Infant Beh Dev* 13:287, 1990.

Fay M: The positive effects of positioning, *Neonatal Network* 7:23, 1988.

Gilfoyle E, Grady A, Moore J: *Children adapt,* 1982, Thorofare, NJ, Slack.

Keefe M et al: A longitudinal comparison of irritable and nonirritable infants, *Nurs Res* 45:4, 1996.

National Center for Clinical Infant Programs: *Diagnostic classification: zero to three diagnostic classification of mental health and developmental disorders in infancy and early childhood,* Virginia, 1994, The Center.

Newman L: Social and sensory environment of low birth weight infants in a special care nursery, *J Nerv Ment Dis* 169:448, 1986.

Semmler C: Positioning and position-inducing deformities. In Semmler C, editor: *A guide to care and management of low birth weight infants: a team approach,* Tucson, 1986, Therapy Skill Builders.

University of Washington, School of Nursing: *NCAST caregiver/parent-child interaction feeding manual,* Seattle, 1994, Nursing Child Assessment Satellite Training.

White-Traut R et al: Patterns of physiologic and behavioral response of intermediate care preterm infants to intervention, *Pediatr Nurs* 19:625, 1993.

Risk for disorganized infant behavior

Mary A. Fuerst-DeWys

Definition   Risk for altered regulation and balanced functioning of the neurobehavioral subsystems (i.e., physiological/autonomic, motor, state, attentional-interaction, self-regulatory systems) that is manifested in disorganized behavioral patterns (modified from NANDA).

Risk Factors

Internal   Pain; hunger; fatigue; respiratory, visceral, or neurological compromise; altered sensory integration; lack of or depletion of energy; pathological condition as a result of prematurity; prenatal exposure to alcohol, cocaine, or multidrug use

External   Overstimulating environment (bright lights, visual clutter, noise levels above 60 decibels), handling when physiologically compromised, care noncontingent to infant state or behavior cues, invasive or painful procedures

Related Factors (r/t)

See Risk Factors

Suggested NIC Interventions

Environmental management, newborn monitoring

Client Outcomes/Goals, Nursing Interventions and Rationales, Client/Family Teaching

See **Disorganized infant behavior**

Ineffective infant feeding pattern

Vicki E. McClurg and Virginia R. Wall

Definition   The state in which an infant demonstrates an impaired ability to suck or coordinate the suck-swallow response

Defining Characteristics

Inability to initiate or sustain an effective suck; inability to coordinate sucking, swallowing, and breathing

Related Factors (r/t)

Prematurity, neurological impairment or delay, oral hypersensitivity, prolonged NPO

Client Outcomes/Goals

- Receives adequate nourishment without compromising autonomic stability (infant)
- Progresses to a normal feeding pattern (infant)
- Learns successful techniques for feeding the infant (family)

Suggested NIC Interventions

Enteral tube feeding, lactation counseling, nonnutritive sucking, tube care: umbilical line

Nursing Interventions and Rationales

- Assess infant's oral reflexes (e.g., root, gag, suck, and swallow).
  These reflexes are necessary for successful oral feedings. Feeding by nipple or breast should be encouraged because it encourages growth and maturity of the gastrointestinal tract and provides comfort for hunger and oral gratification (Danner, 1992b; Siddell, Froman, 1994).
- Determine infant's ability to coordinate suck, swallow, and breathing reflexes.
  As infants develop, they become more able to coordinate breathing with sucking and swallowing (Pickler, Higgins, Crummette, 1993; Siddell, Froman, 1994).
- Collaborate with other health care providers (e.g., physician, neonatal nutritionist, physical and occupational therapists, lactation specialists) to develop a feeding plan.
  Various health care providers contribute expertise to the care of an infant with special needs.
- Implement gavage feedings (or another alternative feeding method) before infant is ready for oral feedings.
  Even after a preterm infant develops the ability to suck and swallow, too much energy

may be required to do so and gavage feedings may be necessary. Serious illness can impair a neonate's ability to suck, and calorie and nutrient needs are increased by the stress of illness (Kinneer, Beachy, 1994).

- Provide opportunities for nonnutritive sucking during gavage feedings (or other alternative feedings) and for 5 minutes prior to initial oral feedings.
  Sucking helps calm infants, which raises the oxygen level and may aid digestion, increase average daily weight gain, and prepare infants for earlier nipple feedings and discharge (Mott, James, Sperhac, 1990; Dickason, Silverman, Schult, 1994).
- Evaluate the feeding environment and minimize sensory stimuli.
  Noxious stimuli must be kept to a minimum to decrease physiological stress on at-risk infants. The neonatal intensive care unit environment can interfere with normal infant development and breast-feeding success and must therefore be modified to enhance attachment and normal development (Meier et al, 1993; Dickason, Silverman, Schult, 1994).
- Position preterm infant in a flexed feeding posture that is similar to the posture used for a full-term infant.
  The "total sucking pattern" of a full-term newborn combines strong physiological flexion and high rib cage position to provide support for the tongue and jaw, which is essential for effective nippling (Shaker, 1990).
- Attempt to nipple-feed baby only when infant is in a quiet-alert state.
  The infant must be able to find and grasp the nipple effectively and then be ready and eager to suck. The quiet-awake state was found to be optimal for feeding preterm infants (Kinneer, Beachy, 1994; McCain, 1992; McCain, 1995).
- Allow appropriate time for nipple feeding to ensure infant's safety without exceeding calorie expenditure.
  Nipple feeding can lead to nutritional deficits because of the increased metabolic demands placed on at-risk infants as a result of thermoregulation, work of respiration and feeding, and decreased ability to absorb nutrients (Dickason, Silverman, Schult, 1994; McCain, 1992; McCain, 1995).
- Monitor infant's physiological condition during feeding.
  Cardiorespiratory and color stability are necessary for nipple feedings (Kinneer, Beachy, 1994).
- Determine infant's active feeding behaviors without prodding.
  Infants must be alert and eager to eat (e.g., rooting, latching on, sucking readily) to ensure a successful feeding. Prodding compromises the infant's safety, interrupts learning, and may give an inaccurate picture of the infant's ability to take in adequate nutrients in preparation for discharge (Shaker, 1990).
- Assess infant's ability to take in enough calories to sustain temperature and growth.
  Calories are needed to sustain basal metabolic rate, activity, digestive and metabolic processes, and growth (Danner, 1992a, Kavanaugh et al, 1995).
- Encourage family to participate in the feeding process.
  Nurses can promote psychosocial development of at-risk infants and their families by encouraging the caretaking ability of the parents (Cusson, Lee, 1994; Meyer et al, 1994).
- Refer to a neonatal nutritionist, physical or occupational therapist, or lactation specialist as needed.
  Collaborative practice with others who are specially trained to meet the needs of this vulnerable population helps ensure feeding and parenting success (Meier et al, 1993).

Client/Family Teaching

- Provide anticipatory guidance for infant's expected feeding course.
  Knowing what to anticipate helps the family feel involved and enhances attachment.
- Teach parents infant feeding methods.
  Parents should be involved in the feeding process as soon as possible so that they can receive positive feedback about their ability to nurture a child and enhance attachment (Dickason, Silverman, Schult, 1994; Meyer et al, 1994).
- Teach parents how to recognize infant cues.
  The parents' understanding of the infant's cues may increase their involvement in infant care by improving their perception of the infant's abilities (Cusson, Lee, 1994).
- Provide anticipatory guidance for the infant's discharge.
  Parents need assistance in assuming responsibility for infant care as the day of discharge approaches (Cusson, Lee, 1994; Kavanaugh et al, 1995).

REFERENCES
Cusson RM, Lee AL: Parental interventions and the development of the preterm infant, *JOGNN* 23:60, 1994.

Danner SC: Breast feeding the neurologically impairment infant, *NAACOG's Clin Issues Perinatal Women Health Nurs* 3:640, 1992.

Danner SC: Breastfeeding the infant with a cleft defect, *NAACOG's Clin Issues Perinatal Women Health Nurs* 3:634, 1992.

Dickason EJ, Silverman BL, Schult MO: *Maternal-infant nursing care,* ed 2, St Louis, 1994, Mosby.

Kavanaugh K et al: Getting enough: Mother's concerns about breastfeeding a preterm infant after discharge, *J Obstet Gynecol Neonatal Nurs* 24:23, 1995.

Kinneer MD, Beachy P: Nipple feeding premature infants in the neonatal intensive-care unit: factors and decisions, *JOGNN* 23:105-112, 1994.

McCain GC: Facilitating inactive awake states in preterm infants: a study of three interventions, *Nurs Res* 41:157, 1992.

McCain GC: Promotion of preterm infant nipple feeding with nonnutritive sucking, *J Ped Nurs* 10:3, 1995.

Meier PP et al: Breastfeeding support services in the neonatal intensive-care unit, *JOGNN* 22:338, 1993.

Meyer EC et al: Family-based intervention improves maternal psychological well-being and feeding interaction of preterm infants, *Pediatrics* 93:241, 1994.

Mott SR, James SR, Sperhac AM: *Nursing care of children and families,* ed 2, Redwood City, Calif, 1990, Addison-Wesley.

Pickler RH, Higgins KE, Crummette BD: The effect of nonnutritive sucking on bottle-feeding stress in preterm infants, *JOGNN* 22:230, 1993.

Pridham KF et al: Nipple feeding for preterm infants with bronchopulmonary dysplasia, *JOGNN* 22:147, 1993.

Shaker CS: Nipple feeding premature infants: a different perspective, *Neonatal Network* 8:9, 1990.

Siddell EP, Froman RD: A national survey of neonatal intensive-care units: criteria used to determine readiness for oral feedings, *JOGNN* 22:147, 1994.

Risk for infection

Gail B. Ladwig

Definition   The state in which an individual is at an increased risk of invasion by pathogenic organisms

Risk Factors

Inadequate primary defenses (e.g., broken skin, traumatized tissue, decrease in ciliary action, stasis of body fluids, change in pH secretions, altered peristalsis), inadequate secondary defenses (e.g., decreased hemoglobin, leukopenia, suppressed inflammatory response); immunosuppression; inadequate acquired immunity; tissue destruction and increased environmental exposure; chronic disease; malnutrition; invasive procedures; pharmaceutical agents; trauma; rupture of amniotic membranes; insufficient knowledge regarding avoidance of exposure to pathogens

Related Factors (r/t)

See Risk Factors

Client Outcomes/Goals

- Remains free from symptoms of infection
- States symptoms of infection to be aware of
- Demonstrates appropriate care of infection-prone site
- Maintains white blood cell count and differential within normal limits
- Demonstrates appropriate hygienic measures such as handwashing, oral care, and perineal care

Suggested NIC Interventions

Immunization/vaccination administration, infection control, infection protection

Nursing Interventions and Rationales

- Observe for signs of infection such as redness, warmth, discharge, and increased body temperature.
  With the onset of infection the immune system is activated and signs of infection appear.
- Assess temperature of neutropenic clients every 4 hours; report a single temperature of greater than 38.5° C or three temperatures of greater than 38° C in 24 hours.
  Neutropenic clients do not produce an adequate inflammatory response, so fever is usually the first and often the only sign of infection (Wujcik, 1993).
- Use an electronic or mercury thermometer to assess temperature.
  When temperature values have important consequences for treatment decisions, use mercury or electronic thermometers with established accuracy (Erickson, Meyer, Moser, 1996).
- Note laboratory values (e.g., white blood cell count and differential, serum protein, serum albumin, cultures).
  Laboratory values are correlated with client's history and physical examination to provide a global view of the client's immune function and nutritional status and develop an appropriate plan of care for the diagnosis (Lehmann, 1991).
- Assess skin for color, moisture, texture, and turgor (elasticity). Keep accurate, ongoing documentation of changes.
  Preventive skin assessment protocol including documentation assists in the prevention of skin breakdown. Intact skin is nature's first line of defense against microorganisms entering the body (Kovach, 1995).
- Carefully wash and pat dry skin, including skinfold areas. Use hydration and moisturization on all at-risk surfaces.
  Maintaining supple, moist skin is the best method of keeping skin intact. Dry skin can lead to inflammation, excoriations, and possible infection episodes (Kovach, 1995) (see **Risk for impaired skin integrity**).
- Encourage a balanced diet emphasizing proteins to feed the immune system.
  Immune function is affected by protein intake (especially arginine), the balance between omega-6 and omega-3 fatty acid intake, and adequate amounts of vitamins A, C, and E and the minerals zinc and iron. A deficiency of these nutrients puts the client at an increased risk of infection (Lehmann, 1991).

- Encourage adequate rest to bolster the immune system.
  Chronic disease and physical and emotional stress increase the client's need for rest (Potter, Perry, 1993).
- Wash hands vigorously with soap for 10 to 30 seconds before and after giving care to client and any time hands become soiled, even if gloves are worn.
  Handwashing is the most important way to prevent and control the spread of infection (McPherson, 1993). When soap is used, the mechanical action of washing and drying removes most of the transient bacteria. Hands should remain in contact with the cleanser for 10 seconds; 20 to 30 seconds would be ideal (Gould, 1994a).
- Hands should be thoroughly dried with paper towels after washing.
  Bacterial transfer occurs more readily between wet surfaces than dry ones (Marples, 1979). More microorganisms were removed with paper towels than with linen. Fecal organisms have been recovered from hands after using hot-air dryers, and bacterial counts are significantly higher than when paper towels are used (Gould, 1994b).
- Follow universal precautions and wear gloves during any contact with body fluids; use goggles and gloves when appropriate.
  Wearing gloves does not obviate the need for scrupulous handwashing. The purpose of wearing gloves is either to protect the hands from becoming contaminated with dirt and microorganisms or prevent the transfer of organisms that are already present on the hands (Smock, Shiel, 1994).
- Sterile technique must be used when inserting urinary catheters. Catheters must be cared for at least every shift.
  The greatest number of nosocomial and home-acquired infections were in patients with Foley catheters (Rosenheimer, 1995).
- Use careful technique when changing and emptying urinary catheter bags; avoid cross-contamination.
  It is during bag changing and emptying that patients are most at risk for cross-infection (Platt et al, 1983; Crow et al, 1993; Roe, 1993).
- Use careful and sterile techniques when using invasive monitoring.
  The invasiveness of venticular assist devices predispose patients to infection. Strict aseptic technique should be maintained (Teplitz, 1990).
- Use careful sterile techniques wherever there is a loss of skin integrity.
  These important measures prevent infection in at-risk patients (Wujcik, 1993).
- Ensure client's appropriate hygienic care with handwashing, bathing, and hair, nail, and perineal care performed by either nurse or client.
  Hygienic care is important to prevent infection in at-risk patients (Wujcik, 1993).

Geriatric
- Recognize that geriatric clients may be seriously infected but have less obvious symptoms.
  The immune system declines with aging. The elderly may present with atypical manifestations of infections (Madhaven, 1994).
- Foot care other than simple toenail cutting should be performed by a podiatrist.
- Observe client for a low-grade temperature or new onset of confusion.
  The elderly can have infections with low-grade fevers. Be suspicious of any temperature rise or sudden confusion—these symptoms may be the only signs of infection (Madhaven, 1994).
- During the peak of the influenza epidemic, limit visits by relatives and friends.
  Hospital and nursing home-acquired influenza A virus infection leads to high mortality in the elderly (Madhaven, 1994).

- Recommend that the geriatric client receive an annual influenza immunization and one-time pneumococcal vaccine.

  Among the many infections to which the aged are susceptible, pneumonia and influenza combined are responsible for the greatest mortality (Madhaven, 1994).

- Recognize that chronically ill geriatric clients have an increased susceptibility to infection; practice meticulous care of all invasive sites.

Home Care Interventions

- Assess home environment for general cleanliness, storage of food items, and appropriate waste disposal. Instruct as necessary in proper disposal and use of disinfecting agents.

  Presence of waste and inappropriate storage of food items can contribute to the presence of pathogens.

- Assess home care environment for appropriate disposal of used dressing materials.

  Used dressing materials may contain or be a primary medium for growth of pathogens.

- Role model all preventive behaviors in care of client (e.g., universal precautions). Do not visit client when you are ill.

  Demonstration is a more effective teaching strategy than verbalization.

- Maintain the cleanliness of all irrigation and cleansing solutions. Change solutions when cleanliness has not been maintained—do not wait to finish bottle.

  Solutions exposed to contaminants provide a medium for growth of pathogens.

- Assess and teach clients about current medications and therapies that promote susceptibility to infection: corticosteroids, immunosuppressants, chemotherapeutic agents, and radiation therapy.

  Knowledge of risk factors promotes vigilance in assessment, prompt reporting, and early treatment.

- Assess client for knowledge of infections that have been drug resistant.

- Instruct client to complete any course of prophylactic antibiotic therapy unless experiencing adverse side effects.

  Prophylactic antibiotic therapy decreases the risk of infection.

Client/Family Teaching

- Teach client and family the symptoms of infection that should be promptly reported to a primary medical caregiver (e.g., redness; warmth; swelling; tenderness or pain; new onset of drainage or change in drainage from wound; increase in body temperature; hepatitis B virus (HBV)/AIDS symptoms: malaise, abdominal pain, vomiting or diarrhea, enlarged glands, rash; TB symptoms: cough, night sweats, dyspnea, changes in sputum, changes in breath sounds; IDDM: sores or wounds that do not heal).

  A high prevalence of HBV/AIDS, an increasing incidence of TB, and the general risk of diabetes are related to increased rate of infection.

- Assess whether client and family know how to read a thermometer; provide instructions if necessary. Chemical dot thermometers are easy to use and decrease risk of infection. Clients need to know that the instructions should be followed carefully, and that electronic or mercury thermometers may be the best choice for accuracy.

  Chemical dot thermometers may underestimate the oral temperature by $-0.4°$ C or more in about 50% of adults and thus lack the sensitivity to screen for fever and provide many false readings. Conversely, they may overestimate axillary temperature by $+0.4°$ C or more in about 50% of adults and some young children and thus lack the specificity to rule out fever and provide many false positive readings (Erickson et al, 1996).

- Instruct client and family about the need for good nutrition (especially protein) and proper rest to bolster immune function.
- If client has AIDS, discuss the continued need to practice safe sex, avoid unsterile needle use, and maintain a healthy life-style to prevent infection.
- Refer client and family to social services and community resources to obtain support in maintaining a life-style that increases immune function (e.g., adequate nutrition, rest, freedom from excessive stress).

REFERENCES   Crow R et al: A study of patients with an indwelling urethral catheter and related nursing practice, Nursing Practice Unit, University of Surrey, 1986. In Roe B: Catheter-associated urinary tract infection: a review, *J Clin Nurs* 2:197, 1993.

Erickson R et al: Accuracy of chemical dot thermometers in critically ill adults and young children, Image 28:23, 1996.

Gould D: Making sense of hand hygiene, *Nurs Times* 90:63, 1994a.

Gould D: The significance of hand-drying in the prevention of infection, *Nurs Times* 90:33, 1994b.

Humphrey C, Milone-Nuzzo P: *Orientation to home care nursing,* Gaithersburg, Md, 1996, Aspen.

Jaffe M, Skidmore-Roth L: *Home health nursing care plans,* ed 2, St Louis, 1993, Mosby.

Kovach T: The barrier defense: skin hydration as infection control, *J Practical Nurs* 45:13, 1995.

Lehmann S: Immune function and nutrition: the clinical role of the intravenous nurse, *J Intraven Nurs* 14:406, 1991.

Madhaven T: Infections in the elderly: Current concepts in management, *Comprehen Ther* 20:465, 1994.

Marples RR, Towers A: A laboratory model for the contact transfer of micro-organisms, *J Hygiene* 82:237, 1979. In Gould D: Making sense of hand hygiene, *Nurs Times* 90:63, 1994.

McPherson M: Handwashing: why, when and how, *Asepsis' Infect Prevent Forum* 15:18, 1993.

Platt R et al: Reduction of mortality associated with nosocomial urinary tract infection, *Lancet* 1:893, 1983.

Potter P, Perry A: *Fundamentals of nursing: concepts, process and practice,* St Louis, 1993, Mosby.

Roe B: Catheter associated urinary tract infection: a review, *J Clin Nurs* 2:197, 1993.

Rosenheimer L: Establishing a surveillance system for infections acquired in home healthcare, *Home Healthcare Nurse* 13:20, 1995.

Smock M, Shiel M: The role of surgeon and procedure gloves in infection control: a closer look at disposable gloves, *Prof Nurse* 9:324, 1994.

Teplitz L: Patients with ventricular assist devices, *Dimens Crit Care Nurs* 9:82, 1990.

Wujcik D: Infection control in oncology patients, *Nurs Clin North Am* 28:639, 1993.

Risk for injury

Betty J. Ackley and Teepa Snow

Definition   The state in which an individual is at risk of injury as a result of the interaction of environmental conditions and the individual's adaptive and defensive resources (NOTE: This nursing diagnosis overlaps with other diagnoses such as **Risk for trauma, Risk for poisoning, Risk for suffocation, Risk for aspiration** and, if the client is at risk of bleeding, **Altered protection.** See these diagnoses if appropriate.)

Risk Factors

Evidence of environmental hazards, lack of knowledge regarding environmental hazards, lack of knowledge regarding safety precautions, history of accidents, impaired mobility, sensory deficit, cerebral dysfunction (modified from Carpenito)

Related Factors (r/t)

See Risk Factors

Client Outcomes/Goals

- Remains free of injuries
- Explains ways to prevent injury

Suggested NIC Interventions

Fall prevention, dementia management, surveillance: safety

Nursing Interventions and Rationales

- Determine risk of falling by using an evaluation tool.

  Risk factors for falling include recent history of falls, depression, altered elimination patterns, dizziness or vertigo, primary cancer diagnosis, confusion, and altered mobility (Hendrich et al, 1995).

- Screen all clients for stability and mobility skills (supine to sit, sitting supported and unsupported, sit to stand, standing, walking and turning around, transferring, stooping to floor and recovering, and sitting down). Use tools such as the Balance Scale by Tinnetti or the Get Up and Go Scale by Mathais.

  It is helpful to determine the client's functional abilities and then plan for ways to improve problem areas or determine methods to ensure safety because of deficits (Lewis et al, 1994).

- Identify clients likely to fall by placing a "Fall Precautions" sign in the room and by keying the Kardex and chart. Use a "high risk fall" arm band and room marker to alert staff for increased vigilance and mobility assistance.

  These steps alert the nursing staff of the increased risk of falls (Cohen, Guin, 1991).

- Evaluate client's medications to determine whether medications increase the risk of falling; consult with physician regarding client's need for medication if appropriate.

- Thoroughly orient client to environment. Place call light within reach and show how to call for assistance; answer call light promptly.

- Keep side rails up using half rails, and maintain bed in a low position. Ensure that wheels are locked on bed and commode. Keep dim light in room at night.

  These safety measures are used as part of a fall-prevention program (Kilpack et al, 1991). Use of full siderails can result in the client climbing over the rails, leading with the head, and sustaining a head injury.

- Routinely assist clients with toileting on their own individual schedules. Always take clients to bathroom when they wake up, before bedtime, and before administering sedatives. Keep the way to the bathroom clear, label the bathroom, and leave the door open.

  The majority of falls are related to toileting. It is more acceptable to fall than to "wet yourself." Studies have indicated that falls are often linked to the need to eliminate in a hurry (Cohen, Guin, 1991).

- Avoid use of restraints; obtain a physician's order if restraints are necessary.

  Restrained elderly clients often experience an increased number of falls, possibly as a result of muscle deconditioning or loss of coordination (Tinetti, Liu, Ginter, 1992). If they are restrained and fall, they can sustain severe injuries, including strangulation, asphyxiation, or head injury from leading with their heads to get out of the bed (DiMaio, Dana, Bix, 1986; Evans, Strumpf, 1990).

- In place of restraints, use the following:
  - Alarm systems with ankle or wrist bracelets
  - Bed or wheelchair alarms

- ▪ Increased observation of client
- ▪ Locked doors to unit
- ▪ Bed with wheels removed to keep bed low (NOTE: May not be acceptable with fire regulations)

These are alternatives to restraints that can be helpful to prevent falls (Commodore, 1995).

- If client is extremely agitated, consider using a special safety bed that surrounds client. If client has a traumatic brain injury, use the Emory cubicle bed.

Special beds can be an effective alternative to restraints and help keep the client safe during periods of agitation (Williams, Morton, Patrick, 1990).

- If clients have a new onset of confusion (delirium), provide reality orientation when interacting with them. Have family bring in familiar items, clocks, watches from home to maintain orientation. If client has chronic confusion with dementia, use validation therapy that reinforces feelings but does not confront reality.

Reality orientation can help prevent or decrease the confusion that increases risk of falling for clients with delirium; validation therapy is more effective for clients with dementia (Fine, 1995). See interventions for **Chronic confusion.**

- Ask family to stay with client to prevent client from accidentally falling or pulling out tubes.
- Remove all possible hazards in environment such as razors, medications, and matches.
- If client is unsteady on feet, use a walking belt; use two nursing staff members when ambulating client.

The client can walk independently with a walking belt, but the nurse can rapidly ensure safety if the knees buckle.

- Place an injury-prone client in a room that is near the nurses' station.

Such placement allows more frequent observation of the client.

- Help clients sit in a stable chair with arm rests. Avoid use of wheelchairs and geri-chairs except for transportation as needed

Clients are likely to fall when left in a wheelchair or geri-chair because they may stand up without locking the wheels or removing the footrests. Wheelchairs do not increase mobility; people just sit the majority of the time (Lipson, Braun, 1993; Simmons et al, 1995).

- Ensure that the chair or wheelchair fits the build, abilities, and needs of the client to ensure propulsion with legs or arms and ability to reach the floor, eliminating footrests and minimizing problems with shearing.

The seating system should fit the needs of the client so that the client can move the wheels, stand up from the chair without falling, and not be harmed by the chair or wheelchair. Footrests can cause skin tears and bruising, as well as postural alignment and sitting posture problems (Lipson, Braun, 1993).

- Refer to physical therapy for strengthening exercises and gait training to increase mobility. Refer to occupational therapy for assistance in helping clients perform activities of daily living (ADLs).

Gait training by physical therapy has been shown to be effective in preventing falls (Galinda-Ciocon, Ciocon, Galinda, 1995).

Geriatric

- Encourage client to wear glasses and hearing aids and use walking aids when ambulating.
- Consider use of a "Merri-walker"—an adult walker that surrounds body if client is mobile but unsafe because of wobbling.

- If client experiences dizziness because of orthostatic hypotension when getting up, teach methods to decrease dizziness, such as rising slowly, remaining seated several minutes before standing, flexing feet upward several times while sitting, sitting down immediately if feeling dizzy, and trying to have someone present when standing. *The elderly develop decreased baroreceptor sensitivity and decreased ability of compensatory mechanisms to maintain blood pressure when standing up, resulting in postural hypotension (Aaronson, Carlon-Wolfe, Schoener, 1991).*

Home Care Interventions

- Assess home environment for threats to safety: clutter, inappropriate storage of chemicals, slippery floors, scatter rugs, unsafe stairs and stairwells, blocked entries, dim lighting, extension cords (across pathway), unsafe electrical or gas connections, unsafe heating devices, unsafe oxygen placement, high beds without rails, excessively hot water, pets and pet excrement. *Clients suffering from impaired mobility, impaired visual acuity, neurological dysfunction, including dementia and other cognitive functional deficits, are all at risk for injury from common hazards.*
- Instruct client and family or caregivers in correcting identified hazards. Refer to occupational therapy services for assistance if needed. Notify landlord or code enforcement office of structural building hazards.
- If client is at risk for falls, use gait belt or additional persons when ambulating. *Gait belts decrease the risk of falls during ambulation.*
- Have client wear supportive shoes when ambulating. *Supportive shoes provide the client with better balance and protect the client from instability on uneven surfaces.*
- Refer to physical therapy services for client and family education in safe transfers and ambulation and for client-strengthening exercises for ambulation and transfers.
- Avoid extreme hot and cold around clients at risk for injury (e.g., heating pads, hot water for baths/showers). *Clients with decreased cognition or sensory deficits cannot discriminate extremes in temperature.*
- Provide a signaling device for clients who wander or are at risk for falls. If client lives alone, provide a Lifeline or similar call device. *Orienting a vulnerable client to a safety net relieves anxiety of the client and caregiver and allows for rapid response to a crisis situation.*
- Provide medical identifications bracelet for clients at risk for injury from dementia, seizures, or other medical disorders.

Client/Family Teaching

- Teach how to safely ambulate at home, including using safety measures such as hand rails in bathroom.
- If client has visual impairment, teach client and caregiver to label significant places in environment that must be easily located with bright colors such as yellow or red (e.g., stair edges, stove controls, light switches).

REFERENCES   Aaronson L, Carlon-Wolfe W, Schoener S: Pressures that fall on rising, *Geriatr Nurs* 12:67, 1991.
Booth DE: Many falls among Alzheimer's patients can be avoided, *Advance* 3:3, 1994.
Bradley L, Siddique CM, Dufton B: Reducing the use of physical restraints in long-term care facilities, *J Gerontol Nurs* 21:21, 1995.

Carpenito LJ: *Nursing diagnosis: application to clinical practice,* ed 6, Philadelphia, 1995, JB Lippincott.

Cohen L, Guin P: Implementation of a patient fall prevention program, *J Neurosci Nurs* 23:315, 1991.

Commodore DI: Falls in the elderly population: a look at incidence, risks, healthcare costs, and preventive strategies, *Rehab Nurs* 20:84, 1995.

DiMaio V, Dana S, Bix R: Death caused by restraint vests, *JAMA* 255:905, 1986.

Evans L, Strumpf N: Myths about elder restraint, *Image J Nurs Scholarship* 22:124, 1990.

Fine JI, Rouse-Bane S: Using validating techniques to improve communication with cognitively impaired older adults, *J Gerontol Nurs* 21:39, 1995.

Galinda-Ciocon DJ, Ciocon JO, Galinda DJ: Gait training and falls in the elderly, *J Gerontol Nurs* 21:11, 1995.

Hendrich A et al: Hospital falls: development of a predictive model for clinical practice, *Appl Nurs Res* 8:129, 1995.

Kilpack V et al: Using research-based interventions to decrease patient falls, *Appl Nurs Res* 4:68, 1991.

Lange M: The challenge of fall prevention in home care: a review of the literature, *Home Healthcare Nurse* 14:199, 1996.

Lewis et al: *The functional tool book,* Washington DC, 1994, Learn.

Lipson J, Braun S: *Toward a restraint-free environment: reducing the use of physical and chemical restraint in long term care and acute settings,* Baltimore, 1993, Health Professions Press.

Malone M et al: The epidemiology of skin tears in the institutionalized elderly, *JAGS* 39:591, 1991.

Miceli DL et al: Prodromal falls among older nursing home residents, *Appl Nurs Res* 7:18, 1994.

Simmons S et al: Wheelchairs as mobility restraints: predictors of wheelchair activity in nonambulatory nursing home residents, *JAGS* 43:384, 1995.

Spellbring AM et al: Improving safety for hospitalized elderly, *J Gerontol Nurs* 14:31, 1988.

Strumpf N, Evans L: Physical restraint of the hospitalized elderly: perceptions of patients and nurses, *Nurs Res* 37:132, 1988.

Tinetti ME, Liu W-L, Ginter SF: Mechanical restraint use and fall-related injuries among residents of skilled nursing facilities, *Ann Intern Med* 116:369, 1992.

Williams LM, Morton GA, Patrick CH: The Emory cubicle bed: an alternative to restraints for agitated traumatically brain injured clients, *Rehab Nurs* 15:30, 1990.

Decreased adaptive capacity: intracranial

Pamela H. Mitchell

Definition   The clinical state in which intracranial fluid dynamic mechanisms that normally compensate for increases in intracranial volumes are compromised, which results in repeated disproportionate increases in intracranial pressure (ICP) in response to a variety of noxious and nonnoxious stimuli (Mitchell, 1993)

Defining Characteristics

Major   Repeated increases in ICP of greater than 10 mm Hg for more than 5 minutes following a variety of external stimuli

Minor   Disproportionate increases in ICP following a single environmental or nursing maneuver stimulus, baseline ICP equal to or greater than 10 mm Hg, decreased compliance as indicated by elevated P_2 component of ICP waveform or wide-amplitude ICP waveform or volume-pressure response elevation (volume-pressure ratio of greater than 2 or pressure-volume index [PVI] of less than 10) (Rauch, Mitchell, Tyler, 1990; Mitchell, 1993)

Related Factors (r/t)

Brain injuries, hydrocephalus, sustained increase in ICP equal to or greater than 10 to 15 mm Hg, decreased cerebral perfusion pressure (CPP) equal to or less than 70 mm Hg, altered cerebral autoregulation

Client Outcomes/Goals

- Experiences fewer than five episodes of disproportionate increases in ICP (DIICP) in 24 hours
- Neurological status changes are not triggered by episodes of DIICP
- CPP remains at or above 70 mm Hg in adults

Suggested NIC Interventions

Cerebral edema management, cerebral perfusion promotion, intracranial pressure (ICP) monitoring, neurologic monitoring

Nursing Interventions and Rationales

For episodes of disproportionate increases in intracranial pressure (DIICP)

- Reverse stimulus if readily apparent:
  - Evaluate position of patient—head should be in midline without neck flexion to prevent intracranial trapping of jugular venous outflow.
    Positional changes of the head and neck are the most consistent triggers of sustained ICP elevations. Both lateral and rotational neck flexion will result in increased ICP until the neck position is restored to a neutral position (Yordy, Hanigan, 1985-1986; Mitchell, Ackerman, 1992; Williams, Coyne, 1993).
  - Return patient to original position if a position change has triggered DIICP.
    No particular body position triggers DIICP unless combined with neck flexion; however, some individuals respond to passive turning to lateral or three-quarters prone positions (Lee, 1989; Mitchell, Ackerman, 1992).
  - Stop suctioning if routine suctioning is triggering DIICP. Follow preventive protocol if future suctioning is indicated.
    A standard series of three suctioning passes can result in stair-step elevation of ICP with each successive pass, even with full hyperoxygenation and hyperinflation prior to suctioning (Kerr et al, 1993).
  - Have clients who can follow directions exhale through their mouth if they are doing a Valsalva maneuver.
    If clients' nonvolitional movements such as posturing and unconscious straining are causing a Valsalva's maneuver, sedation or paralytics with sedation may be indicated (McClelland et al, 1995).
  - Reduce environmental noise and painful or unexpected touching of patient.
    All these factors have been shown to be potent noxious stimuli in individual adults and preterm infants but may not trigger DIICP in the majority of clients (Yordy, Hannigan, 1985-86; Mitchell, Ackerman, 1992).
  - Elevate head of bed *if* the client maintains CPP when ICP is lowered by head elevation.
    Head elevation reduces the average ICP in groups of patients, but individuals may exhibit either no change or even increased ICP (Ropper, O'Rourke, Kennedy, 1982). In addition, when cerebral autoregulation is impaired, even a small systemic blood pressure drop with head elevation may decrease the CPP to an unacceptable level (March et al, 1990).

For DIICP if baseline ICP rises above 15 mm Hg or CPP (mean arterial blood pressure minus mean ICP) is less than 70 mm Hg in adults for 5 minutes or more

- Initiate protocols for lowering ICP according to a collaborative plan with attending physician if ICP remains elevated or CPP decreased outside parameters—usually ICP greater than 15 to 20 mm Hg or CPP less than 60 to 70 mm Hg for 10 or more minutes.

Current recommendations are to manage CPP to maintain pressure equal to or greater than 70 mm Hg for adults based on observations from the Trauma Coma Data Bank indicating CPP as the crucial variable related to outcome (Lang, Chesnut, 1995).

- The plan will vary by region and individual physician preference but may include the following (Ghajar et al, 1995):
  - Cerebrospinal fluid (CSF) drainage via ventriculostomy intermittently to maintain a given ICP level
    CSF drainage will manage CPP by reducing ICP at least temporarily. It does not change adaptive capacity (intracranial compliance) (Chesnut, 1995).
  - Addition of sedation (e.g., morphine, midazolam, propofol) and analgesia with or without paralysis (e.g., atacurium, pavulon) if body movements or fighting respirator continuously stimulate a CPP decrease
    The short-acting agents allow rapid reversal of both sedation and paralysis for short periods to provide periodic neurological examination (McClelland et al, 1995).
  - Bolus administration of osmotic diuretic or other hyperosmotic agent (mannitol, mannitol plus furosemide); may be followed with continuous administration if CPP is not maintained with bolus administration
    Note that it is essential to keep serum osmolality less than 320 mOsm/L to prevent hyperosmolality-related seizures. These agents primarily reduce vascular volume and not cerebral edema. The older practice of keeping clients volume depleted in an attempt to prevent cerebral edema is no longer advocated (Chesnut, 1995).
  - Controlled hyperventilation, maintaining P_{CO_2} of 30 to 35 mm Hg unless ICP continues to be refractory, in which case P_{CO_2} may be briefly decreased below 30 mm Hg if ICP is responsive
    Older standards of early hyperventilation to levels as low as 25 mm Hg have been shown to have poorer outcomes than in similar clients not hyperventilated. Prophylactic use of hyperventilation may induce cerebral ischemia. Although many clinicians continue to use extreme hyperventilation, major trauma centers recommend this only as a last resort in refractory intracranial hypertension (Chesnut, 1995).

To prevent DIICP in patients at risk (clients with elevated P_2 waveforms and ICP of less than 10 mm Hg; clients previously responsive to general stimuli)

- Maintain 15° to 30° head elevation if CPP is maintained at greater than 70 mm Hg.
- Maintain systemic blood pressure adequate to keep CPP at or above 70 mm Hg by body positioning and use of vasoactive protocols.
- Maintain adequate respiratory status; suction if needed but not prophylactically.
- If suctioning required, may use aerosolized lidocaine to reduce associated coughing. Preoxygenate, do not hyperventilate, and limit number of catheter passes to one or two (Kerr et al, 1993).
- Use gentle touching and talking or family visitations.
  These activities rarely stimulate DIICP. Family voices and gentle stroking may help stabilize ICP (Treloar et al, 1991; Mitchell, Ackerman, 1992; Hepworth, Hendrickson, Lopez, 1994).
- Use mechanical turning beds if manual repositioning is a stimulus to DIICP.
  These beds keep the head and neck in a neutral alignment and have been shown not to alter ICP overall (Mitchell, 1993)
- Avoid 90° hip flexion and use of the knee gatch of the bed.

Hip flexion may trap venous blood in the intraabdominal space, increasing abdominal and intrathoracic pressure, which in turn reduces venous outflow from the head (Vos, 1993).

- Sequence nursing care to allow for recovery of baseline ICP between noxious activities such as suctioning and position changes that involve neck flexion.
  Several studies have shown stairstep increases in ICP when a stimulus to DIICP is repeated several times within a short time (Mitchell, Ackerman, 1992; Kerr et al, 1993).

Related to general ICP monitoring

- Monitor ICP and CPP continuously with alarm settings on.
  Secondary brain injury can result from even brief periods of hypoxia and hypotension. Data from the Traumatic Coma Data Bank and international studies have documented that even in well-attended ICUs, periods of more than 5 minutes of systemic hypotension (systolic blood pressure of less than 90 mm Hg) or intracranial hypertension occur in 70% to 90% of clients (Miller, 1993; Jones et al, 1994).
- Notify physician if nursing interventions and collaborative protocols do not maintain a CPP of equal to or greater than 70 mm Hg and an ICP of less than 20 mm Hg for adults; values may be lower for infants.
- Monitor neurological status as well as CPP, including level of arousal, ability to follow commands, response to painful stimuli if arousal is decreased, and brainstem signs (pupil response, respiratory pattern, symmetry of motor response, and vital signs). Notify physician of signs of neurological deterioration regardless of levels of ICP and CPP.
  Brain shift and herniation will be manifested by these changes in neurological status and may occur at any level of ICP. If the client is sedated and paralyzed to control ICP, pupillary changes or changes in response to painful stimuli may be the only available sign of deterioration (Ross et al, 1989; Mitchell, Ackerman, 1993).

Home Care Interventions

NOTE: Clients experiencing potentially rapid changes in ICP are not candidates for home care. However, clients experiencing potentially gradual changes in ICP (i.e., clients with developmental delays due to genetic dysfunction) may be served by home care with the following considerations:

- Identify baseline neurological data prior to discharge from institutional care.
  Baseline data will help to identify changes in status and assist in creating an individualized care plan.
- Evaluate neurological functioning at regular intervals.
  Neurological function improvements require long-term intervention.
- Instruct the caregiver about the client-specific changes that will indicate increased ICP. Examples include changes in speech articulation and eye coordination, decreased ability to focus, increased seizure activity, and decreased coping ability. The nurse is cautioned that changes will be specific to the disability of the client.
  Early reporting of status changes allows for early intervention in neurologically impaired clients.

REFERENCES   Chesnut RM: Medical management of severe head injury: present and future, *New Horiz* 3:581, 1995.
Ghajar J et al: Survey of critical care management of comatose, head-injured patients in the United States, *Crit Care Med* 23:560, 1995.

Hepworth JT, Hendrickson SG, Lopez J: Time series analysis of physiological response durin
West J Nurs Res 16:704, 1994.

Jones PA et al: Measuring the burden of secondary insults in head-injured patients during in
Neurosurg Anesthesiol 6:4, 1994.

Kerr ME et al: Head-injured adults: recommendations for endotracheal suctioning, *J Neuro
1993.

Lang EW, Chesnut RM: Intracranial pressure and cerebral perfusion pressure in severe head injury, *New Horiz*
3:400, 1995.

Lee S: Intracranial pressure changes during positioning of patients with severe head injury, *Heart Lung* 18:411,
1989.

March K et al: Effects of backrest position on ICP and CPP, *J Neurosci Nurs* 22:375, 1990.

McClelland M et al: Continuous midazolam/atacurium infusions for the management of increased intracranial
pressure, *J Neurosci Nurs* 27:96, 1995.

Miller JD: Head injury, *J Neurol Neurosurg Psychiatry* 56:440, 1993.

Mitchell PH: Decreased adaptive capacity. In Kinney MR, Packa DR, Dunbar SB, editors: *AACN's clinical
reference for critical care nursing,* ed 3, St Louis, 1993, Mosby.

Mitchell PH, Ackerman LL: Secondary brain injury reduction. In Bulechek GM, McCloskey JC, editors:
Nursing interventions, ed 2, Philadelphia, 1992, WB Saunders.

Rauch ME, Mitchell PH, Tyler ML: Validation of risk factors for the nursing diagnosis of decreased intracranial
adaptive capacity, *J Neurosci Nurs* 22:173, 1990.

Ropper AH, O'Rourke D, Kennedy SK: Head position, intracranial pressure, and compliance, *Neurology*
32:1288, 1982.

Ross DA et al: Brain shift, level of consciousness and restoration of consciousness in patients with acute
intracranial hematoma, *J Neurosurg* 71:498, 1989.

Treloar DM et al: The effect of familiar and unfamiliar voice treatments on intracranial pressure in head-injured
patients, *J Neuro Nurs* 23(5):295, 1991.

Vos HR: Making headway with intracranial hypertension, *Am J Nurs* 93:28, 1993.

Williams A, Coyne SM: Effects of neck position on intracranial pressure, *Am J Crit Care* 2:68, 1993.

Yordy M, Hanigan WC: Cerebral perfusion pressure in the high-risk premature infant, *Pediatr Neurosci* 12:226,
1985-86.

Knowledge deficit

Suzanne Skowronski

Definition

Absence or deficiency of cognitive information related to a specific topic

Defining Characteristics

Verbalization of the problem, inaccurate follow-through of previous instruction,
inaccurate performance of test, inappropriate or exaggerated behaviors (e.g., hysterical,
hostile, agitated, apathetic)

Related Factors (r/t)

Lack of exposure, lack of recall, information misinterpretation, cognitive limitation, lack
of interest in learning, unfamiliarity with information resources

Client Outcomes/Goals

- Explains disease state, recognizes need for medications, understands treatments
- Explains how to incorporate new health regimen into life-style
- States an ability to deal with health situation and remain in control of life
- Demonstrates how to perform procedure(s) satisfactorily
- Lists resources that can be used for more information or support after discharge

Suggested NIC Interventions

Teaching: disease process, teaching: individual, teaching: infant care

Nursing Interventions and Rationales

- Observe client's ability to learn (e.g., mental acuity, ability to see and hear, no existing pain, emotional readiness, absence of language or cultural barriers).
  Physical and mental readiness are necessary for learning.
- Assess barriers to learning (e.g., perceived change in life-style, financial concerns, cultural patterns, lack of acceptance by peers or coworkers).
  "The initial shock of a diagnosis diminishes a client's cognitive learning capacity" (Camprich, 1992).
- Determine client's previous knowledge of or skills related to their diagnosis and their influence on willingness to learn.
  New information is assimilated into previous assumptions and facts and may involve negotiating, transforming, or stalling.
- When teaching, build on client's literacy skills.
  "Assuming patients can read materials may result in decreased compliance, poor outcomes, or adverse reactions" (Williams, 1995).
- Help client write specific learning objectives.
  Objectives put the content into focus, provide a forum for evaluating outcomes, and ensure continuity. Client involvement improves compliance with the health regimen and makes teaching and learning a partnership.
- Present material that is most significant to client first, such as how to give injections or change dressings; present additional material once client's most pressing educational needs have been met.
  Information building begins with explaining simple concepts and moves on to explanations of complex application situations.
- Determine client's understanding of common medical terminology such as "empty stomach," "emesis," and "palpitation."
  "Clients are expected to read and understand labels on medicine containers, appointment slips, and informed consents, yet an estimated 40 million adults are functionally illiterate" (Williams, 1995).
- Evaluate the readability of the material in pamphlets or written instructions.
  "Consent forms were assessed at grade 13 to 16 level, admission forms grade 11, colon x-rays grade 10 to 12" (Dixon, Park, 1990).
- Conduct a tour of the procedure/treatment room; introduce patient to staff involved in procedure. Provide information on what will be seen, heard, smelled, and felt during the procedure (McCloskey, Bulecheck, 1996).
  "Sensory preparation can decrease stress in clients when they experience the actual sensations" (Johnson, Lauver, 1989).
- Use visual aids such as diagrams, pictures, videotapes, and audiotapes.
  "Audiotapes and videotapes provide an alternative to the written word" (Meade et al, 1994).
- Provide preadmission self-instruction materials to prepare client for postoperative exercises.
  Providing clients with preadmission information about exercises has been shown to increase positive feelings and the ability to perform prescribed exercises (Rice et al, 1992).
- Explain sensations the client will experience during diagnostic procedures or following surgery.

Sensory preparation can decrease distress in clients when they actually experience the sensations (Johnson, Lauver, 1989).

- Identify the primary family support person; be aware of that person's ability to learn and incorporate needed changes.
- Assess willingness of family to incorporate new information, immunizations, medical and dental care, and diet modifications in support of the client.
  "Attention needs to be directed at family adjustment factors. Women recovering from alcohol abuse are at risk for relapse if their spouse continues to drink alcohol" (Murphy, 1993).
- Provide plenty of time for questions, clarification, and reinforcement when teaching family.
  Each family member has a unique learning style. By getting family support for needed changes in diet, stress management, or life-style, the client will be motivated and successful in implementing new information.
- Help client identify community resources for continuing information and support.
  Learning occurs through imitation, so persons who are currently involved in life-style changes can help the client anticipate adjustment issues. Community resources can offer financial and educational support.
- Evaluate client's learning through return demonstrations, verbalizations, or the application of skills to new situations.
  The education process is not complete until the learner successfully implements a skill as a tool for health maintenance.

Geriatric
- Adapt the teaching process for the physical constraints of the aging process (e.g., speak clearly, use a variety of audio-visual-psychomotor methods, use examples, allow time for client to repeat and review).
  Adults are capable of learning at any age. Age modifies but does not inhibit learning (Dellasega et al, 1994).
- Ensure that the client uses necessary reading aids (e.g., glasses, magnifying lenses, large-print texts) or hearing aids.
  Visual and hearing deficits require amplification or clarification of sensory input.
- Use printed material, videotapes, lists, and diagrams that the client can refer to at another time.
  "Audiotapes and videotapes provide an alternative to the written word" (Meade, 1994). They provide a reference that can be used in a less stressful setting, decreasing barriers to learning.
- Assess client's previous knowledge or resistance or blocks to incorporating new information into the current life-style.
  Long-term memory is strong and affects how well new information is interpreted and used.
- Repeat and reinforce information during several brief sessions.
  Understanding past information is essential to acquiring new knowledge. Brief sessions focus attention on essential information.
- Discuss healthy life-style changes that promote wellness for the older adult.
  "It is never too late to stop smoking, lose weight, or modify dietary intake of fats and alcohol. Quality versus quantity of life may be the key issue in teaching self-care health habits" (Walker, 1992).
- Evaluate the readability of the material.
  "Highlight important information, use lists; print should be 8- or 10-point type; use bold face print to accommodate diabetic or cataract patients" (Dixon, Park, 1990).

Home Care Interventions

NOTE: Because home care is an intermittent model of care having a goal of safety and optimal wellness of the client between visits, the importance of teaching (by nurse) and learning (by client) should not be understated. All of the mentioned interventions are applicable to the home setting.

- Select a space and time for teaching in which client and/or caregiver can focus on information to be learned.

  The home setting provides many distractions that may impair the ability of the client to learn.

- Consider the complexity of material or behaviors to be learned. Adjust care plan and respective teaching/learning experiences accordingly to build client confidence in ability to learn (and change).

  Confidence in the ability to learn and change is part of readiness to learn.

- Assess for specific areas of learning that have the potential for strong emotional responses by the client or family/caregiver. Allow time for expression of feelings and encourage acceptance of need for learning.

  Typical client and family responses to emotionally charged learning content include fear, anxiety, helplessness, hopelessness, denial, hostility, rejection, and overprotectiveness (Boehringher, Mannheim Diagnostics, 1983).

- Document client's and caregivers' responses to learning.

  Clear documentation supports continuity in the learning experience.

REFERENCES   Boehringher, Mannheim Diagnostics: *Changing behavior; the dynamics of motivation and adherence in diabetes,* 1983.

Camprich B: A theoretical perspective on attention and patient education, *Adv Nurs Sci* 14:39, 1992.

Dellasega C et al: Nursing process: teaching elderly clients, *J Gerontol Nurs* 31:20, 1994.

Dixon E, Park R: Do patients understand written health information? *Nurs Outlook* 38:278.

Johnson JE, Lauver DR: Alternative explanations of coping with stressful experiences associated with physical illness, *Adv Nurs Sci* 11:39, 1989.

McCloskey J, Bulecheck G: *Nursing interventions classification (NIC),* ed 2, St Louis, 1996, Mosby.

Meade C et al: Educating patients with limited literacy skills: the effectiveness of printed and videotaped material about colon cancer, *Am J Public Health* 84:119, 1994.

Murphy S: Coping strategies of abstainers from alcohol 3 years to post treatment, *Image* 25:32, 1993.

Rice VH et al: Preadmission self-instruction effects on postadmission and postoperative indicators in CABG patients: partial replication and extension, *Res Nurs Health* 15:253, 1992.

Spees C: Knowledge of medical terminology among clients and families, *Image* 23:225, 1990.

Walker S: Wellness for elders, *Holistic Nurs Pract* 7:38, 1992.

Williams M et al: Inadequate functional health literacy among patients at two public hospitals, *JAMA* 274:1677, 1995.

Risk for loneliness

Marty J. Martin

Definition   The subjective state in which an individual is at risk of experiencing vague dysphoria

Risk Factors

Affectional deprivation, physical isolation, cathectic deprivation, social isolation

Related Factors (r/t)

See Risk Factors

Client Outcomes/Goals

- Maintains one or more meaningful relationships (growth enhancing versus codependent or abusive in nature)—relationships allowing self-disclosure—and demonstrates a balance between emotional dependence and independence
- Participates in ongoing positive and relevant social activities and interactions that are personally meaningful
- Demonstrates positive use of time alone when socialization is not possible

Suggested NIC Interventions

Family integrity promotion, socialization enhancement, visitation facilitation

Nursing Interventions and Rationales

- Assess client's perception of loneliness. (Is the person alone by choice, or is the aloneness imposed by others?)

  Social isolation is perceived by others, loneliness is not. See **Social isolation,** *an important nursing diagnosis because it is often a precursor to loneliness (Buchda, 1987).*

- Assist client with identifying loneliness as a feeling and the causes related to loneliness.

  Individuals experiencing loneliness often do not wish to discuss the painful experience and may not recognize its cause. Clients may need assistance in distinguishing between being alone and being lonely.

- Assess client's social support system.

  Use a social support tool or validated assessment tool if possible (e.g., UCLA Loneliness Scale for adolescents [1995]; see reference).

- Assess client's ability and/or inability to meet physical, psychosocial, spiritual, and financial needs and how unmet needs further challenge ability to be socially integrated (e.g., loss of job leading to inability to "afford" usual and familiar social interaction, fatigue; lack of energy necessary for social interaction and personal engagement, impaired skin integument and its relationship to real and/or perceived social isolation).

  NOTE: See **Body image disturbance** if loneliness is associated with impaired skin integument

  Assessment of overall human needs gives direction to the care and treatment of nursing diagnostic categories such as loneliness (O'Brien, Pheifer, 1993). A tool that measures the sense of belonging is important in addressing the relationship between social support and physical illness (particularly cardiac disease) and mortality (Case et al, 1992; House et al, 1988).

- Use active listening skills including assessment and clarification of client's verbal and nonverbal responses and interactions.

  Utilizing therapeutic observation and listening skills helps to accurately assess and validate this diagnosis. Clients are often unable to identify the problems or factors that directly contribute to their sense of isolation (O'Brien, Pheifer, 1993).

- Evaluate client's desire for social interaction in relation to actual social interaction.

  The concept of loneliness involves a discrepancy between the client's desired and achieved level of social interaction (Christian, Dluhy, O'Neill, 1989).

- Assess client's interpersonal skills and address deficits and behaviors that are blocking communication.
- Encourage client to be involved in meaningful social relationships that are characteristic of both giving and receiving support.

It is important to recognize that the positive relevance of social relationships is related to the content and quality of relationships (Gulick, 1994).

- Explore ways to increase client's support system and participation in groups and organizations.
  Studies indicate that people with smaller support systems have higher levels of loneliness (Mahon, 1982).
- Encourage client to practice self-disclosure during conversations.
- Encourage client to develop closeness in at least one relationship.
  Dependence and independence should be balanced in healthy relationships. Previous research has indicated that the development of a balanced level of emotional dependence and the ability to self-disclose are important factors in reducing the risk for loneliness (Mahon, 1982; Mahon, Yarcheski, 1992).

Adolescents
- See references for assessment tool.
- Evaluate the depth and level of character traits, shyness, and self-esteem, particularly of younger and middle adolescent clients.
- Evaluate the family stability of younger and middle adolescent clients, and advocate and encourage healthy, growth-producing relationships with families and support systems.
- For older adolescents, encourage close relationships with peers and involvement in groups and organizations.
  Research indicates that younger adolescents are at a higher risk for loneliness if they are shy or have low self-esteem. Younger adolescents rely more on parental relationships. An expanded set of relationships becomes increasingly important in alleviating loneliness as adolescents mature (Mahon, Yarcheski, 1992).

Geriatric
- Identify community support systems specific to elderly populations.
  Aging is often accompanied by significant losses of family members and other social support systems, which may lead to loneliness and depression.
- Assess clients' adaptive sensory functions or any other health deviations that may limit or decrease their ability to interact with others.
- Assess client's potential or actual hearing loss or hearing impairment.
  Research shows that hearing loss is one of the most prevalent chronic health problems of the elderly in the United States (Christian, Dluhy, O'Neill, 1989). Because of the nature of the sensory deprivation, communication barriers are increased and human intimacy and self-esteem are negatively affected (Chen, 1994). In addition, it is important to note that hearing impairments often go unnoticed and may not be obvious as are more visibly recognized handicaps (Chen, 1994).
- Encourage positive use of solitude to prevent loneliness (e.g., reading, listening to music, enjoying nature).
  The positive use of solitude and a decreased dependence on external stimuli may be particularly important for older individuals who often find themselves alone without external stimuli or social support.
- Provide reading materials for clients who are able to read.
  Older people who enjoyed reading for pleasure were rarely lonely (Rane-Szotak, Herth, 1994).

Home Care Interventions

- If the client is experiencing somatic complaints, evaluate client complaints to assure physical needs are being met, then identify relationship between somatic complaints and loneliness.

Loneliness precipitates somatic complaints and sleeplessness.

- Assist client to identify periods when loneliness is greatest (e.g., certain times of day, anniversaries of past special events). With client permission, refer for services of visiting volunteers.
  The only agenda of visiting volunteers is to meet the social needs of the client. Long-term friendships sometimes develop from volunteer experiences.
- Identify alternatives to eating alone.
  Mealtimes are when clients are often susceptible to loneliness. Loneliness may contribute to nutritional deficiencies or excesses.
- Identify alternatives to being alone (e.g., telephone contact).
- Provide opportunities for the client to contribute to the social well being of others. Homebound clients can contribute via the telephone.
  Contributing to society enhances self-esteem and decreases loneliness. Loss of meaning contributes to loneliness.
- Support religious beliefs.
  Belief in a supreme being provides a feeling of ever-present help and prevents loneliness. If clients have regrets about their life, they may be separated from their usual source of religious comfort.
- Discuss the meaning of death and fears associated with dying alone. Explore the possibility of significant others being with the client at time of death.
  In later stages of life, individuals give significant thought to death and the meaning of their life. If they perceive life as undesirable, they may fear death.

Client/Family Teaching

- Encourage positive use of solitude to prevent loneliness (e.g., reading, listening to music, enjoying nature).
  A positive use of solitude plays a strong role in preventing or alleviating loneliness. The mentioned activities are flow activities—self-directed, independent activities that enhance well-being and decrease feelings of loneliness (Rane-Szotak, Herth, 1994).
- Include the family in all client teaching activities, and give them accurate information regarding the illness severity.
  The family can also experience loneliness. Clients and families often have grossly different perceptions of the severity and threats of illness. The family often perceives the person to be much more ill than the ill person does. A realistic understanding of the person, family, and significant others will decrease the emotional threats of illness (Buchda, 1987).
- Give family members something to do such as holding a hand, applying lotion, or assisting with feeding.
  Facilitation of an individual's sense of relatedness to significant others can reduce loneliness for critically ill clients. Providing a specific task increases the quality of the interaction (Buchda, 1987).
- Encourage family members to express caring by telling the client where they will be and sending messages when they cannot be present.
  Keeping the client informed is a way of expressing caring and helps reduce loneliness (Buchda, 1987).

REFERENCES   Buchda V: Loneliness in critically ill adults, *Dimen Crit Care Nurs* 6:335, 1987.
Case R et al: Living alone after myocardial infarction: impact on prognosis, *JAMA* 267:515, 1992.

Chen H: Hearing in the elderly, relation of healing loss, loneliness, and self-esteem, *J Gerontol Nurs* 20:22, 1994.

Christian E, Dluhy E, O'Neill R: Sounds of silence, *J Gerontol Nurs* 15:4, 1989.

Gulick E: Social support among persons with multiple sclerosis, *Res Nurs Health* 17:195, 1994.

House J, Landis K, Umberson D: Social relationships and health, *Science* 241:540, 1988.

Mahon NE: The relationship of self disclosure, interpersonal dependency, and life changes to loneliness in young adults, *Nurs Res* 31:343, 1982.

Mahon NE, Yarcheski A: Alternate explanations of loneliness in adolescents: a replication and extension study, *Nurs Res* 41:151, 1992.

Mahon NE, Yarcheski T, Yarcheski A: Validation of the revised UCLA loneliness scale for adolescents, *Res Nurs Health* 18:263, 1995.

O'Brien ME, Pheiffer W: Physical and psychosocial nursing care for patients with HIV infection, *Nurs Clin North Am* 28:303, 1993.

Rane-Szotak D, Herth K: A new perspective on loneliness in later life, *Issu Ment Health Nurs* 16:583, 1994.

Rawlins R, Heacock P: *Clinical manual of psychiatric nursing,* ed 2, 1993, St Louis, Mosby.

Impaired memory

Betty J. Ackley

Definition   The state in which an individual experiences the inability to remember or recall bits of information or behavioral skills; may be attributed to either temporary or permanent pathophysiological or situational causes

Defining Characteristics

Major   Observed or reported forgetfulness, inability to determine whether a behavior was performed, inability to learn or retain new skills or information, inability to perform a previously learned skill, inability to recall factual information, inability to recall recent or past events

Minor   Forgets to perform a behavior at a scheduled time

Related Factors (r/t)

Acute or chronic hypoxia, anemia, decreased cardiac output, fluid and electrolyte imbalances, neurological disturbances, excessive environmental disturbances

Client Outcomes/Goals

- Demonstrates use of techniques to help with memory loss
- States having fewer problems with memory loss

Suggested NIC Intervention

Memory training

Nursing Interventions and Rationales

- Assess neurological function; use an assessment tool such as the Mini-Mental Status Examination (MMSE) if possible.
  The MMSE can help determine whether the client has memory loss only or also has delirium or dementia and needs to be referred for further treatment (Breitner, Welsh, 1995).
- Determine whether onset of memory loss is gradual or sudden. If memory loss is sudden, refer client to a physician for evaluation.
  Acute onset of memory loss may be associated with neurological disease, electrolyte disturbances, hypoxia, or many other physiological factors (Vinson, 1989; Breitner, Welsh, 1995).

- Determine amount and pattern of alcohol intake.
  Alcohol intake has been associated with "blackouts"—clients may function but not remember their actions. Long-term alcohol use causes Korsakoff's syndrome with associated memory loss (Vinson, 1989).
- Note client's current medications and intake of any mind-altering substances such as benzodiazepines or marijuana.
  Benzodiazepines can produce memory loss for events that occur after taking the medication; information is not stored in long-term memory (Mejo, 1992). Excessive marijuana use has been shown to result in selective short-term memory deficits in adolescents that continue at least 6 weeks after discontinuing intake of the drug (Schwartz et al, 1989).
- Note client's current level of stress. Ask if there has been a recent traumatic event.
  Posttraumatic stress and anxiety-inducing general life factors can cause memory problems (Mejo, 1992).
- If signs of depression such as weight loss, insomnia, or sad affect are evident, refer client for psychotherapy.
  Depression is commonly associated with memory loss (Mejo, 1992).
- Encourage clients to use a calendar for appointments, keep reminder lists, place a string around finger or rubber band around wrist as reminders, or enlist someone else to remind them of important events.
  Using reminders can serve as cues for memory-impaired clients.
- Help client set up a medication box that reminds client to take medication at needed times; assist client with refilling the box at intervals if necessary.
  Medication boxes are effective because clients will know whether medication has been taken when appropriate compartments are empty.
- If safety is an issue with certain activities (e.g., client forgets to turn off stove after use or forgets emergency telephone numbers), suggest alternatives such as using a microwave or whistling teakettle for heating water and programming emergency numbers in telephone so that they are readily available.
  These measures can increase client safety (Agostinelli et al, 1994).
- Refer client to a memory clinic (if available), a neuropsychologist, or an occupational therapist.
  Memory clinics can help the client learn ways to improve memory. Neuropsychologists have expertise in working with the memory impaired, as do many occupational therapists (Robinson, 1992).
- If stress is associated with memory loss, suggest psychotherapy, exercise, or the use of relaxation techniques.
  Nonpharmacological therapy for treatment of stress syndromes is preferable and less likely to aggravate memory loss than commonly used antianxiety medications (Mejo, 1992).
- Suggest clients use cues, including alarm watches, electronic organizers, or pocket computers, to trigger certain actions at designated times.
  Cues can help remind clients of certain actions (Wilson, Moffat, 1992).
- For clients with memory impairments associated with dementia, see **Chronic confusion.**

Geriatric
- Assess for signs of depression.
  Depression is the most important affective variable for memory loss in the older adult (Byers, 1993; McDougall, 1995).

- Evaluate all medications that client is taking to determine whether they are causing the memory loss.

  Many medications can cause memory loss in the elderly, including anticholinergics, H_2-receptor antagonists, beta-blockers, digitalis, benzodiazapines, barbiturates, and even mild opiates (DeMaagd, 1995).

- Help family develop a memory aid booklet or wallet that contains pictures and labels from client's life.

  Using memory aids helps clients with dementia make more factual statements and stay on topic and decreases the number of confused, erroneous, and repetitive statements (Bourgeois, 1992).

- Help family label items such as the bathroom or sock drawer to increase recall.

  A supportive environment that includes orientation can help increase the client's awareness (Green, Gildemeister, 1994).

Home Care Interventions

- Identify a "checking in" support system (e.g., Lifeline or significant others).

  Checking in ensures client safety.

- Keep furniture placement and household patterns consistent.

  Change increases risk of impaired memory and decreased functioning.

Client/Family Teaching

- When teaching client, determine what the client knows about memory techniques and then build on that knowledge.

  "New material is organized in terms of what already exists, and efficient learning should attempt to take advantage of what is already known in order to graft on new material" (Wilson, Moffat, 1992, p. 21).

- When teaching a skill to client, set up a series of practice attempts. Begin with simple tasks so that clients can be positively reinforced and progress to more difficult concepts.

  Distributed practice with correct recall attempts can be a very effective teaching strategy; practice is widely distributed over time if possible (Wilson, Moffat, 1992).

- Teach clients to use memory techniques, such as repeating information they want to remember, making mental associations to remember information, and placing items in strategic places so that they will not be forgotten.

  These methods increase recall of information the client thinks is important.

REFERENCES   Agostinelli B et al: Targeted interventions: use of the Mini-Mental State Exam, *J Gerontol Nurs* 20:15, 1994.

Bourgeois MS: *Conversing with memory impaired individuals using memory aids: a memory aid workbook,* Gaylord, Mich, 1992, Northern Speech Services.

Breitner JC, Welsh KA: Diagnosis and management of memory loss and cognitive disorders among elderly persons, *Psychiatr Serv* 46:29, 1995.

Byers PH: Older adults' metamemory: coping, depression, and self-efficacy, *Appl Nurs Res* 6:28, 1993.

DeMaagd G: High-risk drugs in the elderly population, *Geriatr Nurs* 16:198, 1995.

Green PM, Gildemeister JE: Memory aging research and memory support in the elderly, *J Neurosci Nurs* 26:241, 1994.

McDougall GJ: Predictors of metamemory in older adults, *Nurs Res* 43:306, 1994.

Mejo SL: Anterograde amnesia linked to benzodiazepines, *Nurse Pract* 17:44, 1992.

Robinson S: Occupational therapy in a memory clinic, *Brit J Occup Ther* 55:394, 1992.

Schwartz RH et al: Short-term memory impairment in cannabis-dependent adolescents, *AJDC* 143:1214, 1989.

Vinson DC: Acute transient memory loss, *Am Fam Physician* 39:249, 1989.

Wilson BA, Moffat N: *Clinical management of memory problems,* San Diego, 1992, Singular.

Impaired physical mobility

Teepa Snow and Betty J. Ackley

Definition   The state in which an individual experiences a limitation of ability for independent physical movement

Defining Characteristics

Inability to purposefully move within the physical environment, including bed mobility, transfer, and ambulation; inability to sit unsupported; reluctance to attempt movement; limited range of motion; decreased muscle strength, control, or mass; imposed restrictions of movement, including mechanical and medical protocol; impaired coordination

Related Factors (r/t)

Intolerance to activity, decreased strength and endurance, pain or discomfort, perceptual or cognitive impairment, neuromuscular impairment, musculoskeletal impairment, depression, severe anxiety

Suggested functional level classifications follow:

0   Completely independent
1   Requires use of equipment or device
2   Requires help from another person for assistance, supervision, or teaching
3   Requires help from another person and equipment device
4   Dependent, does not participate in activity

Client Outcomes/Goals

- Increases physical activity
- Meets mutually defined goals of increased mobility
- Verbalizes feeling of increased strength and ability to move
- Demonstrates use of adaptive equipment (e.g., wheelchairs, walkers) to increase mobility

Suggested NIC Interventions

Exercise therapy: ambulation, exercise therapy: joint mobility, positioning

Nursing Interventions and Rationales

- Screen for mobility skills in the following order: (1) bed mobility, (2) supported and unsupported sitting, (3) transition movements such as sit to stand and sitting down and transfers, and (4) standing and walking activities.
  Screening mobility skills helps provide baselines of performance that can guide mobility-enhancement programming and allows nursing staff to integrate movement and practice opportunities into daily routines and regular and customary care.
- Observe client for cause of impaired mobility. Determine whether cause is physical or psychological.
  Some clients choose not to move because of psychological factors such as an inability to cope or depression. See interventions for **Ineffective individual coping** *or* **Hopelessness.**
- Monitor and record client's ability to tolerate activity and use all four extremities; note pulse rate, blood pressure, dyspnea, and skin color before and after activity. See **Activity intolerance.**
- Observe for and if possible treat pain before activity. Ensure that client is not oversedated.
  Pain limits mobility and is often exacerbated by movement.
- Consult with physical therapy for further evaluation, strength training, gait training, and development of a mobility plan.

- Obtain any assistive devices needed for activity, such as walking belts, walkers, canes, crutches, or wheelchairs, before the activity begins.
  Assistive devices help increase mobility.
- If client is immobile, perform passive range of motion exercises at least twice a day unless contraindicated; repeat each maneuver three times.
  Passive range of motion exercises helps maintain joint mobility, prevent contractures and deformities, increase circulation, and promote a feeling of comfort and well-being (Kottke, Lehman, 1990; Bolander, 1994).
- If client is immobile, consult with physician for a safety evaluation before beginning an exercise program; if program is approved, begin with the following exercises:
  - Active range of motion exercises using both upper and lower extremities (e.g., flexing and extending at ankles, knees, hips)
  - Chin-ups and pull-ups using a trapeze in bed (may be contraindicated in clients with cardiac conditions)
  - Strengthening exercises such as gluteal or quadriceps sitting exercises
  These exercises help reverse weakening and atrophy of muscles.
- Help client achieve mobility and start walking as soon as possible if not contraindicated.
  The longer a client is immobile, the longer it takes to regain strength, balance, and coordination (Bolander, 1994).
- Use a walking belt when ambulating the client.
  The client can walk independently with a walking belt, but the nurse can rapidly ensure safety if the knees buckle.
- Apply any ordered brace before mobilizing client.
  Braces stabilize a body part, allowing increased mobility.
- Increase independence in activities of daily living as client gets stronger; discourage helplessness.
  Providing unnecessary assistance with transfers and bathing activities may promote dependence and a loss of mobility (Mobily, Kelley, 1991).
- If client does not feed or groom self, nurses should sit side-by-side with client, put client's hand over theirs, support client's elbow with their other hand, and help client feed self and comb hair.
  This feeding technique increases client mobility and independence, and clients often eat more food (Pedretti, 1996).

Geriatric
- Initiate a walking program in which clients walk with or without help every day as part of their daily routine.
  Walking programs have been shown to be effective in improving ambulatory status and decreasing disability and the number of falls in the elderly (Koroknay et al, 1995).
- Encourage client to attend a low-intensity aerobic chair exercise class that includes stretching and strengthening chair exercises.
  Chair exercises have been shown to increase flexibility and balance (Mills, 1994).
- Watch for orthostatic hypotension when mobilizing elderly clients.
  Orthostatic hypotension as a result of cardiovascular system changes, chronic diseases, and medication effects is common in the elderly (Mobily, Kelley, 1991).
- Help clients assume the prone position three times per week for 20 minutes each time. If clients are unable to do so, help them turn partially over and assume the position gradually.
  The prone position helps prevent hip deformities that can interfere with balance and walking. This position may be contraindicated in some clients such as morbidly obese clients, respiratory or cardiac clients who cannot lie flat, and neurological clients.

- Do not routinely assist with transfers or bathing activities unless necessary.
  The nursing staff may contribute to impaired mobility by helping too much; encourage client independence (Mobily, Kelley, 1991).
- Use gestures and nonverbal cues when helping clients move if they are anxious or have difficulty understanding and following verbal instructions.
  Nonverbal gestures are part of a universal language that can be understood when the client is having difficulty with communication.
- Ensure that chairs fit clients—chair seat should be 3 inches above the height of the knee. Provide a raised toilet seat if needed.
  Raising the height of a chair can dramatically improve many older people's ability to stand up. Low, deep, soft seats with arm rests that are far apart reduce a person's ability to get up and down without help.
- If client is mainly immobile, provide opportunities for socialization and sensory stimulation (e.g., television and visits). See **Diversional activity deficit.**
  Immobility and a lack of social support and sensory input may result in confusion or depression in the elderly (Mobily, Kelley, 1991). See interventions for **Acute confusion** *or* **Helplessness** *as appropriate.*

Home Care Interventions

- Assess home environment for factors that create barriers to physical mobility. Refer to occupational therapy services if needed to assist client in restructuring home and daily living patterns.
- Refer to home health aide services to support client and family through changing levels of mobility. Reinforce need to promote independence in mobility as tolerated.
  Providing unnecessary assistance with transfers and bathing activities may promote dependence and a loss of mobility (Mobily, Kelley, 1991).
- Assess skin condition at every visit. Establish a skin care program that enhances circulation and maximizes position changes.
  Impaired mobility decreases circulation to dependent areas. Decreased circulation and shearing place the client at risk for skin breakdown.
- Provide support to client and family/caregivers during long-term impaired mobility.
  Long-term impaired mobility may necessitate role changes within the family and precipitate caregiver stress (see **Caregiver role strain).**

Client/Family Teaching

- Teach client to get out of bed slowly when transferring from the bed to the chair.
- Teach client relaxation techniques to use during activity.
- Teach client to use assistive devices such as a cane, a walker, or crutches to increase mobility.
- Teach family members and caregivers to work with clients during self-care activities such as eating, bathing, grooming, dressing, and transferring rather than having client be a passive recipient of care.
  Maintaining as much independence as possible helps maintain mobility skills (Lipson, Braun, 1993).
- Develop a mutually agreed on contract with client regarding goals of increased activity; include measurable landmarks of progress with evaluation dates and sign the contract with the client.

REFERENCES   Bolander VB: Meeting mobility needs. In *Sorensen and Luckmann's Basic nursing: a psychophysiologic approach,* Philadelphia, 1994, WB Saunders.

Hummer A: Get your patient moving, *Am J Nurs* 93:34, 1993.

Kasper CE et al: Alterations in skeletal muscle related to impaired physical mobility: an empirical model, *Res Nurs Health* 16:265, 1993.

Koroknay VJ et al: Maintaining ambulation in the frail nursing home resident: a nursing administered walking program, *J Gerontol Nurs* 21:18, 1995.

Kottke FJ, Lehmann JF: *Krusen's handbook of physical medicine,* ed 4, Philadelphia, 1990, WB Saunders.

Lewis et al: *The functional tool book,* Washington, DC, 1994, Learn.

Lipson J, Braun S: *Toward a restrain-free environment: reducing the use of physical and chemical restraint in long term care and acute settings,* Baltimore, 1993, Health Professions Press.

Mills EM: The effect of low-intensity aerobic exercise on muscle strength, flexibility, and balance among sedentary elderly persons, *Nurs Res* 43:207, 1994.

Mobily PR, Kelley LS: Iatrogenesis in the elderly: factors of immobility, *J Gerontol Nurs* 17:5, 1991.

Ouellet LL, Rush KL: A synthesis of selected literature on mobility: a basis for studying impaired mobility, *Nurs Diag* 3:72, 1992.

Pedretti LW: *Occupational therapy: practice skills for physical dysfunction,* ed 4, St Louis, 1996, Mosby.

Schneider J, Passanisi J: *Exercises for agility, balance, coordination and strength,* 1988, Therapy Skill Builders.

Vorhies D, Riley BE: Deconditioning, *Geriatr Rehab* 9:745, 1993.

Noncompliance

Betty J. Ackley

Definition   An individual's informed decision to not adhere to a therapeutic recommendation

Defining Characteristics

Behavior indicative of failure to adhere (directly observed or verbalized by patient or significant others) *(critical),* objective tests (e.g., physiological measures, detection of markers), evidence of development of complications, evidence of exacerbation of symptoms, failure to keep appointments, failure to progress

Related Factors (r/t)

Patient value system, health beliefs, cultural influences, spiritual values, client-provider relationships, lack of financial resources

Client Outcomes/Goals

- Describes consequence of continued noncompliance with treatment regimen
- States goals for health and the means by which to obtain them
- Communicates an understanding of disease and treatment
- Lists treatment regimens and expectations and agrees to follow through
- Lists alternative ways to meet goals
- Describes the importance of family participation to help client achieve goals

Suggested NIC Interventions

Health system guidance, self-modification assistance

Nursing Interventions and Rationales

- Ask clients why they have not complied with the prescribed treatment—have them "tell their story." Listen nonjudgmentally.
  Compliance assessment should begin with a nonthreatening discussion with the client (Kluckowski, 1992).

- Observe for cause of noncompliance. See related factors previously mentioned. Recognize that noncompliance is very common.
  Rates of noncompliance are estimated at 50% (Kluckowski, 1992).
- Determine client's and family's knowledge of illness and treatment. Teach them about the illness and purpose of the treatment regimen if necessary.
  Knowledge is power and with it comes increased control; the more control clients have, the more likely they are to comply with the prescribed regimen (Kluckowski, 1992).
- Observe client's cultural influences, values, and beliefs regarding illness and whether locus of control is internal or external.
  The client may be unable to assume the sick role because of cultural influences, values, or beliefs and may reject treatment. Clients with an internal locus of control are more compliant (Warren, 1992).
- Monitor client's ability to follow directions, solve problems, concentrate, and read.
  Clients with cognitive impairments may not be able to follow directions and the prescribed treatment regimen.
- Avoid using threats, pressure, and inappropriate fear arousal to increase compliance.
  These measures are unethical and generally ineffective.
- Determine whether client's support system helps or hinders therapy. Bring family members and significant others into the educational process as desired by the client.
  A positive social support system is associated with increased compliance (Warren, 1992).
- Develop a therapeutic relationship based on active listening.
  Good communication has been shown to increase compliance (Crane, 1996).
  Compliance is increased when the client feels that the health care provider is interested in and genuinely cares about the client (Warren, 1992).
- Listen to client's descriptions of their abilities; encourage client to use these abilities in self-care.
- When dealing with complex health care regimens, start client with small behavioral changes (e.g., have chemotherapy client rinse mouth with a saliva substitute twice daily). When one step has been accomplished, add another step.
  The client is often overwhelmed by what is expected and needs help with managing behavioral changes (Boehm, 1992).
- Make client an active partner in the health care team and allow client to give input on which treatments are acceptable and feasible.
  Recognize that clients have absolute power over whether they follow the health care guidelines; health care providers influence behavior.
- Work with client to develop cues that trigger needed health care behaviors (e.g., checking blood sugar before putting on makeup each morning).
  Associating cues with certain behaviors increases the frequency of desired behaviors.
- Work with client to develop an instruction and reminder sheet that fits medications and treatments into the client's life-style.
  Visual reminders help increase compliance.
- For a chronically ill client, develop a multidisciplinary team to provide care, including a nurse, a physician, a pharmacist, a dietitian, and additional therapists as needed. Have team meetings to ensure continuity of care.
  Multidisciplinary team care has been shown to increase compliance (Warren, 1992).

- Develop a mutually agreed on written contract with client regarding needed health care behaviors; give reinforcement as client meets defined goals.
  A client contract that helps the client analyze behaviors and choose behavioral strategies can be very effective in changing health care behaviors (Boehm, 1992).
- Consult with primary care practitioner regarding the possibility of simplifying the health care regimen so that it more easily fits into client's life-style (e.g., taking medications one time per day versus four times per day).
  Complex regimens and inconvenient dose scheduling decrease compliance (Crane, 1996).

Geriatric
- If client has sensory and coordination deficits, use a medication organizer and have the home health nurse or family place client's medications in daily compartments.
  A medication organizer can increase the client's ability to take medications as ordered.
- Help client feel like a partner in managing health care condition—use caring, encouragement, written goals, and a "power with" relationship with nurse.
  These methods have been shown to increase self-efficacy and empower elderly clients to manage their condition (Resnick, 1996).
- Monitor client for signs of depression associated with noncompliance (e.g., refusing to eat or take medications). Refer client for treatment of depression as needed.
  Noncompliance in the elderly may be a form of indirect self-destructive behavior that is associated with depression and leads to suicide (Meisekothen, 1993).
- Use repetition, verbal cues, and memory aids such as picture schedule or reminder sheet when teaching the health care regimen.
  There may be age-related memory deficits that necessitate an increased use of measures that cue the client to perform needed health care behaviors.

Home Care Interventions

NOTE: Because the home care nurse enters the client's home as a guest, the ability of the nurse to establish a supportive, therapeutic relationship is especially important.

- *Before* providing any care, review the home health care Bill of Rights with the client, including the right to refuse treatment.
  Identifying the rights of the client demonstrates respect of the health care system and its representatives for client wishes.
- If included in agency policies and procedures, also review Patient Responsibilities with client (which is often part of printed Bill of Rights).
  Reviewing responsibilities helps client define roles of mutual respect and partnership with the health care provider.
- When clients are noncompliant, redefine personal and health priorities (contract for services) with clients to determine alternative motivational strategies or health actions to meet health goals.
  For clients to carry out desired health actions, they must perceive actions as beneficial to self and the cost of the health action as not being greater than the benefit (Rosenstock, 1974).
- If noncompliant behavior continues, home health care cannot continue to provide services if client chooses not to cooperate with medical regimen.
  Reimbursement guidelines and agency policies do not support the continued use of health care resources when the client makes an informed decision to not follow the prescribed regimen.

- If care is to be terminated, identify all possible alternatives for the client and assist with making an informed choice about future health actions.

  Some regulatory guidelines require health care providers to give written notice of discontinuance of care using established time frames. Noncompliance and a plan for termination of care notwithstanding, it remains the goal and ethical responsibility of home health care providers to promote optimal wellness, independence, and safety.

- Respect the wishes of terminally ill clients to refuse selected aspects of medical regimen. Do not terminate care—provide those aspects of care that client and family or caregivers will accept.

  The goal of hospice care is to provide comfort and dignity in the dying process.

Client/Family Teaching

- Teach clients about medication side effects (e.g., mental changes, sexual dysfunction) so that they understand them and feel comfortable discussing them.

  Many medications can cause side effects such as changes in mental function and impotence, which can lead to noncompliance.

- Teach clients to control their "self-talk" by giving themselves positive messages that will be used to promote desired behaviors such as taking medications and controlling food intake.

  Self-talk has been shown to be a common motivating method for behavior changes (McSweeney, 1993).

  NOTE: The nursing diagnosis **Noncompliance** is judgmental and places blame on the client (Bakker, Kastermans, Dassen, 1995). The author recommends use of the diagnosis **Ineffective management of therapeutic regimen: individual** in place of the diagnosis **Noncompliance.** The diagnosis **Ineffective management of therapeutic regimen: individual** has interventions that are developed by both the health care providers and the client. It is a more respectful and efficacious nursing diagnosis.

REFERENCES   Bakker RH, Kastermans MC, Dassen TW: An analysis of the nursing diagnosis ineffective management of therapeutic regimen compared to noncompliance and Orem's self-care deficit theory of nursing, *Nurs Diagnosis* 6:161, 1995.

Boehm S: Patient contracting. In Bulechek GM, McCloskey JC, editors: *Nursing interventions: essential nursing treatments,* Philadelphia, 1992, WB Saunders.

Cargill JM: Medication compliance in elderly people: influencing variables and interventions, *J Adv Nurs* 17:422, 1992.

Crane K, Kirby B, Kooperman D: Patient compliance for psychotropic medications, *J Psychosoc Nurs* 34:8, 1996.

Foreman L: Medication: reasons and interventions for noncompliance, *J Psychosoc Nurs Ment Health Serv* 31:23, 1993.

Kluckowski JC: Solving medication noncompliance in home care, *Caring* 11:34, 1992.

McSweeney JC: Making behavior changes after a myocardial infarction, *West J Nurs Res* 15:441, 1993.

Meisekothen LM: Noncompliance in the elderly: a pathway to suicide, *J Am Acad Nurs Pract* 5:67, 1993.

Resnick B: Motivation in geriatric rehabilitation, *Image* 28:41, 1996.

Rosenstock I: Health belief model and preventive behavior. In Becker M, editor: *The health belief model and personal health behavior,* Thorofare, NJ, 1974, CB Slack.

Warren JJ: Ethical concerns about noncompliance in the chronically ill patient, *Prog Cardiovasc Nurs* 7:10, 1992.

Altered nutrition: less than body requirements

Carroll A. Lutz

Definition   The state in which an individual experiences an intake of nutrients insufficient to meet metabolic needs

Defining Characteristics

Loss of weight with adequate food intake, body weight 20% or more less than ideal, reported food intake less than recommended daily allowance, weakness of muscles required for swallowing or mastication, reported or evidence of lack of food, aversion to eating, reported altered taste sensation, satiety immediately after ingesting food, abdominal pain with or without pathology, sore and inflamed buccal cavity, hyperactive bowel sounds, lack of interest in food, perceived inability to ingest food, pale conjunctival and mucous membranes, poor muscle tone, excessive hair loss, lack of information, misinformation, misconceptions

Related Factors (r/t)

Inability to ingest or digest food or absorb nutrients as a result of biological, psychological, or economic factors

Client Outcomes/Goals

- Progressively gains weight toward desired goal, maintains weight within normal range for height and age
- Recognizes factors contributing to underweight
- Identifies nutritional requirements
- Consumes adequate nourishment
- Remains free of signs of malnutrition

Suggested NIC Interventions

Eating disorders management, nutrition management, weight gain assistance

Nursing Interventions and Rationales

- Determine healthy body weight for age and height. Refer to dietitian for complete nutrition assessment if 10% less than healthy body weight or if rapidly losing body weight.
  Early diagnosis and a holistic team treatment of eating disorders are desirable.
- Compare usual food intake to food pyramid noting omitted food groups.
  Omission of entire food groups increases risk of deficiencies. Strict vegetarians may be at particular risk of vitamin B_{12} and iron deficiencies.
- Observe clients' ability to eat (time involved, motor skills, visual acuity, ability to swallow various textures of food).
  Poor vision was associated with lower protein and energy (calorie) intakes in home care clients independent of other medical conditions (Payette et al, 1995).
  (NOTE: If client is unable to feed self, see nursing interventions and rationales for **Self-care deficit: feeding.** If client has difficulty swallowing, see nursing interventions and rationales for **Impaired swallowing.**)
- If client lacks endurance, schedule rest periods before meals and open packages and cut up food for client.
  Nursing assistance with activities of daily living (ADLs) will conserve the client's energy for activities the client values. Clients who take longer than 1 hour to complete a meal may require assistance (Evans, 1992).
- Evaluate laboratory studies (serum albumin, serum total protein, serum ferritin, transferrin, hemoglobin, hematocrit, vitamins, and minerals).

An abnormal value in a single diagnostic study may have many possible causes. A prognostic nutritional value index using albumin, transferrin, triceps skinfold, and delayed hypersensitivity was useful in prediction complications after gastrointestinal surgery (Mullen, 1981).

- Be alert for food-nutrient-drug interactions.
  Individuals at greatest risk are those who are malnourished, consume alcohol, are receiving many drugs long term for chronic diseases, or take medications with meals through a feeding tube (Lutz, Prytulski, 1994).
- Assess for recent changes in physiological status that may interfere with nutrition.
  Diarrhea is a precaution for warfarin, possibly causing malabsorption of vitamin K (Black, 1994).
- Consider physiological conditions meriting increased nutriture.
  The Centers for Disease Control (CDC) recommends 0.4 mg folic acid for all women capable of becoming pregnant and 4 mg for women with a history of neural tube defect pregnancies (Centers for Disease Control, 1992).
- Observe client's relationship to food. Attempt to separate physical from physiological causes for difficulty eating.
  It may be difficult to tell if an eating problem is physical or psychological. Refusing to eat may be the only way the client can express some control and may also be a symptom of depression (Evans, 1992).
- Provide companionship at mealtime to encourage nutritional intake.
  Mealtime is usually a time for social interaction (Sanders, 1990).
- Consider six small, nutrient-dense meals to reduce feelings of fullness.
  Eating small frequent meals reduces the sensation of fullness and decreases the desire to vomit (Love, Seaton, 1991).
- Weigh client weekly using same conditions each time.
- Monitor food intake and specify amount of intake (25%, 50%). Consult with dietitian for actual calorie count.
- Monitor state of oral cavity (gums, tongue, mucosa, teeth).
- Provide good oral hygiene before and after meals.
  Good oral hygiene enhances appetite. In addition, the condition of the oral mucosa is critical to the ability to eat. The oral mucosa must be moist with adequate saliva production to facilitate and aid in food digestion (Evans, 1992).
- If a client has anorexia and a dry mouth from medication side effects, offer sips of fluid throughout the day.
  Although artificial salivas are available, more often than not clients prefer to sip water rather than use the more expensive products (Ganley, 1995).
- Determine relationship of eating and other events to onset of nausea, vomiting, diarrhea, or abdominal pain.
- Determine time of day when client's appetite is greatest; offer highest calorie meal at that time.
  Clients with liver disease often have the best appetites at breakfast.
- Offer small volumes of light liquids as an appetizer before meals.
  Small volumes of liquids up to 240 ml stimulate the gastrointestinal tract, which enhances peristalsis and motility (Rogers-Seidel, 1991).
- Administer antiemetics as ordered before meals.
  Antiemetics are more effective when given before nausea occurs.

- Prepare the client for meals—remove unsightly supplies and excretions, and avoid invasive procedures before meals.
  A pleasant environment helps to promote intake.
- If food odors trigger nausea, remove food covers before approaching client's bedside.
  Trapped odors diffuse into air away from client.
- If vomiting is a problem, discourage consumption of favorite foods.
  If clients consume favorite foods and then vomit, the client may later reject them.
- Work with client to develop a plan for increased activity.
  Immobility leads to negative nitrogen balance, which fosters anorexia.
- If client is anemic, offer foods rich in iron, vitamins B_{12} and C, and folic acid.
  Heme iron in meat, fish, and poultry is absorbed more readily than nonheme iron in plants. Vitamin C increases the solubility of iron. Vitamin B_{12} and folic acid are necessary for erythropoiesis.
- If client is lactose intolerant (genetically or following diarrhea), suggest cheeses (natural or processed) with less lactose than fluid milk. Encourage client to identify the extent of the intolerance.
  When lactose intake is limited to the equivalent of 240 ml of milk or less a day, symptoms are likely to be negligible and the use of lactose-digestive aids unnecessary (Suarez, Saviano, Levitt, 1995).
- For agitated clients, offer finger foods (e.g., sandwiches, fresh fruit) and fluids that can be ingested while pacing.
  Food can be consumed if clients are upright, even if they cannot be still.

Geriatric
- Assess components of bone health: calcium intake, vitamin D status, and regular exercise.
  Optimal calcium intake for all men and women more than 65 years of age is 1500 µg/day (NIH Consensus Development Panel, 1994). Vitamin D intakes of 5 µg (200 IU), the current RDA, affect bone loss from the spine and whole body similarly to an intake of 20 µg, but more than 5 µg is needed to limit bone loss from the femoral neck in healthy postmenopausal women at latitude 42° north, in Boston, Massachusetts (Dawson, Hughs, et al, 1995). An 80-year-old person requires almost twice as much time in the sun to produce the same amount of vitamin D as a 20-year-old does (Ryan, Eleazer, Egbert, 1995). A vitamin D supplement should be considered for institutionalized elderly people whose diets do not contain the 300 IU of vitamin D necessary to compensate for lack of sunshine exposure (Lips et al, 1987). Exercise not only increases bone density but also increases muscle mass and improves balance (Nelson et al, 1994).
- Instruct client in correct use of supplements.
  Milk-alkali syndrome has occurred in women ingesting 4 to 12 g of calcium carbonate daily (Beall, Scofield, 1995).
- Consider factors that interfere with nutrition (e.g., lack of transportation, inadequate income).
- Provide appropriate food textures for chewing ease. Insert dentures (if needed) before meals. Assess fit of dentures and refer for dental consultation if needed.
  The bony structure of the jaw changes over time and requires denture adjustment.
  (NOTE: If client is unable to feed self, see nursing interventions and rationales for **Self-care deficit: feeding.**

Home Care Interventions
- Identify appropriate methods for client to meet daily nutritional requirements (i.e., oral intake, TPN, tube feeding).

These data allow for individualized care planning by the nurse.

- Assess the home and economic situations for availability of products to meet nutritional requirements. Refer to medical social services as necessary for assistance with financial or other support in obtaining supplies.
- Assess client and family knowledge of dietary requirements and relationship to previous dietary patterns. Have client keep a weekly diary of nutritional intake.
  Completion of a diary increases client and family awareness of patterns and assists with nutrition planning.
- Include diary information in nutrition planning.
  This allows for plans that more accurately address the client's cultural need and other values surrounding nutrition.
- Encourage social interaction during mealtime, but do discourage chaotic activity or combining mealtimes with other activities.
  Chaotic activity may distract and distress clients, decreasing interest in eating.
- Respect wishes of terminally ill clients to refuse or limit nutrition or request unusual foods.
  The goal of hospice care is to provide comfort and dignity in the dying process. Deny requests for special foods only if they will hasten death or make it more uncomfortable.
  See care plan for **Swallowing, impaired.**
- If client receives nutrients other than orally, assess home for safety in preparation and administration of nutritional supplements (e.g., availability of appropriate storage or mixing space for total parenteral nutrition [TPN], availability of a responsible caregiver for tube feedings or TPN administration).
- Assess caregiver knowledge or ability to learn. Teach procedures as necessary, including central line IV administration and dressing changes.
  Some forms of nutritional intake require special conditions or procedures for administration.
- If caregiver is administering TPN, teach the importance of accuracy in administration and the need to monitor blood values. Draw and monitor blood values per physician order.
  The chemical composition of TPN is patient specific. Its route can impact the well-being of a client in a very short period of time if not administered correctly.

Client/Family Teaching

- Incorporate client and family input into care plan.
  Extrinsic motivators (such as pressure from others) may be less effective than intrinsic motivators (such as beliefs) in promoting healthy behaviors (Patterson et al, 1995).
- Help client and family identify areas in which change will make the greatest contribution to improved nutrition.
  Change is difficult, and multiple changes may be overwhelming.
- Build on strengths in client and family food habits. Adapt to their current practices.
  Accepting client and family preferences shows respect for their culture.
- Select appropriate teaching aids for the client's and family's background.
- Implement an instructional follow-up to answer questions.
- Suggest community resources as suitable (food sources, counseling, Meals on Wheels, senior centers).
- Teach client and family about home tube feeding or ways to manage home parenteral nutrition therapy.

REFERENCES   Alexander D, Ball MJ, Mann J: Nutrient intake and haematological status of vegetarians and age-sex matched omnivores, *Eur J Clin Nutr* 48:538, 1994.

Beall D, Scofield R: Milk-alkali syndrome associated with calcium carbonate consumption, *Medicine* 74:89, 1995.

Black J; Diarrhea, vitamin K and warfarin (letter), *Lancet* 344:1373, 1994.

Centers for Disease Control: Recommendations for the use of folic acid to reduce the number of cases of spina bifida and other neural tube defects, *MMWR* 41(No. RR-14):1, 1992.

Cook JD, Skikne BS, Baynes RD: Iron deficiency: the global perspective. In Hershko C et al, editor: *Progress in iron research,* New York, 1994, Plenum Press.

Dawson-Hughs B et al: Rates of bone loss in postmenopausal women randomly assigned to one of two dosages of vitamin D, *Am J Clin Nutr* 61:1140, 1995.

Evans NJ: Feeding. In Bulechek GM, McCloskey JC, editors: *Nursing interventions: essential nursing treatments,* ed 2, Philadelphia, 1992, WB Saunders.

Ganley BJ: Effective mouth care for head and neck radiation therapy patients, *Medsurg Nurs* 4:133, 1995.

Janelle KC, Barr SI: Nutrient intakes and eating behavior scores of vegetarian and nonvegetarian women, *J Am Diet Assoc* 95:180, 1995.

Khanum S, Ashworth A, Huttly SRA: Controlled trial of three approaches to the treatment of severe malnutrition, *Lancet* 344:1728, 1994.

Lips P et al: Determinants of vitamin D status in patients with hip fracture and in elderly control subjects, *Am J Clin Nutr* 46:1005, 1987.

Love CC, Seaton H: Eating disorders: highlights of nursing assessment and therapeutics, *Nurs Clin North Am* 26:677, 1991.

Lutz CA, Prytulski KR: *Nutrition and diet therapy,* Philadelphia, 1994, FA Davis.

Mullen JL: Consequences of malnutrition in the surgical patient, *Surg Clin North Am* 61:465, 1981.

Nelson ME et al: Effects of high-intensity strength training on multiple risk factors for osteoporotic fractures, *JAMA* 272:1909, 1994.

NIH Consensus Development Panel: Optimal calcium intake, *JAMA* 272:1942, 1994.

Patterson RE et al: Diet-cancer related beliefs, knowledge, norms, and their relationship to healthful diets, *J Nutr Educ* 27:86, 1995.

Payette H et al: Predictors of dietary intake in a functionally dependent elderly population in the community, *Am J Public Health* 85:677-683, 1995.

Rogers-Seidel: *Geriatric nursing care plans,* St Louis, 1991, Mosby.

Ryan C, Eleazer P, Egbert J: Vitamin D in the elderly, *Nutr Today* 30:228, 1995.

Sanders HN: Feeding dependent eaters among geriatric patients, *J Nurs Elderly*, 9:69, 1990.

Small SP, Best DG, Hustins KA: Energy and nutrient intakes of independently-living elderly women, *Can J Nurs Res* 26:71, 1994.

Suarez FL, Savaiano DA, Levitt MD: A comparison of symptoms after consumption of mild or lactose-hydrolyzed milk by people with self-reported severe lactose intolerance, *N Engl J Med* 333:1, 1995.

United States Preventive Services Task Force: Routine iron supplementation during pregnancy policy statement, *JAMA* 270:2846, 1993.

United States Preventive Services Task Force: Routine iron supplementation during pregnancy review article, *JAMA* 270:2848, 1993.

Altered nutrition: more than body requirements

Carroll A. Lutz

Definition   The state in which an individual experiences an intake of nutrients that exceeds metabolic needs

Defining Characteristics

Weight 10% more than ideal for height and frame *(critical),* weight 20% more than ideal for height and frame, triceps skinfold greater than 15 mm in men or 25 mm in women, sedentary activity level, reported or observed dysfunctional eating pattern, pairing of food with other activities, concentration of food intake at the end of day, eating in response to external cues such as time of day or social situation, eating in response to internal cues other than hunger (e.g., anxiety)

Related Factors (r/t)

Excessive intake in relation to metabolic need

Client Outcomes/Goals

- States factors contributing to weight gain
- Identifies behaviors that remain under client's control
- Claims ownership for current eating patterns
- Designs dietary modifications to meet individual long-term goal of weight control using principles of variety, balance, and moderation
- Accomplishes the desired weight loss over a reasonable length of time (1 to 2 lb per week)
- Incorporates appropriate activities requiring energy expenditure into daily life
- Uses sound scientific sources to evaluate need for nutritional supplements

Suggested NIC Interventions

Eating disorders management, nutrition management, weight reduction assistance

Nursing Interventions and Rationales

- Obtain thorough history.
  The most appropriate clients for weight management are adults with no major health problems requiring diet therapy. If a client has a medical condition requiring diet therapy, the assistance of a dietitian may be required (Crist, 1992).
- Evaluate client's psychological status in relation to weight control.
  Children have been included in weight management programs but their growth factor has not, potentially resulting in future growth and health problems. These risks may require the direct attention of dietitians and physicians.
- Determine client's knowledge of a nutritional diet and need for supplements.
  This information is useful in developing an individualized teaching plan based on client's current status.
- Calculate body mass index (BMI) (weight in kilograms divided by height in square meters).
  A normal is 20 to 25 kg/m².
- Compute waist:hip ratio.
  A waist:hip ratio of greater than 0.85 in women and greater than 1 in men indicates increased risk of problems related to obesity (Lutz, Przutulski, 1997).
- Define client's healthy body weight with client, considering experimental and cultural factors.
  Being overweight has been viewed as an individual problem, and treatment has been oriented toward an individual victim-blame model with little consideration of personal context or the influence of cultural values on behavior (Allan, 1994).
- Determine whether client's motivation to lose weight is for appearance or health.
  Female peripheral fat pattern (gynecoid), predominant in most women, is associated with virtually no health impairments (Allan, 1994).
- Observe for behaviors indicating a nutritional intake that is more than body requirements.
  Such observations help paint a clear picture of the client's dietary habits.
- Suggest client keep a diary of food intake and circumstances surrounding its consumption (methods of preparation, duration of meal, social situation, overall mood, activities accompanying consumption).

Self-monitoring helps the client assess adherence to self-determined performance criteria and progress toward desired goals. Self-monitoring serves an important role in the maintenance of internal standards of behavior (Fleury, 1991).

- Adopt a weight loss plan incorporating client's culture and preferences.
  Dramatic weight loss was achieved in Hawaii with a culturally appropriate methodology (Shintani, et al, 1991).
- Advise client to measure food periodically.
  Measuring food makes client aware of normal portion sizes. "Eye-balling" can be extremely inaccurate.
- Review clients' current exercise level. Design a long term exercise program with client and primary health-care provider.
  A health risk appraisal should be performed on all previously sedentary individuals who are beginning a program of exercise (Grubbs, 1993).
- Establish reasonable goal for client's body weight and rate of weight loss (1 to 2 lb per week).
  Height and weight tables have been criticized because they are based on middle-class white men (Allan, 1994).
- Initiate a client contract that involves reinforcing and rewarding the attainment of progressive goals and maintenance of desired weight.
  Patient contracts provide a unique opportunity for patients to learn to analyze their behavior in relationship to the environment and to choose behavioral strategies that will facilitate learning. A series of written contracts provides a history of progress toward desired behaviors (Boehm, 1992).
- Weigh client twice a week using same conditions.
  It is important for the progress of most clients to have the tangible reward that the scale shows. Monitoring twice a week keeps clients on their program by not allowing them to slip into a pattern of eating uncontrollably for a couple of days and then fasting to lose weight (Crist, 1992).
- Instruct client regarding adequate nutritional intake. A total plan permits occasional treats.
  Permanent life-style changes must occur for weight lost to be long lasting. Eliminating all treats is not practical or easily sustained.
- Familiarize client with the following behavior modification techniques (Lutz, Przutulski, 1994):
  - Envision yourself making healthy choices (e.g., a fresh apple rather than apple pie, frozen yogurt rather than ice cream).
  - Eat only in a specific location and position (e.g., sitting at a dining table).
  - Plan food intake for the day.
  - Rearrange schedule to avoid inappropriate eating.
  - Keep a list of activities on refrigerator to avoid boredom.
  - At parties, sit away from snack foods and substitute low-calorie drinks for alcohol.
  - At restaurants, decide before going what to order (side salad, low-fat dressing, low-fat milk, small hamburger [at fast food restaurants]).
  - Avoid other activities (e.g., reading, television) while eating.
  - Drink a glass of water before eating, and drink sips of water between bites of food.
  - Use a small plate.
  - Swallow a bite of food before putting more food on the fork or spoon.
  - Lay fork on plate between bites.

- Pause for a minute during the meal; attempt to increase the pauses.
- Strive to be the last person at the table to finish eating.
- Keep a supply of low-calorie snacks available (e.g., fresh carrots, celery, radishes, peppers, diet soda).
- Plan for treats in advance by saving a portion of calories for a weekly treat.
- Exercise portion control—measure food and avoid second helpings.

- A recommended exercise program involves 45 minutes of exercise five times per week. *As exercise time increases beyond 30 minutes, there is an increased reliance on fat stores for energy (Grubbs, 1993).*
- Assess for use of nonprescription diet aids.
  Ingestion of an herbal supplement containing mahuang, the main plant source of ephedrine, for weight loss caused mania in a client with no history of psychiatric illness (Capwell, 1995). Clinicians should be aware that ostensibly harmless herbal remedies may have potent ingredients that are not subjected to the same scrutiny the Food and Drug Administration (FDA) devotes to prescription drugs (Woolf et al, 1994).
- Observe overuse of particular nutrients.
  Daily digestion of 500 ml of tonic water containing 40 mg of quinine hydrochloride caused photosensitivity. Other conditions associated with tonic water are disseminated intravascular coagulation, recurrent dermatitis, fixed drug eruption, and toxic epidermal necrolysis (Wagner et al, 1994).

Geriatric

- Assess fluid intake.
  The thirst sensation becomes dulled in the elderly.
- Note socioeconomic factors that influence food choices (e.g., intake of carbohydrates because they are less expensive); plan a menu for clients on a fixed income. *Food choices in today's food markets are greatly enhanced, even for those on limited budgets (Love, Seaton, 1991).*
- Suggest a variety of seasonings.
  Sensitivity to sweet and salty tastes are diminished in the elderly.
- Encourage social involvement in activities other than eating.
  Energy needs decrease an estimated 5% per decade after the age of 40.
- Recommend changes judiciously.
  A weight reduction program should be pursued if needed to treat current problems, such as diabetes mellitus or hypertension, but not to prevent new ones (Feldman, 1988).

Home Care Interventions

- Assess client support system. Determine whether significant others will support client efforts at weight loss.
  A positive social support system is associated with increased compliance (Warren, 1992).
- Review client medications. Identify medications that cause fluid retention and stimulants (prescribed or over the counter). Instruct client to review medications with physician before making changes and to avoid stimulants for quick weight loss. *The need for tangible progress in weight loss can precipitate dangerous choices in health practices.*
- Teach client to read food labels when shopping.
  Labels provide additional knowledge that clients can use to make healthy choices.
- Assist client and family with applying and integrating knowledge gained from the mentioned nursing interventions into daily patterns.
  Monitoring and adapting home patterns decreases vulnerability from negative patterns and allows new, healthier patterns to become established.

Client/Family Teaching

- Provide client and family with information regarding the nutritional plan.
  Because the purpose of the plan is to make a permanent change in weight management, decisions regarding treatment plans should be left up to the client and family (Crist, 1992).
- Inform client of health risks associated with obesity.
  Acknowledgment of risks helps the client to verbalize their overall impact.
- Guide client toward changes that will make a major impact on health.
  Even modest weight loss contributes to diabetes and hypertension control.
- Inform client and family of disadvantages of trying to lose weight by dieting only.
  The resting metabolic rate decreases as much as 45% with extreme calorie restriction. The decrease persists after the diet period had ended, leading to the "yo-yo effect." Using only a reduced-calorie diet, as much as 25% of the weight lost can be lean body mass rather than fat. Resting energy expenditure is positively related to lean body mass (Grubbs, 1993).
- Teach the importance of exercise in a weight control program.
  A physically conditioned person uses more fat for energy at rest and during exercise than a sedentary person does (Grubbs, 1993).
- Teach stress-reduction techniques as alternatives to eating.
  Client needs healthy behaviors to substitute for unhealthy behaviors.

REFERENCES   Allan JD: A biomedical and feminist perspective on women's experiences with weight management, *West J Nurs Res* 16:524, 1994.

Boehm S: Patient contracting. In Bulechek GM, McCloskey JC, editors: *Nursing interventions: essential nursing treatments,* ed 2, Philadelphia, 1992, WB Saunders.

Capwell R: Ephedrine-induced mania from a herbal diet supplement (letter), *Am J Psychiatry* 152:647, 1995.

Crist J: Weight management. In Bulechek GM, McCloskey JC, editors: *Nursing interventions: essential nursing treatments,* ed 2, Philadelphia, 1992, WB Saunders.

Feldman EB: *Essentials of clinical nutrition,* Philadelphia, 1988, FA Davis.

Fleury J: Empowering potential: a theory of wellness motivation, *Nurs Res* 40:288, 1991.

Grubbs L: The critical role of exercise in weight control, *Nurse Practitioner* 18:20, 1993.

Love C, Seaton H: Eating disorders: highlights of nursing assessment and therapeutics, *Nurs Clin North Am* 26:677, 1991.

Lutz CA, Przutulski KR: *Nutrition and diet therapy,* Philadelphia, 1994, FA Davis.

Lutz CA, Przutulski KR: *Nutrition and diet therapy,* ed 2, Philadelphia, 1997, FA Davis (In press).

Powers MI et al: All about drugs: adverse effects to watch for, *Am J Nurs* 95:32, 1995.

Powers MI et al: All about drugs: medication administration: how safe is your patient? *Am J Nurs* 95:44, 1995.

Shintani TT et al: Obesity and cardiovascular risk intervention through the ad libitum feeding of traditional Hawaiian diet, *Am J Clin Nutr* 53:1647, 1991.

Wagner G et al: "I'll have mine with a warm twist of lemon." Quinine photosensitivity from excessive intake of tonic water (letter), *Br J Dermatol* 131:734, 1994.

Warren JJ: Ethical concerns about noncompliance in the chronically ill patient, *Prog Cardiovasc Nurs* 7:10, 1992.

Woolf G et al: Acute hepatitis associated with the Chinese herbal product Jin Bu Huan, *Ann Intern Med* 121:729, 1994.

Risk for altered nutrition: more than body requirements

J. Keith Hampton and Gail B. Ladwig, revised by Carroll A. Lutz

Definition

The state in which an individual is at risk of experiencing an intake of nutrients that exceeds metabolic needs.

Risk Factors

Reported or observed obesity in one or both parents, rapid transition across growth percentiles in infants or children, reported use of solid food as major food source before 5 months of age, observed use of food as reward or comfort measure, reported or observed higher baseline weight at beginning of each pregnancy, dysfunctional eating patterns, pairing of food with other activities, concentration of food intake at end of day, eating in response to external cues such as time of day or social situation, eating in response to internal cues other than hunger (e.g., anxiety)

Related Factors (r/t)

See Risk Factors

Client Outcomes/Goals

- Explains concept of a balanced diet
- Compares current eating pattern to a recommended healthy pattern
- Designs dietary modifications to meet individual long-term goal of weight control using principles of variety, balance, and moderation
- Identifies role of exercise in weight control
- Uses sound scientific sources to evaluate need for nutritional supplements

Suggested NIC Interventions

Nutrition management, weight management

Nursing Interventions and Rationales

- See care plan for **Altered nutrition: more than body requirements**
- Observe for presence of risk factors.
- Assess nutritional intake, including the use of supplements.
  Clients may not volunteer information on supplements because they do not consider the supplements pertinent.
- Determine client's knowledge of nutrition.
- Inform client of the health risks associated with overconsumption of nutrients.
  Fetal abnormalities have been related to vitamin A intake. Women who are (or who might become) pregnant should avoid consuming daily supplements containing more than 8000 IU of vitamin A and should consume liver and liver products only in moderation because they contain large amounts of vitamin A (Oakley, Erickson, 1995). The hazard is related to preformed vitamin A in animal product not the provitamin A, carotene, in plants. A client who consumed more than 10 times the RDA for vitamin A for 6 years developed fatal liver toxicity (Kowalski, 1994).
- Discuss wise discontinuation of supplements.
  Rebound scurvy has occurred in clients who suddenly discontinued megadoses (10 times the Recommended Daily Allowance [RDA]) of vitamin C.
- Establish a plan with the client, using techniques in **Altered nutrition: more than body requirements**
  Intervening when client is at risk allows relatively small changes in life-style to be effective.

Geriatric

- Plan to decrease calories in the least disturbing way (e.g., decrease fat in meals rather than eliminating the after-dinner cookie that client has had for years).

- Give client credit for making some wise choices that have allowed them to live to an advanced age.
  Studies show nutrition practices are related to health in certain ways. They are not predictive for individuals.
- Encourage varying food suppliers in the unlikely event of contamination.
  Hypervitaminosis D was caused by inadvertent overfortification of milk by a home-delivery dairy. There were two fatalities—a 72- and an 86-year-old (Blank et al, 1995).

Home Care Interventions

See **Altered nutrition: more than body requirements**

Client/Family Teaching

- Analyze client's nutritional pattern and suggest lower calorie substitutes for high-calorie dishes.
  Ice milk contains 185 cal per cup as compared to 270 cal per cup in ice cream. Low-calorie Italian dressing has 5 cal per tablespoon compared to 80 cal per tablespoon for the regular dressing.
- Demonstrate the use of food labels to make healthy choices. Have the client and family focus on serving sizes, total fat, and simple carbohydrates.
  Standardized food labels in bold type simplify the information search. Some serving sizes listed on labels are unusually small. Fats and sugars contribute least to a healthy diet and most to excessive calorie intake.

REFERENCES   Blank S et al: An outbreak of hypervitaminosis D associated with the overfortification of milk from a home-delivery dairy, *Am J Public Health* 85:656, 1995.

Kowalski T et al: Vitamin A hepatotoxicity: a cautionary note regarding 25,000 IU supplements, *Am J Med* 97:523, 1994.

Lutz CA, Przutulski KR: *Nutrition and diet therapy,* ed 2, Philadelphia, 1997, FA Davis (In Press).

Oakley GP, Erickson JD: Vitamin A and birth defects, *N Engl J Med* 333:1414, 1995.

Small SP, Best DG, Hustins KA: Energy and nutrient intakes of independently-living, elderly women, *Can J Nurs Res* 26:71, 1994.

Altered oral mucous membranes

Diane Krasner and Betty J. Ackley

Definition

The state in which an individual experiences disruptions in the tissue layers of the oral cavity

Defining Characteristics

Oral pain or discomfort, coated tongue, xerostoma (dry mouth), stomatitis, oral lesions or ulcers, lack of or decreased salivation, leukoplakia, edema, hyperemia, oral plaques, desquamation, vesicles, hemorrhagic gingivitis, carious teeth, halitosis

Related Factors (r/t)

Pathological conditions of oral cavity (irradiation to head or neck), dehydration, trauma (e.g., chemical: acidic foods, drugs, tobacco, noxious agents, alcohol; mechanical: ill-fitting dentures, braces, endotracheal or nasogastric tubes); surgery in oral cavity; nothing by mouth (NPO) for more than 24 hours, ineffective oral hygiene, mouth breathing, malnutrition, infection, lack of or decreased salivation, medication

Client Outcomes/Goals

- Maintains intact, moist, oral mucous membranes that are free of ulceration and debris
- Describes or demonstrates measures to regain or maintain intact oral mucous membranes
- Maintains adequate oral intake

Suggested NIC Interventions

Oral health restoration

Nursing Interventions and Rationales

- Inspect oral cavity at least once daily and note any discoloration, lesions, edema, bleeding, exudate, or dryness. Refer to a physician or specialist as appropriate. *Systematic inspection can identify impending problems (Bhaskar, Lilly, Pratt, 1990).*
- Assess for mechanical agents such as ill-fitting dentures or chemical agents such as frequent exposure to tobacco that could cause or increase trauma to oral mucous membranes. *Irritative and causative agents for stomatitis should be eliminated (Rhodes, McDaniel, Johnson, 1995).*
- Monitor client's nutritional and fluid status to determine if adequate. *Dehydration and malnutrition predispose clients to altered oral mucous membranes.*
- Determine client's mental status; if client is unable to care for self, oral hygiene must be provided by nursing personnel. The nursing diagnosis **Bathing/hygiene self-care deficit** is then also applicable.
- Determine client's usual method of oral care and address any concerns regarding oral hygiene. *Whenever possible, build on client's existing knowledge base and current practices to develop an individualized plan of care.*
- If client has no bleeding disorders and is able to swallow, encourage client to brush teeth with a soft toothbrush using a fluoride-containing toothpaste after every meal and floss teeth daily. *The toothbrush is the most important tool for oral care; brushing the teeth is the most effective method for reducing plaque and controlling periodontal disease (Armstrong, 1994; Buglass, 1995).*
- If platelet numbers are decreased or client is unable to swallow, use moistened toothettes for oral care. Avoid using hydrogen peroxide. *A toothbrush can cause soft-tissue injury and bleeding in clients with low numbers of platelets (Armstrong, 1994). Hydrogen peroxide can damage oral mucosa and is extremely foul tasting to clients (Tombes, Gallucci, 1993; Winslow, 1994).*
- Keep inside of mouth moist with frequent sips of water and salt water rinses (½ tsp salt in 8 oz of warm water) or artificial saliva. *Moisture promotes the cleansing effect of saliva and helps avert mucosal drying, which can result in erosions, fissures, or lesions (Rhodes, McDaniel, Johnson, 1995). Sodium chloride rinses have been shown to be effective in prevention and treatment of stomatitis (Feber, 1994).*
- Keep lips well lubricated.
- For clients with stomatitis, increase frequency of oral care up to every hour while awake if necessary. *Increasing the frequency of oral care has been shown to be effective in decreasing stomatitis (Armstrong, 1994).*
- Provide scrupulous oral care to critically ill clients.

Cultures of the teeth of critically ill clients have yielded significant bacterial colonization, which can cause nosocomial pneumonia (Scannapieco, Stewart, Mylotte, 1992).

- If mouth is severely inflamed and it is painful to swallow, contact the physician for a topical anesthetic agent or analgesic order. Modification of oral intake (e.g., soft diet, liquid diet) may also be necessary to prevent friction trauma. The nursing diagnosis **Altered nutrition: less than body requirements** may apply.
- If whitish plaques are present in the mouth or on the tongue and can be rubbed off readily with gauze, leaving a red base that bleeds, suspect a fungal infection and contact the physician for follow-up.
  Oral candidiasis (moniliasis) is extremely common secondary to antibiotic therapy, steroid therapy, HIV infection, diabetes, or immunosuppressive drugs and should be treated with oral or systemic antifungal agents (Bhaskar, Lilly, Pratt, 1990; Sauer, 1991).
- If client is unable to swallow, keep suction nearby when providing oral care.

Geriatric
- Carefully observe oral cavity and lips for abnormal lesions.
  Malignant lesions are more common in the elderly, especially if there is a history of smoking or alcohol use (Sauer, 1991).
- Ensure that dentures are removed and cleaned, preferably after every meal and before bedtime.
  Dentures left in the mouth at night impede circulation to the palate and predispose the client to oral lesions.

Home Care Interventions

- If dryness is a side effect of clients' medications, instruct them in the use of artificial lubricants.
- Monitor sodium intake in hypertensive clients (Humphrey, 1994). Use alternatives to sodium chloride rinses.
  Frequent sodium chloride rinses place the client at risk for exacerbation of hypertension.
- Instruct client to avoid alcohol- or hydrogen peroxide-based commercial products for mouth care and other irritants to the oral cavity (e.g., tobacco, spicy foods).
  Oral irritants can further damage the oral mucosa and increase the client's discomfort.
- Instruct client in ways to soothe the oral cavity (e.g., cool beverages, popsicles, viscous lidocaine) (Jaffe, Roth, 1993).
- If client often breathes by mouth, add humidity to room unless contraindicated.
- If necessary, refer for home health aide services to support family in oral care and observation of the oral cavity.

Client/Family Teaching

- Teach how to inspect the oral cavity and monitor for signs and symptoms of infection, complications, and healing.
- Teach how to implement a personal plan of oral hygiene including a schedule of care.
  Encouragement and reinforcement of oral care are important to oral outcomes (Armstrong, 1994).

REFERENCES   Armstrong TS: Stomatitis in the bone marrow transplant patient, *Cancer Nurs* 17:403, 1994.
Bhaskar SN, Lilly GE, Pratt LW: A practical, high-yield mouth exam, *Patient Care* 24:53, 1990.
Buglass EA: Oral hygiene, *British Journal of Nurs* 4:516, 1995.
Day R: Mouth care in an intensive care unit: a review, *Intensive Crit Care Nurs* 9:246, 1993.
Dose AM: The symptom experience of mucositis, stomatitis, and xerostomia, *Semin Oncol Nurs* 11:248, 1995.

Feber T: Mouth care for patients receiving oral irradiation, *Prof Nurse* 10:666, 1994.

Hatton-Smith CK: A last bastion of ritualized practice? A review of nurses' knowledge of oral healthcare, *Prof Nurse* 9:304, 1994.

Humphrey C, *Home care nursing handbook,* ed 2, Maryland, 1994, Aspen.

Jaffe MS, Skidmore-Roth, L: *Home health care nursing care plans,* ed 2, St Louis, 1993, Mosby.

Rhodes VA, McDaniel RW, Johnson MH: Patient education: self care guide, *Semin Oncol Nurs* 11:298, 1995.

Sauer GC: *Manual of skin diseases,* ed 6, Philadelphia, 1991, JB Lippincott.

Scannapieco FA, Stewart EM, Mylotte JM: Colonization of dental plaque by respiratory pathogens in medical intensive care patients, *Crit Care Med* 20:740, 1992.

Tombes MB, Gallucci B: The effects of hydrogen peroxide rinses on the normal oral mucosa, *Nurs Res* 42:332, 1993.

Treloar DM, Stechmiller JK: Use of a clinical assessment tool for orally intubated patients, *Am J Crit Care* 4:355, 1995.

Winslow EH: Don't use H_2O_2 for oral care, *Am J Nurs* March, 1994, p. 19.

Pain

Christine L. Pasero and Margo McCaffery

Definition Pain is whatever the experiencing persons say it is, existing whenever they say it does (McCaffery, 1968); a state in which an individual experiences and reports the presence of severe discomfort or an uncomfortable sensation (NANDA)

Defining Characteristics

Subjective Pain is always subjective and cannot be proved or disproved. A client's report of pain is the most reliable indicator of pain (Acute Pain Management Guideline Panel, 1992). A client with cognitive ability who can speak or point should use a pain rating scale (e.g., 0 to 10) to identify the current level of pain (self-report) and determine a pain rating goal.

Objective Expressions of pain are extremely variable and cannot be used in lieu of self-report. Neither behavior nor vital signs can substitute for the client's self-report (McCaffery, Ferrell, 1991; McCaffery, Ferrell, 1992). Observable responses to pain are helpful in its assessment, especially in clients who cannot or will not use a self-report pain rating scale. Observable responses may be loss of appetite and inability to deep breathe, ambulate, sleep, or perform activities of daily living. Clients may show guarding, self-protective behavior, self-focusing or narrowed focus, distraction behavior ranging from crying to laughing, and muscle tension or rigidity. In sudden and severe pain, autonomic responses such as diaphoresis, blood pressure and pulse changes, pupillary dilation, or increases or decreases in respiratory rate and depth may be present.

Related Factors (r/t)

Actual or potential tissue damage (biological, chemical, physical)

Client Outcomes/Goals

- Uses a pain rating scale to identify current level of pain and determine a pain rating goal (if client has cognitive abilities)
- Describes how unrelieved pain will be managed
- Reports that pain management regimen relieves pain to a satisfactory level with minimal or manageable side effects
- Performs activities of recovery with a reported acceptable level of pain
- States an ability to obtain sufficient amounts of rest and sleep
- Describes a nonpharmacological method that can be used to control pain

Suggested NIC Interventions

Analgesic administration, conscious sedation, pain management, patient-controlled analgesia (PCA) assistance

Nursing Interventions and Rationales

- Determine whether clients are experiencing pain at the time of the initial interview. If they are, intervene at that time to provide pain relief.
  The intensity of pain and discomfort should be assessed and documented during the initial evaluation of the patient (American Pain Society, 1995).
- Ask clients to describe past experiences with pain and effectiveness of methods used to manage pain, including experiences with side effects, typical coping responses, and how they express pain.
  A number of concerns (barriers) may affect patients' willingness to report pain and use analgesics (Ward et al, 1993).
- Describe adverse effects of unrelieved pain.
  Numerous pathophysiological and psychological morbidity factors may be associated with pain (Puntillo, Weiss, 1994).
- Tell client to report pain location, intensity using a pain rating scale, and quality when experiencing pain.
  The intensity of pain and discomfort should be assessed and documented after any known pain-producing procedure, with each new report of pain, and at regular intervals (American Pain Society, 1995).
- Explore the need for both opioid (narcotic) and nonopioid analgesics.
- Determine client's current medication use.
  To aid in planning pain treatment, obtain a medication history (Acute Pain Management Guideline Panel, 1992).
- Obtain a prescription to administer a nonsteroidal antiinflammatory drug (NSAID), unless contraindicated, on an around-the-clock schedule.
  NSAIDs act mainly in the periphery to inhibit the initiation of pain signals (Dahl, Kehlet, 1991).
- Obtain a prescription to administer opioid analgesia if indicated, orally or intravenously (IV), not intramuscularly, and using a preventive approach to keep pain at or below an acceptable level. Provide IV PCA or other routes of administration when appropriate and available. Because of its fast onset, the IV route is used for control of moderate to severe pain.
  When pain persists or increases, add an opioid to the NSAID. Utilize the simplest analgesic dosage schedules and least invasive pain management modalities first. Avoid the intramuscular route because of unreliable absorption, pain, and inconvenience. Give analgesia around-the-clock (Jacox et al, 1994).
- Discuss client's fears of undertreated pain, overdose, and addiction.
  A number of concerns may affect patients' willingness to report pain and use opioid analgesics (Ward et al, 1993). Because of the many misconceptions regarding pain and its treatment, education about the ability to control pain effectively and correction of myths about the use of opioids should be included as part of the treatment play (Jacox et al, 1994). Addiction is extremely unlikely after clients use opioids for acute pain (Acute Pain Management Guideline Panel, 1992).
- When opioids are administered, assess pain intensity, sedation, and respiratory status at regular intervals.

Opioids may cause respiratory depression because they reduce the responsiveness of carbon dioxide chemoreceptors located in the respiratory centers of the brain. Because even more opioid is required to produce respiratory depression than is required to produce sedation, patients with clinically significant respiratory depression are usually also sedated (Pasero, McCaffery, 1994).

- Review client's flow sheet and medication records to determine overall degree of pain relief, side effects, and analgesic requirements during the past 24 hours.
Systematic tracking of pain appears to be an important factor in improving pain management (Faries et al, 1991).

- Administer supplemental opioid doses as needed to keep pain ratings at or below an acceptable level.
A prn order for a supplementary opioid dose between regular doses is an essential backup (American Pain Society, 1992).

- Obtain prescriptions to increase or decrease opioid doses as needed; base prescriptions on client's report of pain severity and response to the previous dose in terms of relief, side effects, and ability to perform the activities of recovery.
Increase or decrease the dose of opioid based on assessment of the patient's response. Patients' responses and therefore their requirements vary widely, so it is less important to focus on the amount given than on the response (Pasero, McCaffery, 1994).

- Obtain a prescription to change to oral analgesic; use an equianalgesic chart to determine initial dose. See Appendix D for an equianalgesic chart.
The oral route is preferred because it is the most convenient and cost-effective (Jacox et al, 1994).

- In addition to use of analgesics, support client's use of nonpharmacological methods to control pain, such as distraction, imagery, relaxation, massage, and heat and cold application.
Cognitive-behavioral strategies can restore the clients' sense of self-control, personal efficacy, and active participation in own care (Jacox et al, 1994).

- Plan care activities around periods of greatest comfort whenever possible.
Pain diminishes activity (Jacox et al, 1994).

- Ask client to describe appetite, bowel elimination, and ability to rest and sleep. Administer medications and treatments to improve these functions.
Because there is great individual variation in the development of opioid-induced side effects, they should be monitored and, if their development is inevitable, prophylactically treated (Jacox et al, 1994).

Geriatric

- Always take elderly clients' reports of pain seriously and ensure that the pain is relieved.
In spite of what many professionals and, clients believe, pain is not an expected part of normal aging.

- When assessing pain, speak clearly, slowly, and loudly enough for client to hear; repeat information as needed. Be sure client can see well enough to read pain scale and written materials.

- Handle client's body gently. Allow client to move at own speed.

- Watch for side effects when using NSAIDs.

- Elderly clients are at increased risk for gastric and renal toxicity from NSAIDs (Griffin et al, 1991; Acute Pain Management Guideline Panel, 1992). Use NSAIDs with low side-effect profiles (American Pain Society, 1992; Acute Pain Management Guideline Panel, 1992), such as choline and magnesium salicylates (Trilisate), diflunisal (Dolobid), and acetaminophen.

- Use opioids with caution in elderly clients.
  Elderly clients are more sensitive to the analgesic effects of opioid drugs because they experience a higher peak effect and a longer duration of pain relief. Reduce the initial opioid dose by 25% to 50% if the client is frail and debilitated; then increase the dose if safe and necessary (Acute Pain Management Guideline Panel, 1992).

Home Care Interventions

- Review with client and caregivers the cause(s) of pain and the medical regimen specific to the cause. Assess client knowledge and teach disease process as necessary.
  Compliance with the medical regimen for diagnoses involving pain improves the likelihood of successful management (Humphrey, 1994).
- Develop a *full* medication profile including medications prescribed by all physicians and all over-the-counter medications. Assess for drug interactions. Instruct client to refrain from mixing medications without physician approval.
  Pain medications may significantly impact or be impacted by other medications and may cause severe side effects. Some combination of drugs are specifically contraindicated (Jacox et al, 1994).
- Assess client and family knowledge of side effects and safety precautions associated with pain medications (e.g., not driving while using opiates).
  Some terminally ill clients may be receiving high doses of pain medication but still try to be mobile or perform complex tasks.
- If administering medication using highly technological methods, assess home for necessary resources (e.g., electricity), and ensure there will be responsible caregivers to assist client with administration.
  Some routes of medication administration require special conditions and procedures to be safe and accurate.
- Assess knowledge base of client and family for highly technological medication administration. Teach as necessary.
  Appropriate instruction in the home increases the accuracy and safety of medication administration.

Client/Family Teaching

NOTE: To avoid the negative connotations associated with words "drugs" or "narcotics," use the words "pain medicine" when teaching clients.

- Provide written materials on pain control such as the Agency for Health Care Policy and Research (AHCPR) pamphlet, *Pain Control: Patient Guide.*
- Discuss the various discomforts encompassed by the word "pain," and ask client to give examples of previously experienced pain. Explain pain assessment process and purpose of the pain rating scale.
- Teach client to use the pain rating scale to rate intensity of past or current pain. Ask clients to set a pain relief goal by selecting a pain level on the rating scale. If pain is above this level, they should take action that decreases pain or notify a member of the health care team.
- Demonstrate medication administration and use of supplies and equipment. If PCA is ordered, determine client's ability to press appropriate button.
- Reinforce importance of taking pain medications to keep pain under control.
- Reinforce that taking opioids for pain relief is not addiction and that addiction is very unlikely to occur.

- Demonstrate use of appropriate nonpharmacological approaches for controlling pain such as distraction techniques, relaxation breathing, visualization, rocking, stroking, music, and television.

REFERENCES   Acute Pain Management Guideline Panel: *Acute pain management operative or medical procedures and trauma: clinical practice guideline,* Rockville, Md, Feb 1992. Agency for Health Care Policy and Research Pub No 92-0032, Public Health Service, US Department of Health and Human Services.

American Pain Society: *Principles of analgesic use in the treatment of acute pain and cancer pain,* ed 3, Skokie, Ill, 1992, The Society.

American Pain Society Quality of Care Committee: Quality improvement guidelines for the treatment of acute pain and cancer pain, *JAMA* 274:1874, 1995.

Dahl JB, Kehlet H: Non-steroidal anti-inflammatory drugs: rationale for use in severe postoperative pain, *Br J Anaesthesia* 66:703, 1991.

Faries JE et al: Systematic pain records and their impact on pain control, *Cancer Nurs* 14:306, 1991.

Ferrell BR: Pain management in elderly people, *J Am Geriatr Soc* 39:64, 1991.

Griffin MR et al: Nonsteroidal anti-inflammatory drug use and increased risk for peptic ulcer disease in elderly persons, *Annals Internal Med* 114:257, 1991.

Humphrey C: *Home care nursing handbook,* ed 2, Gaithersburg, Maryland, 1994, Aspen.

Jacox A et al: *Management of cancer pain: clinical practice guideline no 9,* Rockville, Md, March 1994, Agency for Health Care Policy and Research Pub No 94-0592 US Department of Health and Human Services, Public Health Service.

McCaffery M: *Nursing practice theories related to cognition, bodily pain and man-environment interactions,* Los Angeles, 1968, University of California at Los Angeles Students' Store.

McCaffery M, Ferrell BR: How would you respond to these patients in pain? *Nursing 91* 21:34, 1991.

McCaffery M, Ferrell BR: How vital are vital signs?, *Nursing 92* 22:42, 1992.

McCaffery M: Analgesics: mapping out pain relief *Nursing 96* 26:41, 1996.

Pasero C, McCaffery M: Avoiding opioid-induced respiratory depression, *AJN* 94:25, 1994.

Puntillo K, Weiss SJ: Pain: its mediators and associated morbidity in critically ill cardiovascular surgical patients, *Nurs Res* 43:31, 1994.

Ward S et al: Patient-related barriers to management of cancer pain, *Pain* 52:319, 1993.

Chronic pain

Christine L. Pasero and Margo McCaffery

Definition   Pain is whatever experiencing persons say it is, existing whenever they say it does (McCaffery, 1968); a state in which an individual experiences pain that continues for more than 6 months in duration (NANDA)

Defining Characteristics

Subjective   Pain is always subjective and cannot be proved or disproved. The client's report of pain is the most reliable indicator of pain. Clients with cognitive abilities who can speak or point should use a pain rating scale (e.g., 0 to 10) to identify their current level of pain (self-report) and determine a pain rating goal.

Objective   Expressions of pain are extremely variable and cannot be used in lieu of self-report. Neither behavior nor vital signs can substitute for the client's self-report (McCaffery, Ferrell, 1991; McCaffery, Ferrell, 1992). Observable responses to pain are helpful in its assessment, especially in clients who cannot or will not use a self-report pain rating scale. Observable responses may be loss of appetite and inability to ambulate, perform activities of daily living (ADLs), work, and sleep. Clients may show guarding, self-protective behavior, self-focusing or narrowed focus, distraction behavior ranging from crying to laughing, and muscle tension or rigidity. In sudden severe pain, autonomic responses such as diaphoresis, blood pressure and pulse changes, pupillary dilation, and increase or decrease in respiratory rate and depth may be present but are usually not present with chronic pain that is relatively stable. Clients with chronic, cancer, or nonmalignant pain may experience threats to self-image, a perceived lack of options for coping, and worsening helplessness, anxiety, and depression. Chronic pain may affect almost every aspect of the client's daily life including concentration, work, and relationships.

Related Factors (r/t)

Actual or potential tissue damage, tumor progression and related pathology, diagnostic and therapeutic procedures (NOTE: The cause of chronic nonmalignant pain may not be known because pain is a new science and an area of diverse types of problems.)

Client Outcomes/Goals

- Uses pain rating scale to identify current level of pain, determines a pain rating goal, and maintains a pain diary (if client has cognitive abilities)
- Describes the total plan for drug and nondrug pain relief, including how to safely and effectively take medicines and integrate nondrug therapies
- Demonstrates ability to pace self, taking rest breaks before they are needed
- Functions on an acceptable ability level with minimal interference from pain and medication side effects

Suggested NIC Interventions

Analgesic administration, pain management, patient-controlled analgesia (PCA) assistance

Nursing Interventions

- Determine whether clients are experiencing pain at time of initial interview. If they are, intervene at that time to provide pain relief.
  The intensity of pain and discomfort should be assessed and documented during the initial evaluation of the patient (American Pain Society, 1995).
- Ask clients to describe past and current experiences with pain and effectiveness of the methods used to manage the pain, including experiences with side effects, typical coping responses, and how they express pain.
  A number of concerns (barriers) may affect clients' willingness to report pain and use analgesics (Ward et al, 1993).
- Describe the adverse effects of unrelieved pain.
  Numerous pathophysiological and psychological morbidity factors may be associated with pain (Puntillo, Weiss, 1994).
- Tell client to report pain location, intensity, and quality when experiencing pain.
  The intensity of pain and discomfort should be assessed and documented after any known pain-producing procedure, with each new report of pain, and at regular intervals (American Pain Society, 1995).
- Ask client to maintain a diary of pain ratings, timing, precipitating events, medications, treatments, and what works best to relieve pain.
  Systematic tracking of pain appears to be an important factor in improving pain management (Faries et al, 1991).
- Explore need for medications from the three classes of analgesics: opioids (narcotics), nonopioids, and adjuvant medications. For chronic neuropathic pain, consider adjuvants such as anticonvulsants and antidepressants that are analgesic.

Some types of pain respond to nonopioid drugs alone; if they do not, consider adding an opioid at increasing doses for increasing pain severity. At any level of pain, analgesic adjuvants may be useful (American Pain Society, 1992). Analgesic combinations may enhance pain relief (McCaffery, 1996).

- Determine client's current medication use.
  To aid in planning pain treatment, obtain a medication history (Acute Pain Management Guideline Panel, 1992).
- Obtain a prescription to administer a nonsteroidal antiinflammatory drug (NSAID), unless contraindicated, on an around-the-clock schedule.
  NSAIDs act mainly in the periphery to inhibit the initiation of pain signals (Dahl, Kehlet, 1991). The analgesic regimen should include a nonopioid drug, even if pain is severe enough to require the addition of an opioid (American Pain Society, 1992).
- For persistent cancer pain, obtain a prescription to administer opioid analgesics.
  When pain persists or increases, an opioid such as codeine or hydrocodone should be added to the NSAID (Jacox et al, 1994).
- If opioid dose is increased, monitor sedation and respiratory status for a brief time.
  Patients receiving long-term opioid therapy generally develop tolerance to the respiratory depressant effects of these agents (Jacox et al, 1994).
- Explain pain management approach that has been ordered, including therapies, medication administration, side effects, and complications.
  One of the most important steps toward improved control of pain is a better client understanding of the nature of pain, its treatment, and the role they need to play in pain control (Jacox et al, 1994).
- Discuss client's fears of undertreated pain, addiction, and overdose.
  A number of concerns (barriers) may affect clients' willingness to report pain and use analgesics (Ward et al, 1993). Because of the many misconceptions regarding pain and its treatment, education about the ability to control pain effectively and correction of myths about the use of opioids should be included as part of the treatment plan. Opioid tolerance and physical dependence are expected with long-term opioid treatment and should not be confused with addiction (Jacox et al, 1994).
- Review client's pain diary, flow sheet, and medication records to determine overall degree of pain relief, side effects, and analgesic requirements over an appropriate time period (e.g., 1 week).
  Systematic tracking of pain appears to be an important factor in improving pain management (Faries et al, 1991).
- Administer supplemental opioid doses as needed to keep pain ratings at or below an acceptable level.
  A prn order for a supplementary opioid dose between regular doses is an essential backup (American Pain Society, 1992).
- Obtain prescriptions to increase or decrease analgesic doses when indicated; base prescriptions on the client's report of pain severity and response to previous dose in terms of relief, side effects, and ability to perform the daily activities and the prescribed therapeutic regimen.
  Opioid doses should be adjusted individually to achieve pain relief with an acceptable level of adverse effects (Jacox et al, 1994).
- If client is receiving parenteral analgesia, use an equianalgesic chart to convert to an oral or another noninvasive route as smoothly as possible.

The oral route is the most preferred because it is the most convenient and cost effective. Avoid the intramuscular route because of unreliable absorption, pain, and inconvenience (Jacox et al, 1994).

- In addition to the use of analgesics, support the client's use of nonpharmacological methods to control pain such as distraction, imagery, relaxation, massage, and heat and cold application.
  Cognitive-behavioral strategies can restore the clients' sense of self-control, personal efficacy, and active participation in their own care (Jacox et al, 1994).
- Plan care activities around periods of greatest comfort whenever possible.
  Pain diminishes activity (Jacox et al, 1994).
- Ask clients to describe their appetite, bowel elimination, and ability to rest and sleep. Administer medications and treatments directed toward improving these functions.
  Because there is great individual variation in the development of opioid-induced side effects, clinicians should monitor and, if development is inevitable, prophylactically treat them (Jacox et al, 1994).
- Explore appropriate resources for management of pain on a long-time basis (e.g., hospice, pain care center).
  Most clients with cancer or chronic nonmalignant pain are treated for pain in outpatient and home care settings. Plans should be made to ensure ongoing assessment of the pain and the effectiveness of treatments in these settings (Jacox et al, 1994).
- If client has progressive cancer pain, assist client and family with handling issues related to death and dying.
  Peer support groups and pastoral counseling may increase the client's and family's coping skills and provide needed support (Jacox et al, 1994).
- If client has chronic nonmalignant pain, assist client and family with minimizing effects of pain on interpersonal relationships and daily activities such as work and recreation.
  Pain reduces clients' options to exercise control, diminishes psychological well-being, and makes them feel helpless and vulnerable. Therefore clinicians should support active client involvement in effective and practical methods to manage pain (Hitchcock, Ferrell, McCaffery, 1994; Jacox, 1994).

Geriatric
- Always take elderly clients' reports of pain seriously, and ensure that the pain is relieved.
  In spite of what many professionals and clients believe, pain is not an expected part of normal aging (Ferrell, 1991).
- Speak clearly, slowly, and loud enough for client to hear. Repeat information as needed.
- Be sure client can see well enough to read pain rating scale and written materials.
  Elderly clients are at increased risk for gastric and renal toxicity from NSAIDs (Griffin et al, 1991; Acute Pain Management Guideline Panel, 1992). Use NSAIDs with low side effect profiles (American Pain Society, 1992; Acute Pain Management Guideline Panel, 1992), such as Trilisate, Dolobid, and acetaminophen.

Home Care Interventions
- Review with client and caregivers the cause of pain and medical regimen specific to cause. Assess client knowledge and teach disease processes as necessary.
  Compliance with the medical regimen for diagnoses involving pain improves the likelihood of successful pain management (Humphrey, 1994).
- Develop a *full* medication profile including medications prescribed by all physicians and all over-the-counter medications. Assess for drug interactions. Instruct client to refrain from mixing medications without physician approval.

Pain medications may significantly impact or be impacted by other medications and may cause severe side effects. Some combinations of drugs are specifically contraindicated (Jacox et al, 1994).

- Assess client and family knowledge of side effects and safety precautions associated with pain medications (e.g., not driving while using opiates).
  Some terminally ill clients may be receiving high doses of pain medication and still try to be mobile or perform complex tasks.
- Collaborate with health care team on an ongoing basis (including client and family) to determine optimal pain control profile. Identify most effective interventions and medication administration routes most acceptable to the family and client.
  Success in pain control is partially dependent on the acceptability of the suggested intervention. Acceptability promotes compliance. Dosages vary among routes and will need to be adjusted accordingly to avoid breakthrough or transitional pain (Bohnet, 1995).
- If administering medication using highly technological methods, assess home for necessary resources (e.g., electricity) and responsible caregivers to assist client with administration.
  Some routes of medication administration require special conditions and procedures to be safe and accurate.
- Assess knowledge base of client and family for highly technological medication administration including the use of PCA pump. Teach as necessary.
  Appropriate instruction in the home increases the accuracy and safety of medication administration.
- Support the client and family in the use of high-dose opiates.
  Well-intentioned friends and family may create added stress by expressing judgment or fears regarding the use of opiates.

Client/Family Teaching

NOTE: To avoid the negative connotations associated with the words "drugs" or "narcotics," use the words "pain medicine" when teaching clients.

- Provide written materials regarding pain control, such as the Agency for Health Care Policy and Research pamphlet, *Managing Cancer Pain, Patient Guide.*
- Discuss the various discomforts encompassed by the word "pain" and ask clients to give examples of pain they have experienced. Explain the pain assessment process and the purpose of the pain rating scale that will be used. Teach clients to use the pain rating scale to rate the intensity of current or past pain. Ask them to set a pain relief goal by selecting a pain rating on the scale; if pain goes above this level, they should take action that decreases pain or notify a member of the health care team.
- Discuss the total plan for drug and nondrug treatment, including medication administration, maintaining a pain diary, and the use of supplies and equipment.
- Reinforce the importance of taking pain medications to keep pain under control.
- Reinforce that taking opioids for pain relief is not an addiction.
- Explain to clients with chronic neuropathic pain the process of taking tricyclic antidepressants; a low dose is used initially and is increased gradually. Emphasize that pain relief is delayed and the drugs must be taken daily. Reassure the patient that although the medicine is an antidepressant, if is for analgesia and not depression. Comparable teaching should take place when an anticonvulsant is prescribed for analgesia.
- Emphasize to clients with chronic nonmalignant pain the importance of participating in the therapeutic regimen (e.g., physical therapy, group therapy).

- Emphasize to clients the importance of pacing themselves and taking rest breaks before they are needed.
- Demonstrate the use of appropriate nonpharmacological approaches for controlling pain.

REFERENCES   Acute Pain Management Guideline Panel: *Acute pain management operative or medical procedures and trauma: clinical practice guideline,* Rockville, Md, 1992, Agency for Health Care Policy and Research Pub No 92-0032, Public Health Service, US Department of Health and Human Services.

American Pain Society: *Principles of analgesic use in the treatment of acute pain and cancer pain,* ed 3, Skokie, Il, 1992, The Society.

American Pain Society Quality of Care Committee: Quality improvement guidelines for the treatment of acute pain and cancer pain, *JAMA* 274:1874, 1995.

Bohnet N: Chronic pain management in the home care setting, *J Wound Ostomy Cont Nurs* 22:135, 1995.

Dahl JB, Kehlet H: Non-steroidal anti-inflammatory drugs: rationale for use in severe postoperative pain, *Br J Anaesthesia* 66:703, 1991.

Faries JE et al: Systematic pain records and their impact on pain control, *Cancer Nurs* 14:306, 1991.

Ferrell BR: Pain management in elderly people, *J Am Geriatr Soc* 39:64, 1991.

Griffin ME et al: Nonsteroidal anti-inflammatory drug use and increased risk for peptic ulcer disease in elderly persons, *Annals Internal Med* 11:257, 1991.

Hitchcock LS, Ferrell BR, McCaffery M: The experience of chronic nonmalignant pain, *J Pain Symptom Manage* 9:312, 1994.

Humphrey C: *Home care nursing handbook,* ed 2, Gaithersburg, Maryland, 1994, Aspen.

Jacox A et al: *Management of cancer pain: Clinical practice guideline no 9,* Rockville, Md, 1994, AHCPR Agency for Health Care Policy and Research, Pub No 94-0592, US Department of Health and Human Services, Public Health Service.

McCaffery M: Analgesics: mapping out pain relief, *Nursing 96* 26:41, 1996.

McCaffery M: Nursing practice theories related to cognition, bodily pain, and man-environment interactions, Los Angeles, 1968, University of California at Los Angeles Students' Store.

McCaffery M, Ferrell BR: How vital are vital signs? *Nursing 92* 22:42, 1992.

McCaffery M, Ferrell BR: How would you respond to these patients in pain? *Nursing 91* 21:34, 1991.

Pasero C, McCaffery M: Avoiding opioid-induced respiratory depression, *Am J Nurs* 94:25, 1994.

Puntillo K, Weiss SJ: Pain: its mediators and associated morbidity in critically ill cardiovascular surgical patients, *Nurs Res* 43:31, 1994.

Ward S et al: Patient-related barriers to management of cancer pain, *Pain* 52:319, 1993.

Risk for altered parent/infant/child attachment

Kathy Wyngarden and Mary A. Fuerst-DeWys

Definition   Disruption of the interactive process between parent/significant other and infant/child that fosters the development of a protective and nurturing reciprocal relationship

Risk Factors   Inability of parents to meet personal needs, anxiety associated with the parent role, substance abuse, premature infant, ill infant or child who is unable to effectively initiate parental contact because of altered behavioral organization, separation, physical barriers, lack of privacy

Parent risk factors

Characteristics during early infancy

Difficulty/inability recognizing infant behavior cues that communicate stress and/or avoidance, approach and/or engagement; hunger, satiety, fatigue; difficulty in alleviating, inability to alleviate distress; inappropriate stimulation; imbalance between disengaging versus engaging behaviors; extreme passivity, intrusiveness, and/or aggression with infant; minimal visiting and/or phone contact during periods of separation

Avoidantly attached characteristics

Emotionally unavailable and/or rejecting, dislikes infant's dependencies, seeks independence, lack of engaging behaviors (e.g., talking, looking, face-to-face looking behaviors, touching, smiling, holding, carrying, cuddling, rocking); depressed or low affect; poor attention during social interactions; inconsistent or no appropriate growth-fostering stimulation

Ambivalently attached characteristics

Displays affection inconsistently; may be attentive but not in tune with child; may be more in touch with child's physical than emotional needs; displays negative or aggressive behaviors toward child; makes negative remarks about child, displays physical aggression; slaps, hits, shakes child

Infant-child risk factors

Avoidantly attached characteristics

Displays significant avoidance/disengagement behaviors toward caregiver (e.g., turning away, avoiding eye contact, stiffening when held), few smiles or social behaviors, avoids mother when upset, may display eating problems, by end of first year seeks little physical contact with mother, displays little displeasure at separation, displays wide range of negative emotions (e.g., anger, sadness, irritability), unresponsive to being held but is upset when put down, demonstrates minimal stranger anxiety, has difficulty with responding or is unable to respond appropriately or predictably to parents' interactional attempts.

Preschool-age characteristics: frequently displays anger or aggression, socially isolated, disliked by peers, stays close to teachers, withdraws when in pain

School-age characteristics: displays absence of warm physical contact with parents and/or aggression toward parents and/or teachers, lacks close friends or has friendships marked by exclusivity and jealousy, may remain isolated from group

Ambivalently attached characteristics

Frequently cries, clingy and demanding, often angry/upset by small separations, chronically anxious in relation to mother, demonstrates limited autonomy and exploration, difficult to soothe after separation while simultaneously displaying anger and seeking comfort, possible bizarre eating and drinking patterns (e.g., refusing food, overeating, hoarding food).

Preschool-age characteristics: anxious, easily overwhelmed; immature and overly dependent on teacher; often avoids mother when upset; may bully or victimize other children.

School-age characteristics: combines intimacy-seeking behavior with hostility, may simultaneously be cute and irritating, is often worried about mother when apart, has trouble functioning in peer groups, difficulty sustaining friendships in large groups

Client Outcomes/Goals

- Maintain infant/child-parent love relationship
- Maintain mutually adaptive infant/child-parent "fit"

Suggested NIC Interventions

Attachment promotion

Nursing Interventions and Rationales

- Establish a trusting relationship with the parents.
  A relationship is primary and trust is the essential component of a therapeutic relationship.

- Assist parents in recognizing behaviors used by infant/child to communicate avoidance/stress and approach/engagement.
  Understanding infant behaviors provides parents with a guide for their own behaviors and gives meaning to their infant's behaviors (Oehler, Hannan, Catlett, 1993).
- Support parent's ability to alleviate infant/child's distress.
  When parents respond quickly to alleviate stress, the child is more likely to calm down rather than be spoiled. The parents are building a foundation for security and trust (Nursing Child Assessment Satellite Training, 1994).
- Assist parents in recognizing how their own interactions affect their infant/child (Hedlund, 1986).
- If necessary, allow mother to verbalize her fears of "ghosts in the nursery" that may influence attachment to her infant/child.
  Ghosts in the nursery are parents' early memories of painful experiences (e.g., unanswered cries, feeling abandoned, being abused) and are real and powerful. "Hearing a mother's cries" is necessary to help her "hear her child's cries," an important aspect of therapeutic healing (Frailberg, Adelson, Shapiro, 1975).
- Listen to the parents' stories to understand their struggle to attach.
  Acknowledge the parents' point of view and stories as worthy of respect; important truths can be learned, such as what they think and how they feel about themselves and their infant (Trout, 1987).
- Assist parents with recognizing how their infant/child learns through senses (e.g., visual, auditory, tactile, kinesthetic) and strategies that can be used, such as timing, intensity, imitation, repetition, to initiate interactions.
  By recognizing infant likes and dislikes based on their behavioral responses to stimuli, parents can generate their own strategies regarding which stimuli is most effective (McCollum, Stayton, 1982).
- Guide parents in adapting to infant/child cues and changing needs.
  Premature infants respond more positively to less intense maternal stimulation (Lozoff et al, 1977).
- Nurture parents so that they in turn can nurture their infant/child.
  Offer a safe, nonjudgmental environment in which parents can express their feelings. If parents are unable to focus on infant, nurse should focus on parents' feelings (Zabielski, 1994).
- Provide guidance in child development.
  Unrealistic expectations of parents regarding infant/child abilities can negatively influence the parent-child relationship.
- Offer another parent as peer support (Lindsey, Roman, 1993).
- Attend to both the parents and infant in an effort to strengthen the early developing attachment relationship.
  Identifying the infant/child's strengths and limitations can provide parents with more information regarding how they can encourage optimal growth and development (Denehy, 1992).
- Encourage parents of hospitalized infants to "personalize" their infant by bringing in baby clothes, pictures of themselves, toys, and tapes of their voices.
  These actions help parents claim the infant as their own.
- Encourage skin-to-skin experience for parents and infants as appropriate.
  Parents who participate in bonding and skin-to-skin activities are less likely to reject their infant (Hamelin, Ramachandran, 1993).

- Acknowledge and support the strengths of the infant/child, parent, and family (Goodfriend, 1993).

REFERENCES   Denehy J: Interventions related to parent-infant attachment, *Nurs Intervent* 27:425, 1992.

Field TM: Effects of early separation, interactive deficits, and experimental manipulation on infant-mother face-to-face interaction, *Child Development* 48:763, 1977.

Frailberg S, Adelson E, Shapiro V: Ghosts in the nursery: a psychoanalytic approach to the problems of impaired infant-mother relationships, *J Am Acad Child Psychiatry* 14:387, 1975.

Goodfriend MS: Treatment of attachment disorders of infancy in a neonatal intensive care unit, *Pediatrics* 91:139, 1993.

Hamelin K, Ramachandran C: Kangaroo care, *Can Nurse* 89:15, 1993.

Hedlund R: Fostering positive social interactions between parents and infants, *Teaching Exceptional Children* 1986, p. 43.

Holaday B: Maternal responses to their chronically ill infants' attachment behavior of crying, *Nurs Res* 30:343, 1981.

Karen R: *Unfolding the mystery of the infant-mother bond and its impact on later life: becoming attached,* New York, 1994, Warner Books.

Klaus M, Kennell J: Mothers separated from their newborn infants, *Pediatr Clin North Am* 17:106, 1970.

Lozoff B et al: The mother-newborn relationship: limits of adaptability, *J Pediatr* 91:1, 1977.

Lyndsay J et al: Creative caring in the NJCO parent to parent support, *Neonatal Network* 12:37, 1993.

McCollum J, Stayton V: Infant/parent interaction: studies and intervention guidelines based on the SIAI model, *J Div Early Childhood* 9:123, 1985.

Oehler J, Hannan T, Catlett A: Maternal views of preterm infants' responsiveness to social interaction, *Neonatal Network* 12:67, 1993.

Trout M: *Working papers on process in infant mental health assessment and intervention,* Champaign, Illinois, 1987, The Infant-Parent Institute.

Zabielski M: Recognition of maternal identity in preterm and fullterm mothers, *Matern Child Nurs J* 22:2, 1994.

Parental role conflict

Peggy Wetsch

Definition

The state in which a parent experiences role confusion and conflict in response to a crisis

Defining Characteristics

Major
Expresses concerns or feelings of inadequacy regarding the ability to provide for child's physical and emotional needs during hospitalization or at home; demonstrates disruption in caretaking routines; expresses concerns about changes in parental role and family functioning, communication, or health

Minor
Expresses concern about perceived loss of control regarding decisions relating to child; reluctant to participate in usual caretaking activities, even with encouragement and support; verbalizes or demonstrates feelings of guilt, anger, fear, anxiety, and frustration concerning the effect of the child's illness on family processes

Related Factors (r/t)

Separation from child as a result of chronic illness, intimidation by invasive or restrictive modalities (e.g., isolation, intubation, specialized care center policies), home care of child with special needs (e.g., apnea monitoring, postural drainage, hyperalimentation), change in marital status, interruptions of family life due to home care regimens (e.g., treatments, caregivers, lack of respite)

Client Outcomes/Goals

- Expresses feelings and perceptions regarding impacts of illness, disability, and/or hospitalization on parental role
- Participates in hospital/home care of as much as they are able given the availability of resources and support systems
- Exhibits assertiveness and responsibility in active family decision-making regarding care of the child
- Describes and selects available resources to support parental management of child/family needs

Suggested NIC Interventions

Crisis intervention, family process maintenance, role enhancement

Nursing Interventions and Rationales

- Assess parent's prior coping behaviors.
  Use of prior effective coping behaviors gives the parent a feeling of competence. Identifying ineffective or absent coping behaviors allows development of interventions. Research indicates that a parent who copes successfully is better able to promote the adjustment and recovery of the child (Ladebauche, 1992).
- Explore parent/family source of stress, usual methods of coping, perceptions of illness/condition and capitalize on strengths identified. Involve both parents in assessment.
  Identification of parents' perceptions of the magnitude of circumstances, degree of perceived adequacy, and usual coping methods can support strategies that promote active constructive coping or develop approaches to build/strengthen coping. Helping the family maintain an optimistic outlook is important for parents who are caring for a chronically ill child at home (Ray, Richtie, 1993; Bond, Phillips, Rollins, 1994; Heaman, 1995; Melnyk, 1995).
- Sustain parental involvement in shared decision-making regarding care by using the following steps:
  - Incorporate parent's information concerning child's typical routines, behaviors, fears, likes and dislikes.
  - Provide clear and direct firsthand information concerning child's condition and progress.
  - Normalize the home/hospital environment as much as possible.
  - Collaborate in care by providing choices when possible.
  Involving parents in a child's caregiving and in decision-making helps increase parental feelings of control and decrease feelings of stress. Noting parents' questions and nonverbal cues to determine need for improved communication is important (Sims, 1992; Shellabarger, Thompson, 1993; Bond, Phillips, Rollins, 1994).
- Seek and support parental participation in care.
  As parents of disabled children gain knowledge and become more involved in caregiving activities, their caregiver identity emerges. Parents eventually emerge as the central persons in their children's lives. Parental participation has been demonstrated to have a positive effect on a child's reactions to procedures, resulting in improved cooperation and decreases in upset behaviors and child's level of activity (Moynihan, Naclerio, Kiley, 1993; Perkins, 1993; Jones, Maestri, McCoy, 1994).
- Provide support for each parent's primary coping strategies.
  Mothers tend to focus more on strategies related to social support, whereas fathers are inclined to analyze situations (Heaman, 1995).

- Offer respite care to assist parents in maintaining sufficient energy and personal resources to continue caregiving responsibilities.
  Medically fragile or technology-dependent children and children with chronic health problems and resultant disabilities receive most of their care at home by family members, frequently at severe economic and psychologic costs (Coffman, Folden, 1992; Folden, Coffman, 1993).
- Determine older than average mother's support systems and self-expectations of motherhood. Pay particular attention to relationships with spouse or partner, family, and friends.
  Social support has a positive influence to early parenting for primiparas more than 35 years of age. Older primiparas with high self-expectations, low satisfaction with parenting, or inadequate social support systems may be at risk (Ferris, Reece, 1994).
- Be available to discuss concerns and be a good listener.
  The parent is more likely to verbalize concerns when the nurse is not hurried. Open communication is essential for the identification of potential coping problems (Ladebauche, 1992).
- Encourage parent to meet own needs of rest, nutrition, and hygiene. Provide facilities so that parent may stay with sick child (e.g., cot, reclining chair). Encourage respite from caregiving duties.
  A parent is unable to meet the child's needs when the basic self-needs are unmet.
- Demonstrate safe places where parent may touch or stroke child. Encourage parent to talk or sing to child. Adjust equipment so that parent is able to hold child; provide a comfortable chair, preferably a rocking chair. Provide opportunities and offer praise for successful caregiving.
  Involvement in child's care will give the parent a sense of control in the hospital environment.
- Refer to available telephone counseling services.
  Telephone counseling services can provide confidential advice to families who might otherwise have no access to help in dealing with a child's problems (Jones, Maestri, McCoy, 1993).

Client/Family Teaching

- Furnish clear explanations about condition, disease or disability, associated treatments, and prognosis. Describe circumstances involving emotional and physical reactions of the child and types of family member reactions that might be anticipated in response to condition or crisis. Provide ample time for skill practice.
  Providing information to families decreases confusion and anxiety, increases understanding, and allows a feeling of competence and control. Providing information about the disease and treatment process helps build the parent's feelings of confidence (Baker, 1994).
- For parents with chronic disabilities, tailor educational opportunities based on the experiential phase (protection, survival, or development of the parent as central person) of the parents as they develop an identity as the central caregiver for their child.
  As parents of physically and/or cognitively disabled children gain knowledge and become more involved in caregiving activities, their caregiver identity emerges (Perkins, 1993).
- Involve parents in formal and/or informal social support situations, including parent-to-parent groups, community agencies and counseling resources.
  Parents of children with special health care needs are uniquely equipped to help each other learn day-to-day coping skills. Utilization of available social supports in the community can make a difference in achieving successful outcomes (Coffman, Folden, 1992; Hartman, Radin, McConnell, 1992).

REFERENCES Baker NA: Avoid collisions with challenging families, *MCN* 19:97, 1994.

Bond N, Phillips P, Rollins JA: Family centered care at home for families with children who are technology dependent, *Pediatr Nurs* 20:123, 1994.

Coffman S, Folden SL: Respite care for medically fragile children, *J Home Health Care Practice* 5:16, 1992.

Ferris A, Reece C: Nutritional consequences of chronic maternal conditions during pregnancy and lactation: lupus and diabetes, *J Clin Nutr* 59:4658, 1994.

Folden SL, Coffman S: Respite care for families of children with disabilities, *J Pediatr Health Care* 7:103, 1993.

Hartman AF, Radin MB, McConnell B: Parent-to-parent support: a critical component of health care services for families, *Issu Comp Pediatr Nurs* 15(1):55, 1992.

Heaman DJ: Perceived stressors and coping strategies of parents who have children with developmental disabilities: a comparison of mothers with fathers, *J Pediatr Nurs* 10:311, 1995.

Jones DC: Effect of parental participation on hospitalized child behavior, *Issue Comp Pediatr Nurs* 17:81, 1994.

Jones LC, Maestri BO, McCoy K: Why parents use the warm line, *MCN* 18:258, 1993.

Ladebauche P: Unit-based family support groups: a reminder, *MCN* 17:18, 1992.

Melnyk BM: Parental coping with childhood hospitalization: a theoretical framework to guide research and clinical interventions, *MCN* 23:123, 1995.

Moynihan P, Nalcerio L, Kiley K: Parent participation, *Nurs Clin North Am* 30:231, 1995.

Perkins MT: Parent-nurse collaboration: using the caregiver identity emergence phases to assist parents of hospitalized children with disabilities, *J Pediatr Nurs* 8:2, 1993.

Ray LD, Ritchie JA: Caring for chronically ill children at home: factors that influence parents' coping, *J Pediatr Nurs* 8:217, 1993.

Shellabarger SG, Thompson TL: The critical times: meeting parental communication needs throughout the NICU experience, *Neonatal Network* 12:39, 1993.

Sims SL et al: Decision making in home health care, *West J Nurs Res* 14:186, 1992.

Altered parenting

Peggy Wetsch

Definition

The state in which a nurturing figure experiences an inability to create an environment that promotes the optimum growth and development of another human being

Defining Characteristics

Abandonment; runaway child; inability to control child; incidence of physical and psychological trauma; lack of parental attachment behaviors; inappropriate visual, tactile, and auditory stimulation; negative identification of infant/child characteristics; negative attachment of meanings to infant/child characteristics; constant verbalization of disappointment about gender or physical characteristics of the infant/child; verbalization of resentment towards the infant/child; verbalization of role inadequacy; inattentiveness to infant/child needs *(critical);* verbal disgust at bodily functions of infant/child; noncompliance with health appointments for self or infant/child; inappropriate caretaking behavior (e.g., toilet training, sleep, rest, or feeding) *(critical);* inappropriate or inconsistent discipline practices; frequent accidents; frequent illnesses; growth and development lag in the child; history of child abuse or abandonment by primary caretakers *(critical);* verbalized desire to have child call parent by first name versus traditional cultural tendencies; care given by multiple caretakers without consideration for the needs of the infant/child; compulsive seeking of role approval from others

Related Factors (r/t)

Lack of available role models; ineffective role models; physical and psychosocial abuse of nurturing figure; lack of support from significant others; unmet social, emotional, and maturational needs of parenting figures; interruption in bonding process (e.g., maternal, paternal); unrealistic expectations of self, infant, or partner; perceived threat to own physical and emotional survival; mental or physical illness; presence of stressors (e.g., finances, legal issues, recent crisis, cultural move); lack of knowledge; limited cognitive functioning; lack of role identity; absent or inappropriate response of child to relationship; multiple pregnancies

Client Outcomes/Goals

- Affirms desire to develop constructive parenting skills to support infant/child growth and development
- Initiates appropriate measures to develop a safe, nurturing environment
- Acquires and displays attentive, supportive parenting behaviors
- Identifies strategies to protect child from harm and/or neglect and initiates action when indicated

Suggested NIC Interventions

Abuse protection: child, attachment promotion, developmental enhancement, family integrity promotion

Nursing Interventions and Rationales

- Use active listening to explore parent's understanding of developmental needs and expectations of child and self within the context of cultural perspectives and influences. *Interviewing with empathy while reserving judgment allows parent to more freely express frustrations and disappointments regarding negative feelings, needs, and parenting skills. Unrealistic expectations may be present when parent does not discern what is normal for the child (Denehy, 1992; Herman-Staab, 1994; Mrazek, Mrazek, Klinnert, 1995).*
- Examine characteristics of parenting style and behaviors including the following:
  - Emotional climate at home
  - Attribution of negative traits to child
  - Failure to support child's increases in autonomy
  - Type of interaction with infant/child
  - Competition with child for spousal/significant other attention
  - Lack of knowledge/concern about health maintenance or behavioral problems
  - Other behaviors or concerns

  Children are at risk for neglect, abuse, and other negative psychosocial outcomes in families with dysfunctions (Mrazek, Mrazek, Klinnert, 1995).
- Institute abuse/neglect protection measures if evidence of inability to cope with family stressors or crisis, signs of parental substance abuse, or significant level of social isolation apparent.
  Risk of abuse/neglect is higher in families with high levels of stress, substance abuse, or lack of social support systems (Devlin, Reynolds, 1994).
- For mothers with toddlers, assess maternal depression, perceptions of difficult temperament in toddler, and low maternal self-efficacy.
  Self-efficacy is defined as one's judgement of how effectively one can execute a task or manage a situation that may contain novel, unpredictable, and stressful elements. A cyclic relationship among depression, perceived difficult temperament, and self-efficacy has been identified. Negative feelings about oneself and one's child are likely to negatively influence the parent-child relationship (Gross et al, 1994).
- Appraise parent's resources and availability of social support systems. Determine single woman's particular sources of support, especially availability of her own mother and partner. Encourage use of healthy, strong support systems.

Before adequate interventions and education can be initiated, understanding of the current support system and concerns must occur. The partner and her mother are often important sources of support (Zacharia, 1994).

- Model age- and cognitively-appropriate caregiver skills by doing the following:
  - Communicating with child at an appropriate cognitive level of development
  - Giving child tasks and responsibilities appropriate to age or functional age/level
  - Instituting safety considerations such as assistive equipment
  - Encouraging child to perform activities of daily living (ADLs) as appropriate.

  These activities illustrate parenting and child-rearing skills and behaviors for parents and family (McCloskey, Bulecheck, 1992).

Client/Family Teaching

- Explain individual differences in child temperaments and compare and contrast with reality of parents expectations. Help parents determine and understand the implications of their child's temperament.

  Promoting parental understanding of temperament facilitates development of more realistic expectations (McClowry, 1992; Melvin, 1995)

- Discuss sound disciplinary techniques, which include "catching" children being good, active listening, conveying positive regard, ignoring minor transgressions, giving good directions, use of praise, and use of time-out.

  Disciplinary methods are subject to a variety of opinions. Proper discipline provides children with security, and clearly enforced rules help them learn self-control and social standards. Parenting classes can be beneficial when parent has had little formal or informal prior preparation (Herman-Staab, 1994).

- Foster acquisition of positive parenting skills.

  Parents may feel powerless. Helping them develop necessary skills or gain knowledge maintains the integrity of the parental role, and parents are then likely to use maladaptive coping styles (Baker, 1994).

- Plan parental education directed towards the following age-related parental concerns:
  - Birth to 2 years   Transition, sleep, aggression
  - 3 to 5 years   Transition, parent-child relationship, sleep
  - 6 to 10 years   School, parent-child relationship, divorce
  - 11 to 18 years   Parent-child relationship, divorce, school

  Parents with children of any age may seek basic information about a variety of concerns, which can be anticipated and addressed by providing ongoing information and support (Jones, Maestri, McCoy, 1993).

- Initiate referrals to community agencies, parent education, stress management training, and social support groups.

  The parent needs support to manage angry or inappropriate behaviors. Use of support systems and social services can provide an opportunity to decrease feelings of inadequacy (Campbell, 1992; Baker, 1994).

- Provide information regarding available telephone counseling services.

  Telephone counseling services can provide confidential advice and support to families who might not otherwise have access to help in dealing with behavioral problems and parenting concerns (Jones, Maestri, McCoy, 1993).

  See **Altered growth and development** for additional teaching interventions.

REFERENCES   Baker NA: Avoid collisions with challenging families, *MCN* 19:97, 1994.

Campbell JM: Parenting classes: focus on discipline, *J Comm Health Nurs* 9:197, 1992.

Denehy JA: Intervention related to parent-infant attachment, *Nurs Clin North Am* 27:425, 1992.

Devlin BK, Reynolds E: Child abuse: how to recognize it, how to intervene, *Am J Nurs* 94:26, 1994.

Herman-Staab B: Screening, management and appropriate referral for pediatric behavior problems, *Nurs Practitioner* 19:40, 1994.

Gross D et al: A longitudinal model of maternal self-efficacy, depression, and difficult temperament during toddlerhood, *Res Nurs Health* 17:207, 1994.

Jones LC, Maestri BO, McCoy K: Why parents use the warm line, *MCN* 18:258, 1993.

McCloskey JC, Bulechek GM, editors: *Nursing interventions classification (NIC),* St Louis, 1992, Mosby.

McClowry SG: Temperament theory and research, *Image* 24:319, 1992.

Melvin N: Children's temperament: intervention for parents, *J Pediatr Nurs* 10:152, 1995.

Mrazek DA, Mrazek P, Klinnert M: Clinical assessment of parenting, *J Am Acad Child Adolesc Psychiatry* 34:272, 1995.

Zachria R: Perceived social support and social network of low-income mothers of infants and preschoolers: pre- and postparenting program, *J Comm Health Nurs* 11:11, 1994.

Risk for altered parenting

Peggy Wetsch

Definition   The state in which a nurturing figure is at risk to experience an inability to create an environment that promotes the optimum growth and development of another human being

Risk Factors

Lack of parental attachment behaviors; inappropriate visual, tactile, or auditory stimulation; negative identification of infant/child characteristics; negative attachment of meanings to infant/child characteristics; constant verbalization of disappointment about gender or physical characteristics of the infant/child; verbalization of resentment toward the infant/child; verbalization of role inadequacy; inattentiveness to infant/child needs *(critical);* verbal disgust at bodily functions of infant/child; noncompliance with health appointments for self or infant/child; inappropriate caretaking behaviors (e.g., toilet training, sleep, rest, feeding) *(critical),* inappropriate or inconsistent discipline practices; frequent accidents; frequent illnesses; growth and development lag in the child; history of child abuse or abandonment by primary caretaker; verbalized desire to have child call parent by first name versus traditional cultural tendencies; care given by multiple caretakers without consideration for the needs of the infant/child; compulsive seeking of role approval from others

Related Factors (r/t)

Lack of available role models; ineffective role models; physical and psychosocial abuse of nurturing figure; lack of support from significant others; unmet social, emotional, or maturational needs of parenting figures; interruption in bonding process (e.g., maternal, paternal); unrealistic expectations for self, infant, or partner; perceived threat to own physical and emotional survival; mental or physical illness; presence of stressor (e.g., finances, legal issues, recent crisis, cultural move); lack of knowledge; limited cognitive functioning; lack of role identity; absent or inappropriate response of child to relationship; multiple pregnancies

Client Outcomes/Goals

- Successfully establishes a nurturing parenting role

Suggested NIC Interventions

Abuse protection: child, attachment promotion, developmental enhancement, family integrity promotion, normalization promotion

Nursing Interventions and Rationales

NOTE: Management of a risk diagnosis necessitates approaches using primary and secondary prevention. Primary prevention interventions, which include such activities as safety instruction, focus on thwarting the development of disease or conditions. Early detection through screening, monitoring, and surveillance is secondary prevention (Shortridge, Valanis, 1992).

- Conduct risk identification noting presence of prior history of abuse, parental/family stressors, strength and adequacy of social support systems, establish coping styles, and other related factors (see related factors).
  Identification of a family at risk signals special teaching and referral needs (McCloskey, Bulecheck, 1992).
- Monitor parent-infant interactions that may signal interrupted or inadequate attachment or other parenting issues.
  Early detection can lead to early intervention and prevent or limit problems (McCloskey, Bulecheck, 1992).

Client/Family Teaching

- Initiate referrals to an appropriate community agency for early follow-up if actual problem is identified. See **Altered parenting** for additional teaching interventions.

REFERENCES   McCloskey JC, Bulechek GM, editors: *Nursing interventions classification (NIC),* St Louis, 1992, Mosby.
Shortridge L, Valanis B: The epidemiological model applied in community health nursing. In Stanhope M, Lancaster J, editors: *Community health nursing: process and practice for promoting health,* ed 3, St Louis, 1992, Mosby.

Risk for perioperative positioning injury

Pamela M. Emery

Definition   A state in which an individual is at risk for injury as a result of the environmental conditions found in the perioperative setting (position selected for surgical clients that provides access to the surgical site, access to the airway for the administration of anesthesia, and maintains normal body alignment and function)

Risk Factors

Age, weight, nutritional status, presence of preexisting conditions such as diabetes, vascular disease, arthritis, or malignancy, effects of anesthesia, and duration of procedure; systems most frequently affected by surgical positioning—the neurological, musculoskeletal, integumentary, respiratory and cardiovascular
May be a potential for impaired tissue perfusion, impaired skin integrity, or neuromuscular or joint injury related to surgical positioning

Complications of surgical positioning

Transient physiological reactions to surgical positioning include skin redness, lumbar backache, stiffness in the limbs and neck, and generalized muscle aches that usually resolve within 24 to 48 hours without treatment (Walsh, 1993). Lumbar back pain, previously considered a transient physiological reaction to positioning may, in some cases, may be persistent in nature (Clark et al, 1993). More serious complications of surgical positioning include pressure ulcers, peripheral nerve injury, deep venous thrombosis, compartment syndrome (impairment of microcirculation in soft tissue), joint injury (Paschal, Strzelecki, 1992; Walsh, 1993). Because compartment syndrome is a reperfusion injury, its signs and symptoms may not be immediately apparent and may develop insidiously (Montgomery, Ready, 1991).

Client Outcomes/Goals

• Remains free of injury related to positioning during the surgical procedure

NOTE: Nursing interventions are based on assessing the client for the existence of or potential for injury to any of the mentioned systems based on observed or elicited risk factors.

Suggested NIC Interventions

Positioning: intraoperative, skin surveillance

Nursing Interventions and Rationales (by surgical position)

Supine position (dorsal recumbent)

• Pad all bony prominences (e.g., head, elbows, sacrum, heels) and positioning devices.

Bony prominences exert pressure on overlying tissue, which predisposes the client to the development of pressure ulcers (Rothrock, 1990; Blaylock, Gardner, 1994). Nerves that pass over or near bony prominences may be injured by compression (Walsh, 1993).

• Support lumbar and popliteal areas.

Maintaining normal lumbar concavity prevents muscle strain. Support under the knees prevents muscle and ligament strain (Rothrock, 1990).

• Use a firm foam rubber support or padded footboard that extends to toes.

A support or footboard prevents plantar flexion and protects the toes from the weight and pressure of draping materials (Meeker, Rothrock, 1995).

• Use padded footboards and shoulder braces when using Trendelenburg's or reverse Trendelenburg's position.

Positioning aids help protect skin from shearing forces, the opposite parallel force between skin and subcutaneous tissue (Rothrock, 1990).

NOTE: Either of these two positions (Trendelenburg or reverse Trendelenburg) may have adverse effects on both the circulatory and respiratory systems, which in most circumstances are monitored and controlled by anesthesia personnel. Modifications of both positions may be suggested and implemented by the nurse in collaboration with the surgeon and anesthesiologist.

• Position client's arms with palms up on armboards at less than a 90° angle to the body with palms up.

Hyperabduction may damage the brachial plexus and stretch the subclavian and axillary vessels (Walsh, 1993; Association of Operating Room Nurses, 1996).

• Position arms at sides of the body with palms against the body, or pronate and secure arms with a broad lift sheet without flexing the elbow.

Tucking the arms prevents compression of the fingers when extending over the edge of the operating table, maintains proper alignment, and prevents compression of the ulnar nerve (Meeker, Rothrock, 1995).

- Protect skin from direct contact with any metal surfaces.
Faulty or improperly grounded electrosurgical units may use alternate pathway through any skin surface in contact with metal and result in an electrical burn (Rothrock, 1990).
- Lift rather than pull or slide client when positioning.
Sliding and pulling increase the incidence of skin injury from shearing and friction.
- Maintain alignment of head with cervical, thoracic, and lumbar vertebrae.
Misalignment, flexion, and twisting may cause muscle and nerve damage as well as airway interference (Meeker, Rothrock, 1995).
- Make sure client's legs are parallel and uncrossed.
Compression from crossed ankles may injure peroneal and tibial nerves and impede circulation (Walsh, 1993).
- Place leg restraint strap (safety belt) 2 inches above knees.
Clients may become disoriented and attempt to change position on the narrow operating table.

Prone position (modification: kneeling, jackknife, or Kraske position)

- Provide an adequate number of personnel to perform a "logroll" turn of the anesthetized client.
Movement and positioning from the supine to the prone position may be safely undertaken by four persons (Meeker, Rothrock, 1995).
- Place chest rolls from clavicles to iliac crests.
Chest rolls allow for lung expansion and free movement of the diaphragm, and they decrease pressure on female breast tissue (Walsh, 1993; Meeker, Rothrock, 1995).
- Place a bolster or pillow under the pelvis.
Support of the pelvis decreases abdominal pressure on the inferior vena cava and male genitalia (Meeker, Rothrock, 1995).
- Place a bolster or pillow under client's ankles.
A cushion prevents plantar flexion and pressure on the toes (Rothrock, 1990).
- Guide client's arms down and forward with elbows flexed and padded and hands placed palm down, to rest on armboards that are extended forward from the operating table.
This movement prevents shoulder dislocation and brachial plexus injury, and padding prevents ulnar and radial nerve compression (Walsh, 1993; Meeker, Rothrock, 1995).
- Place head on foam donut or padded headrest; protect client's ears and eyes.
Ear cartilage may be damaged if the ear folds or is bent. Corneal abrasions may occur if the eyes are not closed and secured during maneuvering and positioning (Meeker, Rothrock, 1995).
- Avoid severe rotation of client's head to one side.
Severe head rotation may stretch skeletal muscles and ligaments, causing postoperative pain and limited motion after surgery (Walsh, 1993).

Lateral position (lateral chest or kidney)

- Provide adequate personnel to properly position client.
Lateral positioning requires a four-person team to safely move the client from the supine position (Rothrock, 1990).
- Use a lift sheet to facilitate the turn.
Lift sheets prevent skin injury resulting from shearing.

- Place a support under the head.
  A pillow or support keeps the head properly aligned with the cervical, spinal, and thoracic vertebrae (Walsh, 1993; Meeker, Rothrock, 1995).
- Flex the bottom leg at the hip and knee.
  Flexing the bottom leg provides a base of support to hold the body in position (Rothrock, 1990).
- Place beanbags, sandbags, or bolsters against the back and abdomen.
  Additional positioning devices provide support and maintain body alignment (Meeker, Rothrock, 1995).
- Pad the lateral aspect of the bottom knee.
  Pressure of the knee against the operating bed may injure the peroneal nerve (Walsh, 1993).
- Place a pillow between the client's legs lengthwise so that the pillow also supports the foot.
  Pressing the bony prominences of one extremity against the other may cause injury to the peroneal and tibial nerves. If the foot extends beyond the pillow it may drop, causing damage to muscles and joints (Walsh, 1993; Meeker, Rothrock, 1995).
- Pad the lower shoulder and bring it forward slightly; the lower arm is extended on a padded armboard.
  All bony prominences should be padded to prevent tissue breakdown. Bringing the shoulder forward relieves pressure on the brachial plexus (Walsh, 1993).
- Place the upper arm on a padded raised armboard or padded Mayo stand.
  Raising the upper arm elevates the scapula and widens the intercostal spaces, which provides access to the upper thoracic cavity (Rothrock, 1990).
- Place an axillary roll at the apex of the scapula in the axillary space of the dependent arm.
  A soft roll relieves pressure on the arm and facilitates chest expansion (Meeker, Rothrock, 1995; Association of Operating Room Nurses, 1996).
  NOTE: Some surgeons prefer the use of wide adhesive tape to secure the hips, arms, and legs. This practice would be contraindicated in clients with tape allergies or in the frail elderly with fragile skin.

Lithotomy position

- Loosely secure the client's arms across the abdomen or extended on padded armboards.
  Arms must not be placed at the client's sides because the table will be "broken" for the procedure, and fingers may extend beyond the break (Rothrock, 1990; Meeker, Rothrock, 1995).
- Pad the sacral area and provide a small lumbar roll.
  Bony prominences must be padded to prevent soft tissue damage. A lumbar roll helps maintain normal lumbar concavity (Meeker, Rothrock, 1995; Association of Operating Room Nurses, 1996).
- Place client's legs in the stirrups simultaneously.
  Raising the legs together requires two persons and helps prevent stress on hip joints (Walsh, 1993).
- Lower client's legs simultaneously and slowly.
  Blood pools result from the stirrup position; lowering the legs slowly helps decrease hypotension (Paschal, Strzelecki, 1992).
- Avoid acute flexion of the thigh.
  Acute flexion of the thigh increases intraabdominal pressure against the diaphragm, thus decreasing tidal volume, which is a more pronounced problem in obese clients

(Meeker, Rothrock, 1995). Severe flexion may also strain the lumbar spine, damage prosthetic hip joints, and cause nerve damage (Walsh, 1993).

- Avoid hyperabduction and excessive external rotation of the hip joint.
  Lumbosacral plexus stretch injury may result from the plexus being stretched and compressed under the inguinal ligament or pubic ramus (Fowl, Skers, Kempczinski, 1992). Femoral myoneuropathy may result from excessive hip abduction and external rotation (Hakim, Katirji, 1993).
- Select lithotomy leg holders with optimal body alignment and weight bearing in mind (e.g., combination knee crutch and boot).
  Product selection and evaluation should be based on identified needs and promote client safety (Association of Operating Room Nurses, 1996).
- Pad all bony prominences and surfaces that may contact the leg support system.
  Pressure on the lateral aspect of the knee may damage the peroneal nerve (Paschal, Strzelecki, 1992). Contact with metal at any point during use of the electrosurgical unit may result in an electrical burn (Rothrock, 1990). Compression of soft tissue may predispose client to venous thrombosis; prolonged compression may result in compartment syndrome (Paschal, Strzelecki, 1992).
- Monitor the length of time the client remains in the lithotomy position.
  Most complications occur following procedures that exceed 5 hours (Fowl, Skers, Kempczinski, 1992). The increased practice of operative laparoscopy, especially in gynecology, has contributed to more prolonged procedures (Schwartz, Stahl, DeCherny, 1993).
  NOTE: If assessment reveals conditions that place the client at increased risk for injury in this position, attempting this position while the client is awake and can report any discomfort may help prevent positioning complications.

REFERENCES

Association of Operating Room Nurses: *AORN standards and recommended practices for perioperative nursing,* Denver, 1996, The Association.

Blaylock B, Gardner C: Measuring tissue interface pressures of two support surfaces used in the operating room, *Ostomy/Wound Manage* 40:42, 1994.

Clark A et al: Role of the surgical position in the development of postoperative low back pain, *J Spinal Disord* 6:238, 1993.

Fowl R, Skers D, Kempczinski R: Neurovascular lower extremity complications of the lithotomy position, *Annals Vasc Surg* 6:4,1992.

Hakim M, Katirji M: Femoral myoneuropathy induced by the lithotomy position: a report of 5 cases with a review of literature, *Muscle Nerve* 16:891, 1993.

Meeker M, Rothrock J: *Alexander's care of the patient in surgery,* ed 10, St Louis, 1995, Mosby.

Montgomery C, Ready L: Epidural opioid analgesia does not obscure diagnosis of compartment syndrome resulting from prolonged lithotomy position, *Anesthesiology* 75:541, 1991.

Paschal C, Strzelecki L: Lithotomy positioning devices: factors that contribute to patient injury, *AORN J* 55:1011, 1992.

Rothrock J: *Perioperative nursing care planning,* St Louis, 1990, Mosby.

Schwartz L, Stahl R, DeCherney A: Unilateral compartment syndrome after prolonged gynecologic surgery in the dorsal lithotomy position, *J Reprod Med* 38:6, 1992.

Walsh J: Postoperative effects of OR positioning, *RN* 56:50, 1993.

Risk for peripheral neurovascular dysfunction

Betty J. Ackley

Definition   The state in which an individual is at risk of experiencing a disruption in circulation, sensation, or motion

Related Factors (r/t)

Fractures, mechanical compression (e.g., tourniquet, cast, brace, dressing, restraints), orthopedic surgery, trauma, immobilization, burns, vascular obstruction

Client Outcomes/Goals

- Maintains circulation, sensation, and movement of an extremity within own normal limits
- Explains signs of neurovascular compromise and ways to prevent venous stasis

Suggested NIC Interventions

Circulatory care, exercise therapy: joint mobility, peripheral sensation management

Nursing Interventions and Rationales

- Perform neurovascular assessment q___h or minutes. Use the five Ps of assessment, which are the following:

  Pain—Assess severity (on scale of 1 to 10), quality, radiation, and relief by medications. *Pain that is unrelieved by medication can be an early symptom of compartment syndrome or may indicate that client needs more effective pain medication (Dykes, 1993).*

  Pulses—Check the pulses distal to the injury. Check uninjured side first to establish a baseline for a bilateral comparison. *An intact pulse generally indicates a good blood supply to the extremity (Dykes, 1993), although compartment syndrome may be present even if the pulse is intact (Gulli, Templeman, 1994).*

  Pallor—Check color and temperature changes below the fracture site. Check capillary refill. *A cold, pale, or bluish extremity indicates arterial insufficiency or arterial damage, and physician should be notified. Normal capillary refill is 3 seconds or less (Dykes, 1993).*

  Parasthesia (change in sensation)—Check by lightly touching the skin proximal and distal to the injury. Refer to the following chart (Dykes, 1993) for guidelines on how to best assess sensation. Ask if client has any unusual sensations such as hypersensitivity, tingling, prickling, decreased feeling, or numbness accompanied by a lack of sensation. *Changes in sensation are indicative of nerve compression and damage and can also indicate compartment syndrome (Dykes, 1993; Gulli, Templeman, 1994).*

  Paralysis—Ask client to do appropriate range of motion exercises in the unaffected and then the affected extremity. Refer to the following chart.

How to Check for Nerve Damage With Common Fractures

Fracture	Nerve damaged	Sensation	Motion
Humerus	Radial	Check over dorsum of index finger	Ask to hyperextend thumb
Radial	Radial	See above	See above
	Medial	Check over palmar surface of fingers	Ask to touch thumb to tip of little finger
Ulnar	Ulnar	Check little finger to ring finger	Ask to spread fingers
Femoral	Peroneal	Check top of foot between first and second toes	Ask to point toes toward head
Fibular	Peroneal	See above	See above
Tibial	Tibial	Ask if medial side of sole of foot feels warm	Ask to point toes downward

- Monitor client for symptoms of compartment syndrome evidenced by decreased sensation, weakness, loss of movement, pain with passive movement, pain greater than expected, pulselessness, and tension in the skin that surrounds the muscle compartment. The symptoms are not always present and can be difficult to assess.
  Compartment syndrome is characterized by increased pressure within the muscle compartment, which compromises circulation, viability, and function of tissues (Andrews, 1993; Gulli, Templeman, 1994).
- Monitor appropriate application and function of corrective device (e.g., cast, splint, traction) q___h.
  An improperly applied device can cause nerve damage, circulatory impairment, or pressure ulcers.
- Position extremity in correct alignment with each position change; check q___h to ensure appropriate alignment.
- Get client out of bed and mobilize as soon as possible after consultation with physician.
  Immobility is a well documented cause of deep vein thrombosis (DVT), in addition to many other complications from bedrest.
- Monitor for signs of DVT, especially in high risk populations of older than 40 years of age, immobility, obesity, taking estrogen or oral contraceptives, history of trauma or surgery, or history of previous DVT, cerebrovascular accident (CVA), varicose veins, malignancy, or cardiovascular disease.
  There are identified risk factors that increase the incidence of DVT and have been validated using a DVT risk scale (Autar, 1996).
- Apply thigh-high graduated compression elastic stockings if ordered; remove daily to give skin care.
  These stockings can be helpful in preventing DVT. If DVT risk is high, consult with physician regarding need for intermittent pneumatic compression of the calves or subcutaneous administration of heparin (Brock, 1994; Ecklund, 1995).
- Watch for signs of DVT evidenced by pain, deep tenderness, swelling in the calf and thigh, and redness in the involved extremity. Take serial leg measurements of the thigh and leg circumferences. In some clients there is a palpable, tender venous cord that can be felt in the popliteal fossa. Do not rely on Homan's sign.
  Thrombosis with clot formation is usually first detected as swelling of the involved leg and then as pain. Leg measurement discrepancies greater than 2 cm warrant further investigation. Homan's sign is not reliable (Slye, 1991; Herzog, 1992). Unfortunately, symptoms of DVTs will not be found on exam of 25% of the clients, even though a DVT is present (Eftychiou, 1996).
- Monitor for any signs of infection (e.g., edema, warmth, drainage, elevated temperature or white blood cell count) if there has been any surgical intervention.
- Help client perform prescribed exercises q___h.
- Provide a nutritious diet and adequate fluid replacement.
  Good nutrition and sufficient fluids are needed to promote healing and prevent complications.

Geriatric
- Use heat and cold therapies cautiously—elderly clients often have decreased sensation and circulation.

Home Care Interventions
- Assess knowledge base of client and family following any institutional care. Teach disease process and care as necessary.

Length of time for institutional care and teaching may have been very short and insufficient for learning.

- If risk is related to fractures and cast care, teach family to complete a neurovascular assessment; it may be as often as every 4 hours but is more commonly two to three times per day. *A risk requiring monitoring more often than every 4 hours for longer than 24 hours indicates a need for institutionally based care.*
- If fracture is peripheral, position the limb for comfort, and change position frequently, avoiding dependent positions for extended periods. *Changes in position enhance circulation.*
- Refer to physical therapy services as necessary to establish exercise program and safety in transfers or mobility within limitations of physical status.
- Establish an emergency plan. *A preset plan will save valuable time in the event of emergency.*

Client/Family Teaching

- Teach client and family to recognize signs for neurovascular dysfunction and report signs immediately to the appropriate person.
- Emphasize proper nutrition to promote healing.
- If necessary, refer client to rehabilitation facility for proper use of assistive devices and measures to improve mobility without compromising neurovascular function.

REFERENCES   Autar R: Nursing assessment of clients at risk of deep vein thrombosis (DVT): the autar DVT scale, *J Adv Nurs* 23:763, 1996.

Brock JC: Compression stockings: do they prevent DVT? *AJN* 11:25, 1994.

Donnor C: Critical difference: detecting venous thrombosis, *AJN* 93:48, 1993.

Dykes PC: Minding the five p's of neurovascular assessment, *Am J Nurs* 93:38, 1993.

Ecklund MM: Optimizing the flow of care for prevention and treatment of deep vein thrombosis and pulmonary embolism, *AACN Clin Issu* 6:588, 1995.

Eftychiou V: Clinical diagnosis and management of the patient with deep venous thromboembolism and acute pulmonary embolism, *Nurse Practitioner* 21:50, 1996.

Gulli B, Templeman D: Compartment syndrome of the lower extremity, *Orthoped Clin North Am* 25:677, 1994.

Herzog JA: Deep vein thrombosis in the rehabilitation client, *Rehab Nurs* 17:196, 1992.

Kayser SR: Management of venous thromboembolic (VTE) disease—Part I: prevention, *Progress Cardiovasc Nurs* 10:31, 1995.

Slye DA: Orthopedic complications: compartment syndrome, fat embolism syndrome, and venous thromboembolism, *Nurs Clin North Am* 26:113, 1991.

Personal identity disturbance

Gail B. Ladwig

Definition

The inability to distinguish between self and nonself

Defining Characteristics

Withdrawal from social contact, change in ability to determine relationship of body to environment, inappropriate or grandiose behavior (Carpenito, 1993)

Related Factors (r/t)

Situational crisis, psychological impairment, chronic illness, pain

Client Outcomes/Goals

- Shows interest in surroundings
- Responds to stimuli with appropriate affect
- Performs self-care and self-control activities appropriate for age
- Acknowledges personal strengths
- Engages in interpersonal relationships
- Verbalizes willingness to change life-style and use appropriate community resources

Suggested NIC Interventions

Decision-making support, self-esteem enhancement

Nursing Interventions and Rationales

- Offer reassurance to the client, and use therapeutic communication at frequent intervals.
  Client reassurance and communication are nursing skills that promote trust and orientation and reduce anxiety (Harvey, 1996).
- Address clients by name; let them know who is approaching and orient them to surroundings.
  These interventions help clients with loss of ego boundaries to identify boundaries between themselves and the environment (Haber et al, 1992).
- Have clients describe their perceptions of the environment as concretely as possible.
  These descriptions provide feedback that confirms the client's existence.
- Give clients permission to share their experiences; they have always lived in secrecy and they are not sure how much is safe to reveal or who believes their illness is an actual illness.
  An average of 6.8 years elapses between the time clients are first assessed and the time they receive an accurate diagnosis (Frye, 1990).
- Use touch only after a thorough assessment and as appropriate.
  Touch, which conveys caring, is an appropriate way of communicating unless it makes the person touched uncomfortable (Wells-Federman et al, 1995). Some clients may touch people to identify separateness from others; other clients experience fusion with others when they touch (Haber et al, 1992).
- Have all team members approach client consistently the same way.
  Consistency promotes trust, which is necessary for establishing a therapeutic relationship that helps the client develop interpersonal relationships.
- Provide time for one-to-one interactions to establish a therapeutic relationship.
  The most critical intervention a nurse can make is to offer to spend time with the client (Harrenstein, 1992).
- Encourage client to verbalize feelings about self and body image; have client make a list of positive strengths.
  These verbalizations help the client recognize the self; listing strengths promotes self-exploration.
- Hold client responsible for age-appropriate behavior; involve client in planning of self-care.
  Involving clients in care gives them a sense of control and helps the client gain ego strength (Preston, 1994).
- Give positive feedback when appropriate self-control is used.
  Positive reinforcement encourages repetition of behavior.
- Encourage participation in group therapy for feedback from others regarding behavior and building relationship skills.

An adaptive narcissistic client's need to depend on other people to feel whole suggests that group therapy could be a powerful tool in treating those who suffer profound wounds to self-esteem (Kurek-Ovshinsky, 1991).

- Use a daily diary to set achievable and realistic goals and monitor successes.
  Journal writing has been found to improve physical and mental health measureably (Wells-Federman et al, 1995).

Geriatric

- Monitor for signs of depression, grief, and withdrawal.
  The personal identity disturbance may mask underlying depression.
- Address clients by their full name preceded by the proper title (Mr., Mrs., Ms., Miss); use nickname or first name only if suggested by the client, and do not use terms of endearment (e.g., "honey").
  Calling a person honey, sweetie, or granny, etc., is demeaning and demoralizing and can increase feelings of loneliness by decreasing a sense of relatedness to self (Buchda, 1987).
- Practice reality orientation principles; ask specifically how the client feels about events that are happening.
  These steps help define ego boundaries.
- Ask client about important past experiences.
  Reconsideration of past experiences, missed opportunities, and mistakes allows older clients to reach ego integrity (Bulechek, McCloskey, 1992).

Home Care Interventions

- Assess client's immediate support system/family for relationship patterns and content of communication.
  Knowledge of relationship dynamics in the client's environment assists the nurse with individualizing care.
- Encourage family to provide support and feedback regarding client identity and ego boundaries.
  The family is a socially significant cultural group that generates behavior, defines roles, and promotes values.
- If client is involved in counseling or self-help groups, monitor and encourage attendance. Help client identify value of group participation after each group encounter.
  Discussion of group participation identifies group feedback and support and reinforces support for change.
- If client is taking prescribed psychotropic medications, assess for understanding of side effects of and reasons for taking medication. Teach as necessary.
- Assess medications for effectiveness and side effects and monitor for compliance.
  Clients with poor ego strength may have difficulty adhering to a medication regimen.

Client/Family Teaching

- Teach stress reduction and relaxation techniques.
  These techniques can be used when the client becomes anxious about the loss of self.
- Refer to community resources or other self-help groups appropriate for the client's underlying problem (e.g., Adult Children of Alcoholics, parent effectiveness group).
  Group therapy provides an arena in which clients can experience the interdependent mode of adaptation without assaults to self-esteem (Kurek-Ovshinsky, 1991).
- Be a role model for family members—talk *to* not *around* the client, give choices to the client when family members may be listening, always address the client by name, and do not interrupt when the client is attempting to communicate.

Role modeling helps to reinstate client individualism and value for a client who has been treated by the family as a "nonperson" (Dolphin, 1984).

- Teach the client appropriate self-care activities, such as dressing and use of assistive devices for eating.

REFERENCES   Buchda V: Loneliness in critically ill adults, *Dimens Crit Care Nurs* 6:335, 1987.

Bulechek G, McCloskey J: *Nursing interventions: essential nursing treatments,* ed 2, Philadelphia, 1992, WB Saunders.

Carpenito JL: *Nursing diagnosis: application to clinical practice,* ed 5, Philadelphia, 1993, JB Lippincott.

Dolphin N: Non-personhood: a nursing diagnosis in the psycho-social realm, *Home Healthcare Nurse* (1-2):16-18, 1984.

Frye B: Art and multiple personality disorder: an expressive framework for occupational therapy, *Am J Occup Ther* 44:1013, 1990.

Haber J et al: *Psychiatric nursing,* ed 4, St Louis, 1992, Mosby.

Harrenstein E: Young women and depression: origin, outcome and nursing care, *Nurs Clin North Am* 26:607, 1992.

Harvey M: Managing agitation in critically ill patients, *Am J Crit Care* 5:7, 1996.

Kurek-Ovshinsky C: Group psychotherapy in an acute inpatient setting: techniques that nourish self-esteem, *Issu Ment Health Nurs* 12:81, 1991.

Preston K: Rehabilitation nursing: a client-centered philosophy, *Am J Nurs* 94:66, 1994.

Wells-Federman C et al: The mind-body connection: the psychophysiology of many traditional nursing interventions, *Clin Nurse Spec* 9:59, 1995.

Risk for poisoning

Catherine Vincent

Definition   Accentuated risk of accidental exposure to or ingestion of drugs or dangerous products in doses sufficient to cause poisoning

Risk Factors
Internal (individual)

Reduced vision, verbalization of an occupational setting that lacks adequate safeguards, lack of safety or drug education, lack of proper precautions, cognitive or emotional difficulties, insufficient finances

External (environmental)

Large supplies of drugs in house, medicines or dangerous products placed or stored within the reach of confused persons, availability of illicit drugs potentially contaminated by poisonous additives, chemical contamination of food and water, unprotected or unventilated areas, presence of poisonous vegetation, presence of atmospheric pollutants

Related Factors (r/t)

See Risk Factors

Client Outcomes/Goals

- Averts inadvertent ingestion or exposures to toxins or poisonous substances
- Explains and undertakes appropriate safety measures to prevent ingestion or exposure to toxins or poisonous substances

Suggested NIC Interventions
Environmental management: safety

Nursing Interventions and Rationales

NOTE: Management of a risk diagnosis necessitates approaches using primary and secondary prevention. Primary prevention interventions, which include such activities as safety instruction, focus on thwarting the development of the disease or condition. Early detection through screening, monitoring, and surveillance is secondary prevention (Shortridge, Valanis, 1992).

- Identify risk factors noting special circumstances in which preventive or protective measures are indicated.
  Identification of family at risk signals special teaching and referral needs (McCloskey, Bulecheck, 1996).
- Evaluate lead exposure risk and consult regarding lead screening measures as indicated (public/ambulatory health).
  Lead poisoning is one of the most common and preventable types of childhood poisoning today. Assessment of exposure risk and blood level testing are important preventive measures (US Department of Health & Human Services, 1994; Agency Toxic Substance & Disease Registry, 1995).
- Properly label medications, including large print for the visually impaired. Supply "Mr. Yuk" labels for families with children.
  Implementing strategies from poisoning prevention programs benefits the client and family (Jones, 1993).
- Detect possible interactions and cumulative or other adverse effects between prescribed medications, self-administered over-the-counter products, and culturally based home treatments.
  Serious consequences may occur if interactions are not identified (Weitzel, 1992).
- Complete exposure history in work environment if toxic exposure occurs (occupational concerns).
  Early exposure detection and treatment and prevention of sequelae are important in the work setting (Agency Toxic Substance & Disease Registry, 1995).

Home Care Interventions

- Prepour medications for clients who are at risk of ingesting too much of a given medication because of mistakes in preparation. Delegate this task to family or caregivers if possible.
  Elderly clients who live alone are at greatest risk.
- Identify poisonous substances in the immediate surroundings of home such as garage or barn: include paints and thinners, fertilizers, rodent and bug control substances, animal medications, gasoline, and oil. Label with name, poison warning sign, and poison control center number. Lock out of the reach of children.
  Poisonous substances of equal danger exist in areas other than the internal home setting. Curious children are at risk for ingesting when exploring.
- Identify risk of toxicity from environmental activities such as spraying trees or roadside shrubs. Contact local departments of agriculture or transportation for Material Substance Data Sheets (MSDS) or to prevent the activity in desired areas.
  Women who are of childbearing age or pregnant and the elderly are at greatest risk.

Client/Family Teaching

Infant/child
- Provide guidance for parents/caregivers regarding age-related safety measures including the following:

- Storing potentially harmful substances in their original containers
- Avoiding storage of medications or toxic substances in food containers
- Placing poisonous houseplants out of the reach of infants and children
- Preventing access to poisonous outdoor plants
- Locking up cleaning agents, disinfectants, and other hazardous materials
- Using extreme caution with pesticides and gardening materials close to children's play areas
- Keeping perfume and makeup out of reach of children

Infants have a high level of hand-to-mouth behavior and will ingest anything. Young children may inadvertently ingest poisonous materials, particularly if they are thought to be food or beverage (Jones, 1993; Mitchell et al, 1995).

- Review necessity of keeping prescription and over-the-counter medications out of reach of children and secure. Lock cupboard if toddler prone to climbing.
  Once infants learn to crawl, they explore and are persistent. When children begin to walk, climb, and develop the concept of object and object permanence, they can reach most heights and open cupboards and unscrew lids. Many toxic substances are not protected with safety caps (Kuhn, 1992; Liebelt, Shannon, 1993; Corbett, 1995).

- Recommend placement of perfumes, ointments, creams, and talcum out of infant/child's reach.
  Even in small quantities, many common over-the-counter remedies and products can be lethal to infants and young children (Liebelt, Shannon, 1993; Morelli, 1993).

- Counsel client and family members regarding medication safety.
  - Avoid sharing prescriptions.
  - Read and follow labeling instructions on all products; adjust dosage for age.
  - Avoid excessive amounts and/or frequency of doses ("if a little does some good . . . a lot should do more").
  - Emphasize avoiding eating or drinking out of containers with the "Mr. Yuk" label (directed at children).

  Prevent overdosing or inadvertent poisoning resulting from inappropriate medication use (Kuhn, 1992).

- Advise family to post first aid charts and poison center instructions in accessible location. Poison control center phone numbers should be posted close to the phone. Poison control should always be called immediately before initiating any first aid measures.
  Rapid initiation of proper treatment reduces mortality and morbidity and decreases emergency room visits and inpatient admissions (Jones, 1993).

- Advise families with young children to prepare a first aid kit for poisoning. Keep syrup of ipecac on hand at all times (two doses per child) and any other supplies recommended by the local poison control center.
  Ipecac induces vomiting; other items will be used to neutralize effects.

- Encourage parents/family to take first aid and other types of safety-related programs.
  The programs extend their level of emergency preparation.

- Initiate referrals to peer group interventions, peer counseling, and other types of substance abuse prevention/rehabilitation programs when substance abuse is identified as a risk factor.
  Clients with substance abuse problems are at risk for contact with tainted substances or for overdose. The peer pressure factor is extremely strong for adolescents;

rehabilitation programs providing nonpunitive and skill-focused approaches are more effective (Anderson, 1996).

Geriatric
- Caution client and family to avoid storing medications with similar appearances close to one another (e.g., nitroglycerin ointment near toothpaste or denture creams). *Confusion and visual impairment can place the older person at risk of incorrectly identifying of contents (Weitzel, 1992).*
- Remind older persons to store medications out of reach when young children come to visit. *Children are inquisitive and may ingest medicines in containers without safety caps (Cudney, Hunter, 1992).*

REFERENCES
Agency Toxic Substance & Disease Registry: Lead toxicity, *AAOHN J* 43:428, 1995.

Agency Toxic Substance & Disease Registry: Taking an exposure history, *AAOHN J* 43:380, 1995.

Anderson NLR: Decisions about substance abuse among adolescents in juvenile detention, *Image* 28:65, 1996.

Corbett JV: Pharmacopeia: accidental poisoning with iron supplements, *MCN* 20:234, 1995.

Cudney SA, Hunter MM: Danger! Grandparents' drugs may be lethal to children: redesigning medicine packages may prevent tragedy, *Geriatr Nurs* 13:222, 1992.

Jones NE: Childhood residential injuries, *MCN* 18:1168, 1993.

Kuhn MM: Drug overdose: salicylates, *Crit Care Nurs* 12:16, 1992.

Liebelt E, Shannon MW: Small doses, big problems: a selected review of highly toxic common medications, *Pediatr Emerg Care* 9:292, 1993.

McCloskey JC, Bulechek GM, editors: *Nursing interventions classifications (NIC),* ed 2, St Louis, 1996, Mosby.

Mitchell A et al: Acute organophosphate pesticide poisoning in children, *MCN* 20:261, 1995.

Morelli J: Pediatric poisoning: the 10 most toxic prescription drugs, *Am J Nurs* 93:26, 1993.

Shortridge L, Valanis B: The epidemiological model applied in community health nursing. In Stanhope M, Lancaster J, editors: *Community health nursing: process and practice for promoting health,* ed 3, St Louis, 1992, Mosby.

US Department of Health and Human Services, US Public Health Service: Put prevention into practice: lead screening in children, *J Am Acad Nurs Prac* 6:379, 1994.

Weitzel EA: Medication management. In Bulechek GM, McCloskey JM, editors: *Nursing interventions: essential nursing treatments,* ed 2, Philadelphia, 1992, WB Saunders.

Post–trauma response

Judith S. Rizzo

Definition
The state in which an individual experiences a sustained painful response to an overwhelming traumatic event; response can occur immediately following an event, years later, or anytime in between

Defining Characteristics
Major
Intrusive responses; reexperiencing the traumatic event, which may be identified in cognitive, affective, behavioral, or sensory motor activities (e.g., flashbacks, intrusive thoughts, repetitive dreams or nightmares); excessive verbalization of the traumatic event; verbalization of survival guilt or guilt about behavior required for survival

Minor
Avoidance responses, psychic or emotional numbness (e.g., impaired interpretation of reality, confusion, dissociation, amnesia, vagueness about traumatic event, constricted affect), altered life-style (self-destructive behaviors such as substance abuse, suicide attempt, or other acting-out behaviors), difficulty with interpersonal relationships,

development of phobia regarding trauma, poor impulse control, irritability, explosiveness, obsessive-compulsive behaviors, panic; most common symptoms—sleeplessness, nightmares of the event, and anxiety, especially immediately following the event

Related Factors (r/t)

Natural or produced disasters, wars, epidemics, rape, assault, torture, catastrophic illnesses or accidents

Client Outcomes/Goals

- Returns to pretrauma level of functioning as quickly as possible
- Acknowledges the traumatic event and begins to work with the trauma by talking about the experience and expressing feelings of fear, anger, anxiety, guilt, and helplessness
- Identifies supports and available resources and is able to connect with them
- Returns to and strengthens coping mechanisms used in prior traumatic event
- Acknowledges event and perceives it without distortions
- Assimilates the event and moves forward to set and pursue life goals

Suggested NIC Interventions

Counseling, support system enhancement

Nursing Interventions and Rationales

- Observe for reaction to traumatic event in all clients regardless of age.
  Groups at risk are those who have a history of emotional problems, are domestic violence victims, have lost a friend or family member by homicide, are homeless, are sexual assault victims (especially those abused as children), and have previous involvement with a traumatic event. Give serious attention to childhood loss (Irwin, 1994). Posttraumatic stress disorder (PTSD) is the expected outcome of youth exposed to suicide, loss, and abuse (Brent, 1995).
- Observe the severity of the client's response and its effect on current functioning.
  The first few days following an event, expect a rollercoaster of emotions. A return to normal can take up to 6 to 8 weeks and for some it can take months (National Organization for Victim Assistance [N.O.V.A.], 1988).
- Provide a safe and therapeutic environment, enabling the client to regain control.
  Safety and empowerment are vital to recovery as are treating person with dignity and sensitivity and being able to tolerate high emotional arousal. Intervention must strike a balance between protection of the victim and confrontation about the reality of the event. A study showed that victims found the confrontational aspects, such as viewing the body, returning to the site, etc. to be helpful (Winje, Ulrick, 1995).
- Remain with client and provide support during periods of overwhelming emotions.
  Being able to withstand a client's strong emotions can be very difficult for an unskilled nurse. The client may initially be in shock and appear dazed or confused.
- Use touch with client's permission (e.g., hand on shoulder, holding hand).
  In a study of personal space invasion in the nurse-client relationship, anxiety scores of the experimental group showed a definite downward trend, indicating that the intrusion of a nurse into a client's space had a calming rather than a stimulating effect (Ricci, 1981).
- Use planned communication to assist client with describing the event and expressing feelings.
  A debriefing model for groups has shown to be effective for traumatized clients (Mitchell, 1988; N.O.V.A., 1988). These models can be modified for individuals.
- Provide opportunities for verbally emotional expression through activities.
  Avoid pressuring clients to express emotions if they are not ready to do so.

- Explore and enhance available support systems.
  Social supports clearly benefit the client. Social support was the most important factor in predicting adaptive coping among family members of seriously mentally ill (Solomon, Draine, 1995). Support systems decrease isolation, encourage communication, and provide diversional activities. Nurses should help traumatized children by strengthening their social relationships and enhancing their ability to self-soothe and process information, which helps them process traumatic memories (Burgess, Hartman, Clements, 1995).
- Assist client with regaining prior sleeping and eating habits.
  Disrupted sleep is the most prevalent symptom following a traumatic event (Schwartz, Kettley, Rizzo, 1992). Consider short-term drug treatment such as short-acting benzodiazepine for first few days following a traumatic event. Imipramine, fluoxetine, clonidine, and carbamazepine have shown promise (Marshall, Kleine, 1995).
- Help client use positive cognitive restructuring to reestablish feelings of self-worth.
  After a traumatic event, thinking often becomes negative and the client feels devalued.
- Normalize symptoms; help client to understand that their feelings and thoughts are a result of the trauma and do not indicate mental illness.
  Many symptoms of a trauma response are mistaken for mental illness, when actually they are normal responses to an abnormal event (Forster, 1994).
- Encourage client to return to normal routine as quickly as possible.
  Nurses can help traumatized children and adolescents relearn flexible responses to begin processing traumatic memories.

Geriatric

- Use environmental assessment skills to identify elderly clients who are traumatized by disaster and/or loss.
  The elderly who live alone are at greatest risk. Early intervention can minimize the response.
- Observe client for concurrent losses that may affect coping skills.
  As the elderly grow older, the number of losses are multiplied and compounded.
- Allow client more time to establish trust and express anger, guilt, and shame about the trauma.
- Review past coping skills and give client positive reinforcement for successfully dealing with other life crises.
  Clients who have adjusted positively to aging and can put events into proper perspective may adjust to loss more positively.
- Monitor client for clinical signs of depression and anxiety; refer to physician for medication if appropriate.
  Depression in the elderly is underestimated in this country.
- Instill hope.
  The therapeutic technique of reminiscence can renew hope (Forbes, 1994). The energy generated by hope can help elderly cope, overcome obstacles, and maintain normal functioning.

Home Care Interventions

- Assess family support and response to client's coping mechanisms. Refer family for medical social services or other counseling as necessary.
  Persons who have not shared the client's traumatic experience may have unrealistic expectations about recovery and recovery time. Support may be denied if the client's response to the trauma does not stay within support system expectations.

- Provide stable routine of day-to-day activities consistent with pretrauma experience. Do not force routine on client.

  Resuming a pretrauma routine can be reassuring to the client and can help place the trauma in perspective. Imposing an undesired routine can further isolate the client.

- If client is receiving medications, assess client's self-medicating ability. Assign a responsible person to administer medications if necessary.

  Crisis creates a feeling of helplessness. The client may be unable to make the simplest decisions (Spradley, 1990).

- Assess the impact of the trauma on significant others (e.g., a father may have to take over his partner's parenting responsibility after she has being raped and injured). Provide empathy and caring to significant others. Refer for additional services as necessary.

  Traumatic events can pose a crisis for significant others as well as the involved client.

Client/Family Teaching

- Explain to client and family what to expect the first few days after the traumatic event and in the future.

  Knowing what to expect can minimize much of the anxiety that accompanies a traumatic response.

- Teach positive coping skills and avoidance of negative coping skills such as alcohol use.

- Teach stress reduction methods such as deep breathing, visualization, meditation, and physical exercise. Encourage use especially when intrusive thoughts or flashbacks occur.

  After a traumatic event, it is tempting for clients to maladaptively cope with their overwhelming emotions, which can establish unhealthy patterns for the future.

- Encourage other healthy living habits with diet, sleep, exercise, family activities, and spiritual pursuits.

- Refer client to peer support groups.

  Peer support decreases sense of social isolation, enhances knowledge, and increases coping skills (Solomon, Draine, 1995).

- Instruct family in ways to be helpful and supportive to the traumatized person. Emphasize importance of listening and "being there" and that there are no magic phrases capable of easing the person's emotional suffering.

REFERENCES
Bille D: Post-traumatic stress disorder: the hidden victim, *J Psychosoc Nurs* 31:19, 1993.

Brent D: Risk factors for adolescent suicide and suicidal behavior, mental and substance abuse disorders, family environmental factors, and life stress, *Suicide Life Threatening Beh* 25 (suppl):52, 1995.

Burgess A, Hartman C, Clements P: Biology of memory and childhood trauma, *J Psychosoc Nurs Ment Health Serv* 33:16, 1995.

Cohen L: Psychiatric hospitalization as an experience of trauma, *Archives Psych Nurs* 8:78, 1994.

Cox H et al: *Clinical applications of nursing diagnosis: adult, child, women's, psychiatric, gerontologic and home health considerations,* ed 2, Philadelphia, 1993, FA Davis.

Forbes S: Hope: an essential human need in the elderly, *J Gerontologic Nurs* 20:5, 1994.

Forster, King: Traumatic stress reactions and the psychiatric emergency, *Psychiatric Ann* 24:603, 1994.

Irwin J: Proneness to dissociation and traumatic childhood, *J Nerv Ment Dis* 182:456, 1994.

Marshall R, Kleine D: Pharmacotherapy in the treatment of post traumatic stress disorder, *Psych Annals* 25:588-97, 1995.

Mitchell J: Stress: development and functions of a critical incident stress debriefing team, *J Emerg Med Serv* 13:43, 1988.

National Organization for Victim Assistance Training Manual (N.O.V.A.): *Coordinating a Community Crisis Response,* 1988, The Organization.

Ricci MS: An experiment with personal space invasion in the nurse-patient relationship and its effect on anxiety, *Issue Ment Health Nurs* 3:203, 1981.

Schwartz J, Kettley J, Rizzo J: Predictors of vulnerability after trauma, unpublished manuscript, 1992.

Solomon P, Draine J: Adaptive coping among family members of persons with serious mental illness, *Psych Serv* 46:1156, 1995.

Spradley B: *Community health nursing, concepts and practice,* ed 3, Glenview, Ill, 1990, Scott Foresman/Little, Brown.

Stern P, Kerry J: Restructuring life after home loss by fire, *Image* 28:11, 1996.

Winje D, Ulvik A: Confrontations with reality: crises intervention services for traumatized families after a school bus accident in Norway, *J Traumatic Stress* 8:429, 1995.

Powerlessness

Gail B. Ladwig

Definition   Perception that one's own actions will not significantly affect an outcome; a perceived lack of control over a current situation or immediate happening

Defining Characteristics

Severe   Verbalized inability to control or influence situation; verbalized inability to control self-care, depression regarding physical deterioration that occurs despite client compliance with regimens, apathy

Moderate   Nonparticipation in care or decision-making when opportunities are provided; verbalized dissatisfaction regarding inability to perform previous tasks or activities; no monitoring of progress; verbalized doubt regarding role performance; reluctance to express true feelings; fear of alienation from caregivers; passivity; inability to seek information regarding care; dependence on others that may result in irritability, resentment, anger, and guilt; no defending of self-care practices when challenged about them

Related Factors (r/t)

Health care environment, interpersonal interactions, life-style of helplessness, illness-related regimen

Client Outcomes/Goals

- States feelings of powerlessness and other feelings related to powerlessness (e.g., anger, sadness, hopelessness)
- Identifies factors that are uncontrollable
- Participates in planning care; makes decisions regarding care and treatment when possible
- Asks questions about care and treatment
- Verbalizes hope for the future

Suggested NIC Interventions

Self-esteem enhancement, self-responsibility facilitation

Nursing Interventions and Rationales

- Observe for factors contributing to powerlessness (e.g., immobility, hospitalization, unfavorable prognosis, no support system, misinformation about situation, inflexible routine).
  Correctly identifying the actual or perceived problem is essential to providing appropriate support measures.

- Establish therapeutic relationship with clients by spending one-to-one time with them, assigning the same caregiver, and keeping commitments (e.g., saying, "I will be back to answer your questions in the next hour").
  The trust and consistency fostered by a therapeutic relationship provides the client with a secure environment in which to deal with problems and develop adaptation skills (Johnson, 1993).
- Allow client to express hope, which may range from "I hope my coffee will be hot," to "I hope I will die with my significant other here." Listen to client's priorities.
  Hope is a way of coping with a stressful situation and motivates the client to continue living. Motivation is necessary in the change process.
- Allow time for questions (15 to 20 minutes each shift); have client write down questions.
  Allowing time for questions encourages the client to take some control of the situation (Roberts, White, 1990).
- Have client assist in planning of care if possible (e.g., determining what time to bathe, taking pain medication before uncomfortable procedures, expressing food and fluid preferences); document specifics in care plan.
  Assisting in care planning also encourages the client to take some control of the situation (Roberts, White, 1990).
- Keep items client uses and needs, such as urinal, tissues, phone, and television controls, within reach.
  Client is able to participate in own care if care devices are accessible. Participation in care enhances a sense of control.
- When dealing with possible long-term deficits, work with the client to set small, attainable goals.
  Clients with spinal-cord injuries focus hope on small gains and take one step at a time. One client stated, "Every little step I took was more important to me than what I had in the end" (Morse, Doberneck, 1995).
- Have client write goals (e.g., dangle legs at bedside 10 minutes for 2 days, then sit in chair 10 minutes for 2 days, then walk to window) and plans to achieve them.
  Active participation enhances a feeling of power.
- Give praise for accomplishments.
  Positive reinforcement encourages repetition of behavior.
- Help clients identify factors not under their control.
  Identifying items with client's control encourages the client to take some control of the situation.
- Keep interactions with client focused on client, not on family or physician; actively listen to client.
  Such a focus helps the client to maintain a sense of self. The client can use a lot of energy by holding in unacceptable or frightening feelings. By listening to the client and allowing these feelings to be expressed, the energy is released and can be used in other ways (Clark, 1993).
- Acknowledge subjective concerns or fears.
  All feelings are personal and have meaning for the client.
- Allow client to take control of as many activities of daily living as possible; keep client informed of all care that will be given.
  Clients are more amenable to therapy if they know what to expect and can perform some tasks independently.

- Develop contract with client that states client's and nurse's responsibilities and privileges.
  A contract helps give a situation structure, clarifies what may or may not happen, and who has responsibility for the client's care.
- See **Hopelessness** and **Spiritual Distress.**

Geriatric

- Explore feelings of powerlessness—the feeling that client's behavior will not affect outcomes
  Quadriplegics and patients more than 60 years of age had higher incidences of feelings of powerlessness (p < 0.5) (Richmond et al, 1992).
- Establish therapeutic relationships by listening; give the client choices and accept the statement of their limitations.
  "Power with" interactions occur when the staff listens to clients: "In therapy, my therapist listened to me. She would not push me if I couldn't do it. She would switch and we would do something else." This factor helped motivate people in a geriatric rehabilitation unit (Resnick, 1996).
- Encourage positive use of solitude—reading, listening to music, enjoying nature—to prevent loneliness.
  A positive use of solitude, with decreased dependence on external stimuli, may be particularly important for older individuals who often find themselves increasingly alone without external stimuli or social support (Rane-Szostak, Herth, 1994).
- Provide reading materials for clients who are able to read.
  Older people who enjoyed reading for pleasure were rarely lonely (Rane-Szostak, Herth, 1994).

Home Care Interventions

NOTE: All of the mentioned nursing interventions are applicable in the home care setting. Include an initial and ongoing assessment and evaluation of potential abuse and neglect. Photograph evidence of abuse or neglect when possible.
  Assault is the single major cause of injury to women (Attala, 1996).
  Chronic abuse and neglect by spouse or other family among the elderly is often hidden until home care is actively involved.

- If neglect or abuse is suspected, identify an emergency plan that addresses the problem immediately and includes a report to the appropriate authorities.
  Client safety is a nursing priority. Reporting is a legal requirement of health care workers.
- Develop a written contract with client that designates what care will be given and responsibility for care elements. Focus should be on care that is controlled by the client.
  A written contract reassures the client that control of care as designated will be honored.
- Empower clients by allowing them to guide specifics of care such as wound care procedures and dressing and grooming details. Confirm client knowledge before empowering and document in chart that client is able to guide procedures. Document in home and in chart preferred approach to procedures. Orient family and caregivers to client role.
  Empowering the client as described motivates the client to actively learn and participate in care. Client values self and perceives power secondary to level of knowledge. Accurate documentation of client knowledge and abilities supports teamwork with health care team and avoids conflict.

Client/Family Teaching

- Explain all procedures, treatments, and expected outcomes.
  Clients are more amenable to therapy if they know what to expect.
- Provide written instructions for treatments and procedures for which the client will be responsible.
  A written record provides a concrete reference so that the client and family can clarify any verbal information that was given. People tend to forget half of what they hear within a few minutes, so it is important for nurses to supplement oral instructions with written material (Wong, 1992).
- Teach stress reduction, relaxation, and imagery. Many cassette tapes are available on relaxation and meditation. Assist the client with relaxation based on the client's preference indicated in the initial assessment.
  Such techniques are useful in combating depression, hopelessness, powerlessness, and poor self-image (Anderson, 1992). Individuals experiencing a sense of powerlessness can use imagery to develop a much needed sense of control (Stephens, 1993).
- Teach cognitive activities, such as using "self talk"—telling self that the situation is under own control and things can change.
  Self-motivation techniques such as "self talk" facilitate lasting behavior change (McSweeney, 1993).
- Help client practice assertive communication techniques.
  Clients with conditions such as quadriplegia need to be assertive so that they can direct their care and be as independent as possible (Bach, McDaniel, 1993).
- Role play (e.g., say, "Tell me what you are going to ask your doctor").
  Role playing is the most commonly used technique in assertiveness training. It deconditions the anxiety that arises from interpersonal encounters.
- Refer to support groups, pastoral care, or social services.
  These services help decrease levels of stress, increase levels of self-esteem, and reassure clients that they are not alone.

REFERENCES

Anderson SB: Guillain-Barre syndrome: giving the patient control, *J Neurosci Nurs* 24:158, 1992.

Attala JM: Detecting abuse against women in the home, *Home Care Provider* 1:1, 1996.

Bach C, McDaniel R: Quality of life in quadriplegic adults: a focus group study, *Rehab Nurs* 18:364, 1993.

Clark S: Challenges in critical care nursing: helping patients and families cope, *Crit Care Nurse* (suppl) 2:3, 1993.

Johnson BS: *Adaptation and growth: psychiatric-mental health nursing,* Philadelphia, 1993, JB Lippincott.

McSweeney J: Making behavior changes after a myocardial infarction, *West J Nurs Res* 15:441, 1993.

Morse J, Doberneck B: Delineating the concept of hope, *Image* 27:277, 1995.

Rane-Szotak D, Herth K: A new perspective on loneliness in later life, *Issu Ment Health Nurs* 16:583, 1994.

Resnick B: Motivation in geriatric rehabilitation, *Image* 28:41, 1996.

Richmond T et al: Powerlessness in acute spinal cord injury patients: a descriptive study, *J Neurosci Nurs* 24:146, 1992.

Roberts S, White BS: Powerlessness and personal control model applied to the myocardial infarction patient, *Prog Cardiovasc Nurs* 5:84, 1990.

Stephens R: Imagery: a strategic intervention to empower clients: Part II—A practical guide, *Clin Nurse Spec* 7:235, 1993.

Wong M: Self-care instructions: do patients understand educational materials? *Focus Crit Care* 19:47, 1992.

Altered protection

Betty J. Ackley

Definition   The state in which an individual experiences a decrease in the ability to guard self from internal or external threats such as illness or injury

Defining Characteristics

Major   Deficient immunity, impaired healing, altered clotting, maladaptive stress response, neurosensory alteration

Minor   Chilling, perspiring, dyspnea, cough, itching, restlessness, insomnia, fatigue, anorexia, weakness, immobility, disorientation, pressure sores

Related Factors (r/t)

Extremes of age, inadequate nutrition, alcohol abuse, abnormal blood profiles (e.g., leukopenia, thrombocytopenia, anemia, coagulation), drug therapies (e.g., antineoplastic, corticosteroid, immune, anticoagulant, thrombolytic), treatments (e.g., surgery, radiation), diseases (e.g., cancer, immune disorders)

Client Outcomes/Goals

- Remains free of infection
- Remains free of any evidence of new bleeding
- Explains precautions to take to prevent infection
- Explains precautions to take to prevent bleeding

Suggested NIC Interventions

Bleeding precautions, infection control, infection protection

Nursing Interventions and Rationales

- Take temperature, pulse, and blood pressure q____h.
  Changes in vital signs can indicate the onset of bleeding or infection.
- Observe nutritional status (e.g., weight, serum protein and albumin, muscle mass size, usual food intake). Work with dietician to increase nutritional status if needed.
  Good nutrition is needed to maintain immune function and support formation of clotting elements.
- Observe sleep pattern; if altered, see nursing interventions and rationales for **Sleep pattern disturbance.**
- Determine amount of stress in client's life. If stress is uncontrollable, see nursing interventions for **Ineffective individual coping.**
  Uncontrolled stress depresses immune system function (Carter, 1993).

Prevention of infection

- Monitor for signs of infection (e.g., fever, chills, flushed skin, drainage, edema, redness, and pain).
  The immune system is stimulated with the onset of infection, resulting in classic signs of infection.
- If immune system is depressed, notify physician of elevated temperature, even in the absence of other symptoms of infection.
  Clients with depressed immune function are unable to mount the usual immune responses to the onset of infection; fever may be the only sign of infection (Wujcik, 1993).
- If white blood cell count is severely decreased (absolute neutrophil count less than 1000 per mm^3), initiate the following precautions:
  - Take vital signs every 4 hours.
  - Complete a head-to-toe assessment twice daily, including inspection of oral mucosa, invasive sites, wounds, urine, and stool; monitor for onset of new complaints of pain.

- Avoid using urinary catheters, injections, or rectal or vaginal procedures.
  Infection can invade when a treatment damages the skin or mucous membranes, which are natural barriers against infection (Flyge, 1993).
- Take meticulous care of all invasive sites.
- Provide frequent oral care.
  The effects of chemotherapy or radiation leave the mouth inflamed; combined with immunosuppression it can result in stomatitis. Good oral care can help prevent this complication (Dose, 1995).
- Have client wear a mask when leaving room.
- Limit and screen visitors to minimize exposure to contagion. Enforce careful handwashing for everyone entering the room.
- Help client bathe daily.
- Serve client a low-microbial cooked food diet, serve well-cooked food only, avoid raw foods, processed meats, soft cheeses, serve sterile water or boiled liquids only (Carter, 1993).
- Help client to cough and deep breathe regularly; maintain appropriate activity level.
- Obtain a private room for client. Take ordered precautions including use of protective isolation or laminar air flow room.
  A private room is always necessary for neutropenic clients. There is no standardization of infection prevention practices nationwide for bone marrow transplant clients (Poe et al, 1994). A client with an absolute neutrophil count of less than 1000 per mm³ is severely neutropenic, has an impaired immune function, and is very prone to infection. Precautions should be taken to limit exposure to pathogens (Wujcik, 1993).
- Watch for signs of sepsis including change in mental status, fever, shaking, chills, and hypotension.
  These are indicators of sepsis (Flyge, 1993).
- See care plan for **Risk for infection** for more interventions regarding prevention of infection.

Prevention of bleeding

- Monitor client's risk for bleeding; evaluate clotting studies and platelet counts.
  Laboratory studies give a good indication of the seriousness of the bleeding disorder.
- Watch for hematuria, melena, hematemesis, hemopytsis, epistaxis, bleeding from mucosa, petechiae, and ecchymoses.
  These areas of bleeding can be detected in a bleeding disorder (Ellenberger et al, 1993; Paschall, 1993).
- Give medications orally or intravenously (IV) only; avoid giving them intramuscularly or subcutaneously. Apply pressure for a longer time than usual to invasive sites such as venipuncture or injection sites.
  Additional pressure is needed to stop bleeding of invasive sites of clients with bleeding disorders.
- Take vital signs frequently; watch for changes associated with fluid-volume loss.
  Excessive bleeding causes a decreased blood pressure and increased pulse and respiratory rates.
- Monitor menstrual flow if relevant; have client use pads instead of tampons.
  Menstruation can be excessive in clients with bleeding disorders. Tampons can increase trauma to the vagina.

- Have client use a moistened toothette instead of a toothbrush. Avoid flossing and use alcohol-free dental products.
  These actions help prevent bleeding in the oral mucosa.
- Ask client to either not shave or only use an electric razor.
  These steps help prevent any unnecessary trauma that could result in bleeding.
- To decrease risk of bleeding, avoid administering salicylates or nonsteroidal antiinflammatory drugs (NSAIDs).
  Salicylates and NSAIDs can cause gastrointestinal bleeding; salicylates interfere with platelet function and can increase bleeding.

Home Care Interventions

- For terminally ill clients, teach and institute all of the mentioned noninvasive precautions that will maintain quality of life. Discuss with client, family, and physician the consequences of contracting infection; determine which precautions do not maintain quality of life and should not be used (e.g., physical assessment twice daily, multiple vital sign assessments).
  Multiple assessments and other invasive procedures are recovery-based, cure-focused activities. The client and physician must agree on an approach to care for the client's remaining life.

Client/Family Teaching

Depressed immune function

- Teach precautions to take to decrease the chance of infection (e.g., avoiding uncooked fruits or vegetables, using appropriate self-care, ensuring a safe environment).
- Teach client and family how to take a temperature. Encourage family to take client's temperature between 3 PM and 7 PM at least once daily.
  The client's temperature is more likely to be elevated in the evening hours because the circadian rhythm peaks during this time (Samples et al, 1985).
- Teach client and family to notify physician of elevated temperature, even in the absence of other symptoms of infection.
  Clients with depressed immune function are unable to mount the usual immune response to the onset of infection; fever may be the only present sign of infection (Wujcik, 1993).
- Teach client to avoid crowds and contact with persons who have infections.
- Teach the need for good nutrition, avoidance of stress, and adequate rest to maintain immune system function.
  Client education to increase nutrition, manage stress, and perform self-care can reduce the risk of neutropenic infection (Carter, 1993).

Bleeding disorder

- Teach client to wear a Medic-Alert bracelet and notify all health care personnel of the bleeding disorder.
- Teach client and family the signs of bleeding, precautions to take to prevent bleeding, and action to take if bleeding begins.
- Caution client to avoid taking over-the-counter medications without permission of physician.
  Medications containing salicylates can increase bleeding.
- Teach client to wear loose-fitting clothes and avoid physical activity that might cause trauma.

REFERENCES   Carter LW: Influences of nutrition and stress on people at risk for neutropenia: nursing implications, *Oncol Nurs Forum* 10:1241, 1993.

Dose AM: The symptom experience of mucositis, stomatitis, and xerostomia, *Semin Oncol Nurs* 11:248, 1995.

Ellenberger BJ, Hass L, Cundiff L: Thrombotic thrombocytopenia purpura: nursing during the acute phase, *Dimens Crit Care Nurs* 12:58, 1993.

Flyge HA: Meeting the challenge of neutropenia, *Nursing* 23:60, 1993.

Paschall FE: Thrombotic thrombocytopenic purpura: the challenges of a complex disease process, *AACN Clin Issu* 4:655, 1993.

Poe SS et al: A national survey of infection prevention practices on bone marrow transplant units, *Oncol Nurs Forum* 21:1687, 1994.

Samples JF et al: Circadian rhythms: basis for screening for fever, *Nurs Res* 34:377, 1985.

Shuey KM: Platelet-associated bleeding disorders, *Semin Oncol Nurs* 12:15, 1996.

Wujcik D: Infection control in oncology patients, *Nurs Clin North Am* 28:639, 1993.

Rape trauma syndrome

Nancee B. Radtke

Definition   The trauma syndrome that develops after actual or attempted forced, violent, sexual penetration against the victim's will and consent.

The syndrome includes an acute phase of disorganization of the victim's life-style and a long-term process of life-style reorganization.

NOTE: Recent research challenges the two-phrase theory of trauma processing that is part of the NANDA diagnosis of **Rape trauma syndrome.** Research found that a victim's level of distress resulting from tension, depression, anger, fatigue, and confusion between 6 and 21 days following trauma was highly predictive of the distress level at 3 months following the trauma; this distress level remained relatively stable up to 4 years (Kilpatrick, Veronen, Best, 1985). This syndrome may include two other components: rape trauma, compound reaction and rape trauma, silent reaction. There are additional nursing care plans for each of these diagnoses.

Defining Characteristics

Acute phase   Emotional reactions (e.g., anger, embarrassment, fear of physical violence and death, humiliation revenge, self-blame), multiple physical symptoms (e.g., gastrointestinal irritability, genitourinary discomfort, muscle tension, sleep pattern disturbance), anxiety, fear, shame, pale complexion, weak pulse, shallow breathing, subdued feelings, numbness, disbelief, slow and inaudible speech, crying

Long-term phase

Changes in life-style (e.g., changing residence, dealing with repetitive nightmares and phobias, seeking family support, seeking social network support)

Rape victims experience emotional, physical, and cognitive reactions to the trauma of rape. During adjustment, clients resume activities, deal with practical matters, deny feelings about rape, experience daydreams and flashbacks, and are less interested in talking about the rape. During integration clients may suddenly become depressed and unable to stop thinking about the rape. Certain experiences trigger memories and nightmares, and clients may experience difficulty working through feelings. The trial of the rapist may also cause problems. As clients recover, they return to their level of functioning before the assault. Unfortunately, persistent depressive symptoms and suicide ideations and attempts are frequent (Tyra, 1993).

Client Outcomes/Goals

- Shares feelings, concerns, and fears
- Recognizes that the rape or attempt was not own fault
- States that no matter what the situation, no one has the right to assault another
- Identifies behaviors and situations within own control to prevent or reduce risk of recurrence
- Describes treatment procedures and reasons for treatment
- Reports absence of physical complications or pain
- Identifies support people and is able to ask them for help in dealing with this trauma
- Functions at same level as before crisis, including sexual functioning
- Recognizes that it is normal for full recovery to take a year.

Suggested NIC Interventions

Crisis intervention, rape-trauma treatment

Nursing Interventions and Rationales

- Observe client's responses including anger, fear, self-blame, sleep pattern disturbances, and phobias.
- Monitor client's verbal and nonverbal psychological state (e.g., crying, wringing hands, avoiding interactions or eye contact with staff).
  The most depressed victims are those most concerned with being stigmatized and blamed for the crime (Frable, Blackstone, Sherbaum, 1990).
- Stay with (or have a trusted person stay with) client initially. If a law enforcement interview is permitted, provide support by staying with client.
  Early crisis intervention involves helping client decide who to tell about the rape and regain the control during the assault.
- Explain each part of treatment. Discuss importance of pelvic examination; if it is the first examination, explain instruments and let client know when and where you will touch.
  Do not wait for the client to ask questions; explain everything you are doing and why it must be done, and when and where you will touch. Eye contact is very important because it helps the client feel worthy and alive (Ruckman, 1992).
- Observe for signs of physical injury. Ask questions such as, "Did he push you?" "Did he hit you?" "Did he choke you?" and "Do you feel sore anywhere?" Instruct client to return for additional photos if bruises become more pronounced in a few days.
  It is important to carefully document that force was used and sexual contact was not consensual. Sore areas are not visible in photos.
- Encourage client to verbalize feelings.
  Listening to clients helps them gain self-control by feeling acceptance from others (Ruckman, 1992).
- Provide privacy so that client can express feelings. Limit the number of nurses present, escort to treatment room as soon as possible, do not question in triage area, close curtains and door, and avoid other interruptions during contact with client (e.g., telephone calls, leaving the room, outside stimuli such as radios).
- Document a one- or two-sentence summary of what happened; getting the details of the sequence of events is the police officer's job.
  If some details that are not in the nurse notes were told to police, the defense attorney may attempt to make this look like a discrepancy in facts, causing reasonable doubt and resulting in an acquittal (Ledry, 1992).

- Enlist the help of supportive counselors who are experienced with rape trauma; refer client to a rape crisis counselor, mental health clinic, or psychotherapist.
  After physical needs are met, the client should be placed in the care of a counselor who can maintain a relationship long after discharge from the emergency department (Ruckman, 1992).
- Instead of asking clients if they want you to call the community rape crisis center, describe it and how their staff will be available after clients go home.
  Clients want control but may have difficulty making decisions during the initial visit to the emergency department. Involvement of social service agencies will help to guarantee a timely follow-up home visit (Jones, 1994).
- Explain collection of specimens for evidence; provide items for self-care after examination (e.g., cleansing the vaginal and rectal area).
  A card with the victim's name and date is held next to the injury in each picture for identification; direct quotes rather than summaries or paraphrases should be used. Most states provide sexual assault evidence collection kits, which prevent any inconsistencies in the collection of evidence that will be used in court.
- Explain that client's undergarments may need to be kept for evidence; instruct client to put other clothing in a paper bag once at home and to not wash it until it is known if it will be needed for evidence.
  Do not place clothes in plastic because moisture may accumulate and cause deterioration. Observe for seminal fluid on body with a Wood's lamp, which shows seminal fluid as flourescent yellow and violet colors in a dark room (Ledray, 1995).
- Discuss the possibility of pregnancy and sexually transmitted diseases (STDs) and the treatments available.
  Administering a urine pregnancy test is routine before giving medications to prevent pregnancy or treat STDs. Most clients prefer to prevent pregnancy rather than face the possibility of terminating it in the future. The risk of human immunodeficiency virus (HIV) exposure is a special concern to rape victims; the nurse should bring the issue up and inform the client of locations and schedules for HIV testing.
- Explain that it is the client's choice whether or not to report the rape.
  The first step in evidence collection is obtaining a signed consent from the client to do an examination and release collected evidence to police.
- Encourage client to report the rape.
  It is important for rape victims to recognize they are victims of a crime that is not their fault (Ledry, 1992). Reporting is an issue separate from prosecution; if victims report, they will not be forced to appear as a witness.
- Discuss client's support system; involve support system if appropriate and client grants permission. Unsupportive and victim-blaming attitudes by significant others are common responses.
  Research indicates that significant others are coping with their own responses to trauma and may be incapable of supporting the victim (Mackey et al, 1992).
- Obtain blood alcohol level if indicated.

Geriatric
- Build a trusting relationship with client.
  Recognize the attitudes and values of an older generation; stigmatization may cause victim to view self with disgust and shame (DeLorey, Wolf, 1993).
- Explain reporting and encourage client to report.
  Embarrassment may prevent reporting; respect client's choice. Older rape victims have

reported having a greater fear of people finding out about their rape than younger women (Tyra, 1993).

- Observe for psychosocial distress (e.g., memory impairment, sleep disturbances, regression, changes in bodily functions).
  Exacerbation of a chronic illness may be a major consequence of sexual assault.
- Identify new injuries related to the assault and their immediate effects on the client's existing health problems (e.g., cardiovascular disease, arthritis, respiratory disease).
  A review of the client's current medications may add to the nurse's understanding of relevant health problems.
- Modify the rape protocol to promote comfort for geriatric clients. Consider positioning female clients with pillows rather than stirrups and consider using a smaller speculum.
  Aging results in decreased muscle tone and thinning of the vaginal wall.
- Assess for mobility limitations and cognitive impairment.
  Elicit information from family or caregivers to verify level of functioning before sexual assault.
- Respect client's need for privacy.
  Older clients may be reluctant to have their children or younger family members present during examination and treatment; give clients a choice.
- Consider arrangements for temporary housing.
  Most sexual assaults of older clients occur in the home.
  NOTE: Older age makes a client more powerless, especially if isolated as a result of living alone. Physical injury can have a much greater effect on older victims, and they may experience a compound reaction because they are older. Sexual violence against an older female is a reflection of antiage and antiwoman attitudes. Sixty percent of sexually assaulted older females are severely injured, 10% are murdered, 7% are stabbed, and 43% are beaten (Delorey, Wolf, 1993).

Male rape
- Reactions to male rape are often either disbelief or an assumption that males who are raped are gay.
  Most females are aware of the possibility that they may be raped, many males are not. The care required is very similar to the care of females who have been raped (Laurent, 1993). Approximately 10% of rape victims who go to rape crisis centers are men (Dunn, Gilchrist, 1993).

Home Care Interventions

- Interact with client nonjudgmentally; it supports the client's self-worth.
  Rape victims usually experience a loss of self-worth.
- Assist the client with realistically assessing the home setting for safety and/or selecting a safe environment in which to live.
  Rape clients may be unable to make a realistic assessment of home safety both immediately after the rape and during long-term recovery.
- Ensure that client has support system in place for long-term support. Instruct family that recovery may take a long time. Refer for medical social work services to assist in setting a support system if necessary. Refer for counseling if necessary.
  The long-term response to rape (up to 4 years) requires ongoing support for the client to reorganize and reintegrate.
- Make sure that physical symptoms from the rape or other physical conditions are followed up.
  Stress response to rape can precipitate reemergence of other physical conditions that may be ignored because of the rape.

Client/Family Teaching

- Provide information on prophylactic antibiotic therapy, hepititis B vaccine, and tetanus prophylaxis for unimmunized patients with trauma.

Prophylaxis for adult victims of sexual assault

Antibiotic prophylaxis
Use one of the following:
Ceftriaxone (250 mg intramuscularly)
Spectinomycin (2 g intramuscularly) plus doxycycline (100 mg orally, twice a day for 7 days)
Azithromycin (1 g orally, single dose) plus metronizadole (2 g orally, single dose)

Prevention of pregnancy
Use one of the following:
Two oral contraceptive tablets (each containing 50 µg of ethinyl estradiol, taken twice 12 hr apart)
Three oral contraceptive tablets (each containing 35 µg of ethinyl estradiol, taken twice 12 hr aprt) plus an antiemetic

---

Prophylactic antibiotic therapy should be prescribed if the assailant is known to be infected, the victim has signs or symptoms of infection, or prophylaxis is requested (Hampton, 1995).
- Discharge instructions should be written for client.
Anxiety can hamper comprehension and retention of information; repeat instructions and provide them in a written form.
- Give instructions to significant others.
Significant others need many of the same supportive and caring interventions as the client; suggest that they too might benefit from counseling.
- Explain purpose of "morning after pill."
The morning after pill—norgestrel (Ovral)—prevents pregnancy and is only used in emergencies. It must be taken within 72 hours (3 days) of sexual contact for it to work. It will not cause a miscarriage if client is already pregnant, but it could harm the baby.
- Explain potential for common side effects related to treatment with norgestrel, such as breast swelling or nausea and vomiting. (Call the emergency department if client vomits within 1 hour of taking pill, because pill may need to be taken again.) The period may take 3 to 30 days to start; if period has not started in 30 days, contact physician.
- Explain potential for severe side effects related to treatment with norgestrel, such as severe leg or chest pain, trouble breathing, coughing up of blood, severe headache or dizziness, and trouble seeing or talking.
- Advise client to call or return if new problems develop.
Physical injuries may not be recognized as a result of client's "numbness" during the initial examination or because client may have forgotten or not understood some of the instructions.

- Teach relaxation techniques.
- Discuss practical life-style changes within client's control to reduce the risk of future attacks.

  Financial limitations can limit some alternatives such as moving to another home. Provide other alternatives such as keeping doors locked, checking car before getting in, not walking alone at night, keeping someone informed of whereabouts, asking someone to check if client has not arrived within reasonable amount of time, keeping lights on in entryway, having keys in hand when approaching car or house, having a remote-key entry car or garage.

- Teach client to use self-defense techniques to surprise attacker and get an opportunity to run for help. Refer client to self-defense school.
- Teach client appropriate outlets for anger.
- Encourage significant other to direct anger at event and attacker, not at the client.
- Emphasize vulnerability of client and ensure that reactions are appropriate for the victim of sexual assault.

  Females are at higher risk for depression than males, and the risk is significantly higher between the ages of 18 and 44 (Mackey et al, 1992).

NOTE: Post-traumatic stress disorder (PTSD) has a high probability of being a psychological sequelae to rape. Research demonstrated two effective treatments for improvement of PTSD in rape victims—prolonged exposure and stress inoculation training (Foa, Steketee, Roghbaum, 1991). Prolonged exposure involves reliving the rape scene by imagining it as vividly as possible, describing it aloud in the present tense, taping this description, and listening to the tape at least once daily. Stress inoculation training uses breathing exercises to diminish anxiety and instruction in coping skills, thought stopping, cognitive restructuring, self-dialogue, and role-playing. Research suggests that a combination of both treatments may provide the optimal effect.

REFERENCES

Attala J: Detecting abuse against women in the home, *Home care provider* 1:1, 1996.

Delorey C, Wolf KA: Sexual violence and older women, *Clin Issu Perinatal Women's Health Nurs* 4:173, 1993.

Dunn S, Gilchrist V: Sexual assault, primary care, *Clin Office Pract* 20:359, 1993.

Foa EB, Skeketee G, Roghbaum BD: Behavioral/cognitive conceptualization of posttraumatic stress disorder, *Behav Ther* 20:155, 1989.

Frable D, Blackstone T, Sherbaum C: Marginal and mindful: deviants in social interaction, *J Pers Soc Psychol* 59:140, 1990.

Hampton H: Care of the woman who has been raped, *N Eng J Med* 322:234, 1995.

Jones J: Elder abuse and neglect: responding to a national problem, *Ann Emerg Med* 23:845, 1994.

Kilpatrick DG, Vereonen LJ, Best CL: Factors predicting psychological distress among rape victims. In Figley GR, editor: *Trauma and its wake: the study and treatment of post-traumatic stress disorder,* New York, 1985, Brunner/Mazel.

Laurent C: Male rape, *Nurs Time* 89:1993.

Ledry L: The sexual assault nurse clinician: a fifteen-year experience in Minneapolis, *JEN* 18:217, 1992.

Mackey T et al: Factors associated with long-term depressive symptoms of sexual assault victims, *Arch Psychiatr Nurs* 6:10, 1992.

Ruckman LM: Rape: how to begin the healing, *Am J Nurs* 92:48, 1992.

Tyra PA: Older women: victims of rape, *J Gerontol Nurs* 1993, p. 7.

Rape trauma syndrome: compound reaction

Nancee B. Radtke

Definition   See **Rape trauma syndrome**

Defining Characteristics

See **Rape trauma syndrome.** Additional characteristics include reactivated symptoms of previous conditions (e.g., physical illness, psychiatric illness, reliance on alcohol or drugs).

Related Factors (r/t)

Rape

Client Outcomes/Goals

See **Rape trauma syndrome**

Suggested NIC Interventions

Counseling, rape-trauma treatment

Nursing Interventions and Rationales

See **Rape trauma syndrome, Powerlessness, Ineffective individual coping, Dysfunctional grieving, Anxiety, Fear, Violence: self-directed,** and **Sexual dysfunction**

Geriatric (risk for compound reaction)

- See **Rape trauma syndrome**

Home Care Interventions

- If client has pursued psychiatric counseling, monitor and encourage attendance.
  Reliving the rape experience and the accompanying feelings is painful. Client may need additional support to continue.
- If client is receiving medications, assess client knowledge base of its purpose, side effects, and interactions with medications for other diagnoses. Monitor for effectiveness, side effects, and interactions.
  Ongoing stress may leave client overwhelmed and less able to cope with impact of changing medical status.
- Establish an emergency plan including hotlines. Contract with the client to use the emergency plan. Role play using the hotlines.
  Having an emergency plan reassures the client and decreases the risk of suicide.
- For other home care and hospice considerations, see **Rape trauma syndrome.**

Client/Family Teaching

- Teach client what reactions to expect during the acute and long-term phases: *acute phase*—anger, fear, self-blame, embarrassment, vengeful feelings, physical symptoms, muscle tension, sleeplessness, stomach upset, genitourinary discomfort; *long-term phase*—changes in life-style or residence, nightmares, phobias, seeking of family and social network support.
  Of assessed rape victims, 16.5% were diagnosed with posttraumatic stress disorder (PTSD) an average of 17 years after the assault (Mackey et al, 1992).
- Encourage psychiatric consultation if client is suicidal, violent, or unable to continue activities of daily living.
  Rape victims are four times more likely to attempt suicide, which is 8.7% higher than nonvictims (Mackey et al, 1992).
- Discuss any of client's current stress-relieving medications that may result in substance abuse.
  The initial response to trauma is for the noradrenergic system to maintain the arousal

state, increase vigilance, and be protective to prevent subsequent trauma. Following massive trauma, neurotransmitters are depleted at the synapse level, which is associated with long-term depression and numbing. This depletion also leaves the client with a different threshold, increasing vulnerability to subsequent stress (Mackey et al, 1992).

REFERENCES   Mackey et al: Factors associated with long-term depressive symptoms of sexual assault victims, *Arch Psychiatr Nurs* 6:10, 1992.

Rape trauma syndrome: silent reaction

Nancee B. Radtke

Definition   See **Rape trauma syndrome**

Defining Characteristics

Abrupt changes in relationships with males, increased nightmares, increased anxiety during interview (e.g., blocking of associations, long periods of silence, minor stuttering, physical distress), pronounced changes in sexual behavior, no verbalization about the rape, sudden onset of phobic reactions

Related Factors (r/t)

Rape

Client Outcomes/Goals

- See **Rape trauma syndrome.**
- Resumes previous level of relationships with significant others
- States improvement in sleep and fewer nightmares
- Expresses feelings about and discusses the rape
  Nondisclosure about a sexual assault may arise out of self-protection, but this defensive coping style acts as a pressure cooker and is associated with more intense depressive symptoms (Mackey et al, 1992).
- Returns to usual pattern of sexual behavior
  Women who are sexually active after the assault report lower levels of depression (Mackey et al, 1992). However, being sexually active cannot be construed to mean that the client has adjusted to or resolved the sexual trauma.
- Remains free of phobic reactions

Suggested NIC Interventions

Counseling, rape-trauma treatment

Nursing Interventions and Rationales

- See nursing diagnoses for **Rape trauma syndrome, Powerlessness, Ineffective individual coping, Dysfunctional grieving, Anxiety, Fear, Violence: self-directed, Sexual dysfunction,** or **Impaired communication.**
- Observe disruptions in relationships with significant others.
  Poorly adjusted clients may elicit unsupportive behavior from others or perceive actions of others in a negative way.
- Monitor for signs of increased anxiety (e.g., silence, stuttering, physical distress, irritability, unexplained crying spells).
  Focus on client's coping strengths.

- Observe for changes in sexual behavior.

  More than 80% of sexually active victims reported some sexual dysfunction as a result of the assault (Mackey et al, 1992). Some victims engage in sexual intimacy to prove to themselves and their partners that they are normal or unaffected by the assault.
- Identify phobic reactions to objects in environment (e.g., strangers, doorbells, being with groups of people, knives).
- Provide support by listening when client is ready to talk.

  Extremely controlled clients may not be believed because they do not fit the stereotypical picture of rape victims.
- Be nonjudgmental when feelings are expressed. Explain that anger is normal and needs to be verbalized. Reassure client with phrases such as, "I'm sorry this happened to you."
- Remain with anxious client even if client is silent. Use gentle speech and actions; move slowly.
- Evaluate somatic complaints.

  Women are at higher risk for depression than men (Mackey et al, 1992).

Geriatric   • See **Rape trauma syndrome**

Home Care Interventions

See **Rape trauma syndrome**

Client/Family Teaching

- See **Rape trauma syndrome.**
- Reassure clients they are not bad and are not at fault. Avoid questions beginning with "why."

  "Why" questions may sound judgmental and feed into self-blame.
- Refer client to sexual assault counselor.

  Long-term counseling may be necessary.
- Offer information about pregnancy, hepatitis B, and sexually transmitted disease testing, treatment, and procedures. Do not wait for victim to request information.

REFERENCES   Mackey et al: Factors associated with long-term depressive symptoms of sexual assault victims, *Arch Psychiatr Nurs* 6:10, 1992.

Relocation stress syndrome

Betty J. Ackley

Definition   Physiological or psychosocial disturbances that result from a transfer from one environment to another

Defining Characteristics

Major   Anxiety, apprehension, increased confusion (elderly), depression, loneliness

Minor   Verbalization of unwillingness to relocate, sleep disturbances, change in eating habits, dependency, gastrointestinal disturbances, increased verbalization of needs, insecurity, lack of trust, restlessness, sad affect, unfavorable comparison of posttransfer and pretransfer staff, verbalization of concern or unhappiness about transfer, vigilance, weight change, withdrawal

Related Factors (r/t)

Past, concurrent, and recent losses; losses involved with the decision to move; feeling of powerlessness; lack of adequate support system; little or no preparation for the impending move; moderate-to-high degree of environmental change; history and types of previous transfers; impaired psychosocial health status; decreased physical health status

Client Outcomes/Goals

- Recognizes and knows the name of at least one staff member
- Expresses concerns about move when encouraged to do so during individual contacts
- Carries out activities of daily living in usual manner
- Maintains previous mental and physical health status (e.g., nutrition, elimination, sleep, social interaction)

Suggested NIC Interventions

Coping enhancement, discharge planning, hope instillation, self-responsibility facilitation

Nursing Interventions and Rationales

- Obtain a history, including reason for the move, client's usual coping mechanisms, history of losses, and family support for the client.
  A history helps determine the amount of support needed and appropriate interventions to decrease relocation stress (Manion, Rantz, 1995).
- If client is an adolescent, try not to move in the middle of the school year, find a "New Comers" club for adolescent to join, and refer for counseling if needed.
  An adolescent who is relocating can experience emotional, social, and cognitive dysfunctions. The interventions listed can be helpful (Puskar, Dvorsak, 1991).
- Observe the following procedures if client is being transferred to a nursing home or adult foster care:
  - Allow client to have a choice of placement and preadmission visits if possible.
    Having some control over the event strengthens problem-solving coping strategies (Oleson, Shadick, 1993). These interventions can help decrease anxiety (Thomasma, Yeaworth, McCabe, 1990.)
  - If client cannot choose placement, arrange for a visit or phone call by a member of the staff to welcome client and show a videotape or at least provide pictures of the new care facility.
  - Have a familiar person accompany client to the new facility.
    This lessens client and family anxiety, confusion, and dissatisfaction (Manion, Rantz, 1995).
  - Validate the caregiver's feelings of difficulty with putting a loved one in a different environment.
    This is a distressing experience, and caregivers feel responsible. Validating their feelings will help establish a trusting relationship (Dellasega, Mastrian, 1995).
- Identify previous routines for activities of daily living (ADLs). Try to maintain as much continuity with previous schedule as possible.
  Continuity of routines has been shown to be a crucial factor in influencing adjustment to a new environment (Manion, Rantz, 1995).
- After the transfer, determine client's mental status; document status and observe for any new onset of confusion.
  Confusion can follow relocation because of the overwhelming stress and sensory overload.
- Use reality orientation if needed (e.g., today is ____, the date is ____, you are at ____ facility). Repeat information as needed, and provide clock or calendar.
  Reality orientation can be helpful to prevent new onset of confusion (Manion, Rantz, 1995).

- Establish the way the client would like to be addressed (Mr., Mrs., Miss, first name, nickname).
  Calling clients by their desired name shows respect.
- Thoroughly orient client to the new environment and routines; repeat directions prn.
  The stress of the move may interfere with client's ability to remember directions (Harkulich, 1992).
- Spend one-to-one time with client. Allow client to express feelings and convey acceptance of them; emphasize that the client's feelings are real and individual and that it is acceptable to be sad or angry about moving.
  Expressing feelings can help the client adjust to the situation.
- Assign the same staff to client; maintain consistency in routines of care.
  Consistency hastens adjustment (Harkulich, 1992).
- Have client state one positive aspect of the new living situation each day.
  Helping the client to focus on the positive aspects of the move can help change attitudes.
- Monitor client's health status and provide appropriate interventions for problems with social interaction, nutrition, sleep, or elimination.
  Stress from the transfer can cause physiological and psychological disturbances (Barnhouse, Brugler, Harkulich, 1992).
- If client is being transferred within a facility, have staff from new unit visit client before transfer.
- Once client is transferred, have previous staff make occasional visits until client is comfortable in new surroundings.
- Watch for coping problems (e.g., withdrawal, regression, or angry behavior) and intervene immediately.
  Failure to cope in a timely manner may cause a permanent pattern of impaired adjustment (Oleson, Shadick, 1993).
- Allow client to grieve for loss of old situation; explain that it is normal to feel sadness over change and loss.
- Allow client to participate in care as much as possible and make decisions when possible (e.g., where to place bed, choice of roommate, bathing routines). Make an effort to accommodate the client.
  Having choices helps prevent feelings of powerlessness that may lead to depression.

Geriatric
- Monitor need for transfer, and transfer only when necessary.
  Elderly clients often adapt poorly to transfer; they can lose normal functioning in certain areas, and relocation may even cause death (Rantz, Egan, 1987).
- Protect client from injuries such as falls.
  Falls and an overall increase in the number of accidents are common with relocation.

Client/Family Teaching
- Teach family about relocation stress syndrome. Encourage them to monitor for signs of the syndrome, that acceptance of the new living situation begins within 6 to 8 weeks after institutionalization, and that adjustment is usually complete within 3 to 6 months (Manion, Rantz, 1995).
- Help significant others learn how to support client with the move by setting up a schedule of visits, dealing with holidays, bringing familiar items from home, and establishing a system for contact when client needs support.

REFERENCES   Barnhouse AH, Brugler CJ, Harkulich JT: Relocation stress syndrome, *Nurs Diag* 3:166, 1992.

Dellasega C, Mastrian K: The process and consequences of institutionalizing an elder, *West J Nurs Res* 17:123, 1995.

Harkulich JT: Relocation stress. In Gettrust K, Brabeck PD, editors: *Nursing diagnosis in clinical practice: guides for care planning,* Albany, NY, 1992, Delmar.

Manion PD, Rantz MJ: Relocation stress syndrome: a comprehensive plan for long-term care admissions, *Geriatr Nurs* 16:108, 1995.

Oleson M, Shadick KM: Application of Moos' and Schaefer's model to nursing care of elderly persons relocating to a nursing home, *J Adv Nurs* 18:479, 1993.

Puskar KR, Dvorsak KG: Relocation stress in adolescents: helping teenagers cope with a moving dilemma, *Pediatr Nurs* 17:295, 1991.

Rantz M, Egan K: Reducing death from translocation syndrome, *Am J Nurs* 87:1351, 1987.

Thomasma M, Yeaworth RC, McCabe BW: Moving day: relocation and anxiety in institutionalized elderly, *J Gerontol Nurs* 16:18, 1990.

Altered role performance

Gail B. Ladwig

Definition   Disruption in the way one perceives one's role performance

Defining Characteristics

Change in self-perception of role, change in others' perception of role, conflict in roles, change in physical capacity to resume role, lack of knowledge regarding role, change in usual patterns of responsibility

Related Factors (r/t)

Health care crisis, change in occupational situation, separation from significant others, change in marital status

Client Outcomes/Goals

- Identifies realistic perception of role
- States personal strengths
- Acknowledges problems contributing to inability to carry out usual role
- Accepts physical limitations regarding role responsibility and considers ways to change life-style to accomplish goals associated with role performance
- Demonstrates knowledge of appropriate behaviors associated with new or changed role
- States knowledge of change in responsibility and new behaviors associated with new responsibility
- Verbalizes acceptance of new responsibility

Suggested NIC Interventions

Role enhancement

Nursing Interventions and Rationales

- Observe client's knowledge of behaviors associated with role.
  Ability to perform perceived roles is easily hampered by illness. It is important to note whether or not the client feels capable of functioning in the usual role.
- Allow client to express feelings regarding the role change.
  The client may experience disappointment and feelings of grief because of a role change. It is therapeutic for the client to express these feelings.
- Ask clients direct questions regarding their new roles and how the health care system can help them continue in their roles.

To maintain self-esteem, it is important to accurately assess the client's needs and ways to meet them; direct questions help elicit factual information.

- Have client make a list of strengths that are needed for the new role. Acknowledge which strengths client has and which strengths need to be developed; work with client to set goals for desired role.
In setting valued goals, people adapt their world to self-generated needs and projects rather than adapting themselves to a given world (Nuttin, 1992). Focusing on strengths helps the client to positively enhance behaviors associated with role performance.

- Have client list problems associated with the new role and identify ways of overcoming them (e.g., if pain is worse late in day, have client complete necessary role tasks early in day).
There are many ways to accomplish tasks; help the client recognize this and make the appropriate accommodations.

- Identify ways to compensate for physical disabilities (e.g., have a ramp built to provide access to house, put household objects within client's reach from wheelchair).
Helping clients to help themselves by modifying the environment enhances self-esteem and fosters a sense of power because they remain able to function in their role.

Geriatric
- Explore community needs after assessing client's strengths; suggest functional activities (e.g., being a foster grandparent or a mentor for small businesses).
If physical strength is declining, activities that require less physical prowess and more mental expertise are sometimes appropriate (Ringsven, Bond, 1991).

- Refer to family counseling as needed for adjustment to role changes.
The family needs to be helped as a system because a change in one person's role affects the entire family.

Home Care Interventions

- Determine the anticipated length of role change.
Knowing the anticipated length of role change helps the client and significant others determine the acceptability of role change, role conflict, and changes in communication patterns.

- Assess family's ability to physically or psychologically assume responsibilities of decrease or change in client's role function.
The health, abilities, or other role expectations of caregivers or significant others may prohibit the assumption of responsibilities once held by the client.

- Offer a referral to medical social services to assist with assessing the short- and long-term impacts of role change.
Collaboration with specialists provides the client with greater resources for adaptation. Terminally ill clients may see the transition of role responsibilities as a task that must be completed before dying. Resolution of role transition will reassure the client, allow remaining energy to be focused elsewhere, and may give client permission to die.

Client/Family Teaching

- Teach significant others about health care changes to expect when the client returns home.
All spouses, male and female, expressed uncertainty about their roles and what their partner could do after discharge (McSweeney, 1993).

- Help client identify resources for assistance in caring for a disabled or aging parent (e.g., adult day care).
There are varying levels of assistance for the aging clients. Clients and their families need assistance in identifying these levels.

- Refer to appropriate community agencies to learn skills for functioning in the new or changed role (e.g., vocational rehabilitation, parenting classes, hospice, respite care). *As one person changes, other family members need to alter their patterns of communication and behavior to maintain balance. Family members also need assistance with developing these new skills (Barry, 1994).*

REFERENCES   Barry P: *Mental health and mental illness,* ed 5, Philadelphia, 1994, JB Lippincott.
McSweeney J: Making behavior changes after a myocardial infarction, *West J Nurs Res* 5:441, 1993.
Nuttin JR: Motivation, intention and volition. In Fleury J, editor: The application of motivational theory to cardiovascular risk reduction, *Image* 24:229, 1992.
Ringsven M, Bond D: *Gerontology and leadership skills for nurses,* Albany, NY, 1991, Delmar.

Self-care deficit, bathing/hygiene

Linda Williams

Definition   The state in which an individual experiences an impaired ability to perform or complete bathing and hygiene activities

Defining Characteristics

Inability to wash body or body parts *(critical),* inability to obtain or get to water source, inability to regulate water temperature or flow

Impaired physical mobility—functional level classification:
- 0   Completely independent
- 1   Requires use of equipment or device
- 2   Requires help from another person for assistance, supervision, or teaching
- 3   Requires help from another person and equipment device
- 4   Dependent, does not participate in activity

Related Factors (r/t)

Intolerance to activity, decreased strength and endurance, pain, discomfort, perceptual or cognitive impairment, neuromuscular impairment, musculoskeletal impairment, depression, severe anxiety

Client Outcomes/Goals

- Remains free of body odor, maintains intact skin
- States satisfaction with ability to use adaptive devices to bathe
- Bathes with assistance of caregiver as needed without anxiety
- Explains and uses methods to bathe safely and with minimal difficulty

Suggested NIC Interventions

Bathing, self-care assistance: bathing/hygiene

Nursing Interventions and Rationales

- Observe for cause of inability to bathe; see related factors.
  Self-care requires multisystem competence. Restorative program planning is specific to problems that interfere with self-care.
- Assess client's ability to bathe self, noting specific deficits.
  Functional assessment provides analysis data for activities of daily living tasks to be used in goal and intervention planning.

- Ask clients for input on bathing habits such as whether they prefer a shower or tub bath and timing of bath desired.
  Providing the client with opportunities for guiding own care increases control and prevents learned helplessness (LeSage et al, 1989). Creating opportunities for guiding personal care honors long-standing routines and increased control, prevents learned helplessness, and preserves self-esteem (Miller, 1994).
- Request referrals for occupational and physical therapy.
  Collaboration and correlation of activities with interdisciplinary team members increases the client's mastery of self-care tasks.
- Plan activities to prevent fatigue during bathing.
  Energy conservation increases activity tolerance and promotes self-care.
- Provide medication for pain 45 minutes before bathing if needed.
  Pain relief promotes participation in self-care.
- Place all bathing equipment within easy reach.
  Environmental modifications promote safety and conserve energy.
- Use any necessary adaptive bathing equipment (e.g., long-handled brushes, soap-on-a-rope, washcloth mitt, wall bars, tub bench, shower chair, commode chair without pan in shower).
  Adaptive devices extend the client's reach, increase speed and safety, and decrease exertion.
- Provide privacy; have only one caregiver providing bathing assistance, encourage a traffic-free bathing area, and post privacy signs.
  Towel bathing increases privacy, which conveys respect during bathing (Wright, 1990). The client perceives less privacy if more than one caregiver participates and a central bathing area in a high-traffic location that allows staff to enter freely during care is used (Miller, 1994).
- Keep client warmly covered.
  Clients, especially elderly clients, who are prone to hypothermia may experience evaporative cooling during and after bathing, which produces an unpleasant cold sensation (Miller, 1994).
- Allow client to participate as able in bathing. Smile and provide praise for accomplishments in a relaxed manner.
  The client's expenditure of energy provides the caregiver the opportunity to convey respect for a well-done task, which increases the client's self-esteem. Smiling and being relaxed are associated with a calm, functional client response (Burgener et al, 1992).
- Inspect skin condition during bathing.
  Observation of skin allows detection of skin problems.
- Use or encourage caregiver to use an unhurried, caring touch.
  The basic human need of touch offers reassurance and comfort.
- If client is bathing alone, place assistance call light within reach.
  A readily available signaling device promotes safety and provides reassurance for the client.
- Monitor client for fatigue, frustration, or inability to complete bathing tasks and assist client as needed.
  Bathing can produce atypical responses in acutely ill patients (Robichaud-Ekstrand, 1991).

Geriatric
- Provide same type of bathrobe and bathing articles, such as scented dusting powder and bath oil, that client used previously.

Use of sensory channels to stimulate memory may help foster understanding of bathing and self-care (Danner et al, 1993).

- Assess for grieving resulting from loss of function.
  Grief resulting from loss of function can inhibit relearning of self-care.
- Arrange bathing environment to promote sensory comfort: reduce noise of voices and water, and decrease glare from tiles, white walls, and artificial lights.
  Noise discomfort can result from high-echo tiled walls, loud voices, and running water. Glare can cause visual discomfort, especially in clients with visual changes or cataracts (Miller, 1994).
- Allow client or caregiver adequate time to complete the bathing activity.
  Significant aging increases the time required to complete a task, so elderly individuals with a self-care deficit require more time to complete a task.
- Use only mild soap on genital and axillary areas; rinse well.
  Soap can alter skin pH and may increase skin dryness that results from decreased oil and perspiration production in the elderly.
- Limit bathing to once or twice a week; provide a partial bath at other times.
  Frequent bathing promotes skin dryness.
- Use tepid water; test water temperature before use.
  Hot water promotes skin dryness and may burn a client with decreased sensation.
- Use a gentle touch when bathing; avoid vigorous scrubbing motions.
  Aging skin is thinner, more fragile, and less able to withstand mechanical friction.
- Apply an emollient to wet skin after bathing.
  Applying an emollient to wet skin decreases skin dryness by preventing the loss of moisture that occurs during bathing (Fenske, Grayson, Newcomer, 1989).

Home Care Interventions

- Based on functional assessment and rehabilitation capacity, refer for home health aide services to assist with bathing and hygiene.
  Support by home health aides preserves the energy of the client and provides respite for caregivers.
- Cue cognitively impaired clients in steps of hygiene.
  Cognitively impaired clients can successfully participate in many activities with cueing. Participation in self-care can enhance the self-esteem of cognitively impaired clients.
- Respect the preference of terminally ill clients to refuse or limit hygiene care.
  Maintaining hygiene, even with assistance, may require excessive energy demands from terminally ill clients. Pain on touch or movement may be intractable and not resolved by medication.
- If a terminally ill client requests hygiene care, make an extra effort to meet request and provide care when client and family will most benefit (e.g., before visitors, at bedtime, in early morning).
  When desired, improved hygiene greatly boosts the morale of terminally ill clients.
- Maintain temperature of home at a comfortable level when providing hygiene care to terminally ill clients.
  Terminally ill clients may have difficulty with thermoregulation, which will add to the energy demand or decrease comfort during hygiene care.

Client/Family Teaching

- Teach how to use adaptive devices for bathing.
  Adaptive devices can provide independence, safety, and speed.

- Teach bathing techniques that promote safety (e.g., getting into tub before filling it with water, emptying water before getting out, using an antislip mat, wall-grab bars, tub bench). *Safety devices decrease fear of injury and increase independence.*
- Teach client and family an individualized bathing routine that includes a schedule, privacy, skin inspection, soap or lubricant, and chill prevention. *Understanding the client's needs and teaching the methods to meet these needs increases the client's satisfaction with the bathing experience.*

REFERENCES   Burgener S et al: Caregiver and environmental variables related to difficult behaviors in institutionalized, demented elderly persons, *J Gerontol* 47:242, 1992.

Danner C et al: Cognitively impaired elders: using research findings to improve nursing care, *J Gerentol Nurs* 19:5, 1993.

Fenske N, Grayson L, Newcomer V: Common problems of aging skin, *Patient Care* 23:225, 1989.

LeSage J et al: Learned helplessness, *J Gerontol Nurs* 15:9, 1989.

Miller R: Managing disruptive responses to bathing elderly residents, *J Gerontol Nurs* 20:35, 1994.

Robichaud-Ekstrand S: Shower versus sink bath: evaluation of heart rate, blood pressure and subjective response of the patient with myocardial infarction, *Heart Lung* 20:375, 1991.

Wright L: Bathing by towel, *Nurs Time* 86:36, 1990.

Self-care deficit, dressing/grooming

Linda Williams

Definition   The state in which an individual experiences an impaired ability to perform or complete dressing and grooming activities

Defining Characteristics

Impaired ability to put on or take off necessary items of clothing *(critical),* impaired ability to obtain or replace articles of clothing, impaired ability to fasten clothing, inability to maintain appearance at a satisfactory level

Related Factors (r/t)

Intolerance to activity, decreased strength and endurance, pain, discomfort, perceptual or cognitive impairment, neuromuscular impairment, musculoskeletal impairment, depression, severe anxiety

Client Outcomes/Goals

- Dresses and grooms self to optimal potential
- Uses adaptive devices to dress and groom
- Explains and uses methods to enhance strengths during dressing and grooming
- Dresses and grooms with assistance of caregiver as needed

Suggested NIC Interventions

Dressing, haircare, self-care assistance: dressing/grooming

Nursing Interventions and Rationales

- Observe for cause of inability to dress and groom self; see related factors. *Self-care requires multisystem competence. Restorative program planning is specific to problems that interfere with self-care.*
- Assess client's ability to dress and groom self; note specific deficits. *Functional assessment provides activities of daily living task analysis data for goal and intervention planning.*

- Identify and include client's strengths in dressing and grooming.
  Incorporating the client's strengths into a dressing and grooming program increases self-care independence.
- Ask client for input on clothing choices and how to increase the ease of dressing.
  Providing the client with opportunities for guiding own care increases control and prevents learned helplessness (LeSage et al, 1989).
- Request referrals for occupational and physical therapy.
  Collaboration and correlation of activities with interdisciplinary team members increases the client's mastery of self-care tasks.
- Provide medication for pain 45 minutes before dressing and grooming if needed.
  Pain relief promotes participation in self-care.
- Plan activities to prevent fatigue while dressing and grooming.
  Energy conservation increases activity tolerance and promotes self-care.
- Help client store clothing and grooming devices within easy reach; closet rods or drawers between eye and hip level and turntables are helpful.
  Environmental modifications minimize bending and conserve energy (Lorig, Fries, 1990).
- Select larger-sized clothing and clothing with elastic waistbands, Velcro fasteners, or wide sleeves and pant legs.
  Simplifying clothing choices promotes independence.
- Use adaptive dressing and grooming equipment as needed (e.g., long-handled brushes, grasping devices, Velcro closures, zipper pulls, button hooks, elastic shoelaces, large buttons, soap-on-a-rope, suction holders).
  Adaptive devices increase speed and safety and decrease exertion.
- Lay clothing out in the order that it will be put on by the client.
  Simplifying dressing tasks increases self-care ability.
- Encourage client to dress appropriately for time of day.
- Perform dressing and grooming activities in a consistent sequence each day.
  An established routine of waking and dressing provides a sense of normalcy and increases motivation to perform self-care. Prolonged repetition promotes increased relearning of self-care tasks (Giles, Shore, 1989).
- Encourage participation; guide client's hand through task if necessary.
  Experiencing the normal process of a task through guided practice facilitates optimal relearning.

Geriatric
- Assess for grieving resulting from loss of function.
  Grief resulting from loss of function can inhibit relearning of self-care tasks.
- Frequently assess client's pain; provide pain relief as needed before dressing and grooming activities.
  Elderly people have twice the incidence of pain of younger people; they often have more than one pain source, which commonly includes arthritis (Acute Pain Management Guideline Panel, 1992).
- Assess tasks client can complete.
  Assessing what the client can do decreases caregiver responsibility and allows caregiver to give positive reinforcement to client.
- Allow client or caregiver adequate time to complete dressing (e.g., do not insist that client is dressed at an early hour).
  Significant aging increases the time required to complete a task; elderly clients with a self-care deficit requires more time to complete a task.

Home Care Interventions

- Based on functional assessment and rehabilitation capacity, refer for home health aide services to assist with dressing and grooming.
  Support by home health aides preserves the energy of the client and provides respite for caregivers.
- Cue cognitively impaired clients in steps of dressing and grooming.
  Cognitively impaired clients can participate successfully in many activities with cueing. Participation in self-care can enhance the self-esteem of cognitively impaired clients.
- Respect the preference of the terminally ill client to refuse dressing and limit grooming.
  Dressing and grooming, even with assistance, may require excessive energy demands from the terminally ill. Pain on touch or movement may be intractable and not resolved by medication.
- If terminally ill clients request dressing and grooming, make an extra effort to meet request and provide care when client and family will most benefit (e.g., before visitors, in early morning).
  When desired, dressing and grooming are a great boost to the morale of terminally ill clients and their families.
- Maintain the temperature of the home at a comfortable level when dressing terminally ill clients.
  Terminally ill clients may have difficulty with thermoregulation, which will add to the energy demand or decrease comfort during hygiene activities.

Client/Family Teaching

- Teach client to dress the affected side first, then the unaffected side.
  Dressing the affected side first allows for easier manipulation of clothing.
- Teach the simplest step in a task until mastered, and then proceed to more complicated steps.
  Simplifying dressing and grooming tasks that consist of many small steps promotes mastery.
- Teach how to use adaptive devices for dressing and grooming.
  Assistive devices can provide independence, safety, and speed.
- Teach client and family to select clothes appropriate for the season, temperature, and weather.
  Clients with altered sensation need to understand the factors that influence body temperature and the environment.

REFERENCES   Acute Pain Management Guideline Panel: *Acute pain management: operative or medical procedures and trauma,* Clinical Practice Guideline, Rockville, Md, 1992, Agency for Health Care Policy and Research, Pub No 92-0032, Public Health Service, US Department of Health and Human Services.

Giles G, Shore M: A rapid method for teaching severely brain injured adults how to wash and dress, *Arch Phys Med Rehab* 70:156, 1989.

LeSage J et al: Learned helplessness, *J Gerontol Nurs* 15:9, 1989.

Lorig K, Fries J: *The arthritis helpbook,* ed 3, Reading, Mass, 1990, Addison-Wesley.

Self-care deficit, feeding

Linda Williams

Definition   The state in which an individual experiences an impaired ability to perform or complete feeding activities for oneself

Defining Characteristics

Inability to bring food from a receptacle to the mouth

Related Factors (r/t)

Intolerance to activity, decreased strength and endurance, pain, discomfort, perceptual or cognitive impairment, neuromuscular impairment, musculoskeletal impairment, depression, severe anxiety

Client Outcomes/Goals

- Feeds self
- States satisfaction with ability to use adaptive devices for feeding
- Provides assistance with feeding when necessary (caregiver)

Suggested NIC Interventions

Feeding, self-care assistance: feeding

Nursing Interventions and Rationales

- Observe for cause of inability to feed self independently; see related factors.
  Self-care requires multisystem competence. Restorative program planning is specific to problems that interfere with self-care.
- Assess client's ability to feed self. Test gag reflex bilaterally, and note specific deficits.
  Functional assessment provides ADL task analysis data for matching client's ability to feed self with caregiver's level of assistance (Van Ort, Phillips, 1995).
- Ask client for input on methods to facilitate eating and feeding (e.g., cultural foods, other food and fluid preferences).
  Providing the client with opportunities for guiding personal care increases control and prevents learned helplessness (LeSage et al, 1989).
- Request referral for occupational and physical therapy; request a dictician.
  Collaboration and correlation of activities with interdisciplinary team members increases the client's mastery of self-care tasks.
- Use any necessary adaptive feeding equipment (e.g., rocker knives, plate guards, suction mats, built-up handles on utensils, scoop dishes, large-handled cups).
  Adaptive devices increase independence.
- Ensure that client has dentures, hearing aids, and glasses in place.
  Adaptive devices increase opportunity for self-care.
- Seat client at table using name card and placement as appropriate with meal in visual range.
  Familiar feeding patterns and cues increase self-feeding (Van Ort, Phillips, 1995).
- Help client into sitting position; ensure that client's head is flexed slightly forward and shoulders are supported while eating and for 1 hour after a meal.
  Gravity assists with swallowing, and aspiration is decreased when sitting upright.
- Prepare meal items before client begins eating.
  Preparing items for the client conserves energy for hand-to-mouth activities.

- Provide small portions of favorite foods at proper serving temperature.
  Functional feeding can be improved by altering the physical context of the meal to appeal to the client (Jaeger, 1989).
- Provide consistency in caregiver and meal activities.
  Mutual increases in subtle cue interpretation occur between the consistent caregiver and client, which fosters self-care (Athlin, Norberg, 1987).
- Caregiver should sit beside client (on client's unaffected side).
  Sitting beside the client makes the caregiver more comfortable and less likely to hurry and encourages the client to eat more (Kolodny, Malek, 1991).
- Caregiver should sit at a half circle table if interacting with a group of clients and remain with clients until meal is completed.
  Environmental strategies that reduce interruptions and distractions increase self-care (Hogstel, Robinson, 1989).
- Encourage participation; guide client's hand through task if needed.
  Experiencing the normal process of a task through guided practice facilitates optimal relearning (Tappen, 1994).
- Allow client to participate in feeding as able, and provide praise for all feeding attempts; increase tasks as able.
  The client should be an active participant in feeding instead of a passive recipient of food (Osborn, Marshall, 1993).
- Provide praise for all feeding attempts; increase tasks as able.
  Client's expenditure of energy provides caregiver the opportunity to convey respect for a well-done task, which increases self-esteem.
- Plan activities to prevent fatigue before meals.
  Energy conservation increases activity tolerance and promotes self-care.
- Provide medication for pain before meals if needed.
  Pain relief promotes participation in self-care.
- Provide client with a pleasant meal environment. Keep the environment free of toileting devices and odors, avoid painful procedures before meals, remove lids from tray, provide clean utensils for separate courses, and maintain a social environment.
  Attention to the aesthetics of feeding increases feeding success.
- Encourage client to keep food on the unaffected side of mouth with a rocking motion to deposit the food.
  Keeping food away from the affected side of the mouth prevents pocketing of food (Donahue, 1990).
- Be prepared to intervene if choking occurs; have suction equipment readily available and know the Heimlich maneuver.
  Dysphagia increases the risk of choking (Donahue, 1990).
- Provide oral hygiene after eating and check for pocketing of food.
  Aspiration can occur from food left in the mouth.

Geriatric

- Allow client with dentures adequate time to chew.
  Chewing with dentures takes four times longer to reach a certain level of mastication than chewing with natural teeth.
- Choose soft foods rather than liquids or use dietary thickeners.
  Choking occurs more easily with clear liquids than solid or soft foods (Hogstel, Robinson, 1989).
- Provide finger foods.

Finger foods can be nutritious as well as allowing independence and the choice of what and when to eat.

- Use intermittent positive verbal encouragement and gentle touch on patient's forearm to encourage feeding.

Verbal cueing and touch used in combination increase nutritional intake (Lange-Alberts, Shott, 1994).

Home Care Interventions

- Based on functional assessment and rehabilitation capacity refer for home health aide services to assist with feeding.

Support by home health aides preserves the energy of the client and provides respite for caregivers.

- Cue cognitively impaired clients when feeding.

Cognitively impaired clients can participate successfully in many activities with cueing. Participation in self-care can enhance the self-esteem of cognitively impaired clients.

- Respect the preference of terminally ill clients to refuse nutrition or assistance with eating. Refer to care plans for **Nutrition, alteration in; Nutrition, less than body requirements; and Swallowing, impaired.**
- If terminally ill clients request nutrition, take special care to provide foods and assistive devices that protect the client from aspiration, minimize energy requirements, and meet the client's taste preferences.

Terminally ill clients have altered taste and other sensations, which impact their willingness to eat or to invest time or energy in eating.

Client/Family Teaching

- Teach client how to use adaptive devices.

Adaptive devices increase independence.

- Teach clients with hemianopsia to turn their head so that the plate is in the line of vision.

Compensation for hemianopsia is done by turning head to place items in line of vision (Needham, 1993).

- Teach visually impaired clients to locate foods according to numbers on a clock.
- Teach caregiver feeding techniques that prevent choking (e.g., sitting beside client on the unaffected side, feeding client slowly, checking food temperature, providing fluid between bites, establishing a method to communicate readiness for next bite, limiting conversation while chewing).

Sitting beside the client makes the caregiver more comfortable and less likely to hurry (Kolodny, Malek, 1991).

REFERENCES   Athlin E, Norberg A: Caregiver's attitudes to and interpretations of the behavior of severely demented patients during feeding in a patient assignment care system, *Int J Nurs Stud* 24:145, 1987.

Decastro J, Decastro E: Spontaneous meal patterns of humans: influence of the presence of other people, *Am J Clin Nutrition* 50:237, 1989.

Donahue P: When it's hard to swallow: feeding techniques for dysphagia management, *J Gerontol Nurs* 16:6, 1990.

Hogstel M, Robinson N: Feeding the frail elderly, *J Gerontol Nurs* 15:16, 1989.

Jaeger M: Providing nutritional support, *Nursing 89* 19:100, 1989.

Kolodny V, Malek A: Improving feeding skills, *J Gerontol Nurs* 17:20, 1991.

Lange-Alberts M, Shott S: Nutritional intake, *J Gerontol Nurs* 20:36, 1994.

LeSage J et al: Learned helplessness, *J Gerontol Nurs* 15:9, 1989.

Needham J: *Gerontological nursing: a restorative approach,* Albany, NY, 1993, Delmar.

Osborn C, Marshall M: Self-feeding performance in nursing home residents, *J Gerontol Nurs* 19:7, 1993.

Phaneuf C: Screening elders for nutritional deficits, *Am J Nurs* 96:58, 1996.

Tappen R: The effect of skill training on functional abilities of nursing home residents with dementia, *Res Nurs Health* 17:159, 1994.

Van Ort S, Phillips L: Nursing interventions to promote functional feeding, *J Gerontol Nurs* 21:6, 1995.

Self-care deficit, toileting

Linda Williams

Definition   The state in which an individual experiences an impaired ability to perform or complete toileting activities for oneself

Defining Characteristics

Inability to get to toilet or commode *(critical),* inability to sit on or rise from toilet or commode *(critical),* inability to manipulate clothing for toileting *(critical),* inability to carry out proper toileting hygiene *(critical),* inability to flush toilet or commode

Related Factors (r/t)

Impaired transfer ability, impaired mobility status, intolerance to activity, decreased strength and endurance, pain, discomfort, perceptual or cognitive impairment, neuromuscular impairment, musculoskeletal impairment, depression, severe anxiety

Client Outcomes/Goals

- Remains free of incontinence and impaction with no urine or stool on skin
- States satisfaction with ability to use adaptive devices for toileting
- Explains and uses methods to be safe and independent in toileting

Suggested NIC Interventions

Environmental management, self-care assistance: toileting

Nursing Interventions and Rationales

- Observe cause of inability to toilet independently; see related factors.
  Self-care requires multisystem competence. Restorative program planning is specific to problems that interfere with self-care.
- Assess ability to toilet; note specific deficits.
  Functional assessment provides analysis data for activities of daily living tasks for use in goal and intervention planning.
- Ask client for input on toileting methods and timing and how to better provide toileting activity assistance.
  Providing the client with opportunities for guiding own care increases control and prevents learned helplessness (LeSage et al, 1989).
- Assess client's usual bowel and bladder toileting patterns and the terminology used for toileting.
  Individuals develop a unique pattern of toileting over time for faster, normal elimination.
- Request referral for occupational and physical therapy for help in working with client to transfer from bed to commode.
  Collaboration and correlation of activities with interdisciplinary team members increases the client's mastery of self-care tasks.

- Use any necessary assistive toileting equipment (e.g., toilet risers, raised toilet seat, suction mats, spill-proof urinals, support rails next to toilet, toilet safety frames, Sanifems [allow a woman to void standing], fracture bedpans).
  Adaptive devices promote independence and safety.
- Provide privacy.
  Privacy can prevent suppression of elimination resulting from embarrassment about noise and odor.
- Schedule toileting to occur when defecation urge is strongest or voiding is likely (e.g., in the morning, every 2 hours, after meals, at bedtime). Assist client until self-care ability increases.
  The defecation urge is strongest in morning or within 1 hour after meals or warm beverages. Approximately 50 to 75 ml of urine are produced hourly, the urge to void occurs when 200 ml has accumulated, so a 2-hour schedule can reduce incontinence.
- Allow client to participate as able in toileting, and provide praise for accomplishments. Increase tasks as client is able, and work with client to aim toward independence in toileting.
  Client's expenditure of energy provides caregiver the opportunity to convey respect for a well-done task, which increases self-esteem.
- Obtain a bedside commode if necessary; avoid bedpans if possible. If client is acutely ill, provide bedpan at appropriate intervals.
  A sitting position uses gravity and is more conducive to normal elimination.
- Make assistance call button readily available to client, and answer light promptly; remove environmental barriers to toilet.
  To decrease incontinence, the client needs rapid access to toileting facilities; navigational barriers can increase incontinence episodes (Noelker, 1987).
- Assess and remove physical barriers to toilet such as cluttered walkways.
  Environmental assessment identifies barriers that can increase incontinence episodes (Penn et al, 1996).
- Keep toilet paper and handwashing items within easy reach of client.
- Inspect skin condition.
  Observation of skin allows detection of skin problems.
- Provide prompt skin care and linen changes after incontinence episodes.
  The presence of urine or stool on the skin leads to skin breakdown.

Geriatric
- Assess client's pain frequently and provide pain relief as needed before dressing/grooming activities.
  Elderly persons have twice the incidence of pain that younger persons have and often more than one pain source, which commonly includes arthritis (Acute Pain Management Guideline Panel, 1992).
- Assess client's mobility status and speed of movement.
  Elderly women with slower mobility have more incontinent episodes (Wyman, Eiswick, 1993).
- Reassure client that call light will be answered promptly.
  The elderly cannot respond quickly to the urge to void as a result of limited functional ability and environmental barriers; they are also unable to delay voiding as a result of decreased muscle tone and neurological changes (Palmer, 1994).
- Provide a small footstool in front of toilet or commode.
  Intraabdominal pressure is increased by elevating knees above the hips, which facilitates elimination in elderly persons with weak abdominal muscles.

- Assess client's functional ability to manipulate clothing for toileting. If necessary, modify clothing with Velcro fasteners and elastic waists.
  Delays caused in manipulating zippers and buttons may cause functional incontinence (Penn et al, 1996).
- Avoid use of indwelling or condom catheters if possible.
  An indwelling urinary catheter is a source of infection and keeps the bladder empty, which reduces bladder capacity and decreases the opportunity for independent toileting.
- Help clients develop a regular toileting schedule. Verbally prompt them as a reminder.

Home Care Interventions

- Based on functional assessment and rehabilitation capacity, refer for home health aide services to assist with toileting.
  Support by home health aides preserves the energy of the client and provides respite for caregivers.
- Cue cognitively impaired clients in steps of toileting.
  Cognitively impaired persons can participate successfully in many activities with cueing. Participation in self care can enhance the self-esteem of cognitively impaired clients.
- Avoid the use of medications which place undue toileting stress on the client who is terminally ill.
- Provide pain medication for terminally ill clients 20 to 45 minutes before toileting in anticipation of possible pain (e.g., in coordination with a bowel stimulation program). See plan for **Constipation.**
  Pain from touch or movement may be intractable and not resolved by medication, but medication may decrease the pain enough to allow limited movement and passing of stool.
- Consider use of an indwelling catheter when terminally ill clients are in too much pain to move and hygiene and skin integrity are difficult to maintain.
  The goal of hospice care is to promote comfort and dignity in the dying process.

Client/Family Teaching

- Teach client and family how to toilet client with adaptive and safety devices.
  Adaptive devices can provide independence, safety, and speed.
- Prepare client for toileting needs by teaching the action of medications such as diuretics.
  Medications that promote elimination require prompt responses to toileting needs.
- Teach family how to help client toilet, including the use of a bedpan, commode, and appropriate toileting schedule.

REFERENCES   Acute Pain Management Guideline Panel: *Acute pain management operative or medical procedures and trauma,* Clinical practice guideline, Agency for Health Care Policy and Research Pub No 92-0032, Rockville, Md, 1992, Public Health Service, US Department of Health and Human Services.

Jirovec M: The impact of daily exercise on the mobility, balance and urine control of the cognitively impaired nursing home residents, *Int J Nurs Stud* 28:145, 1991.

LeSage J et al: Learned helplessness, *J Gerontol Nurs* 15:9, 1989.

Noelker L: Incontinence in elderly cared for by the family, *Gerontologist* 27:194, 1987.

Palmer M: Level 1: Basic assessment and management of urinary incontinence in nursing homes, *Nurs Pract Forum* 5:152, 1994.

Penn C et al: Assessment of urinary incontinence, *J Gerontol Nurs* 22:8, 1996.

Wyman J, Eiswick R: Influence of functional, urological and environmental characteristics on urinary incontinence in community-dwelling older women, *Nurs Res* 42:270, 1993.

Chronic low self-esteem

Helen Kelley

Definition   Long-standing negative self-evaluations and feelings about self or capabilities

Defining Characteristics

Major   Self-negating verbalizations, expressions of shame or guilt, evaluation of self as unable to deal with events, rationalization or rejection of positive feedback about self, exaggeration of negative feedback about self, hesitancy about new things or situations

Minor   Frequent lack of success in work or other life events, excessive adherence to or dependency on others' opinions, lack of eye contact, nonassertive or passive nature, indecisiveness, excessive searches for reassurance

Related Factors (r/t)

Childhood abuse or neglect (physical, sexual, or emotional), abusive adult relationships, elder abuse, mental illness (especially depression), drug or alcohol use or dependence, eating disorders

Client Outcomes/Goals

- Demonstrates improved ability to interact with others (e.g., maintains eye contact, expresses feelings)
- Verbalizes increased self-acceptance through use of positive self-statements
- Identifies personal strengths
- Sets small, achievable goals
- Attempts independent decision making

Suggested NIC Interventions

Self-esteem enhancement

Nursing Interventions and Rationales

- Actively listen to and respect the client.
  An attentive attitude conveys acceptance (Norris, 1992).
- Assist patient with identifying and confronting problems of not valuing self or enduring abuse from others.
  Tolerance of abusive or violent behavior may be developed over time (Norris, 1992).
- Assess existing strengths and coping abilities, and provide opportunities for their expression and recognition.
  Self-esteem is enhanced by the ability to perform competently (Coopersmith, 1981).
- Reinforce the personal strengths and positive self-perceptions that client identifies.
  This is effective in enhancing global self-worth (Manus, Killeen, 1995).
- Identify and limit client's negative self-assessments.
  Limitations disrupt the pattern of negative distortion.
- Encourage realistic and achievable goal setting; recognize the value of attempts and accomplishments.
  Reframe "failures" as opportunities to learn and change tactics.

- Demonstrate and promote effective communication techniques.
  Effective communication increases the opportunity to receive positive validation from others.
- Encourage independent decision-making by reviewing options and their possible consequences with client.
  Autonomy enhances self-esteem (Crouch, Straub, 1983).
- Assist patient to challenge negative perceptions of self and performance.
  Use "failure" as an opportunity to provide valuable feedback (Grainger, 1991).
- Promote a positive environment and activities that enhance self-esteem.
  Self-esteem is correlated with the ability to meet self-care requirements (Connelly, 1995; Bailey, 1996).
- Assist patient with evaluating the impact of family and peer group on feelings of self-worth.
  Peer group and family may be factors in reinforcing feeling of guilt, blame, and shame (Bennett, 1995).
- Support socialization and communication skills.
  Increases opportunities for support and validation from others.

Geriatric
- Support client in identifying and adapting to functional changes. Accurate evaluation allows client to establish realistic expectations of self.
- Use reminiscence therapy to identify patterns of strength and accomplishment.
  Identifying strengths and accomplishments counteracts pervasive negativity.
- Encourage participation in peer group activities.
  Withdrawal and social isolation are detrimental to feelings of self-worth.

Home Care Interventions

- Assess client's immediate support system/family for relationship patterns and content of communication.
  Knowledge of client relationships assists the nurse with individualizing care.
- Encourage family to provide support and feedback regarding client value or worth.
  The family is a socially significant cultural group that generates behavior, defines roles, and promotes values.
- Refer to medical social services to assist the family in pattern changes that could benefit the client.
  The best nursing plan may be to access specialty services for the client and family.
- If client is involved in counseling or self-help groups, monitor and encourage attendance. Help client identify value of group participation after each group encounter.
  Discussion about group participation clarifies and reinforces group feedback and support.
- If client is taking prescribed psychotropic medications, assess for knowledge of medication side effects and reasons for taking medication. Teach as necessary.
  Understanding the medical regimen supports compliance.
- Assess medications for effectiveness and side effects and monitor client for compliance.
  Clients with poor ego strength may have difficulty adhering to a medication regimen.

Client/Family Teaching

- Refer to community agencies for psychotherapeutic counseling
- Refer to psychoeducational groups on stress reduction and coping skills.

REFERENCES   Bailey BJ: Meditators of depression in adults with diabetes, *Clin Nurs Research* 5:28, 1992.
Bennett LA: Accountability for alcoholism in American families, *Soc Sci Med* 40:15, 1995.
Connelly CE: An empirical study of a model of self-care in chronic illness, *Clin Nurs Spec* 7:247, 1993.
Coopersmith S: *The antecedents of self-esteem,* Palo Alto, Calif, 1981, Consulting Psychologist Press.
Crouch MA, Straub V: Enhancement of self-esteem in adults, *Fam Comm Health* 6:65, 1983.
Grainger RD: Dealing with feelings of guilt and shame, *Am J Nurs* 9:12, 1991.
Manus HE, Killeen MR: Maintenance of self-esteem by obese children, *J Child Adolescent Psych Nurs* 8:17, 1995.
Norris J: Nursing interventions for self-esteem disturbance, *Nurs Diag* 3:48, 1992.

Self-esteem disturbance

Helen Kelley

Definition   Negative self-evaluation and negative feelings about self or capabilities, which may be directly or indirectly expressed

Defining Characteristics

Self-negating verbalization, expressions of shame or guilt, evaluation of self as unable to deal with events, rationalization or rejection of positive feedback about self, exaggeration of negative feedback about self, rationalization of personal failures, hesitancy about new things or situations, denial of problems obvious to others, projection of blame or responsibility for problems, hypersensitivity to slight criticism, grandiosity

Client Outcomes/Goals

- Accurately assesses own strengths and weaknesses
- Admits own error without excessive guilt or defensiveness
- Accept compliments
- Takes risks and tries new things or puts self in new situations
- Accepts responsibility for own actions
- Accepts criticism and attempts to correct problems

Suggested NIC Interventions

Self-esteem enhancement

Nursing Interventions and Rationales

- Ask clients to list one positive attribute for each negative attribute they generate.
  The list promotes a realistic and balanced self-perspective.
- Treat client nonjudgmentally; acknowledge client's right to have personal values and beliefs.
  Nonjudgmental treatment encourages honesty and shows appreciation for client's unique qualities (Norris, 1992).
- Help client identify origins of self-esteem.
  Self-esteem is learned behavior and can be changed.
- Have client participate in a daily grooming routine.
  Positive feelings are generated when a person is well groomed.
- Reframe mistakes and errors (own and others') as natural and human experiences.
  Modeling acceptance of self and others lessens the need for defensive responses when errors are made.
- Have client practice making positive statements about self and responding in a positive way when compliments are given; role playing may be used.

- Encourage a problem-solving approach rather than an approach emphasizing doubt or defensiveness.
  A problem-solving approach promotes constructive action.
- Encourage client to ask for feedback rather than silently worry about criticism.
  Feedback promotes self-control.
- Give recognition for appropriate risk-taking attempts and encourage the practice of new behaviors.
  Change requires a willingness to tolerate the discomfort of unfamiliar behavior and responses for a period of time (Wilson, Kneisel, 1992).
- Convey genuine acceptance and respect for the client.
  Self-worth is influenced by the respect and recognition of others (Norris, 1992).
- Assist in identification of strengths and provide recognition when they are used.
  Recognition reinforces feelings of competence.
- Provide positive reinforcement for achievements and progress toward goals.
  A self-portrayal decreases the impact of self-criticism.
- Encourage self-responsibility through realistic identification of capabilities as well as needs.
  Identification of needs and abilities promotes appropriate expression of independence as well as dependence on others.
- Encourage communication and expression of feelings through active listening and empathic responses.
  Active listening reinforces the values and rights of a person.
- Support a realistic self-appraisal of abilities and competence.
  Positive feedback corrects predominantly negative self-perceptions.

Geriatric
- Promote a positive self-image—compliment clients on appearance, and help them look their best.
- Do not appear rushed; encourage verbalization of client's fears about the illness or dysfunction.
  An elderly client's response time may be slower. Multiple losses lead to fear about the illness or dysfunction.
- Help client to review life and identify successes. Encourage participation in support/reminiscence groups.
  Reminiscence is very therapeutic for elderly clients.
- Promote honest expression of perceptions.
  Elderly clients experiencing multiple losses may develop a fear of the illness or dysfunction.
- Assist in planning a schedule for regular visits by family and significant others.

Home Care Interventions
See care plan for **Self-esteem, chronic, low.**

Client/Family Teaching
- Teach that self-esteem is learned and can be changed.
- Refer client to community agencies, self-help groups, or counseling as needed.
- Instruct parents to provide clearly defined expectations and limits.
  Expectations and limits contribute to higher levels of self-esteem.
- Instruct parents to encourage independent functioning as appropriate.
  Autonomy contributes to promotion of self-esteem in children (Coopersmith, 1981).

REFERENCES   Bulechek G, McCloskey J: *Nursing interventions: essential nursing treatments,* Philadelphia, 1992, WB Saunders.

Coopersmith S: *The antecedents of self esteem,* Palo Alto, Calif., 1981, Consulting Psychologist Press.

Norris J: Nursing intervention for self-esteem disturbance, *Nurs Diag* 3:48, 1992.

Wilson HS, Kneisel CR: *Psychiatric nursing,* Menlo Park, Calif, 1992, Addison-Wesley.

Situational low self–esteem

Helen Kelley

Definition   Negative self-evaluation of feelings about self that develop in response to a loss or change in an individual who previously had a positive self-evaluation

Defining Characteristics

Major   Episodic occurrence of negative self-appraisal in response to life events in a client with a previously positive self-appraisal

Minor   Self-evaluation, verbalization of negative feelings about the self (e.g., helplessness, uselessness), expressions of shame or guilt, evaluation of self as unable to handle situations or events, difficulty making decisions

Related Factors (r/t)

Situational crisis, significant losses, numerous or changing roles, stressful changes, work, family, body image and appearance, health problems, disability

Client Outcomes/Goals

- States effect of life events on feelings about self
- Recognizes personal strengths
- Acknowledges presence of guilt and does not blame self if an action was related to another person's appraisal
- Seeks help when necessary

Suggested NIC Interventions

Self-esteem enhancement

Nursing Interventions and Rationales

- Actively listen to, demonstrate respect for, and accept client.
  Clarification of thoughts and feelings promotes self-acceptance (LeMone, 1991).
- Assist in the identification of problems and situational factors that contribute to problems.
  Identification validates problems.
- Help clients recognize that only they can control themselves by using statements such as "No one can make you feel guilty without your consent."
- Mutually identify strengths, resources, and previously effective coping strategies.
  Acknowledgement of competence enhances self-esteem (Miller, 1983) and reinforces previously intact self-esteem (Anderson, 1995).
- Have client list strengths.
- Accept client's own pace in working through grief or crisis situations.
  Pressuring the client to prematurely resolve feelings increases the client's sense of inadequacy (Kus, 1985). Adjustment to loss or change can have detrimental effects on the entire concept of self (Drench, 1994).

- Accept the client's own defenses in dealing with the crisis.
  Denial protects the self-concept by distorting reality in a self-enhancing way (Russell, 1993).
- Assess client for symptoms of depression and potential for suicide or violence; immediately notify appropriate personnel of symptoms (see **Risk for violence**).
  Safety measures and psychiatric interventions are essential when a risk for violence is present. Coping attempts may be ineffective during time of crisis.
- Provide information about support groups of people who have experiences or interests in common.
  Support groups provide an opportunity to both give and receive support and understanding.
- Support problem-solving strategies but discourage decision-making when in crisis.
  Crisis is a time of increased tension and disorganization.
- Explore constructive outlets for frustration.
  Exploration expands strategies for coping.
- Encourage objective appraisal of self and life events and challenge negative or perfectionistic expectations of self.
  A positive adjustment to illness may be the result of the ability to lower ideal self-expectations (Heidrich, 1992).
- See **Self-esteem disturbance** and **Chronic low self-esteem.**

Home Care Interventions

- Establish an emergency plan and contract with the client for its use.
  Knowing an emergency plan is reassuring to the client. Establishing a contract validates the worth of the client and provides a caring link between the client and society.
- See **Self-esteem, chronic, low.**

Client/Family Teaching

- Assess person's support system (family, friends, community) and involve if desired.
- Educate client and family regarding the grief process.
  Understanding this process normalizes responses of sadness, anger, guilt, and helplessness.
- Teach client and family that the crisis is temporary.
  Knowing that the crisis is temporary provides a sense of hope for the future.
- Refer to appropriate community resources or crisis intervention centers.

REFERENCES   Anderson KL: The effect of chronic obstructive pulmonary disease on quality of life, *Res Nurs Health* 18:547, 1995.
Drench ME: Changes in body image secondary to disease and injury, *Rehab Nurs* 19:31, 1994.
Heidrich SM, Ward SE: The role of the self in adjustment to cancer in elderly women, *Oncol Nurs Forum* 19:1491, 1992.
Kus RJ: Crisis intervention. In Bulechek GM, McCloskey JC, editors: *Nursing interventions: treatments for nursing diagnoses,* Philadelphia, 1985, WB Saunders.
LeMone P: Analysis of a human phenomenon: self-concept, *Nurs Diag* 2:126, 1991.
Miller JF: *Coping with chronic illness: overcoming powerlessness,* Philadelphia, 1983, FA Davis.
Russell GC: The role of denial in clinical practice, *J Adv Nurs* 18:938, 1993.

Risk for self-mutilation

Gail B. Ladwig

Definition   The state in which an individual is at high risk to perform a deliberate act on the self with the intent not to kill but to injure, which produces immediate tissue damage to the body

Risk Factors (r/t)

Inability to properly cope with increased psychological or physiological tension; feelings of depression, rejection, self-hatred, separation anxiety, guilt, and depersonalization; fluctuating emotions; command hallucinations; need for sensory stimuli; parental emotional deprivation; dysfunctional family

Groups at risk Clients with borderline personality disorders (especially females 16 to 25 years of age), clients in a psychotic state (frequently males in young adulthood), emotionally disturbed or battered children, mentally retarded and autistic children, clients with a history of self-injury

Client Outcomes/Goals

- States appropriate ways to cope with increased psychological or physiological tension
- Expresses feelings.
- Seeks help when having hallucinations.
- Uses appropriate community agencies when caregivers are unable to attend to emotional needs

Suggested NIC Interventions

Anger control assistance, behavior management: self-harm, environmental management

Nursing Interventions and Rationales

- Assessment data may have to be gathered at different times; allowing a family member or trusted friend to be present during the assessment may be helpful.
  Self-mutilation sometimes occurs if clients have been victims of sadistic ritual abuse. They may react intensely and irrationally to routine office visits. Rather than postponing treatment, using the listed interventions may be helpful (Young, 1993).
- Assess for family history of substance abuse.
  Self-mutilation and heavy use of mental health services have been correlated with having an alcoholic parent (Rose, Peabody, Strategies, 1991).
- Monitor client's behavior using 15-minute checks at irregular times so that client does not notice a pattern.
  When there is lack of control, client safety is an important issue and close observation is essential. Not following a pattern prevents clients from being self-abusive when they know a caregiver will not be present.
- Secure a written or verbal contract from client to notify staff when experiencing the desire to self-mutilate.
  Discussing feelings of self-harm with a trusted person provides relief for the client. A contract gets the subject out in the open and places some of the responsibility for safety with the client.
- Help the client identify cues that precede impulsive behavior
  Often, supposedly impulsive events are preceded by tension and unrecognized impulse control (Gallop, 1992).
- Give praise when client identifies urges and delays self-destructive behavior.
  Delaying destructive behavior and increasing awareness of urges to be self-destructive should both be acknowledged as progress (Gallop, 1992).

- Monitor for presence of hallucinations. Ask specific questions, such as "Do you hear voices that other people do not hear?"
  Brief, reversible psychotic episodes tend to occur as a response to stress (First et al, 1994). An accurate assessment of the client's contact with reality is important in planning care; acknowledging that the client may hear something that others do not may open up communication and help establish trust.
- Assure clients that they will not be alone and will be safe during hallucinations. Provide referrals for medication.
  Hallucinations can be very frightening, so clients needs reassurance that they will not be left alone.
- Be extremely cautious about touching clients when they are experiencing an *abreaction* (reenactment of precipitating trauma). Sometimes physically holding a client is necessary to prevent self-injury.
  Touch may be intrepreted as coming from an abuser and could result in aggressive acting out. Even well-intentioned or consoling touching may further upset the client. A therapist who is attempting to be consoling should always ask abreacting clients whether they can be touched. Clients may initially refuse, but they generally appreciate the offer. An offer may be repeated several times and clients may eventually agree to be touched or held. If clients must be held to prevent self-injury, explain why it is necessary before touching them (Fike, 1990).
- If self-mutilation does occur, care for the wounds in a matter-of-fact way.
  This approach does not promote inappropriate attention-getting behavior and may decrease repetition of behavior.
- When client is experiencing extreme anxiety, use one-to-one staffing.
  The presence of a trusted individual may calm fears about personal safety.
- Reinforce alternative ways of dealing with anxiety such as exercise, engaging in unit activities, or talking about feelings.
  With practice, clients can substitute other behaviors when feeling anxious. If inappropriate ways of handling life situations can be learned, appropriate ways can also be learned.
- Keep environment safe; remove all harmful objects from the area. Use of unbreakable glass is recommended for clients at risk for self-injury.
  Client safety is a nursing priority. Putting a hand through a window was the most frequent self-injuring behavior in this study. Unbreakable glass would eliminate this type of injury (Callias, Carpenter, 1994).
- If client is unable to control behavior, provide interactive supervision, not isolation.
  Isolation and deprivation take away individuals' coping abilities and place them at risk for self-harm. Implementing seclusion for clients who have injured themselves in the past may actually facilitate self-injury. "Despite finding themselves lodged within spartan rooms cleared of artifacts, having had personal clothing removed, and having been searched, clients showed an extraordinary 'morbid resourcefulness' for inflicting injury" (Burrow, 1992).
- Involve client in planning of care and emphasize that client can make choices.
  Problem solving is a way to gain better emotional control by assisting clients with seeing the connection between problems and emotions (Miller, Eisner, Allport, 1994).
- Emphasize that client must comply with the rules of the unit. Give positive reinforcement for compliance and minimize attention paid to disruptive behavior.
  It is important to reinforce appropriate behavior to encourage repetition.

- Involve the client in group therapy.
  Group members learn to identify patterns of behavior that were acquired as a result of painful past events. The past is not trivialized but acknowledged as leading to patterns that now influence all interactions (Gallop, 1992).
- Use group therapy to exchange information about methods of coping with loneliness, self-destructive impulses, and interpersonal relationships, as well as housing, employment, and health care system issues directly and noninterpretively.
  Data suggest that an important component of effective group treatment for a seriously ill person with borderline personality disorder is the meaningful exchange of information. The degree of structure may be a necessary condition for positive outcomes (Nehls, 1992).
- Concentrate on client's strengths. Have client visualize the word "STOP" when negative self-talk begins, and replace the negativity with an affirmation or positive statement.
  Individuals with borderline personality disorder commonly engage in self-talk that is invalid and self-deprecating (Miller, Eisner, Allport, 1994).
- Refer to protective services if there is evidence of abuse.
  It is the nurse's legal responsibility to report abuse.

Home Care Interventions

- Assess the family and caregiving situation for ability to protect the client.
  Client safety between home visits is a nursing priority.
- Establish an emergency plan including when to use hotlines and 911. Develop a contract with the client on use of the emergency plan. Role play access to the emergency resources with the client and caregivers.
  Having an emergency plan reassures the client and caregivers and promotes client safety. Contracting gives guided control to the client and enhances self-esteem.
- Assess the home environment for harmful objects. Have family remove or lock objects as able.
  Client safety is a nursing priority.
- If client behaviors intensify, refer for mental health intervention.
  The degree of disturbance and the ability to manage care safely at home determines the level of services needed to protect the client.
- Refer for homemaker or psychiatric home health aide services for respite and client reassurance.
  Responsibility for a person at high risk for self-mutilation provides high caregiver stress. Respite decreases caregiver stress; the presence of caring individuals is reassuring to both the client and caregivers, especially during periods of client anxiety.
- If client is on psychotropic medications, assess client and family knowledge of medication administration and side effects. Teach as necessary.
  Knowledge of the medical regimen promotes compliance.
- Evaluate the effectiveness and side effects of medications.
  Accurate clinical feedback improves physician ability to prescribe an effective medical regimen specific to client needs.

Client/Family Teaching

- Suggest feasible activities for the client and significant others (simple tasks like washing dishes, taking out the garbage). Performance of complex previous tasks such as bill paying may not be possible until therapy is complete. Client and family need to know this is a temporary situation.

The education of clients with multiple personality disorder and their significant others is both critical and practical. Teaching helps to reduce anxiety and gives them strategies for coping with their distress (Fike, 1990).

- Teach stress reduction techniques such as imagery and controlled breathing (breathing in on "re" and out on "lax"); teach client to sustain the breathing-out phase.
  Imagery is effective in helping clients adjust to the demands of chronic illness (Stephens, 1993).
- Provide client and family with phone numbers of appropriate community agencies for therapy and counseling.
  Continuous follow-up care may be necessary, so the method to access this care must be given to the client.
- Give client positive things on which to focus by referring to appropriate agencies for job-training skills or education.
  Alternative coping skills and the means to access them are essential for continued good mental health.

REFERENCES   Burrow S: The deliberate self-harming behavior of patients within a British special hospital, *J Adv Nurs* 17:138, 1992.

Callias M, Carpenter M: Self-injurious behavior in a state psychiatric hospital, *Hosp Community Psychiatry* 45:170, 1994.

Fike ML: Considerations and techniques in the treatment of persons with multiple personality disorder, *Am J Occup Ther* 44:999, 1990.

First MB et al: Changes in mood, anxiety, and personality disorders, *Psychiatr Nurs* 1994, p. 1.

Gallop R: Self-destructive and impulsive behavior in the patient with a borderline personality disorder: rethinking hospital treatment and management, *Arch Psychiatr Nurs* 6:178, 1992.

Miller C, Eisner W, Allport C: Creative coping: A cognitive-behavioral group for borderline personality disorder, *Arch Psychiatr Nurs* 8:280, 1994.

Nehls N: Group therapy for people with borderline personality disorder: interventions associated with positive outcomes, *Issu Ment Health Nurs* 13:255, 1992.

Rose SM, Peabody CG, Strategies B: Undetected abuse among intensive case management clients, *Hosp Community Psychiatry* 42:5, 1991.

Stephens R: Imagery: a strategic intervention to empower clients. Part II—a practical guide, *Clin Nurs Spec* 7:235, 1993.

Young W: Sadistic ritual abuse: an overview in detection and management, *Primary Care* 20:447, 1993.

Sensory/perceptual alterations (specify): visual, auditory, kinesthetic, gustatory, tactile, olfactory

Betty J. Ackley

Definition   The state in which an individual experiences a change in the amount or patterning of oncoming stimuli accompanied by a diminished, exaggerated, distorted, or impaired response to such stimuli

Defining Characteristics

Major   Disorientation regarding time, place, or persons; altered abstraction; altered conceptualization; change in problem-solving abilities; reported or measured change in sensory acuity; change in behavior pattern; anxiety; apathy; change in usual response to stimuli; indication of body image alteration; restlessness; irritability; altered communication patterns

Minor   Complaints of fatigue, alterations in posture, changes in muscular tension, inappropriate responses, hallucinations

Related Factors (r/t)

Altered, excessive, or insufficient environmental stimuli; altered sensory reception, transmission, or integration; endogenous chemical alterations (e.g., electrolytes), exogenous chemical alterations (e.g., drugs); psychological stress

Client Outcomes/Goals

- Demonstrates understanding by a verbal, written, or signed response
- Demonstrates relaxed body movements and facial expressions
- Explains plan to modify life-style to accommodate visual or hearing impairment
- Remains free of physical harm resulting from decreased balance or a loss of vision, hearing, or tactile sensation
- Maintains contact with appropriate community resources

Suggested NIC Interventions

Communication enhancement: hearing deficit, reality orientation, surveillance: safety

Nursing Interventions and Rationales

Sensory deprivation/overload

- Observe for factors that can cause sensory/perceptual alterations (e.g., insufficient sleep, sensory deprivation, sensory overload with excessive noise and stimuli, substance abuse, medications, electrolyte imbalance, normal aging process). *Sensory/perceptual alterations are common in clients' critical and surgical care (especially cardiac surgery) and in hospitalized elderly clients (Wilson, 1993).*
- Assess orientation, attention, concentration, memory, ability to think, overall appearance, body movements, speech, use of appropriate language, mood, and affect. *A complete bedside assessment is necessary to determine the presence of sensory/perceptual alteration (Inaba-Roland, Maricle, 1992). Symptoms of sensory deprivation or overload include changes in attention span, confusion, emotional lability, talking to self, and changes in visual routines.*

Sensory deprivation

- Help clients out of bed and into a different environment at intervals. Use a "stretcher chair" if client is unable to transfer. *Spending large amounts of time isolated in bed has been shown to result in sensory disturbances in healthy people. Elderly people who are ill can develop confusion from sensory deprivation (Downs, 1974).*
- Orient client to time, place, and person. Inform client of current weather, news items, family visits, or telephone calls. *Reality orientation can help prevent onset of confusion.*
- Converse with client when entering the room, touch client as appropriate and according to client's cultural norms, and explain all procedures. Do not discuss client's situation with physician or fellow staff without including client in the conversation. *Meaningful human contact within the framework of the client's culture may help decrease the incidence of confusion (Kloosterman, 1991).*
- Provide radio, television, clocks, and calendars. *These items will help maintain orientation and increase sensory stimuli.*
- Encourage visits from significant others. Encourage client to keep pictures of family and friends at bedside. *Hospitalized clients who have less contact with significant others have an increase in sensory/perceptual alterations (Foreman, 1986).*

- If client has hearing or vision loss, see section of nursing care plan on this area. Both vision and hearing loss can increase sensory deprivation.

Sensory overload

- Recognize that pain, lack of sleep, worry, and effects of medications can aggravate the effects of sensory overload.
- Help clients maintain their "humanness" by showing compassion, using touch as appropriate, treating them with respect and dignity, and communicating before giving all care.
  In high-technology environments, clients become depersonalized and overwhelmed by multiple stimuli and need "high touch care" to deal with the high-technology environment (Halm, Alpen, 1993).
- Decrease noise pollution as much as possible (e.g., place pulse oximeter away from client's head, turn off suction when not in use, hang IVs before alarm sounds).
  Constant noxious noise can lead to sensory overload and ICU psychosis and impede healing (Griffin, 1992; Halm, Alpen, 1993). Constant noise also makes the nurse less caring and more aggressive in nature (Grummet, 1993).
- Cluster activities to provide rest periods; morning naps are especially helpful. Ensure at least 2 hours of uninterrupted sleep at night. See nursing interventions for **Sleep pattern disturbance.**

Auditory—hearing loss

- Keep background noise to a minimum. Turn off television and radio when communicating with client.
  Background noise significantly interferes with hearing in the hearing-impaired client.
- Stand or sit directly in front of client when communicating. Make sure adequate light is on nurse's face, avoid covering mouth or face with hands while speaking, establish eye contact, and use nonverbal gestures.
  These measures make it easier to read lips and see nonverbal communication, which is a large component of all communication.
- Speak distinctly in lower voice tones if possible. Do not overenunciate or shout at client.
  In many kinds of hearing loss, clients lose the ability to hear higher-pitched tones but can still hear lower-pitched tones. Overenunciating makes it difficult to read lips. Shouting makes the words less clear and frightens the client.
- If necessary, provide a communication board or personnel who know sign language.
  Alternative forms of communication help decrease social isolation.
- Try inserting the earpieces of the stethoscope into the client's ears, and talking into diaphragm.
  Stethoscopes magnify sound and can help some clients hear better.
- Refer to appropriate resources such as a speech and hearing clinic, audiologist, or ear, nose, and throat physician.
  Hearing loss can be treated with medical or surgical interventions or use of a hearing aid.
- Observe emotional needs and encourage expression of feelings.
  Hearing impairments may cause frustration, anger, fear, and self-imposed isolation (Taylor, 1993).

Visual—loss of vision

- Identify name and purpose when entering client's room.
  Identification when entering the room helps the client feel secure and decreases social isolation.

- Orient to time, place, person, and surroundings. Provide a radio or talking books.
  These actions help client remain oriented and provide sensory stimulation.
- Keep doors completely open or closed. Keep furniture out of path to bathroom and do not rearrange furniture.
  These steps help maintain a safe environment for the client (Beaver, Mann, 1995).
- Feed client at mealtimes if blindness is temporary.
- Keep siderails up for client's safety; explain this precaution to client.
- Converse with and touch client frequently during care if frequent touch is within client's cultural norm.
  Appropriate touch can decrease social isolation.
- Walk client by having client grasp nurse's elbow and walk partly behind nurse. Walk a frightened or confused client by having client put both hands on nurse's shoulders; nurse backs up in desired direction while holding client around the waist.
  These methods help the client feel secure and ensures safety.
- Keep call light button within client's reach; check location of call light button before leaving the room.
- Ensure access to eyeglasses or magnifying devices.
- Pay attention to client's emotional needs. Encourage expression of feelings and expect grieving behavior.
  Blind people grieve the loss of vision and experience a loss of identity and control over their lives (Vader, 1992).
- Refer to optometrist, ophthalmologist, or specialist in vision loss for vision care if needed.
  Treatment of diabetic retinopathy can greatly reduce the incidence of blindness (Winslow, 1994). Many clients with eye disorders need frequent medical care to maintain vision.

NOTE For **Sensory perceptual alteration: kinesthetic and tactile,** see **Risk for injury.** For **Sensory perceptual alteration: olfactory and gustatory** see **Altered nutrition: less than body requirements.**

Geriatric
- Keep environment quiet, soothing, and familiar. Use consistent caregivers.
  These measures are comforting to the elderly and help decrease confusion.
- Avoid providing extremely hot or cold foods or using hot bathwater if client has decreased sensation in mouth, hands, or feet.
- If client has a sensory deprivation, encourage family to provide sensory stimulation with music, voices, photographs, touch, and familiar smells.
- If client has a hearing or vision loss, work with client to ensure contact with others and to strengthen the social network.
  Severe loneliness can accompany hearing or vision loss in the elderly as a result of self-imposed isolation (Christian, Dluhy, O'Neill, 1989; Foxall et al, 1992).

Home Care Interventions

The listed interventions are applicable in the home care setting

Client/Family Teaching

- For low-vision elderly clients with macular degeneration or cataract formation, teach client/family methods to increase independence and prevent injury including the following:
  - Put red or yellow identifiers on important items that need to be seen such as a red strip at the edge of steps, red behind a light switch, or a red dot on a stove or washing machine to indicate how far to turn knob.
  - Use a watch or clock that verbally tells time and a phone with large numbers and emergency numbers programmed in.

- ▪ Use low-vision aids including magnifying devices, a closed-circuit television that magnifies print, a special lens for close and distant vision, and guides for writing checks and envelopes.
  - ▪ Increase lighting in the home, and decrease glare where light reflects on shiny surfaces. Use motion lights that come on automatically when a person enters the room.
- Teach family how to provide appropriate stimuli in the home environment to prevent sensory/perceptual alterations.
- Teach blind client how to feed self; associate food on plate with hours on a clock so that client can identify location of food.
- Refer to community agencies for help in dealing with sensory/perceptual losses.

REFERENCES   Beaver KA, Mann WC: Overview of technology for low vision, *Am J Occup Ther* 49:913, 1995.

Christian E, Dluhy N, O'Neill R: Sounds of silence: coping with hearing loss and loneliness, *J Gerontol Nurse* 15:4, 1989.

Cropp AJ et al: Name that tone: the proliferation of alarms in the intensive care unit, *Chest* 105:1217, 1994.

Downs FS: Bedrest and sensory disturbances, *AJN* 3:434, 1974.

Foreman M: Acute confusional states in hospitalized elderly: a research dilemma, *Nurs Res* 35:34, 1986.

Foxall MJ et al: Predictors of loneliness in low vision adults, *West J Nurs Res* 14:86, 1992.

Griffin JP: The impact of noise on critically ill people, *Holistic Nurse Pract* 6:53, 1992.

Grumet GW: Pandemonium in the modern hospital, *New Engl J Med* 328:433, 1993.

Halm MA, Alpen MA: The impact of technology on patients and families, *Adv Clin Nurs Res* 28:443, 1993.

Inaba-Roland K, Maricle R: Assessing delirium in the acute care setting, *Heart Lung* 21:48, 1992.

Kloosterman ND: Cultural care: the missing link in severe sensory alteration, *Nurs Sci Q* 4:119, 1991.

Taylor KS: Geriatric hearing loss: management strategies for nurses, *Geriatr Nurs* 14:74, 1993.

Vader LA: Vision and vision loss, *Nurs Clin North Am* 27:705, 1992.

Wilson LD: Sensory perceptual alteration: diagnosis, prediction and intervention in the hospitalized adult, *Nurs Clin North Am* 28:747, 1993.

Winslow EH: Laser treatment prevents blindness, *AJN* 3:19, 1994.

Sexual dysfunction

Gail B. Ladwig

Definition   The state in which an individual experiences a change in sexual function that is unsatisfying, unrewarding, and inadequate

Defining Characteristics

Verbalization of problem, alteration in achieving perceived sex role, actual or perceived limitation imposed by disease or therapy, value conflict, alteration in achieving sexual satisfaction, inability to achieve desired satisfaction, seeking of confirmation of desirability, alteration in relationship with significant other, change of interest in self and others

Related Factors (r/t)

Biopsychosocial alteration of sexuality, ineffectual or absent role models, physical abuse, psychosocial abuse (e.g., harmful relationships), vulnerability, value conflict, lack of privacy, lack of significant other, altered body structure or function (e.g., pregnancy, recent childbirth, drugs, surgery, anomalies, disease process, trauma, irradiation), misinformation, knowledge deficit

Client Outcomes/Goals

- Identifies individual cause of sexual dysfunction
- Identifies stressors that contribute to dysfunction
- Discusses alternative, satisfying, and acceptable sexual practices for self and partner
- Discusses with partner concerns about body image and sex role

Suggested NIC Interventions

Sexual counseling

Nursing Interventions and Rationales

- Gather client's sexual history, noting normal patterns of functioning and client's vocabulary.

  Sexual problems can result from biological, intrapersonal, and interpersonal distress. Generally, several of these factors combine to produce sexual dysfunction. Nurses can prevent some sexual dysfunctions from developing by being prepared and willing to empathetically discuss sexuality with their clients and provide them with accurate information. Sexuality and sexual behavior must be assessed on an individual basis (Fontaine, 1991).

- Determine client's and partner's current knowledge and understanding.

  One of the most important nursing interventions is giving practical information (Laurent, 1994). If unsure of a client's sexuality, use the term partner, which helps avoid making any assumptions or judgments about a relationship. A sexual relationship may be heterosexual or homosexual, and nurses must not lose sight of this (Taylor, 1994).

- Observe for stress, anxiety, and depression as a possible cause of dysfunction.

  Sexual dysfunction can be attributed to many psychological factors.

- Observe for grief related to loss (e.g., amputation, mastectomy, ostomy).

  *A change in body image often precedes sexual dysfunction (see **Body image disturbance**).*

- Explore physical causes such as diabetes, arteriosclerotic heart disease, drug or medication side effects, or smoking (males).

  Researchers have shown that sexual difficulties often occur as a result of cardiovascular disease. In fact, at least 25% to 50% of men and women who have suffered a previous myocardial infarction (MI) never regain their earlier frequency of sexual activity, and some do not resume any sexual activity at all (Papadopoulos, 1991).

- Provide privacy and be verbally and nonverbally nonjudgmental.

  Privacy is important in ensuring confidentiality. To facilitate communication, it is also vital that the nurse clarify personal values and remain nonjudgmental.

- Provide privacy to allow sexual expression between client and partner (e.g., private room, Do Not Disturb sign for a specified length of time).

  The hospital setting has little opportunity for privacy, so the nurse must ensure that it is available.

- Explain need for client to share concerns with partner.

  Regardless of sexual function and activities, maintaining the relationship is important for meeting intimacy needs (Lemone, 1991).

- Validate clients' feelings, let them know they are normal, and correct misinformation.

  A sensitive nurse who has an understanding of sexual health, functioning, and interferences can direct those who need help toward treatment (Lewis, 1992).

Geriatric
- Discuss with client and partner their present role adjustments.

  This discussion assists client and partner with coping.

- Teach about normal changes that occur with aging: *female*—reduction in vaginal lubrication, decrease in the degree and speed of vaginal expansion, reduction in duration and resolution of orgasm; *male*—increase in time required for erection, increase in erection time without ejaculation, less firm erection, decrease in volume of seminal fluid, increase in time another erection can occur (12 to 24 hours).
  The older adult experiences a number of physiological changes; these changes are gradual and vary from person to person (Shell, Smith, 1994).
- Suggest the following to enhance sexual functioning: *female*—use water-based vaginal lubricant, increase foreplay time, avoid direct stimulation of the clitoris if painful (clitoris may be exposed because of atrophy of the labia), practice Kegel exercises (alternately contracting and relaxing the muscles in the pelvic area), urinate immediately after coitus because of irritation to the urethra and bladder, and consult with a physician about use of systemic estrogen therapy or topical estrogen cream; *male*—have female partner try a new coital position by bending her knees and placing a pillow under her hips to elevate pelvis, (will more easily accommodate a partially erect penis), massage penis down using pressure at base, which puts pressure on major blood vessel and keeps blood in the penis; ask the female partner to literally push the penis into the vagina herself and flex her vaginal muscles that have been strengthened by Kegel exercises; if one of the partners has a protruding abdomen, experiment to find a position that allows the penis to reach the vagina (have woman lie on her back with legs apart and knees sharply bent while the man places himself over her with his hips under the angle formed by the raised knees); consult with a physician about use of penis self-injection with phentolamine/papaverine, which will elicit an erection that lasts about 1 hour.
  These gender-specific sexual interventions for the elderly may help maintain sexual functioning (Shell, Smith, 1994).
- Assess the possibility of erectile dysfunction.
  Erectile dysfunction occurs in men of any age but is more common in older men. Sexual functioning can almost always be restored, but many men never seek help (Lewis, 1992).
- Explore with client and partner various sexual gratification alternatives (e.g., caressing, sharing feelings).
  There are many satisfying alternatives for expressing sexual feelings. The many losses associated with aging leave the elderly with special needs for love and affection.
- Discuss the difference between sexual function and sexuality.
  All individuals possess sexuality from birth to death, regardless of the changes that occur over the life span.
- If prescribed, teach how to use nitroglycerin before sexual activity.
  Pain inhibits satisfying sexual activity.
- See **Altered sexuality pattern.**

Home Care Interventions

- Assist the client and significant other with identifying place and time in home and daily living for privacy in sharing sexual or relationship activity. If necessary, assist clients in communicating need for privacy to other family members. Consider periodic escapes to desirable surroundings.
  The home setting can be one that affords little if any privacy without conscious effort of the members of the home.

- Confirm that physical reasons for dysfunction have been addressed. Encourage participation in support groups or therapy if appropriate.
  Clients often express embarrassment at continuing medical intervention or participation in groups once they are back in the community and know that peers may judge their activities.
- Reinforce or teach client about sexual functioning, alternative sexual practices, necessary sexual precautions. Update teaching as client status changes.
  If the client and/or significant other have received information during an institutional stay, other stressors may have made the information a temporarily low priority or may have impaired learning. Depending on the cause for dysfunction, the client may experience changing status or feelings about the problem.

Client/Family Teaching

- Teach the importance of resting before sexual activity. For some clients, mornings are the best time for sexual activity.
  Clients may have a more satisfying experience if they are not tired.
- Teach the client to resume intimate physical contact by using mutual touching 3 to 6 weeks after an MI.
  Sexual activity after an MI should not be demanding, so mutual touching is recommended (Papadopoulos, 1991).
- Teach client to begin vigorous sexual activity after an MI when client can walk rapidly for 10 minutes and then climb two flights of stairs in 10 seconds.
  If this can be done without shortness of breath or other symptoms, then the client is ready to begin preestablished levels of sexual activity (Papadopoulos, 1991).
- Teach client to take prescribed pain medications before sexual activity.
  Pain inhibits satisfying sexual activity.
- Teach possible need for modifying positions (e.g., side-to-side, limited resting on arms, heavier person on bottom).
  Changes in position can enhance satisfaction and comfort.
- Refer to appropriate community resources such as a clinical specialist, family counselor, or sexual counselor; if appropriate, include both partners in the discussion.
  A high percentage of women report a need for more information after a cancer surgery that affected their sexual response. They also express a need for partners to be included in the discussions (Corney et al, 1992).
- Teach vaginal dilation to prevent stenosis and to expect a bit of spotting after first session of intercourse.
  Clients with gynecological cancer and surgery, particularly cervical cancer, could reduce the number of physical problems if the preceding information was taught (Laurent, 1994).
- Teach how drug therapy affects a sexual response, such as the possible side effects and the need to report them.
  Some drugs used for multiple sclerosis (MS) may impair sexual functioning. Antispastic drugs (e.g., methantheline, baclofen) may reduce libido, and tranquilizing drugs (e.g., diazepam, barbiturates) may interfere with emission and ejaculation in men. Tricyclic antidepressant drugs (e.g., imipramine, amitriptyline) may interfere with erection in men and with vaginal lubrication, clitoral engorgement, and orgasm in women (Dupont, 1995).

- Teach the importance of diabetic control and its effect on sexuality to clients with insulin-dependent diabetes.
  Sexual functioning may be changed by alterations in glucose levels, infections that affect comfort during sexual intercourse, changes in vaginal lubrication and penile erection, and changes in sexual desire and arousal (Lemone, 1993).
- Teach specifics if client has a stoma: do not substitute the stoma for an anus, and substitute for the natural body lubricant should be used. (Saliva can be applied with fingers.)
  If a stoma is abused in this way, it can become traumatized and need further surgery. Clients may have decreased natural lubrication; they have complained that synthetic lubricants become dry and tangled in the pubic hairs causing discomfort (Taylor, 1994).
- See geriatric interventions if there is a problem with erection associated with stoma surgery.

REFERENCES Corney R et al: The care of patients undergoing surgery for gynecological cancer: the need for information, emotional support and counseling, *J Adv Nurs* 17:667, 1992.
Dupont S: Multiple sclerosis and sexual functioning—a review, *Clin Rehab* 9:135, 1995.
Fontaine K: Unlocking sexual issues, *Nurs Clin North Am* 26:737, 1991.
Laurent C: Talking treatment. Therapy for cervical cancer has left some women with severe sexual problems, *Nursing Times* 90:14, 1994.
Lemone P: Human sexuality in adults with insulin-dependent diabetes mellitus, *Image* 25:101, 1993.
Lemone P: *Transforming: patterns of sexual function in adults with insulin-dependent diabetes mellitus,* Birmingham, 1991, University of Alabama.
Lewis JH: Treatment options for men with sexual dysfunction, *J ET Nurs,* 19:131, 1992.
Papadopoulos C: Sex and the cardiac patient, 1994. *Med Aspects Hum Sexuality* 24:55, 1991. In Quadagno D et al: Cardiovascular disease and sexual functioning, *Appl Nurs Res* 8:143, 1995.
Shell J, Smith C: Sexuality and the older person with cancer, *Oncol Nurs Forum* 21:553, 1994.
Stuart G, Sundeen S: *Pocket guide to psychiatric nursing,* ed 2, St Louis, 1991, Mosby.
Taylor P: Beating the taboo, *Nursing Times* 90:51, 1994.

Altered sexuality pattern

Gail B. Ladwig

Definition   The state in which an individual expresses concern regarding own sexuality

Defining Characteristics
Reported difficulties, limitations, or changes in sexual behaviors or activities

Related Factors (r/t)
Knowledge or skill deficit regarding alternative responses to health-related transitions, altered body functioning or structure, illness or medical cause, lack of privacy, lack of significant other, ineffective or absent role models, conflicts with sexual orientation, variant preferences, fear of pregnancy or of acquiring a sexually transmitted disease, impaired relationship with significant other

Client Outcomes/Goals
- States knowledge of difficulties, limitations, or changes in sexual behaviors or activities
- States knowledge of sexual anatomy and functioning
- States acceptance of altered body structure or functioning

- Describes acceptable alternative sexual practices
- Identifies importance of discussing sexual issues with significant other
- Describes practice of "safe sex" in regard to pregnancy and avoidance of sexually transmitted diseases

Nursing Interventions and Rationales

- After establishing rapport or a therapeutic relationship, give client permission to discuss issues dealing with sexuality; ask client specifically, "Have you been or are you concerned about functioning sexually because of your health status?"
  Sexual problems can result from biological, intrapersonal, and interpersonal distress. Generally, several of these factors combine to produce sexual dysfunction. Nurses can prevent some sexual dysfunctions from developing by being prepared and willing to empathetically discuss sexuality with their clients and provide them with accurate information. Sexuality and sexual behavior must be assessed on an individual basis (Fontaine,1991).
- Determine client's and partner's current knowledge and understanding.
  One of the most important nursing interventions is giving practical information (Laurent, 1994).
- Discuss alternative sexual expressions for altered body functioning or structure; closeness and touching are other forms of expression, and some clients choose masturbation for sexual release.
  Masturbation is one of the most common sexual expressions but at the same time is one of the least acknowledged (Fontaine, 1991).
- If mutual masturbation is a choice of expression, provide latex gloves.
  Latex gloves prevent possible exposure to infection through cuts on hands (Tucker et al, 1996).
- Discuss modifying positions to accommodate the altered physical state; instruct in the use of pillows for comfort.
  Modified positions can enable and enhance sexual satisfaction otherwise impeded by physical disability.
- Encourage client to discuss concerns with their partner.
  If unsure of a client's sexuality, use the term partner *to avoid making any assumptions or judgments about the relationship. A sexual relationship may be heterosexual or homosexual, and nurses must not lose sight of this (Taylor, 1994).*
- Provide the client privacy for sexual expression (e.g., closed door when significant other visits, "Do Not Disturb" sign on door).
  The hospital environment needs to allow for sexual expression between partners.

Geriatric
- Help client redefine sexuality in broader terms such as sharing, communication, and intimacy.
  Sexuality is a primary part of being human and does not cease after age 65. Elderly individuals need to continue to view themselves as masculine or feminine (Shell, Smith, 1994).
- Allow client to verbalize feelings regarding loss of sexual partner or significant other. Acknowledge problems such as disapproval from children, lack of available partners for women and environmental variables that will make forming new relationships difficult.
  Many individuals face loneliness when they lose a partner, and the loss of interpersonal intimacy is a sensitive problem. After a loss of this magnitude, elderly people often find that forming new relationships is difficult. Privacy is also a problem (Shell, Smith, 1994).

- Provide a milieu that allows for discussion of sexual issues and a higher level of sexual satisfaction. Allow couples to room together and bring in double beds from home. Place signs on the door to ensure privacy.
  Environmental variables have an impact on elderly people's ability to freely express sexuality (Shell, Smith, 1994).
- Provide clients with the following information:
  - Exercise, such as walking, swimming, cycling, and riding a stationary bike, will help control flabby thighs and weak musculature and make people feel more sexually attractive.
  - Overindulgence in food or alcohol can affect sexual activity (see **Altered nutrition: less than body requirements**
  - Resting and sleeping on a firm mattress may augment sexual desire.
  - Femininity and masculinity are still important.
  - Pay attention to cleanliness, skin care and clothing.
  - Change environment.
  - Experiment with position changes.
    Because the majority of the elderly population maintains sexual interest, desire, and functioning, the mentioned interventions may be helpful during the rehabilitation process. Older adults may exercise aerobically 3 to 5 times a week for 15 to 30 minutes depending on physical status and treatment regimen (Steinke, Bergen, 1986).
- See **Sexual dysfunction.**

Home Care Interventions

- Assist client and significant other with identifying place and time in the home and daily living for privacy in sharing sexual or relationship activity. If necessary, assist clients with communicating the need for privacy to other family members. Consider periodic escapes to desirable surroundings.
  The home setting can be one which affords little if any privacy without conscious effort of the members of the home.
- Confirm that physical reasons for dysfunction have been addressed. Encourage participation in support groups or therapy if appropriate.
  Clients express embarrassment at continuing medical intervention or participation in groups once they are back in the community and know that peers may judge their activities.
- Reinforce or teach about sexual functioning, alternative sexual practices, necessary sexual precautions. Update teaching as client status changes.
  If the client or significant other has received information during an institutional stay, other stressors may have made the information a temporarily low priority or may have impaired learning. Depending on the cause for dysfunction, the client may experience changing status or feelings about the problem.

Client/Family Teaching

- Refer to appropriate community agencies (e.g., certified sex counselor, Reach to Recovery, Ostomy Association).
  There may be needs that either are beyond the nurse's skill and ability to address or are related to a particular situation (e.g., presence of an ostomy that requires intervention from specialized sources) (Lewis, 1992).
- Provide information regarding self-care (e.g., *Beauty and Cancer* [Noyes, Mellodey, 1988]) and positioning (e.g., *Sexuality and Cancer: for the woman who has cancer and her partner,* Schover, 1988).

Couples may hesitate to change their routines. Providing this kind of information in a sensitive way often gives permission to change (Shell, Smith, 1994).

- Discuss contraceptive choices. Refer to appropriate health professional (e.g., gynecologist, nurse practitioner).
  Specialists may be needed for complex situations.
- Teach safe sex, which includes using latex condoms, applying spermicide with nonoxynol 9 inside and outside of the condom (which appears to give added protection if the condom breaks), washing with soap immediately after sexual contact, not ingesting semen, avoiding oral-genital contact, not exchanging saliva, avoiding multiple partners, abstaining from sexual activity when ill, and avoiding recreational drugs and alcohol when engaging in sexual activity.
  Accurate information regarding safe sex is essential for sexually active clients (Tucker et al, 1992).

REFERENCES   Fontaine K: Unlocking sexual issues, *Nurs Clin North Am* 26:737, 1991.

Laurent C: Talking treatment: therapy for cervical cancer has left some women with severe sexual problems, *Nursing Times* 90:14, 1994.

Lewis JH: Treatment options for men with sexual dysfunction, *J ET Nurs* 19:131, 1992.

Noyes D, Mellodey P: *Beauty and cancer,* Los Angeles, 1988, AC Press.

Schover L: *Sexuality and cancer: for the woman who has cancer and her partner,* New York, 1988, American Cancer Society.

Shell J, Smith C: Sexuality and the older person with cancer, *Oncol* 21:553, 1994.

Taylor P: Beating the taboo, *Nursing Times* 90:51, 1994.

Tucker M et al: *Patient care standards: collaborative practice planning,* ed 6, St Louis, 1996, Mosby.

Impaired skin integrity

Diane Krasner

Definition

The state in which an individual's skin is adversely altered

Defining Characteristics

Disruption of skin surface, destruction of skin layers

Related Factors (r/t)

External (environmental)

Hyperthermia, hypothermia, chemical substance, mechanical factors (e.g., friction, shearing forces, pressure, restraint), irradiation, physical immobilization, humidity

Internal (somatic)

Medication, altered nutritional state (e.g., obesity, emaciation), altered metabolic state, altered circulation, altered sensation, altered pigmentation, skeletal prominence, developmental factors, immunological deficit, altered skin turgor (change in elasticity)

Client Outcomes/Goals

- Regains integrity of skin surface
- Reports any altered sensation or pain at site of skin impairment
- Demonstrates understanding of plan to heal skin and prevent reinjury
- Describes measures to protect and heal the skin and to care for any skin lesion

Suggested NIC Interventions

Incision site care, pressure ulcer care, skin care: topical treatments, skin surveillance, wound care

Nursing Interventions and Rationales

- Assess site of skin impairment and determine etiology (e.g., acute or chronic wound, burn, dermatological lesion, pressure ulcer, skin tear).
  Prior assessment of wound etiology is critical for proper identification of nursing interventions (van Rijswijk, 1996).
- Determine that skin impairment involves skin damage only (e.g., partial-thickness wound, stage-I or stage-II pressure ulcer). Classify superficial pressure ulcers in the following manner:
  - Stage I: Nonblanchable erythema of intact skin, heralding lesion of skin ulceration
  - Stage II: Partial-thickness skin loss involving epidermis or dermis, superficial ulcer that appears as an abrasion, blister, or shallow crater (National Pressure Ulcer Advisory Panel, 1989)
- For wounds deeper into subcutaneous tissue, muscle, or bone (stage III or stage IV pressure ulcers), see the nursing diagnosis **Impaired tissue integrity.**
- Monitor site of skin impairment at least once a day for color changes, redness, swelling, warmth, pain, or other signs of infection. Determine whether client is experiencing changes in sensation or pain. Pay special attention to high-risk areas such as bony prominences, skinfolds, the sacrum, and heels.
  Systematic inspection can identify impending problems early (Bryant, 1993).
- Monitor client's skin care practices, noting type of soap or other cleansing agents used, temperature of water, and frequency of skin cleansing.
  Individualize plan according to client's skin condition, needs, and preferences. Avoid harsh cleansing agents, hot water, extreme friction or force, or cleansing too frequently (Panel for the Prediction and Prevention of Pressure Ulcers in Adults, 1992).
- Monitor client's continence status, and minimize exposure of skin impairment and other areas to moisture from incontinence, perspiration, or wound drainage.
- If client is incontinent, implement an incontinence management plan to prevent exposure to chemicals in urine and stool that can strip or erode the skin; refer to a physician (e.g., urologist, gastroenterologist) for an incontinence assessment (Doughty, 1991; Wound, Ostomy, and Continence Nurses Society, 1992, 1994; Fantl et al, 1996).
- For clients with limited mobility, use a risk-assessment tool to systematically assess immobility-related risk factors.
  A validated risk-assessment tool such as the Norton or Braden Scale should be used to identify clients at risk for immobility-related skin breakdown (Panel for the Prediction and Prevention of Pressure Ulcers in Adults, 1992).
- Do not position client on site of skin impairment. If consistent with overall client management goals, turn and position client at least every 2 hours; transfer client with care to protect against the adverse effects of external mechanical forces such as pressure, friction, and shear.
  If the goal of care is to keep a client (e.g., a terminally ill client) comfortable, turning and repositioning may not be appropriate. Maintain the head of the bed at the lowest possible degree of elevation to reduce shear and friction, and use lift devices, pillows, foam wedges, and pressure-reducing devices in the bed. Evaluate for the use of specialty mattresses or beds as appropriate (Panel for the Prediction and Prevention of Pressure Ulcers in Adults, 1992; Wilson, 1994).

- Implement a written treatment plan for topical treatment of the site of skin impairment.
  A written plan ensures consistency in care and documentation (Maklebust, Sieggreen, 1996). Topical treatments must be matched to the client, wound, and setting (Krasner, 1996).
- Select a topical treatment that will maintain a moist wound-healing environment and is balanced with the need to absorb exudate.
  Caution should always be taken not to dry out the wound (Bergstrom et al, 1994).
- Avoid massaging around the site of skin impairment and over bony prominences.
  Research suggests that massage may lead to deep-tissue trauma (Panel for the Prediction and Prevention of Pressure Ulcers in Adults, 1992; Ortiz, 1992).
- Assess client's nutritional status; refer for a nutritional consult and/or institute dietary supplements.
  Inadequate nutritional intake places individuals at risk for skin breakdown and compromises healing (Bahl, 1995).

Home Care Interventions

- Identify client's phase of wound healing (inflammation, proliferation, maturation) and stage of injury.
  Accurate understanding of tissue status combined with knowledge of underlying diagnoses and product validity provide a basis for determining appropriate treatment objectives (Rolstad, 1990). There is no single wound dressing appropriate for all phases of wound healing (Rolstad, 1990).
- Instruct and assist client and caregivers to remove or control impediments to wound healing (e.g., management of underlying disease, improved approach to client positioning, improved nutrition).
  Wound healing can be delayed or fail totally if impediments are not controlled (Rolstad, 1990).
- Initiate a consultation in a case assignment with an enterostomal therapy (ET) nurse to establish a comprehensive plan as soon as possible.
  In studies of clients with comparable wound care problems, ET nurses were more than twice as successful as non-ET home care nurses in accomplishing wound healing (Arnold, Weir, 1994).

Client/Family Teaching

- Teach skin and wound assessment and ways to monitor for signs and symptoms of infection, complications, and healing.
  Early assessment and intervention helps prevent serious problems from developing.
- Teach client to use a topical treatment that is matched to the client, wound, and setting.
  The topical treatment must be adjusted as the status of the wound changes (van Rijswijk, 1995; Krasner, 1996).
- If consistent with overall client management goals, teach how to turn and reposition at least every 2 hours.
  If the goal of care is to keep a client (e.g., terminally ill client) comfortable, turning and repositioning may not be appropriate (Panel for the Prediction and Prevention of Pressure Ulcers in Adults, 1992).
- Teach client to use pillows, foam wedges, and pressure-reducing devices to prevent pressure injury.

REFERENCES   Arnold N, Weir D: Retrospective analysis of healing in wounds cared for by ET nurses versus staff nurses in a home setting, *J Wound Ostomy Cont Nurs* 21:4, 1994.

Bahl SM: Nutritional considerations in wound management. In Gogia PP: *Clinical wound management,* Thorofare, NJ, 1995, Slack.

Bergstrom N et al: *Treatment of pressure ulcers,* Clinical Practice Guideline No 15, Agency for Health Care Policy and Research, Pub No 95-0652, Rockville, Md, 1994, Public Health Service, US Department of Health and Human Services.

Bryant R: *Acute and chronic wounds,* St Louis, 1993, Mosby.

Doughty D: *Urinary and fecal incontinence: nursing management,* St Louis, 1991, Mosby.

Fantl JA et al: *Urinary incontinence in adults: acute and chronic management,* Clinical Practice Guideline, No 2, 1996 Update. Agency for Health Care Policy and Research, No 96-0682, Rockville, Md, 1996, US Department of Health and Human Services. Public Health Service.

Krasner D: Dressing decisions for the twenty-first century: on the cusp of a paradigm shift, *Wound* 8:16, 1996.

Maklebust J, Sieggreen M: *Pressure ulcers: guidelines for prevention and nursing management,* ed 2, Springhouse, Pa, 1996, Springhouse.

National Pressure Ulcer Advisory Panel, *Consensus development conference statement,* Buffalo, NY, 1989, The Panel.

Ortiz M: Massage message, *AJN* 92:24C, 1992.

Panel for the Prediction and Prevention of Pressure Ulcers in Adults: *Pressure ulcers in adults: prediction and prevention,* Clinical Practice Guideline No 3, Agency for Health Care Policy and Research, Pub No 92-0047, Rockville, Md, 1992, US Department of Health and Human Services, Public Health Service.

Rolstad B: Treatment objectives in chronic wound care, *Home Healthcare Nurse* 9:6, 1990.

Suntken G et al: Implementation of a comprehensive skin care program across care settings using the AHCPR pressure ulcer prevention and treatment guidelines, *Ostomy Wound Manage* 42:2, 1996.

van Rijswijk L: General principles of wound management. In Gogia PP: *Clinical wound management,* Thorofare, NJ, 1995, Slack.

van Rijswijk L: Wound assessment and documentation. In Krasner D, Kane D: *Chronic wound care: a clinical source book for health care professionals,* ed 2, Wayne, Pa, 1996, Health Management Publications.

Wilson S: Mattresses that spell relief, *AJN* 94:48, 1994.

Wound, Ostomy, and Continence Nurses Society: *Standards of care: patient with urinary incontinence,* Costa Mesa, Calif, 1992, The Society.

Risk for impaired skin integrity

Diane Krasner

Definition   The state in which an individual's skin is at risk of being adversely altered

Risk Factors
External (environmental)
Hypothermia, hyperthermia, chemical substance, mechanical factors (e.g., shearing forces, pressure, restraint), irradiation, physical immobilization, humidity

Internal (somatic)
Medication, altered nutritional state (e.g., obesity, emaciation), altered metabolic state, altered circulation, altered sensation, altered pigmentation, skeletal prominence, developmental factors, immunological deficit, altered skin turgor (change in elasticity), psychogenic factors, immunological deficit

Related Factors (r/t)
See Risk Factors

Client Outcomes/Goals
- Reports altered sensation or pain at risk areas
- Demonstrates understanding of personal risk factors for impaired skin integrity
- Verbalizes a personal plan for preventing impaired skin integrity

Suggested NIC Interventions

Pressure management, pressure ulcer prevention, skin surveillance, positioning

Nursing Interventions and Rationales

- Monitor skin condition at least once a day for color or texture changes, dermatological conditions, or lesions. Determine whether client is experiencing loss of sensation or pain. *Systematic inspection can identify impending problems early (Krasner, Kane, 1996).*
- Identify clients at risk for impaired skin integrity as a result of compromised perfusion, immunocompromise, or chronic medical conditions such as diabetes mellitus or renal failure.
  These patient populations are known to be at high risk for impaired skin integrity (Bergstrom et al, 1987; Stotts, Wipke-Tevis, 1995).
- Monitor client's skin care practices, noting type of soap or other cleansing agents used, temperature of water, and frequency of skin cleansing.
  Individualize plan according to client's skin condition, needs, and preferences. Avoid harsh cleansing agents, hot water, extreme friction or force, or too-frequent cleansing (Panel for the Prediction and Prevention of Pressure Ulcers in Adults, 1992).
- Monitor client's continence status and minimize exposure of the site of skin impairment and other areas to moisture from incontinence, perspiration, or wound drainage.
  If client is incontinent, implement an incontinence management plan to prevent exposure to chemicals in urine and stool that can strip or erode the skin; refer to a physician (e.g., urologist, gastroenterologist) for an incontinence assessment (Doughty, 1991; Wound, Ostomy and Continence Nurses Society, 1992, 1994; Fantl et al, 1996).
- For clients with limited mobility, monitor condition of skin over bony prominences.
  Pressure ulcers usually occur over bony prominences such as the sacrum, coccyx, trochanter, and heels as a result of unrelieved pressure between the prominence and support surface (Maklebust, Sieggreen, 1996).
- Use a risk-assessment tool to systematically assess immobility-related risk factors.
  A validated risk-assessment tool such as the Norton or Braden Scale should be used to identify clients at risk for immobility-related skin breakdown (Bergstrom et al, 1987; Panel for the Prediction and Prevention of Pressure Ulcers in Adults, 1992).
- Implement a written prevention plan.
  A written plan ensures consistency in care and documentation (Maklebust, Sieggreen, 1996).
- If consistent with overall client management goals, turn and position client at least every 2 hours; transfer client with care to protect against the adverse effects of external mechanical forces (e.g., pressure, friction, shear).
  If the goal of care is to keep the client (e.g., a terminally ill client) comfortable, turning and repositioning may not be appropriate. Maintain the head of the bed at the lowest possible degree of elevation to reduce shear and friction and use lift devices, pillows, foam wedges, and pressure-reducing devices in the bed (Panel for the Prediction and Prevention of Pressure Ulcers in Adults, 1992).
- Avoid massaging over bony prominences.
  Research suggests that massage may lead to deep-tissue trauma (Ortiz, 1992; Panel for the Prediction and Prevention of Pressure Ulcers in Adults, 1992).
- Assess client's nutritional status; refer for a nutritional consult and/or institute dietary supplements.

Inadequate nutritional intake places individuals at risk for skin breakdown and compromises healing (Bahl, 1995).

Geriatric
- Limit number of complete baths to two or three per week and alternate them with partial baths. Use a tepid water temperature (between 90° F and 105° F) for bathing. *Excessive bathing, especially in hot water, depletes aging skin of moisture and increases dryness.*
- Use superfatted soaps such as Dove, Tone, or Caress. *Superfatted soaps help retain moisture in dry, aging skin (Hardy, 1992).*
- Increase fluid intake within cardiac and renal limits to a minimum of 1500 ml per day. *Dry skin is caused by loss of fluid; increasing fluid intake hydrates the skin.*
- Increase humidity in the environment, especially during the winter, by using a humidifier or placing a container of water on a warm object. *Increasing the moisture in the air helps keep moisture in the skin (Fenske, Grayson, Newcomer, 1989).*

Home Care Interventions
- See care plan for **Skin integrity, impaired.**
- Assess caregiver vigilance and ability. *In a limited study of the Braden Scale, caregiver vigilance and ability were recognized as potentially significant variables in determining risk of developing pressure sores (Ramundo, 1995).*
- Initiate a consultation in a case assignment with an enterostomal therapy (ET) nurse to establish a comprehensive plan as soon as possible. *In studies of clients with comparable wound care problems, ET nurses were more than twice as successful as non-ET home care nurses in accomplishing wound healing (Arnold, Weir, 1994).*

Client/Family Teaching
- Teach client skin assessment and ways to monitor for impending skin breakdown. *Early assessment and intervention help prevent the development of serious problems (Murray, Blaylock, 1994).*
- If consistent with overall client management goals, teach how to turn and reposition client at least every 2 hours. *If the goal of care is to keep the client (e.g., a terminally ill client) comfortable, turning and repositioning may not be appropriate (Panel for the Prediction and Prevention of Pressure Ulcers in Adults, 1992).*
- Teach client to use pillows, foam wedges, and pressure-reducing devices to prevent pressure injury (Bryant, 1993).

REFERENCES   Arnold N, Weir D: Retrospective analysis of healing in wounds cared for by ET nurses versus staff nurses in a home setting, *J Wound Ostomy Cont Nurs* 21:4, 1994.

Bahl SM: Nutritional considerations in wound management. In Gogia PP: *Clinical wound management,* Thorofare, NJ, 1995, Slack.

Bergstrom N et al: The Braden scale for prediction of pressure sore risk, *Nurs Res* 36:205, 1987.

Bryant R: *Acute and chronic wounds,* St Louis, 1993, Mosby.

Doughty D: *Urinary and fecal incontinence: nursing management,* St Louis, 1991, Mosby.

Fantl JA et al: *Urinary incontinence in adults: acute and chronic management,* Clinical Practice Guideline No 2, 1996 Update, Agency for Health Care Policy and Research. Pub No 96-0682, Rockville, Md, 1996, US Department of Health & Human Services, Public Health Service.

Fenske NA, Grayson LD, Newcomer VD: Common problems of aging skin, *Patient Care* 23:225, 1989.

Hardy MA: Dry skin care. In Bulechek GM, McCloskey JC, editors: *Nursing interventions: essential nursing treatments,* ed 2, Philadelphia, 1992, WB Saunders.

Krasner D, Cuzzell J: Pressure ulcers. In Gogia PP: *Clinical wound management,* Thorofare, NJ, 1995, Slack.

Krasner D, Kane D: *Chronic wound care: a clinical source book for healthcare professionals,* Wayne, Pa, 1996, Health Publications.

Maklebust J, Sieggreen M: *Pressure ulcers: guidelines for prevention and nursing management,* ed 2, Springhouse, Pa, 1996, Springhouse.

Murray M, Blaylock B: Maintaining effective pressure ulcer prevention programs, *Med Surg Nurs* 3:85-92, 1994.

Ortiz M: Massage message, *AJN* 92:24C, 1992.

Panel for the Prediction and Prevention of Pressure Ulcers in Adults: *Pressure ulcers in adults: prediction and prevention,* Clinical Practice Guideline No 3, Agency for Health Care Policy and Research, Pub No 92-0047, Rockville, Md, 1992, US Department of Health and Human Services, Public Health Service.

Ramundo J: Reliability and validity of the Braden Scale in the home care setting, *J Wound Ostomy Cont Nurs* 22:3, 1995.

Rolstad BS: Treatment objectives in chronic wound care, *Home Healthcare Nurse* 9:6, 1990.

Singh P: Wound healing in the home health arena, *Home Healthcare Nurse* 12:1, 1993.

Stotts NA, Wipke-Tevis: Co-factors in impaired wound healing, *Ostomy Wound Manage,* vol 42, 1996.

Suntken G et al: Implementation of a comprehensive skin care program across care settings using the AHCPR pressure ulcer prevention and treatment guidelines, *Ostomy Wound Manage* 42:2, 1996.

Wound, Ostomy, and Continence Nurses Society: *Standards of care: dermal wounds: pressure ulcers,* Costa Mesa, Calif, 1992, The Society.

Wound, Ostomy, and Continence Nurses Society: *Standards of care: patient with fecal incontinence,* Costa Mesa, Calif, 1994, The Society.

Wound, Ostomy, and Continence Nurses Society: *Standards of care: patient with urinary incontinence,* Costa Mesa, Calif, 1992, The Society.

Sleep pattern disturbance

Gwethalyn B. Edwards and Betty J. Ackley

Definition   Disruption of sleep time that causes discomfort or interferes with desired life-style

Defining Characteristics

Verbal complaints of difficulty falling asleep *(critical),* awakening earlier or later than desired *(critical),* interrupted sleep *(critical),* verbal complaints of not feeling well-rested *(critical),* changes in behavior and performance (e.g., increasing irritability, restlessness, disorientation, lethargy, listlessness), physical signs (e.g., mild or fleeting nystagmus, slight hand tremor, ptosis of eyelid, expressionless face, dark circles under eyes, frequent yawning, changes in posture), thick speech with mispronunciation and incorrect words

Related Factors (r/t)

Sensory alterations: internal (e.g., illness, psychological stress), external (e.g., environmental changes, social cues)

Client Outcomes/Goals

- Wakes up less frequently during night
- Awakens refreshed and is less fatigued during day
- Falls asleep without difficulty
- Verbalizes plan to implement bedtime routines

Suggested NIC Interventions

Sleep enhancement

Nursing Interventions and Rationales

- Assess client's sleep patterns and usual bedtime rituals and incorporate these into the plan of care.

Usual sleep patterns are individual; data collected through a comprehensive and holistic assessment are needed to determine the etiology of the disturbance (Spenceley, 1993). Staff nurses' evaluation of client's sleep states are usually valid (Edwards, Schuring, 1993).

- Observe for underlying physiological or psychological illnesses causing insomnia (e.g., hyperthyroidism, nocturia occurring with benign hypertrophic prostatitis, depression). *Symptomology of disease states and depression can cause insomnia (Evans, Rogers, 1994).*

- Determine level of anxiety; if client is anxious, see nursing interventions and rationales for **Anxiety.**
Anxiety interferes with sleep. Interventions such as relaxation training can help clients reduce anxiety (Hyman et al, 1989).

- Observe client's medication, diet, and caffeine intake. Look for hidden sources of caffeine such as over-the-counter medications.
Difficulty sleeping can be a side effect of medications such as bronchodilators; caffeine can also interfere with sleep.

- Provide measures to assist with sleep such as quiet time before bed, warm milk, or a back massage.
Simple measures can increase quality of sleep. Research has shown back massage to be effective (Richards, 1994).

- Provide pain relief shortly before bedtime and position client comfortably for sleep.
Clients have reported that uncomfortable positions and pain are the most likely factors to disturb sleep (Reimer, 1987).

- Monitor for presence of sleep apnea as evidenced by loud snoring and periods of apnea; obtain a referral for sleep studies from a physician.

- Keep environment quiet (e.g., avoid use of intercoms, lower volume on radio and television, keep beepers on nonaudio mode, anticipate alarms on IV pumps, talk quietly on unit).
Excessive noise causes sleep deprivation that can result in ICU psychosis (Barr, 1993). Health volunteers exposed to recorded critical care noise levels experienced poor sleep (Topf, 1992).

- Use soothing sound generators with sounds of the ocean, rainfall, or waterfall to induce sleep, or use "white noise" such as a fan to block out other sounds.
Ocean sounds promoted sleep for a group of postoperative open-heart surgery clients (Williamson, 1992).

- For hospitalized stable clients, consider instituting the following sleep protocol to foster sleep:
  - *Night shift*—Give client the opportunity for uninterrupted sleep from 1:00 AM to 5:00 AM. Keep environmental noise to a minimum.
  - *Evening shift*—Limit napping between 4:00 PM and 9:00 PM. At 10:00 PM turn lights off, provide sleep medication according to individual assessment, and keep noise and conversation on the unit to a minimum.
  - *Day shift*—Encourage short naps before 11:00 AM. Enforce a physical activity regimen as appropriate. Schedule newly ordered medications to avoid waking client between 1:00 AM and 5:00 AM.
Critical care nurses can take action to promote sleep (Edwards, Schuring, 1993).

Geriatric
- Observe elimination patterns. Have client decrease fluid intake in the evening, and ensure that diuretics are taken early in the morning.
  Many elderly people void during the night; increasing water intake at night or taking diuretics late in the day increases nocturia, which results in disrupted sleep.
- If client is waking frequently during the night, consider the presence of sleep apnea problems and refer to a sleep clinic for evaluation.
  Sleep apnea in the elderly may be caused by changes in the respiratory drive of the central nervous system or may be obstructive and associated with obesity (Foyt, 1992).
- Encourage social activities. Help elderly get outside for increased light exposure and to enjoy nature.
  Exposure to light and social interactions influence the circadian rhythms that control sleep (Elmore, Betrus, Burr, 1994).
- Suggest light reading or nonexcitable television as an evening activity.
  Soothing activities decrease stimulation of the reticular activating system and help sleep come naturally.
- Increase daytime physical activity.
- Avoid use of hypnotics and alcohol to sleep.
  Long-term use of hypnotics can induce a drug-related insomnia. Alcohol also disrupts sleep and can exacerbate sleep apnea (Evans, Rogers, 1994).
- Reduce daytime napping in the late afternoon; limit naps to short intervals as early in the day as possible.
  The majority of elderly nap during the day (Evans, Rogers, 1994). Avoiding naps in the late afternoon makes it easier to fall asleep at night.

Home Care Interventions
- Provide support to the family of clients with chronic sleep pattern disturbance.
  Ongoing sleep pattern disturbances can disrupt family patterns and cause sleep deprivation in the client or family members, which creates increased stress on the family.

Client/Family Teaching
- Encourage client to avoid coffee and other caffeinated foods and liquids.
  Caffeine intake increases the time it takes to fall asleep and increases awake time during the night (Evans, Rogers, 1994).
- Teach relaxation techniques, pain relief measures, or the use of imagery before sleep.
- Encourage client to develop a bedtime ritual that includes quiet activities such as reading, television, or crafts.
- Teach the following guidelines for improving sleep habits:
  - Go to bed only when sleepy.
  - When awake in the middle of the night, go to another room, do quiet activities, and go back to bed only when sleepy.
  - Use the bed only for sleeping, not for reading or snoozing in front of the television.
  - Avoid afternoon and evening naps.
  - Get up at the same time every morning.
  - Recognize that not everyone needs 8 hours of sleep.
  - Do not associate lulls in performance with sleeplessness; sleeplessness should not be blamed for everything that goes wrong during the day.
    These guidelines have been effective in improving quality of sleep (Morin, 1993).

REFERENCES   Barr WJ: Noise notes: working smart, *Am J Nurs* 93:16, 1993.

Edward GB, Schuring LM: Pilot study: validating staff nurses' observations of sleep and wake states among critically ill patients, using polysomnography, *Am J Crit Care* 2:125, 1993.

Edwards GB, Schuring LM: Sleep protocol: a research-based practice change, *Crit Care Nurse* 13:84, 1993.

Elmore SK, Betrus PA, Burr R: Light, social zeitgebers, and the sleep-wake cycle in the entrainment of human circadian rhythms, *Res Nurs Health* 17:471, 1994.

Evans BD, Rogers AE: 24-Hour sleep/wake patterns in healthy elderly persons, *Appl Nurs Res* 7:75, 1994.

Foyt MM: Impaired gas exchange in the elderly, *Geriatr Nurs* 13:262, 1992.

Hyman RB et al: The effects of relaxation training on clinical symptoms: a meta-analysis, *Nurs Res* 38:216, 1989.

Jensen DP, Herr KA: Sleeplessness, *Nurs Clin North Am* 28:385, 1993.

Morin C: Cognitive behavior therapy for late-life insomnia, *J Consult Clin Psychol* 61:137, 1993.

Reimer M: Sleep pattern disturbance: nursing interventions perceived by patients and their nurses as facilitating nocturnal sleep in hospital. In *Classification of Nursing Diagnoses: Proceedings of the Seventh Conference,* 1987, North American Nursing Diagnosis Association.

Richards KC: Sleep promotion in the critical care unit, *AACN Clin Issu* 5:152, 1994.

Simpson T, Rayshan Lee E, Cameron C: Patients' perceptions of environmental factors that disturb sleep after cardiac surgery, *Am J Crit Care* 5:173, 1996.

Spenceley SM: Sleep inquiry: a look with fresh eyes, *Image* 25:249, 1993.

Topf M: Effects of personal control over hospital noise on sleep, *Res Nurs Health* 15:19, 1992.

Williamson J: The effect of ocean sounds on sleep after coronary artery bypass graft surgery, *Am J Crit Care* 1:91, 1992.

Impaired social interaction

Pam B. Schweitzer

Definition   The state in which an individual participates insufficiently, excessively, or ineffectively in social exchange

Defining Characteristics

Major   Verbalized or observed discomfort in social situations; verbalized or observed inability to receive or communicate a satisfying sense of belonging, caring, interest, or shared history; observed use of unsuccessful social interaction behaviors, dysfunctional interactions with peers, family, or others

Minor   Family report of change in interaction patterns

Related Factors (r/t)

Knowledge or skill deficit regarding ways to enhance mutuality, communication barriers, self-concept disturbance, absence of significant other or peers, limited physical mobility, therapeutic isolation, sociocultural dissonance, environmental barriers, altered thought processes

Client Outcomes/Goals

- Identifies barriers that cause impaired social interactions
- Discusses feelings that accompany impaired and successful social interactions
- Uses available opportunities to practice interactions
- Uses successful social interaction behaviors
- Reports increased comfort in social situations
- Communicates, states feelings of belonging, demonstrates caring and interest in others
- Reports effective interactions with client (family)

Suggested NIC Interventions
Socialization enhancement

Nursing Interventions and Rationales

- Observe for cause of discomfort in social situations; ask client to explain when discomfort began and identify any losses (e.g., loss of health, job, or significant other; aging) and changes (e.g., marriage, birth or adoption of a child, change in body appearance).
  Individualized assessment indicates specific interventions (Warren, 1993).
- Have client list behaviors that are associated with being disconnected, and discuss alternative responses that may increase comfort.
  Connections occur when a person is actively involved with another person, object, group, or environment; such involvement promotes a sense of comfort, well-being, and anxiety reduction (Hagerty et al, 1993).
- Monitor client's use of defense mechanisms, and support healthy defenses (e.g., client focuses on present and avoids placing blame on others for personal behavior).
  Positive reinforcement of strengths perpetuates them.
- Have client list behaviors that cause discomfort. Discuss alternative ways to alleviate discomfort (e.g., focusing on others and their interests, practicing making caring statements such as, "I understand you are feeling sad").
- Encourage client to express feelings to others (e.g., "I feel sad also").
  Self-expression invites involvement and increases connectedness (Hagerty et al, 1993).
- Identify client strengths; have client make a list of strengths and refer to it when experiencing negative feelings. Client may find it helpful to put the list on a note card to carry at all times.
  Being aware of strengths when they are needed can increase successful interactions.
- Have group members identify each others' strengths in a group setting.
  This exercise encourages individuals to practice relating to each other on a more intimate level (Drew, 1991).
- Role play comfortable and uncomfortable social interactions with the client and appropriate responses (e.g., acknowledging a friendly greeting, responding to rude remarks with an "I" statement, such as, "I understand you may feel that way, but this is how I feel").
  Role plays may help the client develop social interaction skills and identify feelings associated with isolation (Warren, 1993).
- Model appropriate social interactions. Give positive verbal and nonverbal feedback for appropriate behavior (e.g., make statements such as, "I'm proud that you made it to work on time and did all the tasks assigned to you without saying that your supervisor was picking on you," make eye contact). If not contraindicated, touch client's arm or hand when speaking.
  One way to learn social skills is to observe the productive interactions of others (Drew, 1991).

Geriatric
- Avoid assuming that social isolation is normal for elderly clients.
  Caregiver bias and elderly client bias lead to a lack of recognition and treatment of the client's mental health needs (Dellasega, 1991).
- Monitor for depression, a particular risk in the elderly.
  Age and its associated losses may cause formerly socially active people to be alone. Loneliness contributes to depression and social withdrawal (Warren, 1993).

- Provide group situations for client.

Group settings are necessary for the client to practice new skills.

Home Care Interventions

- Assess family or living environment for social dynamics. Refer for medical social services to assist with family dynamics if appropriate.

The family is a socially significant cultural group that generates behavior, defines roles, and promotes values.

- Avoid contact with negative persons.

Negative interactions reinforce undesired patterns.

- Identify activities that client does alone and assist client with balancing solitary and social activities.

A healthy balance of social and private time supports positive coping.

- Establish pattern of care and daily activities that involves client socially (e.g., Meals on Wheels, home health aide visits). Give supportive feedback for positive and appropriate interactions.

The assumption of new patterns of interaction requires practice in safe situations. Feedback reinforces desired behaviors.

- Refer to or support involvement with supportive groups and counseling.

Group settings provide the opportunity to practice new skills. Counseling assists the client with defining appropriate actions and is a source of support.

Client/Family Teaching

- Help client accept responsibility for own behavior. Have client keep a journal; and review it together at prescheduled intervals. Give client positive feedback for appropriate behaviors, and suggest alternative approaches for behaviors that do not enhance social interaction.

Positive reinforcement perpetuates appropriate behaviors.

- Teach social interaction skills for use in actual situations the client is faced with daily.

Through productive connections with others, social skills are learned and a repertoire of roles for many social situations is developed, which leads to an increase in self-esteem and the capacity to interact with others (Drew, 1991).

- Practice social skills one-to-one and, when the client is ready, in group sessions.

Practice improves performance and comfort level.

- Refer to appropriate social agencies for assistance (e.g., family therapy, self-help groups, crisis intervention).

REFERENCES   Coco P: When should I use the nursing diagnosis of "impaired social interactions related to grief and loss" and how should I intervene? *Adv Clin Care* 5:45, 1990.

Damrosch S: General strategies for motivating people to change their behavior, *Nurs Clin North Am* 26:833, 1991.

Dellasega C: Meeting the mental health needs of elderly clients, *J Psychosoc Nurs Ment Health Serv* 29:10, 1991.

Drew N: Combatting the social isolation of chronic mental illness, *J Psychosoc Nurs Ment Health Serv* 29:14, 1991.

Hagerty BM et al: An emerging theory of human relatedness, *Image* 25:291, 1993.

Heineken J: Disconfirmation in dysfunctional communication, *Nurs Res* 31:211, 1982.

Lee H, Coenen A, Heim K: Island living: the experience of loneliness in a psychiatric hospital, *Appl Nurs Res* 7:7, 1994.

Tilden VP, Nelson CA, May BA: The IPR inventory: development and psychometric characteristics, *Nurs Res* 39:337, 1990.

Walton CG et al: Psychological correlates of loneliness in the older adult, *Arch Psychiatr Nurs* 5:165, 1991.
Warren BJ: Explaining social isolation through concept analysis, *Arch Psychiatr Nurs* 7:270, 1993.

Social isolation

Gail B. Ladwig

Definition	Aloneness experienced by the individual and perceived as imposed by others and as a negative or threatened state

Defining Characteristics

Objective   Absence of supportive significant others (e.g., family, friends, group) *(critical),* sad or dull affect, inappropriate or immature interests and activities for developmental age or stage, uncommunicative or withdrawn behavior, lack of eye contact, preoccupation with own thoughts, repetitive and meaningless actions, hostility in voice or behavior, desire to be alone, existence in a limited subculture, evidence of physical or mental handicap or altered state of wellness, behavior that is unaccepted by dominant cultural group

Subjective   Feelings of aloneness imposed by others *(critical),* feelings of rejection, feelings of difference from others, inadequacy in or absence of a significant purpose in life, inability to meet expectations of others, insecurity in public, expression of values acceptable to the subculture but unacceptable to the dominant cultural group, expression of interests inappropriate to the developmental age or state

Related Factors (r/t)

Factors contributing to the absence of satisfying personal relationships such as a delay in accomplishing developmental tasks, immature interests, alterations in mental status, unacceptable social behavior, unacceptable social values, altered state of wellness, inadequate personal resources, or an inability to engage in satisfying personal relationships

Client Outcomes/Goals

- Identifies the reasons for feelings of isolation
- Practices the social and communication skills needed to interact with others
- Initiates interactions with others, sets and meets goals
- Participates in activities and programs at level of ability and desire
- Describes feelings of self-worth

Suggested NIC Interventions

Socialization enhancement

Nursing Interventions and Rationales

- Observe for barriers to social interaction (e.g., illness; incontinence; decreasing ability to form relationships; lack of transportation, money, support system, or knowledge). *Each individual may have different etiologies of social isolation; therefore adequate information must be gathered so that appropriate interventions can be planned (Badgor, 1990).*
- Note risk factors (e.g., ethnic/cultural minority, chronic physiological or psychological illness or deformities, elderly). *These clients may be at risk for social isolation (Warren, 1993).*
- Discuss causes of perceived or actual isolation. *The individual's experience of illness, the mediating circumstances of everyday life that*

influence quality of life, and emotions, fears, and concerns all have a bearing on the way illness is managed (Anderson, 1991).

- Promote social interactions. Support grieving and verbalization of feelings.
  Women in this study needed counseling about the management of illness, but some said they would have benefited from psychological counseling as well. They needed help with the emotional aspects of living with a chronic illness (Anderson, 1991).
- Establish trust one-on-one and then gradually introduce client to others.
  The first step in reversing social isolation is developing the ability to relate to one person. As this skill is accomplished, the client can gradually learn to relate to others.
- Use active listening skills; establish a therapeutic relationship and spend time with the client.
  Spending time with the client enhances self-esteem.
- Help client experience success by working together to establish easily attainable goals (e.g., 10 minutes conversing with peer).
  Success encourages repetition of behaviors, and setting small achievable goals is more likely to help the client be successful.
- Provide positive reinforcement when client seeks out others.
  Receiving instrumental social support such as practical help, advice, and feedback significantly contributes to positive well-being (White, 1992).
- Help client identify appropriate diversional activities to encourage socialization.
  Active participation by the client is essential for behavioral changes.
- Encourage physical closeness (e.g., use touch) if appropriate.
  Touch can be therapeutic and healing.
- Identify available support systems and involve them in client care.
  Clients cope more successfully with stressful life events if they have support (White, 1992).
- Encourage liberal visitation for hospitalized clients.
  Frequent contact with support persons decreases feelings of isolation.
- Help client identify role models and others with similar interests.
  Sometimes the client needs someone to model appropriate behavior.
- See nursing diagnosis **Risk for loneliness**.

Geriatric

- Observe for aggression or other interpersonal problems, poor self-image or signs of powerlessness, confusion of the past with the present, complaints about feeling confined or deserted, or difficulty setting goals and making decisions.
  Social isolation should be considered as a nursing diagnosis when the mentioned behaviors are observed (Copel, 1988; Meddaugh, 1991).
- Assess for hearing deficits; provide aids and use adaptive techniques such as facing the individual when speaking, speaking slowly, lowering the pitch of the voice, and enunciating clearly.
  There is a relationship between hearing acuity and loneliness. Hearing loss is one of the most prevalent chronic health problems of older adults, especially the very old (i.e., an average age of 83). Adaptive techniques that facilitate communication must be used (Dugan, Kivett, 1994).
- If clients are in a health-care facility, visit them for at least 10 minutes every 2 to 3 hours.
  The presence of a trusted individual provides emotional security for the client.
- Involve nonprofessionals in activities, projects, and goal setting with the clients.
  Practice interdisciplinary management for unit-based activities: crafts, art and sewing, videos, large-print books, magazines, games, musical instruments, and assistive listening devices.

Nursing assistants are frequently concerned about the social support of residents, so they can be a valuable resource for generating intervention ideas. (Alterations in job descriptions would be required.) Enjoyable interactions between nursing assistants and residents would provide the assistants with diversion and rest from the strenuous aspects of personal care and might have a positive effect on the resident/assistant relationship. Residents with visual, hearing, cognitive, and mobility impairments will participate more readily in events that involve a smaller number of people and in which the staff takes initiative and establishes rapport with each resident (Windriver, 1993).

- Offer client choice of activities and people with whom to sit and socialize. Introductions to strangers may need to be repeated several times.
  A recognized intervention for loneliness is to provide opportunities and assistance for making choices, setting goals, and making decisions. Cognitively impaired clients may require several repetitions (Windriver, 1993).
- Put clients in groups according to activity preferences, abilities, age, life situations, personal and cultural characteristics, and social networks.
  Positive social interactions are enhanced by the mentioned interventions (Windriver, 1993).
- Develop and display a seating chart for the common areas of each personal care unit and a process for both identifying needed changes and executing them promptly.
  Personality factors that are difficult to predict affect the success of social groupings (Windriver, 1993).
- Consider use of simulated presence therapy (see **Hopelessness).**
  Simulated presence therapy appears to be most effective in treating social isolation (Woods, Ashley, 1995).
- Refer to programs such as Foster Grandparents and Senior Companions.
  Emotional isolation leads to social isolation. Social programs help increase contact with peers and decrease isolation. Programs to alleviate emotional isolation should focus on attachment loss (Dugan, Kivett, 1994).

Home Care Interventions

- Confirm that the home setting has a telephone. Obtain one if necessary for medical safety. If client lives alone, set up a "lifeline" safety system that requires the client to answer the telephone.
  A lifeline can be a safety net for physical and psychological safety.
- Encourage family involvement in daily life in small, nonthreatening activities, short outings, assistance with shopping, and asking for input from isolated person in decision making.
  Reversing social isolation is a gradual process.
- Establish pattern of care and daily activities to involve the client socially (e.g., Meals on Wheels, home health aide visits).
  Pattern changes encourage new behaviors.
- Have client keep a diary of social experiences. Discuss diary during visits.
  A review of social experiences helps client identify those that are most comfortable.
- Identify activities that client does alone. Assist client with balancing solitary and social activities, keeping alone time at a minimum.
  A healthy balance of social and private time supports positive coping.
- Refer for visiting volunteer services.
  Spending time with the client enhances client self-esteem.

- When clients are ready, encourage them to volunteer for short periods with community agencies in which contact is positive and nonthreatening (e.g., with hospitalized elders for 1 hour per week).
  Contributing to the welfare of others enhances self-esteem.
- Assess options for living that allow client privacy but not isolation (e.g., boarding home, congregate living).
  Group living can provide a safety net for clients predisposed to isolation and depression.

Client/Family Teaching

- Teach skills related to problem solving, communication, social interaction, activities of daily living, and positive self-esteem.
  All of these skills are necessary to change isolating behavior.
- Teach role playing (practicing communication skills in specific situations).
  Role playing may help clients develop social interaction skills and identify feelings associated with their isolation (Warren, 1993).
- Encourage client to initiate contacts with self-help groups, counselors, and therapists.
  If adjustment is to be successful and maintained, management of a chronic illness cannot occur in isolation; it requires a complex interaction of resources (White, 1992).
- Provide information to client about senior citizen services, housesharing, pets, daycare centers, churches, and community resources.
  The well-documented negative effect of social isolation suggests that clients without confidants and supportive others must be referred to alternative sources, such as cardiac rehabilitation programs, support groups, and community agencies (McCauley, 1995).
- Refer socially isolated *caregivers* to appropriate support groups as well.
  Identification and recognition of the overwhelming task of caregiving are needed so that the caregiver does not suffer in silence. Alzheimer's disease support groups offer participants an opportunity to share troubles and triumphs with others who truly understand the turmoil of caregiving (Bergman-Evans, 1994) (see **Caregiver role strain).**

REFERENCES   Anderson JM: Immigrant women speak of chronic illness: the social construction of the devalued self, *J Adv Nurs* 16:710,717, 1991.

Badgor VA; Men with cardiovascular diseases and their spouses, coping health and marital adjustment, *Arch Psychiatr Nurs* 4:1990.

Bergman-Evans BF: Alzheimer's and related disorders: loneliness, depression, and social support of spousal caregivers, *J Gerontol Nurs* 20:6, 1994.

Copel LC: Loneliness: a conceptual model, *J Psychosoc Nurs Ment Health Serv* 26:14, 1988.

Dugan E, Kivett V: The importance of emotional and social isolation to loneliness among very old rural adults, *Gerontologist* 34:340, 1994.

McCauley K: Assessing social support in patients with cardiac disease, *J Cardiovasc Nurs* 10:73, 1995.

Meddaugh DJ: Before aggression erupts, *Geriatr Nurs* 12:114, 1991. In Windriver W: Social isolation: unit-based activities for impaired elders, *J Gerontol Nurs* 19:15, 1993.

Warren B: Explaining social isolation through concept analysis, *Arch Psychiatr Nurs* 7:270, 1993.

White NE: Coping, social support and adaptation to chronic illness, *West J Nurs Res* 14:2, 1992.

Windriver W: Social isolation: unit-based activities for impaired elders, *J Gerontol Nurs* 19:15, 1993.

Woods P, Ashley J: Simulated presence therapy: using selected memories to manage problem behaviors in Alzheimer's disease patients, *Geriatr Nurs* 16:9, 1995.

Spiritual distress (distress of the human spirit)

Gail B. Ladwig

Definition   A disruption in the life principle that pervades a person's being and integrates and tran-scends one's biological and psychosocial nature

Defining Characteristics

Expresses concern with meaning of life and death and with belief systems *(critical);* expresses anger toward God; questions the meaning of suffering; verbalizes inner conflict about beliefs; verbalizes concern about relationship with deity; questions meaning of own existence; unable to participate in usual religious practices; seeks spiritual assistance; questions moral and ethical implications of therapeutic regimen; uses gallows humor; demonstrates displacement of anger toward religious representatives; describes nightmares and sleep disturbances; shows alterations in behavior or mood evidenced by anger, crying, withdrawal, preoccupation, anxiety, hostility, or apathy

Related Factors (r/t)

Separation from religious or cultural ties, challenged belief and value system as a result of either intense suffering or the moral and ethical implications of therapy

Client Outcomes/Goals

- States conflicts or disturbances related to practice of belief system
- Discusses beliefs about spiritual issues
- States feelings of trust in self, God, or other belief systems
- Continues spiritual practices not detrimental to health
- Discusses feelings about death
- Displays a mood appropriate for the situation

Suggested NIC Interventions

Spiritual support

Nursing Interventions and Rationales

- Observe client for self-esteem, self-worth, feelings of futility, or hopelessness.
  Verbalizations of feelings of low self-esteem, low self-worth, and hopelessness may indicate a spiritual need.
  Monitor support systems. Be aware of own belief systems and accept client's spirituality. To effectively help a client with spiritual needs, an understanding of own spiritual dimension is essential (Highfield, Carson, 1983).
- Be physically present and available to help client determine religious and spiritual choices.
  Physical presence can decrease separation and aloneness, which clients often fear (Dossey et al, 1988).
- Provide quiet time for meditation, prayer, and relaxation.
  Clients need time to be alone during times of health change.
- Help client make a list of important and nonimportant values.
  Individual clients are experts on their own paths, and knowing their values helps in exploring their uniqueness (Dossey et al, 1988).
- Ask how to be most helpful; actively listen, reflect, and seek clarification.
  Listening attentively and being physically present can be spiritual (Berggren-Thomas, Griggs, 1995). Obtain permission from the client to respond to spiritual needs from own spiritual perspective (Smucker, 1996).
- If client is comfortable with touch, hold client's hand or place hand gently on arm.
  Touch makes nonverbal communication more personal.

- Help client develop and accomplish short-term goals and tasks.
  Accomplishing goals increases self-esteem, which may be related to the client's spiritual well-being.
- Help client find a reason for living and be available for support.
  "The need for a positive attitude for optimum healing was by far the most frequently mentioned subtheme by these participants and the strongest area of literature" (Criddle, 1993).
- Listen to client's feelings about death. Be nonjudgmental and allow time for grieving.
  All grief work takes time and is unique. Acceptance of client differences is essential to open communication.
- Help client develop skills to deal with an illness or life-style changes. Include client in planning of care.
  Clients perceived the experience of healing as an active process and expressed a desire to take conscious control (Criddle, 1993).
- Provide appropriate religious materials, artifacts, or music as requested.
  Helping a client incorporate rituals, sacraments, reading, music, imagery, and meditation into daily life can enhance spiritual health (Conrad, 1985).
- Provide privacy for client to pray with others or to be read to by members of own faith.
  Privacy shows respect for and sensitivity to the client.
- See **Potential for enhanced spiritual well-being.**

Geriatric
- Assist client with a life review and help client identify noteworthy experiences.
- Discuss personal definitions of spiritual wellness with client.
  Listening attentively and helping elderly clients identify past coping strategies are part of helping with life review and finding meaning in life (Berggren-Thomas, Griggs, 1995).
- Identify clients' past sources of spirituality. Help clients explore their lives and identify those experiences that are noteworthy. Clients may want to read the Bible or have it read to them.
  Older adults frequently identified spirituality as a source of hope (Gaskins, Forte, 1995).
- Discuss the client's perception of God in relation to the illness.
  Different religions view illness from different perspectives.
- Offer to pray with client or caregivers.
  Prayer was described as an important part of spirituality by caregivers (Kaye, Robinson, 1994).
- Offer to read from the Bible or other book chosen by client.
  A religious ritual may comfort the client.

Home Care Interventions
- All of the mentioned nursing interventions apply in the home setting.

Client/Family Teaching
- Encourage family and friends to visit and show their concern.
  Social networks support spiritual well-being (Young, Dowling, 1987).
- Encourage family and friends to support client's belief through prayer.
  Positive effects of prayer include rapid recovery and prevention of complications (Byrd, 1988).
- Include directions to hospital chapel when orienting client and family to hospital unit.
  Attendance at services and a visit to the chapel may be important to the client and family.

- Refer client to spiritual advisor of choice. Prepare for chosen religious rituals.
  Some religions may have ceremonies associated with healing and illness.
- Refer to counseling, therapy, support groups, or hospice.
  The client may need more support and ongoing spiritual assistance.

REFERENCES   Berggren-Thomas P, Griggs M: Spirituality in aging: spiritual need or spiritual journey? *J Gerontol Nurs* 21:5, 1995.

Byrd RC: Positive therapeutic effects of intercessory prayer in a coronary care unit population, *South Med J* 81:826, 1988.

Conrad NJ: Spiritual support for the dying, *Nurs Clin North Am* 20:415, 1985.

Criddle L: Healing from surgery: a phenomenological study, *Image* 25:208, 1993.

Dossey M et al: *Holistic nursing: a handbook for practice,* Rockville, Md, 1988, Aspen.

Gaskins S, Forte L: The meaning of hope: implications for nursing practice and research, *J Gerontol Nurs* 21:17, 1995.

Highfield M, Carson C: Spiritual needs of patients: are they recognized? *Cancer Nurs* vol 6, 1983.

Kaye J, Robinson K: Spirituality among caregivers, *Image* 26:218, 1994.

Smucker C: A phenomenological description of the experience of spiritual distress, *Nurs Diag* 7:81, 1996.

Young G, Dowling W: Dimensions of religiosity in old age: accounting for variation in types of participation, *J Gerontol* 42:376, 1987.

Potential for enhanced spiritual well-being

Gail B. Ladwig

Definition   The process of an individual's developing and unfolding of mystery through harmonious interconnectedness that springs from inner strengths

Defining Characteristics

Inner strengths as evidenced by a sense of awareness, self-consciousness, a sacred source, a unifying force, an inner core, and transcendence; unfolding mystery regarding experience with life's purpose, meaning, mystery, uncertainty, and struggles; harmonious interconnectedness as evidenced by relatedness, connectedness, and harmony with self, others, higher power, God, and the environment

Client Outcomes/Goals

- States recognition of inner strengths
- States purpose and meaning for life
- Expresses feelings of hope
- Lists values harmonious with inner core
- States harmony with self, others, higher power, God, and the environment

Suggested NIC Interventions

Spiritual support

Nursing Interventions and Rationales

- Perform a spiritual assessment that includes client's relationship with God, purpose and direction in life, religious affiliation, and any other significant beliefs.
  A spiritual assessment is a part of holistic evaluation and needs to include the mentioned information (Fehring, Frenn, 1987).
- Assist clients with values clarification; have them list values that are important and on which they are willing to consistently act.

Values clarification is a nursing activity that promotes spiritual health and wellness (Boss, Corbett, 1990).

• Promote support from family members and significant others by encouraging family visits, phone calls, and involvement in care.

These strategies help maintain social support networks to foster hope and spiritual well-being (Farran, McCann, 1989).

• Help arrange visits with clergy, and allow private time for prayer and family participation in spiritual reading.

Adults prefer this type of spiritual care (Reed, 1991).

• Set mutual times to sit and talk with client; suggest 30 minutes twice a day. If client does not wish to talk, just sit with client.

The nurse's presence and willingness to listen contribute to a sense of hope or well-being (Clark, Heidenreich, 1995). Hope is necessary for life; "without hope we begin to die" (Simsen, 1988).

• Offer to pray with or for client.

Spiritual needs can be met by praying with or for the client (Dettmore, 1984).

• Offer to read to client.

Some clients cannot read because they are illiterate, have a pathological problem that prevents reading, or are taking medications that cause visual problems or drowsiness. Reading to clients, whether or not it is religious, is caring because time is being spent with them (Bolander, 1994).

• See care plan for **Spiritual distress (distress of the human spirit).**

Home Care Interventions

• All of the mentioned nursing interventions apply in the home setting.

Client/Family Teaching

• Help client obtain religious rites or spiritual guidance.

Spiritual support (belief in a divine being or God) was identified as a factor that contributed to initiation and maintenance of behavior changes after an illness (McSweeney, 1993). The nurse is rarely the client's primary spiritual caregiver. No single approach to spiritual care is satisfactory for all clients; many kinds of resources are needed (Bolander, 1994).

• Assist clients with developing spirituality. List the most valuable qualities they can bring from within, circumstances most helpful for unfolding these qualities, and ways of incorporating these circumstances into their life-styles.

Interventions assist clients with bringing forth courage, compassion, inner peace, and creative insight (spirituality) (Macrae, 1995).

REFERENCES   Bolander V: *Sorensen and Luckmann's basic nursing: a psychophysiologic approach,* Philadelphia, 1994, WB Saunders.

Boss JA, Corbett T: The developing practice of the parish nurse: an inner-city experience. In Solari-Twadell PA, Djupe AM, McDermott MA, editors: *Parish nursing: the developing practice,* Park Ridge, Ill, 1990, National Parish Nurse Resource Center.

Clark C, Heidenreich T: Spiritual care for the critically ill, *Am J Crit Care* 4:77, 1995.

Dettmore D: Spiritual care: remembering your patients' forgotten needs, *Nursing* 14:46, 1984.

Farran CJ, McCann J: Longitudinal analysis of hope in community-based older adults, *Psychiatr Arch Nurs* 3:272, 1989.

Fehring RJ, Frenn M: Holistic nursing care: a church and university join forces, *J Christ Nurs* 4:25, 1987.

Macrae J: Nightingale's spiritual philosophy and its significance for modern nursing, *Image* 27:8, 1995.

McSweeney J: Making behavior changes after a myocardial infarction, *West J Nurs Res* 15:441, 1993.

Reed P: Preferences for spiritually related nursing interventions among terminally ill and nonterminally ill hospitalized adults and well adults, *Appl Nurs Res* 4:122, 1991.

Simsen B: Nursing the spirit, meeting patients' spiritual needs, *Nurs Times* 84:31, 1988.

Risk for suffocation

Peggy Wetsch

Definition   Accentuated risk of accidental suffocation (inadequate air available for inhalation)

Risk Factors

Internal (individual)

Reduced olfactory sensation, reduced motor abilities, lack of safety education, lack of safety precautions, cognitive or emotional difficulties, disease or injury process

External (environmental)

Pillow placed in infant's crib; propped bottle in infant's crib; vehicle warming in closed garage; children playing with plastic bags or inserting small objects into their mouths or noses; discarded or unused refrigerators or freezers with doors; children left unattended in or near bathtubs, pools, or hot tubs; household gas leaks; smoking in bed; use of fuel-burning heaters not vented to outside; low-strung clotheslines; pacifier hung around infant's head; eating large mouthfuls of food

Related Factors (r/t)

See Risk Factors

Client Outcomes/Goals

- Explains and undertakes appropriate measures to prevent suffocation
- Demonstrates correct techniques for emergency rescue maneuvers (i.e., Heimlich maneuver, rescue breathing, cardiopulmonary resuscitation [CPR]), and describes situations that necessitate them

Suggested NIC Interventions

Airway management, environmental management: safety, respiratory monitoring

Nursing Interventions and Rationales

NOTE: Management of a risk diagnosis necessitates approaches using primary and secondary prevention. Primary prevention interventions, which include such activities as safety instruction, focus on thwarting the development of disease or condition. Early detection through screening, monitoring and surveillance is secondary prevention (Shirtridge, Valanis, 1992).

- Conduct risk factor identification noting special circumstances in which preventive or protective measures are indicated. Note presence of environmental hazards including the following:
  - Plastic bags (e.g., dry cleaner's bags, bags used for mattress protection)
  - Cribs with slats wider than 2⅜ inches
  - Ill-fitting crib mattresses that can allow infant to become wedged
  - Pillows in cribs
  - Abandoned large appliances such as refrigerators, dishwashers, or freezers
  - Clothing with cords or hoods that can become entangled
  - Bibs, pacifiers on a string, drapery cords, pull-toy strings

- Earth cave-ins
- Food items

    Suffocation by airway obstruction is a leading cause of death in children less than age 6. Cords longer than 12 inches can lead to strangulation. Identification of clients and families at risk signals special teaching and referral needs (Rivara, Bergman, LoGero, 1982; Green, 1993; Jones, 1993; McCloskey, Bulechek, 1992).

- Identify hospitalized clients at particular risk for suffocation, including the following:
    - Clients with altered level of consciousness
    - Infants or young children
    - Clients with developmental delays
- Institute safety measures such as proper positioning and feeding precautions. See **Risk for aspiration, impaired swallowing** for additional interventions.

    Vigilance and special protective measures are necessary for clients at greater risk for suffocation (Green, 1993).

Geriatric
- Observe client for pocketing of food in side of mouth; remove food as needed.
- Position client in high Fowler's position when eating and for a half hour afterward.

Home Care Interventions

- Assess home for potential safety hazards in systems that are not likely to be fixed (e.g., faulty pilots or gas leaks in gas stoves, carbon monoxide release from heating systems, kerosene fumes from portable heaters). Assist family with having these areas assessed and making appropriate safety arrangements (i.e., installing detectors, making repairs).

    Assessment and correction of system problems prevents accidental suffocation.

- Use care in pillow placement when positioning frail elderly clients who are bedbound.

    Frail elderly clients are at risk for suffocation if pillows become lodged in the bed and the client cannot reposition because of weakness.

Client/Family Teaching

- Counsel families on the following:
    - General safety practices such as not smoking in bed, proper disposal of large appliances, using properly functioning heating systems and ventilation, having functional smoke detectors, and opening garage doors when warming up a car
    - Safety measures appropriate to the functional or developmental age of the client (with emphasis on crib safety in particular)
    - Sleeping precautions such as not sleeping next to small infants, which places them at a greater risk of smothering

    Legislated countermeasures have led to decreased suffocation incidences with the exception of mechanical crib strangulation. Families and caregivers need to continue to be attentive and aware of potentially dangerous situations (National Safety Council, 1992; Green, 1993).

- Advise parents to avoid food that can be inhaled (e.g., peanuts, popcorn, hard candy, gum, whole or large pieces of hot dog, whole grapes). Nonfood items smaller than 1¼ inches in diameter (e.g., latex balloons, small parts on toys) also present a hazard.

    Rigid items that are spherical or cylindrical shape can cause upper airway occlusion. Mechanical suffocation and asphyxia resulting from foreign objects in the respiratory tract are the leading cause of death in children less than 1 year of age. Children less than 2 years of age have high level of hands-to-mouth behavior. Combined with a lack of fear, they are at risk even in a child-safe environment (Carson, 1992; Green, 1993; Holida, 1993).

- Provide information to parents about obtaining the "no choke test tube" if desired.
  This tube teaches parents about safe sizes of toys and other small objects (Jones, 1993).
- Stress water and pool safety precautions including vigilant, uninterrupted parent supervision.
  An intense drive for exploration combined with a lack of awareness of danger makes drowning a threat. A child's high center of gravity and poor coordination make buckets and toilets a threat because a child looking inside can fall over and become lodged (Green, 1993; Jones 1993).
- Underscore the necessity of not allowing children to play with or near electric garage doors and keeping garage door openers out of reach of young children.
  Children close to the ground may not be large enough to trigger reversal mechanisms on the door and may become entrapped.
- Recommend that families who are seeking daycare or in-home care for children, geriatric family members, or at-risk family members with developmental or functional disabilities to inspect environment for hazards and examine first aid preparation and vigilance of providers.
  Many working families must trust others to care for family members.
- Involve family members in learning and practicing rescue techniques, including treatment of choking, breathing, and CPR. Initiate referral to formal training classes.
  Family members need adequate preparation to deal with emergency situations (Green, 1993).

REFERENCES   Carson L: Triage decisions: an 11-month-old with unexplained respiration distress, *J Emerg Nurs* 18:82, 1992.

Green PM: High risk for suffocation. In McFarland GK, McFarlane EA, editors: *Nursing diagnosis and intervention,* St Louis, 1993, Mosby.

Holida DL: Latex balloons: they can take your breath away, *Pediatr Nurs* 19:39, 1993.

Jones NE: Childhood residential injuries, *MCN* 18:168, 1993.

McCloskey JC, Bulechek GM, editors: *Nursing interventions classification (NIC),* St Louis, 1992, Mosby.

McFadden EA: Product safety alert: syringe cap aspiration, *J Pediatr Nurs* 8:52, 1993.

National Safety Council: *Accident facts,* Itasca Ill, 1992, The Council.

Rivara FP, Bergman AB, LoGero JP: Epidemiology of childhood injuries II: sex differences in injury rates, *Am J Dis Child* 13:502, 1982.

Shirtridge L, Valanis B: The epidemiological model applied in community health nursing. In Stanhope M, Lancaster J, editors: *Community health nursing: process and practice for promoting health,* ed 3, St Louis, 1992, Mosby.

Impaired swallowing

Roslyn Fine and Betty J. Ackley

Definition   The state in which an individual has a decreased ability to voluntarily pass fluids or solids from the mouth to the stomach via the esophagus.

Defining Characteristics

Observed evidence of a swallowing difficulty (e.g., stasis of food in oral cavity, coughing, choking, wet or gurgly voice, spitting of food, major delay in swallowing, double swallowing, drooling, watering eyes, nasal drainage, evidence of aspiration)

Related Factors (r/t)

Neuromuscular impairment (e.g., decreased or absent gag or swallow reflex, decreased strength or excursion of muscles involved in mastication, perceptual impairment, facial paralysis), mechanical obstruction (e.g., edema, tracheostomy tube, laryngeal or oral cancer), fatigue, limited awareness, red or irritated oropharyngeal cavity

Client Outcomes/Goals

- Demonstrates effective swallowing and swallowing without choking or coughing
- Remains free from aspiration (e.g., lungs clear, temperature within normal range)

Suggested NIC Interventions

Aspiration precautions, swallowing therapy

Nursing Interventions and Rationales

- Assess ability to swallow by positioning examiner's thumb and index finger on client's laryngeal protuberance. Ask client to swallow; feel larynx elevate. Ask client to cough; test for a gag reflex on both sides of posterior pharyngeal wall (lingual surface) with a tongue blade. Do not rely on presence of gag reflex to determine when to feed.
  Normally the time taken for the bolus to move from the point at which the reflex is triggered to the esophageal entry (pharyngeal transit time) is 1 second or less (Logeman, 1983). Cardiovascular accident (CVA) clients with prolonged pharyngeal transit times (prolonged swallowing) have a greatly increased chance of developing aspiration pneumonia (Johnson, McKenzie, Sievers, 1993). Clients can aspirate even if they have an intact gag reflex (Baker, 1993; Lugger 1994).
- Observe for signs associated with swallowing problems (e.g., coughing, choking, spitting of food, drooling, difficulty handling oral secretions, double swallowing or major delay in swallowing, watering eyes, nasal discharge, wet or gurgly voice, decreased ability to move tongue and lips, decreased mastication of food, decreased ability to move food to the back of the pharynx, slow or scanning speech).
  These are all signs of swallowing impairment (Baker, 1993; Lugger, 1994).
- Evaluate medications clients are presently taking, especially elderly clients. Consult with the pharmacist for assistance in monitoring for incorrect doses and drug interactions that could result in dysphagia.
  Dysphagia is more prevalent in the elderly because of the coexistence of a variety of neurological, neuromuscular, or oncological conditions. Most elderly clients take numerous medications, which when taken individually, can slow motor function, cause anxiety and depression, and reduce salivary flow. When taken together, these medication interactions can result in impaired swallowing function. Drugs that reduce muscle tone for swallowing and can cause reflux include calcium channel blockers and nitrates. Drugs that can reduce salivary flow include antidepressants, antiparkinsonism drugs, antihistamines, antispasmodics, antipsychotic agents or major tranquilizers, antiemetics, antihypertensives, and drugs for treating diarrhea and anxiety (Sonies, 1992; Sliwa, Lis, 1993).
- If client has impaired swallowing, refer to speech and language pathologist for bedside evaluation and use dysphagia team.
  The dysphagia team is composed of a rehabilitation nurse, speech and language pathologist, dietician, physician, and radiologist who work together to help the client learn to swallow safely and maintain a good nutritional status.
- If client has impaired swallowing, do not feed until an appropriate diagnostic workup is completed. Ensure proper nutrition by consulting with physician for enteral feedings.
  Feeding a client who cannot adequately swallow results in aspiration and possibly death.

- If client has an intact swallowing reflex, attempt to feed. Observe the following feeding guidelines:
  - Position client upright at a 90° angle with the head flexed forward at a 45° angle. *This position forces the trachea to close and esophagus to open, which makes swallowing easier and reduces the risk of aspiration.*
  - Ensure client is awake, alert, and able to follow sequenced directions before attempting to feed. *As the client becomes less alert the swallowing response decreases, which increases the risk of aspiration.*
  - Begin by feeding client ⅓ tsp applesauce. Provide sufficient time to masticate and swallow.
  - Place food on unaffected side of tongue.
  - During feeding, give client specific directions (e.g., "Open your mouth, chew the food completely, and when you are ready, tuck your chin to your chest and swallow").
  - Watch for uncoordinated chewing or swallowing, coughing immediately after eating or delayed coughing (which may indicate silent aspiration), pocketing of food, wet-sounding voice, sneezing when eating, delay of more than 1 second in swallowing, or a change in respiratory patterns. If any of these signs are present, put on gloves, remove all food from oral cavity, stop feedings, and consult with a speech and language pathologist and a dysphagia team. *These are signs of impaired swallowing and possible aspiration (Donahue, 1990; Baker, 1993).*
- If client tolerates single-textured foods such as pudding, Cream of Wheat, or strained baby food, advance to a soft diet with guidance from the dysphagia team. Avoid foods such as hamburgers, corn, and pastas that are difficult to chew. Also avoid sticky foods such as peanut butter and white bread. *The dysphagia team should determine the appropriate diet for the client on the basis of progression in swallowing as well as ensuring that the client is nourished and hydrated.*
- Avoid providing liquids until client is able to swallow effectively. Add a thickening agent to liquids to obtain a soft consistency that is similar to honey or pudding (depending on degree of swallowing problems). *Thickened liquids form a cohesive bolus that the client can swallow with increased efficiency (Langmore, Miller, 1994).*
- Work with client on swallowing exercises prescribed by dysphagia team (e.g., touching palate with tongue, stimulating tonsillar arch and soft palate with a cold metal examination mirror or cotton swab [thermal stimulation]). *Swallowing exercises can improve the client's ability to swallow (Langmore, Miller, 1994).*
- Provide meals in a quiet environment away from excessive stimuli such as a community dining room. *A noisy environment can be an aversive stimuli and decrease effective mastication and swallowing.*
- Have suction equipment available during feeding. If choking occurs and suctioning is necessary, discontinue oral feeding until client is safely assessed with a videofluoroscopic swallow study. *Suctioning may be necessary if the client is choking on food and could aspirate.*

- Check oral cavity for proper emptying after client swallows and after client finishes meal. Provide oral care at end of meal. It may be necessary to manually remove food from client's mouth; use latex gloves and keep client's teeth apart with a padded tongue blade.
  Food may become pocketed in the affected side and cause stomatitis and tooth decay and may be aspirated later.
- Praise client for successfully following directions and swallowing appropriately.
  Praise reinforces behavior and sets up a positive atmosphere in which learning takes place.
- Keep client in an upright position for 30 to 45 minutes following a meal.
  An upright position ensures that food stays in the stomach until it has emptied and decreases the chance of aspiration following meals.
- Auscultate lung sounds after feeding; note new crackles or wheezing and elevated temperature or white blood cell count.
  The presence of new crackles or wheezing and elevated temperature or white blood cell count could indicate aspiration of food, so the physician should be notified.
- Keep a record of food intake.
  A food intake record will allow the nurse, speech and language pathologist, and dietician to determine the adequacy of nutritional intake (Beadle, Townsend, Palmer, 1995).
- Evaluate nutritional status daily. If not adequately nourished, work with dysphagia team to determine whether client needs to avoid oral intake (be NPO) with therapeutic feeding only or needs enteral feedings until client can swallow adequately.
  Enteral feedings can maintain nutrition if client is unable to swallow adequate amounts of food (Grant, Rivera, 1995).

Client/Family Teaching

- Teach client and family exercises prescribed by dysphagia team.
- Teach client a step-by-step method of swallowing effectively.
- Educate client and family about rationales for food consistency and choices.
- Teach family how to monitor client to prevent aspiration during eating.

REFERENCES Baker DM: Assessment and management of impairments in swallowing, *Nurs Clin North Am* 28:793, 1993.

Beadle L, Townsend S, Palmer D: The management of dysphagia in stroke, *Nurs Stand* 9:37, 1995.

Donahue PA: When it's hard to swallow: feeding techniques for dysphagia management, *J Gerontol Nurs* 16:6, 1990.

Grant MM, Rivera LM: Anorexia, cachexia, and dysphagia: the symptom experience, *Semin Oncol Nurs* 11:266, 1995.

Hufler DR: Helping your dysphagic patient eat, *RN* 1987, p. 36.

Johnson ER, McKenzie SW, Sievers A: Aspiration pneumonia in stroke, *Arch Phys Med Rehabil* 74:973, 1993.

Langmore SE, Miller RM: Behavioral treatment for adults with oropharyngeal dysphagia, *Arch Phys Med Rehab* 75:1154, 1994.

Logemann JA: *Evaluation and treatment of swallowing disorders,* San Diego, 1983, College Hill.

Lugger KE: Dysphagia in the elderly stroke patient, *J Neurosci Nurs* 26:78, 1994.

Richter JE, Schechter GL: A new, commonsense approach to dysphagia, *Patient Care* 26:87, 1992.

Sliwa JA, Lis S: Drug-induced dysphagia, *Arch Phys Med Rehab* 74:445, 1993.

Sonies BC: Oropharyngeal dysphagia in the elderly. In Baum BJ, editor: *Clinics in geriatric medicine,* Philadelphia, 1992, WB Saunders.

Williams MJ, Walker GT: Managing swallowing problems in the home, *Caring* 11:59, 1992.

Risk for altered body temperature

Sandra K. Cunningham

Definition   The state in which an individual is at risk for failure to maintain body temperature within a normal range

Risk Factors

Extremes of age or weight, exposure to cool/cold or hot/warm environments, dehydration, inactivity or vigorous activity, medications that cause vasoconstriction or vasodilatation, altered metabolic rate, sedation, clothing inappropriate for environmental temperature, illness or trauma that affects body temperature regulation

Related Factors (r/t)

See Risk Factors

Client Outcomes/Goals

- Maintains temperature within normal range
- Explains measures needed to maintain normal temperature
- Explains symptoms of hypothermia or hyperthermia

Suggested NIC Interventions

Temperature regulation, temperature regulation: inoperative, vital signs monitoring

Nursing Interventions and Rationales

- Monitor temperature every _____ hour(s) or use continuous temperature monitoring as appropriate.
  Normal adult body temperature is 96.8° F (36° C) to 100.4° F (38° C). (Black, Matassarin-Jacobs, 1993). Disease, injury, or pharmacological agents may impair risk for altered body temperature (Holtzclaw, 1993; Dennison, 1995).
- Take vital signs every _____ hour(s), noting signs of hypothermia (e.g., decreased pulse, respiration, blood pressure) or hyperthermia (e.g., rapid, bounding pulse; increased respiratory rate).
  Consistent monitoring promotes prevention and early intervention in clients with altered cardiopulmonary status associated with hypothermia or hyperthermia.
- Monitor client for signs of hypothermia (e.g., shivering, cool skin, piloerection, pallor, slow capillary refill, cyanotic nailbeds, decreased mentation, coma).
  Monitoring for defining characteristics of hypothermia allows for prevention and/or early intervention.
- Monitor client for signs of hyperthermia (e.g., visual disturbances, headache, nausea and vomiting, muscle flaccidity, absence of sweating, delirium, coma).
  Monitoring for defining characteristics of hyperthermia allows for prevention and/or early intervention.
- Maintain a consistent room temperature (from 68° F to 72° F).
  A consistent temperature limits environmental effects on thermoregulation.
- Promote adequate nutrition and hydration.
  This will help maintain a normal body temperature.
- Adjust clothing to facilitate passive warming or cooling as appropriate.
  This will help maintain a normal body temperature.
- Avoid sedatives that depress cerebral function and circulation.
  This practice limits the risk factors associated with a risk for altered body temperature.

- Refer to social services and a dietician as appropriate.
  Adequate nutrition, hydration, environment, and clothing decrease the risk of hypothermia or hyperthermia.
- See nursing interventions and rationales for **Hypothermia** or **Hyperthermia** as appropriate.

Geriatric
- Older adults have a decreased ability to adapt to temperature extremes and need protection from extreme environmental temperature. Be aware of factors such as room temperature (heating/air conditioning), clothing (layered/loose), and fluid intake.
  Older adults have a higher threshold of central temperature for sweating, diminished or absent sweating, impaired warmth or cold perception, an impaired shiver response, diminished thermogenesis, an abnormal peripheral blood flow response to warmth or cold, and a compromised cardiovascular reserve (Robbins, 1989).
- Assess medication profile for potential risk of drug-related altered body temperature.
  Anesthetics, barbiturates, salicylates, nonsteroidal antiinflammatory drugs (NSAIDs), diuretics, antihistamines, anticholinergics, beta blockers, and thyroid hormones have been linked to altered body temperatures (Miller, 1991).

Pediatric
- Recognize that pediatric clients have a decreased ability to adapt to temperature extremes.
  The combination of a relatively larger body surface area, smaller body-fluid volume, less well-developed temperature control mechanisms, and a smaller amount of protective body fat limits the pediatric client's ability to maintain normal temperatures (Henderson, 1990; Roncoli, Medoff-Cooper, 1992).

Home Care Interventions

All of the mentioned nursing interventions are applicable in the home setting.

Client/Family Teaching

- Teach client and family ways to prevent hypothermia or hyperthermia.
- Teach client and family signs of hypothermia and hyperthermia and appropriate interventions.
  Adequate teaching improves compliance and reduces anxiety.
- Teach client and family proper method for taking temperature.
  Optimal placement of the appropriate device is essential for accurate monitoring.
- Teach client and family of medications associated with altered body temperature as appropriate.
  Appropriate teaching prevents potential hypothermic or hyperthermic event.

REFERENCES   Black JM, Matassarin-Jacobs E: *Luckmann and Sorensen's Medical-surgical nursing: a psychophysiologic approach,* Philadelphia, 1993, WB Saunders.

Dennison D: Thermal regulation of patients during the perioperative period, *AORN J* 61:827, 1995.

Henderson DP: Pediatric update: hypothermia and the pediatric patient, *J Emerg Nurs* 16:411, 1990.

Holtzclaw BJ: Monitoring body temperature, *AACN Clin Issu Crit Care Nurs* 4:44, 1993.

McCloskey JC, Bulecheck GM: *Nursing interventions classification (NIC),* ed 2, St Louis, 1996, Mosby.

Miller CA: Driving the temperatures up and down, *Geriatric Nurs* 12:44, 1991.

Miller CA: Nursing care of older adults: theory and practice, Glenview, Ill, 1990, Scott Foresmann/Little Brown.

Robbins AS: Hypothermia and heat stroke: protecting the elderly patient, *Geriatrics,* vol 44, 1989.

Roncoli M: Medoff-Cooper B: Thermoregulation in low-birth-weight infants, *NAACOG's Clin Issues* 3:25, 1992.

Whaley LF, Wong DL: *Essentials of pediatric nursing,* St Louis, 1989, Mosby.

Ineffective management of therapeutic regimen: families

Margaret Lunney

Definition   A pattern of regulating and integrating into family processes a program for treatment of illness and its sequelae that is unsatisfactory for meeting specific health goals

Defining Characteristics

Major   Inappropriate family activities for meeting the goals of a treatment or prevention program

Minor   Lack of family attention to illness and its sequelae, acceleration of illness symptoms of a family member, verbalized desire to manage the treatment of illness and prevent its sequelae, verbalized difficulty with regulation or integration of one or more prescribed regimens, verbalized neglect of family actions to reduce risk factors for progression of illness and sequelae

Related Factors (r/t)

See **Ineffective management of therapeutic regimen: individual**

Client Outcomes/Goals

- Make adjustments in usual activities (e.g., diet, activity, stress management) to incorporate the therapeutic regimens of family members
- Reduce illness symptoms of family members
- Desire to manage the therapeutic regimens of its members
- Verbalize that some of the difficulties of managing therapeutic regimens are decreased
- Describe actions to reduce risk factors

Suggested NIC Interventions

Family involvement, family mobilization, family process maintenance

Nursing Interventions and Rationales

- Establish an open and trusting relationship with family members.

  If trust is established with family members, they are more likely to openly share the real difficulties of integrating therapeutic regimens with family process (Friedman, 1992).
- Ensure that all strategies for working with family are culturally appropriate.

  Cultural competence is needed to work with culturally diverse families (Degazon, 1996).
- Review with family members congruence and incongruence of family behaviors and health-related goals.

  To attain the motivation that is needed for changes in daily habits, family members should understand the relationship of daily habits to health-related goals (Miller, 1992). Family goals are stable and take precedence over health-related goals.
- Help family members make decisions regarding ways to integrate therapeutic regimens with daily living. Provide advice or suggestions as solicited and accepted by family.

  Decisions made by the family, rather than by health providers or others, guide everyday actions (Friedman, 1992). Advice from others, including nurses, will not be followed unless it is valued and respected by the family.
- Demonstrate respect for and trust in family decisions.

  People make decisions that they believe are appropriate. Families who believe they are respected and trusted by health providers are more likely to collaborate effectively with them.
- Acknowledge the challenge of integrating therapeutic regimens with family behaviors.

  Therapeutic regimens require modifications of daily activities that have already been established based on family values and beliefs (Miller, 1992). Acknowledging the difficulty of changing family habits supports families during the process.

- Review symptoms of illness(es) and work with family toward a development of greater awareness of symptoms.
  Knowledge and awareness of symptoms improve families' abilities to adjust behaviors to prevent and manage symptoms (Lubkin, 1994).
- Provide sufficient knowledge to support family decisions regarding therapeutic regimens.
  Knowledge deficits can be a major obstacle to effectively managing therapeutic regimens (Fujita, Duncan, 1994).
- Selectively support family decisions to adjust the therapeutic regimens as indicated.
  Sometimes families do not have access to health providers or need to make independent decisions because of side effects or adverse effects of therapeutic regimens. Family members need to make informed decisions that are in their best interests (Miller, 1992; Lubkin, 1994). Providing support for appropriate decisions improves the ability of the family to make such decisions.
- Advocate for family in negotiating therapeutic regimens with health providers.
  Illness regimens are generally not arbitrary or absolute; therefore modifications can be discussed as needed to fit in with family life-styles (Miller, 1992; Lubkin, 1994).
- Help family mobilize social supports.
  Increased social support helps families meet health-related goals (Miller, 1992; Pender, 1996).
- Help family members modify perceptions as indicated.
  Individual perceptions regarding the seriousness, susceptibility, and threat of illness may be distorted or inaccurate but may be modified with new information (Pender, 1996).
- Use one or more family theories (e.g., from theorists such as Bowen, Satir, Minuchin) to describe, explain, or predict family dynamics.
  Family systems are complex and may not be understood by the nurse without adequate knowledge of family theories (Friedman, 1992).
- Collaborate with nurses or other consultants regarding strategies for working with families.
  For some families the knowledge and skills of nurses with advanced degrees or of other specialists may be needed to design effective interventions (Kang, Barnard, Oshio, 1994).

Home Care Interventions

- Assess cultural, social, and family influences on achievement of health goals or regimen.
  "Cultural lifeways are shared among members of the group and understood, often without persons being aware that their world view differs from another. Symptoms are perceived, labeled and reacted to in ways that make sense within the culture" (Wenger, 1993, p. 22).
- Assess family for need of assistance with management and evaluation (M & E) of care plan.
  "The focus of the nurse's skill in M & E is on the . . . supervision of the delivery of care by multiple caregivers . . . [and] is usually found with overlapping medical conditions . . . [The] numerous diagnoses and care provided is of such complexity that the client's medical condition would be jeopardized if not managed by a skilled nurse" (Humphrey, Milone-Nuzzo, 1996, pp. 66-67).

- Assist family with obtaining the necessary supplies or personnel support to manage therapeutic regimen as they would choose if possible.
  This kind of support demonstrates respect for and trust in family decision-making. Family decisions can be reconsidered if previous decisions are not feasible.

Client/Family Teaching

- Teach about all aspects of therapeutic regimens. Provide as much knowledge as family will accept. Adjust instruction to account for what family already knows, and provide information in a culturally congruent manner.
- Teach ways to adjust family behaviors for inclusion of therapeutic regimens.
- Teach safety in taking medication.
- Teach family members to act as self-advocates with health providers who prescribe therapeutic regimens.

REFERENCES   Degazon C: Cultural diversity and community health nursing practice. In Stanhope M, Lancaster J, *Community health nursing: promoting health of aggregates, families, and individuals,* ed 4, St Louis, 1996, Mosby.

Friedman MM: *Family nursing: theory and practice,* ed 3, Norwalk, Conn, 1992, Appleton & Lange.

Fujita LJ, Duncan J: High risk for ineffective management of therapeutic regimen: a protocol study, *Rehab Nurs* 19:75, 1994.

Humphrey C, Milone-Nuzzo P: *Orientation to home care nursing,* Gaithersburg, Md, 1996, Aspen.

Kang R, Bernard K, Oshio S: Description of the clinical practice of advanced practice nurses in family-centered early intervention in two rural settings, *Public Health Nurs* 11:376, 1994.

Lubkin IM: Chronic illness: impact and interventions, ed 3, Boston, 1994, Jones & Bartlett.

Lubkin IM: Chronic illness: impact and interventions, ed 2, Boston, 1990, Jones & Bartlett.

Miller JF: *Coping with chronic illness: overcoming powerlessness,* ed 2, Philadelphia, 1992, FA Davis.

Pender NJ: *Health promotion in nursing practice,* ed 3, Norwalk, Conn, 1996, Appleton & Lange.

Stetz KM, Lewis FM, Houck GM: Family goals as indicants of adaption during chronic illness, *Public Health Nurs* 11:385, 1994.

Wenger F: Cultural meaning of symptoms, *Holistic Nurs Pract* 22:7, 1993.

Effective management of therapeutic regimen: individual

Margaret Lunney

Definition

A pattern of regulation and integrating into daily living a program for treatment of illness and sequelae that is satisfactory for meeting specific health goals

Defining Characteristics

Appropriate choices of daily activities for meeting the goals of a treatment or prevention program, illness symptoms are within a normal range of expectation, verbalized desire to manage the treatment of illness and sequelae, verbalized intent to reduce risk factors for progression of illness and sequelae

Client Outcomes/Goals

- Acknowledges appropriateness of choices for meeting goals of treatment or prevention programs
- Agrees to continue making appropriate choices
- Verbalizes intent to contact health provider(s) for additional information, support, or resources as needed
- States knowledge of risk factors

Suggested NIC Interventions

Anticipatory guidance, health system guidance

Nursing Interventions and Rationales

- Acknowledge congruence of activities of daily living with health-related goals.
  Support from health provider in efforts made to manage therapeutic regimens may motivate individuals to continue these efforts despite encountered difficulties (Miller, 1992).
- Support decisions regarding methods of integrating therapeutic regimens with daily living.
  Support from health providers for previous decisions provides evidence of continued ability to successfully manage therapeutic regimens (Miller, 1992).
- Provide information on possible illness trajectories so that client can plan for future management.
  Knowledge and awareness of illness trajectories enables the individual to plan for future management of therapeutic regimens (Lubkin, 1990).
- Review methods of contacting health provider(s) as needed for changes in therapeutic regimen and/or methods of incorporating therapeutic regimens with activities of daily living (ADLs).
  Although interventions for problems in managing therapeutic regimens may not be needed at the present time, individuals should know how to obtain such support if needed in the future.
- Record client effectiveness of managing therapeutic regimens.
  Health providers may continue to assess and diagnose ineffective management unnecessarily. The health care system saves time, effort, and money if an assessment and diagnosis of effective management are communicated to other health providers.

Home Care Interventions

- Assess family for need of assistance with management and evaluation (M & E) of care plan.
  "The focus of the nurse's skill in M & E is on the . . . supervision of the delivery of care . . . by multiple caregivers . . . [and] is usually found with overlapping medical conditions . . . [The} numerous diagnoses and care provided is of such complexity that the client's medical condition would be jeopardized if not managed by a skilled nurse" (Humphrey, Milone-Nuzzo, 1996, pp. 66-67).
- Assist family with obtaining the necessary supplies or personnel support to manage therapeutic regimen as they would choose if possible.
  This kind of support demonstrates respect for and trust in family decision-making. Family decisions can be reconsidered if early decisions are not workable.

Client/Family Teaching

- Teach management of future problems if needed.

REFERENCES   Bakker RH, Kastermans MC, Dassen TWN: An analysis of the nursing diagnosis: ineffective management of therapeutic regimen compared to noncompliance and Orem's self-care deficit theory of nursing, *Nurs Diag* 6:161, 1995.

Degazon C: Cultural diversity and community health nursing practice. In Stanhope M, Lancaster J: *Community health nursing: promoting health of aggregates, families, and individuals.* ed 4, St Louis, 1996, Mosby.

Fujita LJ, Duncan J: High risk for ineffective management of therapeutic regimen: a protocol study, *Rehab Nurs* 19:75, 1994.

Humphrey C, Milone-Nuzzo P: *Orientation to home care nursing,* Maryland, 1996, Aspen.

Lubkin IM: *Chronic illness: impact and interventions,* ed 3, Boston, 1994, Jones & Bartlett.

Lumney M: *The concept of management and therapeutic regimen: validation of four nursing diagnoses,* Unpublished paper submitted to NANDA, 1991.

Northrup D: Self-care myth reconsidered, *Adv Nur Sci* 15:59, 1993.

Ineffective management of therapeutic regimen: individual

Margaret Lunney

Definition   A pattern of regulating and integrating into daily living a treatment program for an illness and its aftereffects that is unsatisfactory for meeting specific health goals

Defining Characteristics

Major   Choices of daily living ineffective for meeting the goals of a treatment or prevention program

Minor   Acceleration (expected or unexpected) of illness symptoms, verbalized desire to manage the treatment of illness and prevention of sequelae, verbalized difficulty with regulation/integration of one or more prescribed regimens for treatment of illness and its effects or prevention of complications, verbalized that action not taken to reduce risk factors for prevention of illness and sequelae

Related Factors (r/t)

Complexity of health care system, complexity of therapeutic regimen, decisional conflicts, economic difficulties, excessive demands on individual or family, family conflict, family patterns of health care, inadequate number and types of cues to action, knowledge deficits, mistrust of regimen or health care personnel, perceived seriousness, perceived susceptibility, perceived barriers, perceived benefits, powerlessness, social support deficits

Client Outcomes/Goals

- Describes daily food and fluid intake that meets therapeutic goals
- Describes activity/exercise patterns that meet therapeutic goals
- Describes scheduling of medications to meet therapeutic goals
- Verbalizes ability to manage therapeutic regimens
- Collaborates with health providers to decide on a therapeutic regimen that is congruent with health goals and life-style

Suggested NIC Interventions

Behavior modification, self-modification assistance

Nursing Interventions and Rationales

NOTE: This diagnosis does *not* have the same meaning as the diagnosis **Noncompliance.** This diagnosis is made with the client; if the client does not agree with the diagnosis, it should not be made (Lumney, 1991; Bakker, Kastermans, Dassen, 1995).

- See **Effective management of therapeutic regimen: individual** and **Ineffective management of therapeutic regimen: families.**
- Establish a collaborative partnership with client so that meeting health-related goals can be met.
  Partnerships with health care consumers are different than traditional roles in health care. Partnerships enable the consumer to take an active role in decision-making regarding the therapeutic regimen (Lumney, 1991; Courtney et al, 1996).

- Discuss all strategies with client in context of client's culture.
  Culture affects all decisions for meeting therapeutic goals (Degazon, 1996).
- Identify daily actions that are not therapeutic.
  The client and nurse or provider should agree on which actions are not therapeutic as a basis for intervention.
- Identify reasons for nontherapeutic actions and discuss alternatives.
  There are many possible reasons for actions that do not meet therapeutic goals. Reasons can change with increased knowledge and different perceptions.
- Explain rationales for specific therapeutic regimens that meet health-related goals.
  Clients take responsibility for therapeutic regimens that they understand.
- Provide information about the therapeutic regimen in various formats (e.g., brochure, video, other written instructions).
  People learn in various ways (e.g., visual learners, auditory learners). Therapeutic regimens that are prescribed by health providers are often harder to learn than providers realize. Adequate resources are needed to enhance learning (Lubkin, 1994; Miller, 1992).
- Discuss possible changes that will allow client to meet therapeutic goals.
  Although decisions about actions to meet therapeutic goals are made by the client, the collaborative nature of a nurse-client relationship can help the client with decision-making.
- Encourage critical thinking to consider strategies for changes in behavior.
  Habits that are unhealthy such as overeating and smoking are difficult to change. Although the impetus for change must come from the client, the nurse can prompt the client to change by suggesting alternative strategies.
- Develop a contract with client to maintain motivation for changes in behavior.
  Development of a contract between nurses and clients or clients and themselves provides a concrete way to keep track of actions that meet health-related goals.
- Review methods of contracting health providers as needed for changes in therapeutic regimen.
  People with chronic illnesses need to know a way to obtain resources that may be needed in the future.

Home Care Interventions

All of the mentioned nursing interventions are applicable in the home setting (see **Therapeutic regimen, effective management, individual**).

Client/Family Teaching

- Teach about all aspects of the therapeutic regimens. Provide as much knowledge as person will accept. Adjust instruction to account for what family already knows and provide information in a culturally congruent manner.
- Teach ways to adjust daily activities for inclusion of therapeutic regimens.
- Teach safety in taking medications.
- Teach client to act as self-advocate with health providers who prescribe therapeutic regimens.

REFERENCES   Bakker RH, Kastermans MC, Dassen TWN: An analysis of the nursing diagnosis: Ineffective management of therapeutic regimen compared to noncompliance and Orem's self-care deficit theory of nursing, *Nurs Diag* 6:161, 1995.

Courtney R et al: The partnership model: working with individuals, families, and communities towards a new vision of health, *Public Health Nurs* 13:177, 1996.

Degazon C: Cultural diversity and community health nursing practice. In Stanhope M, Lancaster J: *Community health nursing: promoting health of aggregates, families, and individuals,* ed 4, St Louis, 1996, Mosby.

Fujita LJ, Duncan J: High risk for ineffective management of therapeutic regimen: a protocol study, *Rehab Nurs* 19:75, 1994.

Lubkin IM: Chronic illness: impact and interventions, ed 3, Boston, 1994, Jones & Bartlett.

Lumney M: *The concept of management of therapeutic regimen: validation of four nursing diagnoses,* Unpublished paper submitted to NANDA, 1991.

Miller JF: *Coping with chronic illness: overcoming powerlessness,* ed 2, Philadelphia, 1992, FA Davis.

Northrup D: Self-care myth reconsidered, *Adv Nurs Sci* 15:59, 1993.

Stanhope M, Lancaster J: *Community health nursing: promoting health of aggregates, families, and individuals,* ed 4, St Louis, 1996, Mosby.

Ineffective thermoregulation

Sandra K. Cunningham

Definition The state in which an individual's temperature is unable to maintain a stable, normal core body temperature; temperature fluctuation between hypothermia and hyperthermia

Defining Characteristics
Major Fluctuations in body temperature above or below the normal range (see defining characteristics for **Hypothermia** and **Hyperthermia**)

Related Factors (r/t)
Trauma, illness, immaturity, aging, fluctuating environmental temperature

Client Outcomes/Goals
- Maintains temperature within a normal range
- Exhibits no signs of compromised status
- Explains measures needed to maintain normal temperature
- Explains symptoms of hypothermia or hyperthermia

Suggested NIC Interventions
Temperature regulation, temperature regulation: intraoperative

Nursing Interventions and Rationales
- Monitor temperature at least every 2 hours as needed.
  A normal temperature is between 96.8° F (36° C) and 100.4° F (38° C) (Black, Matassarin-Jacobs, 1993).
- Monitor blood pressure, pulse, and respiration rate, noting signs of hypothermia—decreased pulse, respiration, and blood pressure—or hyperthermia—rapid bound pulse and increased respiratory rate.
- Monitor for other signs of hypothermia, such as shivering, cool skin, piloerection, pallor, slow capillary refill, cyanotic nailbeds, decreased mentation, a comatose state.
- Monitor for other signs of hyperthermia, such as visual disturbances, headache, nausea and vomiting, muscle flaccidity, absence of sweating, delirium, a comatose state.
  Monitoring promotes early identification of ineffective thermoregulation.
- Adjust environmental temperature to client's needs.
  Controlled temperatures limit the environmental effects on thermoregulation (Robbins, 1989, Meyer-Pahoulis et al, 1993; Dennison, 1995).
- Adjust clothing to facilitate passive warming or cooling as needed.
  This step assists in maintaining a normal body temperature (Dennison, 1995).

- Refer to social services or a dietician as appropriate.
  A preventive approach with an adequate environment and proper nutrition, hydration, and clothing decreases the risk of hypothermia or hyperthermia.
- If client is hypothermic, see nursing interventions for **Hypothermia.**
- If client is hyperthermic, see nursing interventions for **Hyperthermia.**

Home Care Interventions
All of the mentioned nursing interventions apply to the home setting.

Client/Family Teaching
- Teach client and family an age-appropriate method for taking temperature.
  Age-appropriate measurement techniques improve accuracy of readings (Finke, 1991; Bliss-Holtz, 1993).
- Teach client and family importance of thermoregulation and possible negative effects of excessive heat or cold.
- Teach client and family signs of prevention and treatment of hypothermia/hyperthermia.
  Appropriate teaching improves compliance and reduces anxiety.

REFERENCES   Black JM, Matassarin-Jacobs E: *Luckmann and Sorensen's Medical-surgical nursing: a psychophysiologic approach,* Philadelphia, 1993, WB Saunders.
Bliss-Holtz J: Determination of thermoregulatory state in full-term infants, *Nurs Res* 42:204, 1993.
Dennison D: Thermal regulation of patients during the perioperative period, *AORN J* 61:827, 1995.
Finke CT: Measurement of the thermoregulatory response: a review, *Focus Crit Care* 18:408, 1991.
Meyer-Pahoulis E et al: The pediatric patient in the post anesthesia care unit, *Nurs Clin North Am* 28:519, 1993.
Robbins AS: Hypothermia and heat stroke: protecting the elderly patient, *Geriatrics* 44:73, 1989.

Altered thought processes

Helen Kelley

Definition
The state in which an individual experiences a disruption in cognitive operations and activities

Defining Characteristics
Inaccurate interpretation of environment, cognitive dissonance, distractibility, memory deficits or problems, hypervigilance, hypovigilance, inappropriate or nonreality-based thinking

Related Factors (r/t)
Head injury, mental disorder, personality disorder, organic mental disorder, substance abuse, severe interpersonal conflict, sleep deprivation, sensory deprivation or overload, impaired cerebral perfusion, metabolic or electrolyte imbalances

Client Outcomes/Goals
- Remains oriented to time, place, and person; demonstrates improved cognitive function
- Remains free from physical harm
- Performs activities of daily living appropriately and independently
- Identifies community resources for help after discharge

Suggested NIC Interventions
Delusion management, dementia management

Nursing Interventions and Rationales

- Observe for causes of altered thought processes (see related factors).
- Monitor and record client's neurological status (level of consciousness, increased intracranial pressure), mental status (memory, cognition, judgment, concentration), vital signs, laboratory results, and ability to follow commands.
  This examination helps identify pathophysiological or psychiatric symptoms.
- Report any new onset or sudden increase in confusion.
  A substantial proportion of postsurgical patients suffer an abnormal temporary change in mental status that can have adverse effects on their recovery (Platzer, 1989).
- Adjust communication style to client. Speak slowly and calmly; use short phrases and concrete, nontechnical words; use writing if appropriate; allow time for thinking; use face-to-face communication; listen carefully; and seek clarification.
  Effective communication promotes understanding.
- Assess pain and promptly provide comfort measures.
  Confused clients cannot accurately report pain; untreated pain increases anxiety and agitation (Foreman, 1989a).
- Identify and remove potentially dangerous items in the environment.
  Cognitive impairment can result in a number of problems, such as communication difficulties, compromised safety, self-care deficits, and behavioral problems.
- Limit use of sedatives and drugs affecting the nervous system.
  Higher medication usage is correlated with more frequent onset of confusion (Foreman, 1989b; Dellasega, Stricklin, 1993).
- Use soft restraints with discretion and physician order.
  Restraints may exacerbate confusion (Yorker, 1988).
- Orient client—call client by name; introduce self on each contact; frequently mention time, date, and place; prominently display a clock and calendar that are easy to read in room and refer to them; and request family to bring in familiar pictures and articles from home.
  These steps help reinforce reality and provide cues that maintain orientation. External, written reminders are more effective than verbal reinforcement for memory aids (McDougall, 1995).
- Stay with clients if they are agitated and likely to be injured.
- Establish predictable care routines; maintain continuity of client's nursing staff.
  Routines promote feelings of security.
- Frequently check on client and have brief interactions to prevent sensory deprivation.
- Avoid an overstimulated or a sensory-deprived environment. Provide adequate lighting that is not too bright. Alternate short, frequent visits with defined rest periods. Monitor noise levels.
  Excessive environmental stimuli can adversely affect client's level of orientation and increase disorganization.
- Assist client with daily hygiene as needed; encourage self-care.
  Good hygiene and self-care increase self-esteem and autonomy.
- Provide support to family during client's period of disorientation. Involve family in current care and planning of postdischarge care.
  Family involvement promotes continuity of care.
- Initiate a social service referral to find help for client following discharge.

- Observe for hallucinations as evidenced by inappropriate laughter, slow verbal responses, lip movements without sound, smiling at inappropriate times, or grimacing.
- Ask direct questions such as, "Are you seeing or hearing something now?" or "Do you sometimes hear or see things that other people don't hear or see?"
- Do not attempt to argue or change client's beliefs, but do not imply agreement. *These actions encourage the client to hold more rigidly to beliefs.*
- Accept clients are seeing or hearing things that are not there, but tactfully tell clients that only they are hearing or seeing these things. Focus on feelings that accompany hallucinations and delusions rather than content (e.g., "You look frightened"). *Acceptance promotes trust and understanding.*
- Set limits on delusional conversations (e.g., "We discussed that; let's talk about what is happening now on the unit").
- Ask for clarification when necessary.
- Help client state needs and ask for assistance.
- Involve client in short activities.
- See **Risk for violence** for further nursing interventions and rationales.

Geriatric
- Monitor for dementia, as evidenced by its gradual onset and a progressive deterioration, or for delirium, as evidenced by its acute onset and generally reversible course. *States of confusion require careful assessment (Vermeersch, 1990).*
- Focus on feelings associated with hallucinations and delusions rather than content. *Tuning into disoriented clients' feelings is more important than rigidly insisting that they share the nurse's reality. Be comforting and understanding when client has processing difficulties (Bleathman, Morton, 1992).*

Home Care Interventions
- Assess family knowledge of disease process and plan of care; teach as necessary. Encourage participation. *Involving significant others in caregiving often helps them cope with the stress of the client's health problem (Stuart, Sundeen, 1991).*
- If client's condition deteriorates, seek acute medical health intervention immediately.
- Identify an emergency plan and criteria for use with family or caregivers. *An appropriate level of clinical intervention supports client and family well-being.*
- Identify responsible caregiver for medication administration. Teach purpose, administration, and side effects of medications based on level of knowledge. *Clients with altered thought process cannot perform health-related care tasks with consistency.*
- Identify cultural variables that affect client responses to stimuli. Use cultural information to provide support to client. Avoid reference to threatening cultural values. *Familiar patterns provide a sense of security for cognitively impaired persons (Stuart, Sundeen, 1991).*
- Use a night light. *Night lights help clients reorient themselves and decrease fear if clients awaken during the night.*
- Allow clients control over aspects of their environment as they are able. *Although sometimes only for a short time, control enhances self-esteem.*
- Identify client's interests and skills. Provide an opportunity to use them without taxing client judgment and cognitive ability. *Diversional activities decrease anxiety and give meaning to life.*

Client/Family Teaching

- Teach family reorientation techniques and need to frequently repeat instructions.
- Help family identify coping skills, environmental supports, and community services for dealing with chronically mentally ill clients.
- Discuss caregiver's need for respite; offer support, encouragement, and information for meeting those needs.

REFERENCES   Algase DL, Beel-Bates CA: Everyday indicators of impaired cognition: development of a new screening scale, *Res Nurs Health* 16:57, 1993.

Bleathman C, Morton I: Validation therapy: extracts from 20 groups with dementia sufferers, *J Adv Nurs* 17:658, 1992.

Coyle MK: Organic illness mimicking psychiatric episodes, *J Gerontol Nurs* 13:31,1987.

Dellasega C, Stricklin ML: Cognitive impairment in elderly home health clients, *Home Health Care Serv Quart* 14:81, 1993.

Foreman M: Complexities of acute confusion, *Geriatr Nurs* 3:136, 1989a.

Foreman M: Confusion in the hospitalized elderly: incidence onset and associated factors, *Res Nurs Health* 12:21, 1989b.

Inaba-Roland T, Maricle S: Assessing delirium, *Heart Lung* 19:45, 1992.

McDougall GC: Memory strategies used by cognitively intact and cognitively impaired older adults, *J Am Acad Nurs Pract* 7:369, 1995.

Platzer H: Post-operative confusion in the elderly—a literature review, *Int J Nurs Stud* 26:367, 1989.

Stuart G, Sundeen S: *Pocket guide to psychiatric nursing,* ed 2, St Louis, 1991, Mosby.

Vermeersch PE: Clinical assessment of confusion, *Appl Nurs Res* 1990, p. 28.

Wilson HS, Kneisel CR: *Psychiatric nursing,* Menlo Park, Calif, 1992, Addison-Wesley.

Yorker BC: The nurse's use of restraint with a neurologically impaired patient, *J Neurosci Nurs* 20:390, 1988.

Impaired tissue integrity

Diane Krasner

Definition

The state in which an individual experiences damage to tissues such as subcutaneous tissue, fascia, or muscle

Defining Characteristics

Destruction of skin surface (full thickness), disruption or destruction of body tissues

Related Factors (r/t)

Altered circulation, nutritional deficit or excess, fluid deficit or excess, knowledge deficit, impaired physical mobility, chemical irritants (including body excretions, secretions, medications), thermal factors (temperature extremes), mechanical factors (pressure, shear, friction), irradiation (including therapeutic irradiation)

Client Outcomes/Goals

- Reports any altered sensation or pain at site of tissue impairment
- Demonstrates understanding of plan to heal tissue and prevent injury
- Describes measures to protect and heal the tissue, including wound care

Suggested NIC Interventions

Wound care

Nursing Interventions and Rationales

- Assess site of impaired tissue integrity and determine etiology (e.g., acute or chronic wound, burn, dermatological lesion, pressure ulcer, leg ulcer).

Prior assessment of wound etiology is critical for proper identification of nursing interventions (Van Rijswijk, 1996).

- Determine size and depth of wound (e.g., full-thickness wound, stage III or stage IV pressure ulcer).
  Wound assessment is more reliable when performed by the same caregiver, the client is in the same position, and the same techniques are used (Krasner, 1992; Miller, 1994).
- Classify pressure ulcers in the following manner:
  - *Stage III:* Full-thickness skin loss involving damage to or necrosis of subcutaneous tissue that may extend down to but not through underlying fascia; ulcer appears as a deep crater with or without undermining of adjacent tissue
  - *Stage IV:* Full-thickness skin loss with extensive destruction, tissue necrosis, or damage to muscle, bone, or supporting structures (e.g., tendons, joint capsules) (National Pressure Ulcer Advisory Panel, 1989).
- Monitor site of impaired tissue integrity at least once daily for color changes, redness, swelling, warmth, pain, or other signs of infection. Determine whether client is experiencing changes in sensation or pain. Pay special attention to all high-risk areas such as bony prominences, skinfolds, sacrum, and heels.
  Systematic inspection can identify impending problems early (Bryant, 1993).
- Monitor status of skin around wound; monitor client's skin care practices, noting type of soap or other cleansing agents used, temperature of water, and frequency of skin cleansing.
  Individualize plan according to client's skin condition, needs, and preferences. Avoid harsh cleansing agents, hot water, extreme friction or force, or cleansing too frequently (Panel for the Prediction and Prevention of Pressure Ulcers in Adults, 1992).
- Monitor client's continence status and minimize exposure of skin impairment site and other areas to moisture from incontinence, perspiration, or wound drainage.
  If client is incontinent, implement an incontinence management plan to prevent exposure to chemicals in urine and stool that can strip or erode the skin; refer to a physician (e.g., urologist, gastroenterologist) for an incontinence assessment (Doughty, 1991; Wound, Ostomy, and Continence Nurses Society, 1992, 1994; Fante et al, 1996).
- Monitor for correct placement of tubes, catheters, and other devices. Assess skin and tissue affected by the tape that secures these devices.
  Mechanical damage to skin and tissues as a result of pressure, friction, or shear is often associated with external devices.
- In orthopedic clients, check every 2 hours for correct placement of footboards, restraints, traction, casts, or other devices, and assess skin and tissue integrity. Be alert for symptoms of compartment syndrome (see **Risk for peripheral neurovascular dysfunction).**
  Mechanical damage to skin and tissues (pressure, friction, or shear) is often associated with external devices.
- For clients with limited mobility, use a risk assessment tool to systematically assess immobility-related risk factors.
  A validated risk assessment tool such as the Norton or Braden Scale should be used to identify clients at risk for immobility-related skin breakdown (Bergstrom et al, 1987; Panel for the Prediction and Prevention of Pressure Ulcers in Adults, 1992).
- Implement a written treatment plan for topical treatment of the skin impairment site.
  A written treatment plan ensures consistency in care and documentation (Maklebust, Sieggreen, 1996). Topical treatments must be matched to the client, wound, and setting (Bolton, Van Rijswijk, 1991; Hess, 1995; Krasner, 1996).

- Identify a plan for debridement if necrotic tissue (eschar or slough) is present and if consistent with overall client management goals.

  Healing does not occur in the presence of necrotic tissue (Pressure Ulcer Treatment Guideline Panel, 1994; Cuzell, Krasner, 1995).
- Select a topical treatment that maintains a moist wound-healing environment that is balanced with the need to absorb exudate and fill dead space.

  Caution should always be taken to not dry out the wound (Pressure Ulcer Treatment Guideline Panel, 1994; Krasner, Kane, 1996).
- Do not position client on site of impaired tissue integrity. If consistent with overall client management goals, turn and position client at least every 2 hours, and carefully transfer client to avoid adverse effects of external mechanical forces (pressure, friction, and shcar).

  Evaluate for use of specialty mattresses of beds as appropriate (Ketts, 1995; Wilson, 1994). If the goal of care is to keep the client (e.g., a terminally ill client) comfortable, turning and repositioning may not be appropriate. Maintain the head of the bed at the lowest degree of elevation possible to reduce shear and friction, and use lift devices, pillows, foam wedges, and pressure-reducing devices in the bed (Panel for the Prediction and Prevention of Pressure Ulcers in Adults, 1992).
- Avoid massaging around site of impaired tissue integrity and over bony prominences.

  Research suggests that massage may lead to deep-tissue trauma (Ortiz, 1992; Panel for the Prediction and Prevention of Pressure Ulcers in Adults, 1992).
- Assess client's nutritional status; refer for a nutritional consultation and/or institute dietary supplements.

  Inadequate nutritional intake places the client at a risk for skin breakdown and compromises healing (Bahl, 1995).

Home Care Interventions

- Assess client's current phases of wound healing (inflammation, proliferation, maturation) and stage of injury.

  Accurate understanding of tissue status combined with knowledge of underlying diagnoses and product validity provide a basis for determining appropriate treatment objectives (Rolstad, 1990). There is no single wound dressing appropriate for all phases of wound healing (Rolstad, 1990).
- Instruct and assist client and caregivers with removing or controlling impediments to wound healing (e.g., management of underlying disease, improvement in approach to client positioning, improved nutrition).

  Wound healing can be delayed or fail totally if impediments are not controlled (Rolstad, 1990).
- Initiate a consultation in a case assignment with an enterostomal therapy (ET) nurse to establish a comprehensive plan as soon as possible.

  In studies of clients with comparable wound care problems, ET nurses were more than twice as successful as non-ET home care nurses in accomplishing wound healing (Arnold, 1994).

Client/Family Teaching

- Teach skin and wound assessment and ways to monitor for signs and symptoms of infection, complications, and healing.

  Early assessment and intervention helps prevent the development of serious problems (Van Rijswijk, 1996).

- Teach use of a topical treatment that is matched to client, wound, and setting.
  The topical treatment needs to be adjusted as the status of the wound changes (Krasner, 1996).
- If consistent with overall client management goals, teach how to turn and reposition client at least every 2 hours.
  If the goal of care is to keep the client (e.g., a terminally ill client) comfortable, turning and repositioning may not be appropriate (Panel for the Prediction and Prevention of Pressure Ulcers in Adults, 1992).
- Teach use of pillows, foam wedges, and pressure-reducing devices to prevent pressure injury.

REFERENCES

Arnold N, Weir D: Retrospective analysis of healing in wounds cared for by ET nurses versus staff nurses in a home setting, *J Wound Ostomy Cont Nurs* 21:4, 1994.

Bahl SM: Nutritional considerations in wound management. In Sogra PP: *Clinical wound management,* Thorofare, NJ, 1995, Slack.

Bergstrom N et al: The Braden scale for prediction of pressure sore risk, *Nurs Res* 36:205, 1987.

Bolton L, Van Rijswijk L: Wound dressings: meeting clinical care and biological needs, *Dermatological Nurs* 3:146, 1991.

Bryant R: *Acute and chronic wounds,* St Louis, 1993, Mosby.

Cuzzell J, Krasner D: Wound dressings. In Sogra PP: *Clinical wound management,* Thorofare, NJ, 1995, Slack.

Doughty D: *Urinary and fecal incontinence: nursing management,* St Louis, 1991, Mosby.

Fante JA et al: Urinary incontinence in adults: acute and chronic management, *Clin Practice* vol 2, 1996 update.

Hess CT: *Wound care: nurse's clinical guide,* Springhouse, Pa, 1995, Springhouse.

Ketts R: Low-air-loss-beds: an effective tool, *AJN* 95:53, 1995.

Krasner D: Dressing decisions for the twenty-first century: on the cusp of a paradigm shift, *Wounds* 8:16, 1996.

Krasner D: Wound measurement: some tools of the trade, *AJN* 1992.

Krasner D, Kane D: *Chronic wound care: a clinical sourcebook for healthcare professionals,* ed 2, Wayne, Pa, Health Management Publications, 1996.

Maklebust J, Sieggreen M: *Pressure ulcers: guidelines for prevention and nursing management,* ed 2, Springhouse, Pa, 1996, Springhouse.

Miller P: Grids beat tape for measuring wounds, *AJN* 94:25, 1994.

National Pressure Ulcer Advisory Panel: *Consensus development conference statement,* Buffalo, NY, 1989, The Panel.

Ortiz M: Massage message, *AJN* 92:42C, 1992.

Panel for the Prediction and Prevention of Pressure Ulcers in Adults: *Pressure ulcers in adults: prediction and prevention,* Clinical Practice Guideline, No 3, Agency for Health Care Policy and Research Pub No 92-0047, Rockville, Md, 1992, US Department of Health and Human Services, Public Health Service.

Rolstad BS: Treatment objectives in chronic wound care, *Home Healthcare Nurse* 9:6, 1990.

Singh: Wound healing in the home health arena, *Home Healthcare Nurse* 12:1, 1993.

Suntken Gwen et al: Implementation of a comprehensive skin care program across care settings using the AHCPR pressure ulcer prevention and treatment guidelines, *Ostomy Wound Manage* 42:2, 1996.

Van Rijswijk L: Wound assessment and documentation. In Krasner D, Kane D: *Chronic wound care: a clinical sourcebook for healthcare professionals,* ed 2, Wayne, Pa, Health Management Publications, 1996.

Wilson S: Mattresses that spell relief, *AJN* 94:48, 1994.

Wound, Ostomy, and Continence Nurses Society: *Standards of care: dermal wounds: pressure ulcers,* Costa Mesa, Calif, 1992, The Society.

Wound, Ostomy, and Continence Nurses Society: *Standards of care: patient with fecal incontinence,* Costa Mesa, Calif, 1994, The Society.

Altered tissue perfusion (specify type): cerebral, renal, cardiopulmonary, GI, peripheral

Betty J. Ackley

Definition   The state in which an individual experiences a decrease in nutrition and oxygenation at the cellular level as a result of a deficit in capillary blood supply

Defining Characteristics

Cold extremities; dependent, blue, or purple skin color; leg is pale when elevated and color does not return when leg is lowered *(critical);* diminished arterial pulsations *(critical);* shiny skin; lack of lanugo; round scars covered with atrophied skin; gangrene; slow-growing, dry, thick, and brittle nails; claudication; blood pressure changes in extremities; bruits; slow-healing lesions

Related Factors (r/t)

Interruption of arterial flow, interruption of venous flow, exchange problems, hypovolemia, hypervolemia

Client Outcomes/Goals

- Demonstrates adequate tissue perfusion as evidenced by palpable peripheral pulses, warm and dry skin, adequate urinary output, and the absence of respiratory distress
- Verbalizes knowledge of treatment regimen, including medications and their actions and possible side effects
- Lists any suggested life-style changes
- Identifies factors causing decreased tissue perfusion
- Demonstrates adequate cerebral perfusion as evidenced by improved mentation, normal vital signs, and freedom from neurological dysfunction

Suggested NIC Interventions

Circulatory care

Nursing Interventions and Rationales

Cerebral perfusion

- See **Decreased adaptive capacity: intracranial; Risk for injury**

Peripheral perfusion

- Check dorsalis pedis and posterior tibial pulses bilaterally; if unable to find them, use a Doppler stethoscope.
  Diminished or absent peripheral pulses indicate arterial insufficiency (Harris, 1996).
- Note skin color and temperature.
  Skin pallor or mottling, cool or cold skin temperature, or an absent pulse can signal arterial obstruction, which is an emergency that requires immediate intervention. Rubor (reddish-blue color accompanied by dependency) indicates dilated or damaged vessels. Brownish discoloration of skin indicates chronic venous insufficiency (Bright, Georgi, 1992).
- Check capillary refill.
  Nailbeds usually return to a pinkish color within 3 seconds after nailbed compression.
- Note skin texture and the presence of hair, ulcers, or gangrenous areas on the legs or feet.
  Thin, shiny, dry skin with hair loss and brittle nails is seen in clients with arterial insufficiency, in addition to gangrene, or ulcerations, on toes and anterior surfaces of the foot. If ulcerations are on the side of the leg, they are usually venous in nature.

- Note presence of edema in extremities and rate it on a 4-point scale. Measure circumference of ankles and calf at the same time each day in the early morning (Cahall, Spence, 1995).
- Assess for pain in extremities, noting severity, quality, timing, and exacerbating and alleviating factors.
  In clients with venous insufficiency the pain lessens with elevation of the legs and exercise. In clients with arterial insufficiency the pain increases with elevation of the leg and exercise (Black, 1995). Some clients have both arterial and venous insufficiency. Arterial insufficiency is associated with pain when walking (claudication) that is relieved by rest. Clients with severe arterial disease have feet pain while at rest, which keeps them awake at night. Venous insufficiency is associated with aching, cramping, and discomfort (Bright, Georgi, 1992).

Arterial insufficiency

- Do not elevate legs above the level of the heart.
  With arterial insufficiency, leg elevation decreases arterial blood supply to the legs.
- For early arterial insufficiency, encourage excercise such as walking or riding an exercise bicycle working up to 30 minutes per day.
  Exercise enhances the development of collateral circulation, strengthens muscles, and provides a sense of well-being (Cahall, Spency, 1995).
- Help keep clients warm, and have them wear socks and shoes or sheepskin-lined slippers when mobile. Do not apply heat.
  Clients with arterial insufficiency complain of being constantly cold; therefore keep extremities warm to maintain vasodilation and blood supply. Heat application can easily damage ischemic tissues (Creamer-Bauer, 1992).
- Pay meticulous attention to foot care. Refer to podiatrist if client has a foot or nail abnormality.
  Ischemic feet are very vulnerable to injury; careful foot care can prevent further injury.
- If client has ischemic arterial ulcers, see **Impaired tissue integrity,** but use occlusive dressings with caution.
  Occlusive dressings should be used with caution in clients with arterial ulceration because of the increased risk for cellulitis (Cahall, Spence, 1995).

Venous insufficiency

- Elevate edematous legs as ordered and ensure that there is no pressure under the knee, which decreases venous circulation.
  Elevation increases venous return and helps decrease edema.
- Apply support hose as ordered.
  Support hose help decrease edema. Studies have demonstrated that thigh-high compression stockings can be effective in decreasing the incidence of deep vein thrombosis (Brock, 1994).
- Encourage client to walk with support hose on and perform toe up and point flex exercises.
  Exercise helps increase venous return, build up collateral circulation, and strengthen the calf muscle pumps (Cahall, Spence, 1995).
- Observe for signs of deep vein thrombosis of pain, tenderness, swelling in the calf and thigh, redness in the involved extremity. Take serial leg measurements of the thigh and leg circumferences. In some clients there is a palpable, tender venous cord that can be felt in the popliteal fossa. Do not rely on Homan's sign.

Thrombosis with clot formation is usually first detected as swelling of the involved leg and then as pain. Leg measurement discrepancies greater than 2 cm warrant further investigation. Homan's sign is not reliable (Herzog, 1992). Unfortunately symptoms of already-developed deep vein thrombosis will not be found in 25% of the clients' exams (Eftychiou, 1996).

Geriatric
* Change positions slowly when getting client out of bed.
The elderly have increased postural hypotension resulting from age-related losses of cardiovascular reflexes.

Home Care Interventions

* Differentiate between arterial and venous insufficiency
Accurate diagnostic information clarifies clinical assessment and allows for more effective teaching.
* Assess client knowledge of the underlying disease process. Teach as necessary.
* Assess client nutritional status, paying special attention to obesity and malnutrition.
Malnutrition contributes to anemia, which further compounds the lack of oxygenation to tissues. Obese patients encounter poor circulation in adipose tissue, which can create increased hypoxia in tissue (Rolstad, 1990).
* Assess for symptoms of cellulitis.
Cellulitis often accompanies peripheral vascular disease and is related to poor tissue perfusion (Marrelli, 1994).

Client/Family Teaching

* Explain importance of good foot care. Recommend that diabetic client wear padded socks, special insoles, and jogging shoes.
Cushioned footwear can decrease pressure on feet, decrease callus formation, and save the feet (George, 1993).
* Stress importance of not smoking, following a weight loss program (if client is obese), carefully controlling diabetic condition, controlling hyperlipidemia and hypertension, and reducing stress.
All of these risk factors for atherosclerosis can be modified (Bright, Georgi, 1992).
* Teach client to avoid exposure to cold, limit exposure to brief periods if going out in cold weather, and wear warm clothing.
* Teach to recognize the signs and symptoms that need to be reported to a physician (e.g., change in skin temperature, color, or sensation).
NOTE: If client is receiving anticoagulant therapy, see **Altered protection.**

REFERENCES   Black SB: Venous stasis ulcers: a review, *Ostomy Wound Manage* 41:20, 1995.
Bright LD, Georgi S: Peripheral vascular disease, is it arterial or venous? *Am J Nurs* 92:34, 1992.
Brock JD: Compression stockings: do they prevent DVT? *Am J Nurs* 11:25, 1994.
Cahall E, Spence RK: Practical nursing measures for vascular compromise in the lower leg, *Ostomy Wound Manage* 41:16, 1995.
Creamer-Bauer C: Tissue perfusion, altered peripheral. In Gettrust KV, Brabec PD, editors: *Nursing diagnosis in clinical practice: guidelines for planning care,* Albany, NY, 1992, Delmar.
Eftychiou V: Clinical diagnosis and management of the patient with deep venous thromboembolism and acute pulmonary embolism, *Nurse Practitioner* 21:50, 1996.
George NE: Give 'em the old soft shoe: working smart, *Am J Nurs* 93:16, 1993.
Harris AH, Brown-Etris M, Troyer-Caudle J: Managing vascular leg ulcers, *Am J Nurs* 1:38, 1996.
Herzog JA: Deep vein thrombosis in the rehabilitation client, *Rehab Nurs* 17:196, 1992.
Marrelli TM: *Handbook of home health standards and documentation guidelines for reimbursement,* ed 2, St Louis, 1994, Mosby.
Rolstad BS: Treatment objectives in chronic wound care, *Home Healthcare Nurse* 9:6, 1990.

Risk for trauma

Gail B. Ladwig

Definition   Accentuated risk of accidental tissue injury (e.g., wound, burn, fracture)

Risk Factors
Internal (individual)

Weakness, balancing difficulties, reduced temperature or tactile sensation, reduced large- or small-muscle coordination, reduced hand-eye coordination, lack of safety education, lack of safety precautions, insufficient finances to purchase safety equipment or do repairs, cognitive or emotional difficulties, history of previous trauma

External (environmental)

Slippery floors (e.g., wet or highly-waxed); snow or ice collected on stairs or walkways; unanchored rugs; bathtub without hand grips or antislip equipment; unsteady ladders or unanchored electrical wires; litter or liquid spills on floors or stairways; high beds; children playing without gates at the top of the stairs; obstructed passageways; unsafe window protection in homes with young children; inappropriate call-for-aid mechanisms for client on bedrest; pot handles facing toward front of stove; very hot bath water (e.g., unsupervised bathing of young children); potentially ignitable gas leaks; delayed lighting of gas burner or oven; experimentation with chemicals or gasoline; unscreened fires or heaters; plastic aprons or flowing clothes around an open flame; children playing with matches, candles, or cigarettes; inadequately stored combustible items or corrosives (e.g., matches, oily rags, lye); contact with rapidly moving machinery, industrial belts, or pulleys; coarse bed linen; struggles within bed restraints; faulty electrical plugs, frayed wires, or defective appliances; contact with acids or alkalis; fireworks; radiotherapy; use of cracked dishware or glasses; knives stored uncovered; guns or ammunition stored unlocked; large icicles hanging from the roof; exposure to dangerous machinery; children playing with sharp-edged toys; high-crime neighborhood and vulnerable clients; driving a mechanically unsafe vehicle; driving under the influence of alcoholic beverages or drugs; driving at excessive speeds; driving without necessary visual aids; children riding in the front seat in car; smoking in bed or near oxygen; overloaded electrical outlets, grease waste collected on stoves; use of thin or worn potholders; misuse of necessary headgear for motorized cyclists; carrying young children on adult bicycles; unsafe road or road-crossing conditions; playing or working near vehicle pathways (e.g., driveways, laneways, railroad tracks); nonuse or misuse of seatbelts

Related Factors (r/t)

See Risk Factors

Client Outcomes/Goals

- Remains free from trauma
- Explains actions that can be taken to prevent trauma

Suggested NIC Interventions

Environmental management; safety, skin surveillance

Nursing Interventions and Rationales

- Provide vision aids for visually impaired clients.
  A client with a sensory loss must be protected from injury; therefore the visually impaired client must wear vision aids (Potter, Perry, 1993).
- Assist client with ambulation.
- Have family member evaluate water temperature for client.

A client with a tactile sensory impairment resulting from age or psychological or physiological factors needs to be protected from burns.

- Assess client for causes of impaired cognition.
Confusion from delirium and depression is reversible, but dementia is not reversible and has implications for long-term safety (Holt, 1993).
- Use reality orientation to improve client's cognition.
Focusing on what is real helps decrease clients' delusions and hallucinations and helps prevent them from acting out and injuring themselves.
- Make a social service referral for financial assistance.
- Teach safety measures to prevent trauma; ensure that client can read if using written materials.
Health care professionals have a legal and ethical obligation to provide clients with self-care instructions they can understand (Wong, 1992).
- Keep walkways clear of snow, debris, and household items.
Such measures prevent trauma from falls.
- Provide assistive devices in bathrooms (e.g., handrails, nonslip decals on floor of shower and bathtub).
These measures also prevent trauma from falls (Whirret, Wooldridge, 1992).
- Ensure that call-light systems are functioning and that client is able to use them.
Hospital injuries often result from a client's attempt to get out of bed and use the bathroom when caregiver cannot be contacted.
- Never leave young children unsupervised around water or cooking areas.
Young children are at risk for drowning even in small amounts of water. Heat and fire from cooking are a hazard to young children.
- Keep flammable and potentially flammable articles out of the reach of young children.
- Lock up harmful objects such as guns.
Accidental discharge of guns is a major cause of trauma.
- Teach to observe safety in high-crime neighborhoods (e.g., lock doors, do not leave home at night without a companion, keep entry ways well lit).
Adequate lighting helps protect the home and its inhabitants from crime (Potter, Perry, 1993).
- Instruct clients not to drive under the influence of alcohol or drugs. Assess for problems and refer to appropriate resources regarding drug and alcohol education.
A well-supported relationship exists between alcohol consumption and traumatic deaths from falls, fires, burns, and motor vehicle crashes.
- See nursing interventions and rationales for **Risk for injury, Impaired home maintenance management, Risk for poisoning, Risk for aspiration, and Risk for suffocation.**

Geriatric
- Perform a home safety assessment and recommend following preventions: keep electrical cords out of flow of traffic; remove small rugs or make sure they are slip resistant; increase lighting in hallways and other dark areas; place a light in bathroom; keep towels, curtains, and other things that might catch fire away from stove; store harmful products away from food products; provide at least one grab bar in tubs and showers; check prescribed medications for appropriate labels; store medications in original containers or in a dispenser of some type (i.e., egg carton, seven-day plastic dispenser); if the client cannot administer medications according to directions, secure someone to administer medications.

Injuries and accidents are among the major causes of death and chronic debilitation for older adults. The listed interventions are recommended (Whirret, Wooldridge, 1992).

- Mark stove knobs with bright colors; outline step borders.
  Easily visible markings are helpful for clients with decreased depth perception (Potter, Perry, 1993).
- Discourage driving at night.
  A decline in depth perception, slower recovery from glare, and night blindness are common in the elderly and make night driving a difficult and unsafe task (Ringsven, Bond, 1991).
- Encourage family members to reminisce with agitated clients.
  Agitation was the second most common behavior among 1000 residents sampled in 42 skilled nursing homes. Agitated individuals are prone to injury. Reminiscence by a special family member was the only intervention that effectively calmed severely agitated clients observed over a 24-hour period (Woods, Ashley, 1995).

Client/Family Teaching

- Educate family regarding age-appropriate child safety, environmental safety precautions, and intervening in an emergency.
- Teach family to assess day care center's or babysitter's knowledge regarding child safety, environmental safety precautions, and assisting a child in an emergency.
- Discuss various ways an adolescent can protect self from trauma while maintaining peer relationships.
- See **Risk for poisoning, Risk for aspiration, Risk for suffocation, Risk for injury, and Impaired home maintenance management.**

REFERENCES   Holt J: How to help confused patients, *Am J Nurs* 93:32, 1993.
Potter A, Perry A: *Fundamentals of nursing: concepts, process & practice,* St Louis, 1993, Mosby.
Ringsven M, Bond D: *Gerontology and leadership skills for nurses,* Albany, NY, 1991, Delmar.
Whirret T, Wooldridge P: Home safety & older adults, *Caring Magazine* 56, Dec 1992.
Wong M: Self-care instructions: do patients understand educational materials? *Focus Crit Care* 19:47, 1992.
Woods P, Ashley J: Simulated presence therapy: using selected memories to manage problem behaviors in Alzheimer's disease patients, *Geriatr Nurs* 16:9, 1995.

Unilateral neglect

Leslie Kalbach and Betty J. Ackley

Definition   The state in which an individual is perceptually unaware of and inattentive to one side of the body

Defining Characteristics

Major   Consistent inattention to stimuli on an affected side

Minor   Inadequate self-care, positioning or safety precautions in regard to affected side, failure to look toward affected side, food left on plate on affected side

Related Factors (r/t)

Effects of disturbed perceptual abilities (e.g., hemianopia, one-sided blindness, neurological illness, trauma)

NOTE: Because the right hemisphere is dominant in directing attention, unilateral neglect is more common if neurological pathology occurs in the right hemisphere of the brain, which results in left-sided neglect. Also unilateral neglect frequently occurs with parietal lesions (Herman, 1992; Kalbach, 1991).

Client Outcomes/Goals

- Demonstrates techniques that can be used to minimize unilateral neglect
- Cares for both sides of the body appropriately and keeps affected side free from harm

Suggested NIC Interventions

Unilateral neglect management

Nursing Interventions and Rationales

- Monitor client for signs of unilateral neglect (e.g., not washing, shaving, or dressing one side of the body; sitting or lying inappropriately on affected arm or leg; failing to respond to stimuli on the contralateral side of lesion; eating food on only one side of plate; or failing to look to one side of the body).
  Looking, listening, touching, and searching deficits occur on the affected side of the body and may or may not be associated with a loss of vision, sensation, or motion on the affected side (Kalbach, 1991; Herman, 1992).
- If available, use the "star cancellation test" to evaluate presence of unilateral neglect.
  The star cancellation test consists of a series of big and little stars and words scattered on a page. When directed to cross out all the little stars, clients with unilateral neglect will miss stars on one side of the paper (Halligan, Marshall, Wade, 1987; Taylor, Ashburn, Ward, 1994).
- Provide a safe, well-lit, and clutter-free environment. Place call light on unaffected side. Keep siderails up when client is in bed. Cue client to environmental hazards when mobile.
  Cognitive impairment may accompany neglect, so safety is of paramount importance.
- Nursing interventions for clients with unilateral neglect should be implemented in the following stages as client progresses:

Stage I—Focus attention mainly on nonneglected side.
  - Set up environment so that most activity is on unaffected side.
  - Keep client's personal items within view and on unaffected side.
  - Position client's bed so that activity is on unaffected side.
    The initial priority is client safety (Kalbach, 1991).

Stage II—Help client develop an awareness of neglected side.
  - Gradually focus client's attention on affected side.
  - Gradually move personal items and activity to affected side.
  - Stand on client's affected side when assisting with ambulation or activities of daily living.
    The goal is now for the client to develop an awareness of the neglected side (Kalbach, 1991).

Stage III—Help client develop ability to compensate for neglect.
  - Encourage client to bathe and groom affected side first.
  - Focus touch and talking on affected side; use a positive approach (e.g., "Mary, turn your head to the left and you'll see your grandchildren" [Carnevali, Patrick, 1993]).
  - Use constant and positive reminders to keep client scanning entire environment.
  - Use bright yellow or red stickers on outer margins in reading or writing exercises. Have client look for the sticker before reading or writing.
    Use cues and anchors to promote attention to the neglected side and help the client develop compensatory mechanisms to deal with the neglect syndrome (Kalbach, 1991; Cooke, 1992; Riddoch, Humphreys, Bateman, 1983).

- Refer to a rehabilitation nurse specialist, neuropsychologist, or occupational therapist for continued help in dealing with unilateral neglect. Include visual stimuli and eye-patching techniques.
  Monocular patching with lateralized visual stimulation may significantly reduce neglect in daily activities (Butter, Kirsch, 1992); The neuropsychologist can be helpful to ameliorate symptoms of unilateral neglect (Riddoch et al, 1995).

Home Care Interventions

Several of the listed interventions may be adapted for use in the home care setting.

Client/Family Teaching

- Explain pathology and symptoms of unilateral neglect.
- Teach client how to scan regularly to check the position of body parts and to regularly turn head from side to side for safety when ambulating.
- Teach caregivers positive cueing (reminders to help client remember to interact with entire environment).

REFERENCES   Butter CM, Kirsch N: Combined and separate effects of eye patching and visual stimulation on unilateral neglect following stroke, *Arch Phys Med Rehab* 73:1133, 1992.
Carnevali DL, Parick M: *Nursing management for the elderly,* ed 3, Philadelphia, 1993, JB Lippincott.
Cooke D: Remediation of unilateral neglect: what do we know? *Aust Occ Th J* 39:19, 1992,
Halligan PW, Marshall JC, Wade DT: Visuospatial neglect: underlying factors and test sensitivity, *Lancet* ii(8668):908, 1989.
Herman EW: Spatial neglect: new issues and their implications for occupational therapy practice, *Am J Occup Ther* 46:207, 1992.
Kalbach LR: Unilateral neglect: mechanisms and nursing care, *J Neurosci Nurs* 23:125, 1991.
Riddoch MF, Humphreys GW: The effect of cueing on unilateral neglect, *Neuropsychologist* 21:589, 1983.
Riddoch MF, Humphreys GW, Bateman A: Cognitive deficits following stroke, *Physiotherapy* 81:465, 1995.
Taylor D, Ashburn A, Ward CD: Asymmetrical trunk posture, unilateral neglect and motor performance following stroke, *Clin Rehab* 8:48, 1994.

Altered urinary elimination

Mikel Gray

Definition   The state in which an individual experiences a disturbance in urine elimination
NOTE: This is a broad diagnosis covering many dysfunctional voiding conditions. See **Functional incontinence, Reflex incontinence, Stress incontinence, Total incontinence, Urge Incontinence,** and **Urinary retention** for information on these more specific diagnoses.

Defining Characteristics

Irritative voiding symptoms: dysuria, diurnal urinary frequency, nocturia, urgency; incontinence: urine loss with exertion (stress incontinence), urine loss with hyperactive detrusor contractions (urge or reflex incontinence), urine loss from extraurethral source or continuous leakage (total incontinence), or urine loss because of inability to gain toilet access or cognitive issues (functional incontinence); urinary retention: obstructive symptoms including poor stream force, intermittent urine flow, postvoid dribbling, feelings of incomplete bladder evacuation; acute urinary retention: sudden incomplete inability to urinate

Related Factors (r/t)

Irritative voiding symptoms: urinary infection, inflammatory lesions of the bladder or urethra, urge incontinence, low bladder wall compliance; incontinence (see specific diagnosis); urinary retention (see specific diagnosis); acute urinary retention (see **Urinary retention**)

Client Outcomes/Goals

- Maintains diurnal frequency of no more than every 2 hours
- Maintains nocturia frequency of no more than 1 time per night (adults less than 70 years of age) and no more than twice per night (clients older than 70 years of age)
- Postpones voiding until toileting facility is accessed, clothing removed
- Maintains postvoiding residual volumes less than 100 ml or 25% of total bladder capacity
- Remains free of pain during bladder filling and when urinating

Suggested NIC Interventions

Urinary elimination management

Nursing Interventions and Rationales

- Assess bladder function using the following:
  - Focused history including duration of altered urine elimination symptoms, characteristics of symptoms, patterns of diurnal and nocturnal urination patterns, frequency and volume of urine loss, alleviating and aggravating factors, and exploration of possible causative factors
  - Focused physical assessment of perineal skin integrity, vaginal vault and evaluation of urethral hypermobility, neurological evaluation including bulbocavernosus reflex and perineal sensations
  - Review results of urinalysis for presence of urinary infection, polyuria, hematuria, proteinuria, and other abnormalities (or obtain urine for analysis)

  A history, focused physical assessment, and urinalysis comprise the basic, essential components of evaluation for any patient with dysfunctional voiding complaints (Urinary Incontinence Guideline Panel, 1996; Karlowicz, 1995).
- Complete a more detailed assessment on selected patients including a bladder log and functional/cognitive assessment (see **Functional incontinence, Reflex incontinence, Stress incontinence, Total incontinence,** and **Urge incontinence**).
- Assess client for urinary retention (see **Urinary retention**).
- Teach client general guidelines for bladder health:
  - Avoid dehydration and its irritative effects on the bladder. Fluid consumption should be 30 ml/kg of body weight (National Academy of Sciences, Food and Nutrition Board, 1980).
  - Clients with irritative voiding symptoms should reduce or eliminate bladder irritants including caffeine, aspartame, carbonated beverages, and alcohol from diet. (Intake of citrus juices, all coffee or tea, and chocolates may be reduced or eliminated if clients have severe symptoms of interstitial cystitis.)
  - Avoid constipation by adequate consumption of dietary fluids and fiber, exercise, and regular bowel elimination patterns.
  - Avoid or stop smoking.

    Dehydration increases irritative voiding symptoms and may enhance the risk of urinary infection. Constipation predisposes the individual to urinary retention and increases the risk of urinary infection. Smoking may increase the severity or risk of stress incontinence and is clearly linked with an increased risk for bladder cancer (Pearson, Larson, 1992; Karlowicz, 1995).
- Consult physician for culture and sensitivity testing and antibiotic treatment in clients with evidence of a urinary infection.

Urinary tract infections are transient, reversible conditions that frequently lead to irritative voiding symptoms and urge incontinence in susceptible persons (Urinary Incontinence Guideline Panel, 1996).

- Refer clients with irritative symptoms, chronic, burning bladder, and urethral pain to a urologist or specialist in the management of pelvic pain.
  Bladder pain and irritative voiding symptoms in the absence of an acute urinary infection may indicate the presence of interstitial cystitis, a chronic condition requiring ongoing treatment (Gillenwater, Wein, 1987).
- Teach client to recognize symptoms (dysuria, cloudy, odorous urine, suprapubic discomfort, with or without fever) and manage a urinary tract infection.
- Teach client to recognize and seek help promptly should hematuria occur.
  Hematuria in the presence of irritative voiding symptoms typically indicates urinary tract infection; however, gross painless hematuria (and bleeding with irritative symptoms) may indicate a bladder cancer (Gray, 1992).
- Assist the individual with urinary leakage to select a product that adequately contains urine, avoids soiling clothing, is not apparent when worn under clothing, and protects the underlying skin (see **Total incontinence).**
- Teach perineal care, including judicious use of soaps and use of vaginal douches only in special circumstances.
  Fastidious organisms of the vaginal, rectal, and perineal area may promote dysuria and frequency or may lead to a clinically significant urinary tract infection (Maskell, 1986).

Geriatric
- Provide an environment that encourages toileting for elderly clients cared for in home and in acute care, long-term care, or critical care units.
  Insufficient toileting opportunities, medications, acute or chronic illnesses, and other environmental factors may contribute to functional incontinence or exacerbate other forms of urinary leakage in elderly clients (Jirovec, Wells, 1990; Morris, Browne, Saltmarche, 1992; Gray, Burns, 1996).
- Perform urinalysis on all elderly clients who have a sudden change in urine elimination patterns, lower abdominal discomfort, acute confusion, or a fever of unclear origin.
  The common symptoms of a urinary infection, particularly dysuria and suprapubic discomfort, are frequently not apparent in elderly clients (Urinary Incontinence Guideline Panel, 1996).
- Encourage elderly women to drink at least 10 oz of cranberry juice daily.
  Cranberry juice has been reported to exert a bacteriostatic effect on Escherichia coli, *the most common pathogen associated with urinary infection among community dwelling adult women (Avorn et al, 1994).*

Home Care Interventions
- If client is using a Foley or suprapubic catheter, teach catheter hygiene.
  Good catheter hygiene techniques decrease the risk of infection.
- For clients with spinal cord injuries and with physician orders, instruct clients to follow a urinary elimination program similar to the following:
  - Maintain fluid intake of up to 125 ml/hr when awake. Do not exceed recommended intake.
    Maintaining fluid intake flushes the urinary system. Higher intake than noted increases the risk for related urinary tract problems in clients with spinal cord injuries (Hammond et al, 1989).

- Empty bladder routinely.

  Regular emptying of the bladder prevents urine pooling and increases the ability of bladder cells to resist infection.

- If catheterizing clients, use clean technique.

  Catheterizations provide a portal of entry for bacteria. Using clean technique reduces the risk for infections.

- Take urinary tract medications at times they are prescribed (Hammond et al, 1989).

  Medications may be ordered at specified intervals to keep urine acidic or maintain an antibiotic blood level that will decrease infection (Hammond et al, 1989).

Client/Family Teaching

- Provide all clients with the basic principles for optimal bladder function.
- Teach health care providers and community that urinary incontinence is not a normal part of aging and can be corrected or managed with proper evaluation and care.
- Provide information to health care providers and community about signs, symptoms and management of urinary tract infections and interstitial cystitis.
- Teach client and family signs and symptoms of urinary tract infection and its management.
- Teach client and family to recognize hematuria and promptly seek care should this symptom occur.

REFERENCES

Avorn J et al: Reduction of bacteriuria and pyuria after ingestion of cranberry juice, *JAMA* 271:751, 1994.

Gillenwater JY, Wein AJ: Summary of the National Institute of Arthritis, Diabetes, Digestive and Kidney Diseases workshop on interstitial cystitits, *J Urol* 140:203, 1987.

Gray ML: *Genitourinary disorders,* St Louis, 1992, Mosby.

Gray ML, Bruns SB: Continence management, *Crit Care Clin North Am* 8:29, 1996.

Hammond Margaret et al, editors: *Yes you can. A guide to self care for persons with spinal cord injury,* 1989, Paralyzed Veterans of America.

Jirovec MM, Wells TJ: Urinary incontinence in nursing home residents with dementia: the mobility-cognition paradigm, *Appl Nurs Res* 3:11, 1990.

Karlowicz KA, editor: *Urologic nursing: principles and practice,* Philadelphia, 1995, WB Saunders.

Maskell R: Are fastidious organisms an importance cause of dysuria and frequency? The care for. In Asscher AW, Brumfitt W, editors: *Microbial diseases in nephrology,* London, 1986, John Wiley & Sons.

Morris A, Browne G, Saltmarche A: Urinary incontinence among cognitively impaired elderly veterans, *J Gerontol Nurs* 18:33, 1992.

Pearson BD, Larson J: Improving elders continence state, *Clin Nurs Res* 1:430, 1992.

Urinary Incontinence Guideline Panel, *Urinary incontinence in adults,* Clinical Practice Guideline, Rockville, Md, Agency for Health Care Policy and Research, ed 2, 1996.

Urinary retention

Mikel Gray

Definition

The state in which an individual experiences incomplete bladder evacuation

Defining Characteristics

Major

Measured urinary residual greater than 100 ml or 25% of total bladder capacity

Obstructive voiding symptoms: poor stream force, intermittency of stream, hesitancy of urination, postvoiding dribbling, feelings of incomplete bladder emptying

Minor   Irritative voiding symptoms: urgency to urinate, diurnal frequency of urination, nocturia
               Overflow incontinence (dribbling urine loss caused when intravesical pressure
               overwhelms the sphincter mechanism)

Related Factors

Bladder outlet obstruction: benign prostatic hyperplasia, prostate cancer, prostatitis, urethral
stricture, bladder neck dyssynergia, bladder neck contracture, detrusor striated sphincter
dyssynergia, obstructing cystocele or urethral distortion, urethral tumor, urethral polyp,
posterior urethral valves, postoperative complication; deficient detrusor contraction strength:
sacral level spinal lesions, cauda equina syndrome, peripheral polyneuropathies, herpes zoster
or simplex affecting sacral nerve roots, injury or extensive surgery causing denervation of
pelvic plexus, medication side effect, complication of illicit drug use, impaction of stool

Client Outcomes/Goals

- Completely and regularly eliminates urine from the bladder; maintains measured
  urinary residual volume of less than 100 ml or 25% of total bladder capacity (voided
  volume plus urinary residual volume)
- Corrects or relieves obstructive symptoms
- Corrects or alleviates irritative symptoms
- Remains free of upper urinary tract damage (renal function remains sufficient, absence
  of febrile urinary infections)

Suggested NIC Interventions

Urinary catheterization, urinary retention care

Nursing Interventions/Rationales

- Obtain a focused urinary history emphasizing character and duration of symptoms.
  Inquire about obstructive as well as irritative symptoms, complications including
  episodes of acute urinary retention, and aggravating and alleviating symptoms.
  *A focused nursing history provides clues to the likely etiology of retention and its
  management.*
- Question the client concerning specific risk factors for urinary retention including the
  following:
  - Neurological disorders affecting the sacral spinal cord
  - Metabolic disorders such as diabetes mellitus and related conditions associated with
    polyuria and peripheral polyneuropathies
  - Medications including antispasmodics/parasympatholytics, alpha adrenergics,
    antidepressants, sedatives, narcotics, psychotropic medications, illicit drugs
  - Bowel elimination patterns, predisposition toward impaction
  - Acute illness, acute loss of mobility
  *Urinary retention is related to multiple factors affecting either detrusor contraction
  strength or urethral (bladder outlet) flow resistance (Gray, 1992).*
- Perform a focused physical assessment (or review results of a recent physical)
  including perineal skin integrity; inspection, percussion, and palpation of the lower
  abdomen for obvious bladder distention; a neurological exmination including perineal
  skin sensation and the bulbocavernosus reflex; and a vaginal vault examination in
  women and a digital rectal examination in men.
  *The physical assessment provides clues to the likely etiology of urinary retention and
  its management.*
- Determine urinary residual volume by catheterizing the patient immediately after
  urination or by obtaining a bladder ultrasound following micturition.

Catheterization provides the most accurate method for determining urinary residual volume, but the procedure is invasive, carries a risk of infection, and may be uncomfortable for the patient. A bladder ultrasound is not as accurate as catheterization, nonetheless it is adequate for making clinical judgments and is noninvasive (Chan, 1993; Lewis, 1995).

- Complete a bladder log including patterns of urine elimination and urine loss (if present), nocturia, and volume and type of fluids consumed.
  The bladder log provides an objective verification of urine elimination patterns and allows comparison of fluids consumed versus urinary output over a 24-hour period (Gray, 1992).
- Consult with physician concerning eliminating or altering medications suspected of producing or exacerbating urinary retention.
  Medication side effects may cause or greatly exacerbate urinary retention in susceptible individuals (Urinary Incontinence Guideline Panel, 1996).
- Assess severity of retention and its impact on quality of life using a symptom score such as the American Urological Association (AUA) Prostate Symptom Score (BPH Guideline Panel, 1994).
  A symptom allows rating of the severity of obstructive and irritative symptoms, providing baseline assessment and evaluation of the efficacy of management.
- Teach clients with mild to moderate obstructive symptoms to double void by urinating, staying in the rest room for 3 to 5 minutes, and then making a second effort to urinate.
  Double voiding promotes more efficient bladder evacuation by allowing the detrusor to contract initially and then rest and contract again (Gray, 1992).
- Teach clients with urinary retention and infrequent voiding to urinate at scheduled times.
  Timed or scheduled voiding may reduce urinary retention by preventing bladder overdistension.
- Advise male clients with urinary retention related to benign prostatic hyperplasia to use the following guidelines for prevention of acute urinary retention:
  - Avoid taking over-the-counter cold remedies containing decongestants (alpha adrenergic agonists).
  - Avoid taking over-the-counter dietary medications (which frequently contain alpha adrenergic agonists)
  - Discuss voiding problems with a health care provider before beginning new prescription medications.
  - After prolonged exposure to cool weather, warm body before attempting to urinate.
  - Avoid overfilling bladder by establishing regular urination patterns and refraining from excessive intake of alcohol.
    These manageable factors predispose the patient to acute urinary retention by overdistending the bladder and compromising detrusor contraction strength or by increasing outlet resistance (Gray, 1992).
- Teach clients who are unable to void specific strategies to manage this potential medical emergency, including the following:
  - Drink a cup of hot tea or coffee.
  - Attempt to urinate in complete privacy.
  - Place feet solidly on floor.
  - If unable to avoid using previous strategies, take a warm sitz bath or shower and void (if possible) while still in tub or shower.
  - If unable to void within 6 hours or if bladder distention is producing significant pain, seek urgent or emergency care.

A warm cup of coffee or tea stimulates the bladder and may promote voiding. Attempting to urinate in complete privacy and placing the feet solidly on the floor help relax the pelvic muscles and encourage voiding. Warm water also stimulates the bladder and may produce voiding; the cooling experienced by leaving the tub or shower may again inhibit the bladder (Gray, 1992).

- Remove indwelling urethral catheter at midnight in the hospitalized patient to reduce the risk of acute urinary retention.
  Removal of indwelling catheters at night has several advantages over morning removal, including a larger initial voided volume.

- Consult physician about bladder stimulation in patient with urinary retention caused by deficient detrusor contraction strength.
  Electrical stimulation of the bladder neck has been reported to be beneficial among persons with urinary retention resulting from deficient detrusor contraction strength (Moore et al, 1993).

- Teach clients with significant urinary retention to perform self-intermittent catheterization as directed.
  Intermittent catheterization allows regular, complete bladder evacuation without serious complications (Horsley, Crane, Reynolds, 1982).

- Use indwelling catheters for clients with urinary retention who are not suitable candidates for intermittent catheterization.
  An indwelling catheter provides continuous drainage of urine; however, the risk of serious urinary complications with prolonged use is significant (Anson, Gray, 1993; Stickler, Zimakoff, 1994).

- Advise clients managed by indwelling catheters that bacteria in urine is an almost universal finding after catheters have remained in place for a period of weeks or months and that only symptomatic infections warrant treatment.
  The indwelling catheter is associated with frequent bacterial colonization. Most bacteriuria does not produce significant infection and attempts to eradicate it often produce subsequent morbidity because resistant bacteria are encouraged to reproduce while more easily managed strains are eradicated (Moore, Rayome, 1995; White, Ragland, 1995).

Geriatric

- Aggressively assess elderly patients, particularly those with dribbling urinary incontinence, urinary tract infections, and related conditions for urinary retention.
  Elderly clients may experience urine retention of 1500 ml or more with few or no apparent symptoms. A urinary residual volume and related assessments are necessary to determine the presence of retention in this population (Williams, Wallhagen, Dowling, 1993).

- Assess elderly clients for impaction when urinary retention is documented or suspected.
  Impaction is a reversible factor that is commonly associated with urine loss and retention among elderly persons (Urinary Incontinence Guideline Panel, 1996).

- Assess elderly males for retention related to benign prostatic hyperplasia or prostate cancer.
  The incidence of urinary retention related to benign prostatic hyperplasia and prostate cancer increase with age (BPH Guideline Panel, 1994).

Home Care Interventions

- If client is using a Foley or suprapubic catheter, teach client and/or caregivers catheter hygiene.
  Good catheter hygiene reduces the chance of infection and the need for extra recatheterizations resulting from obstruction.

- If client has a spinal cord injury, teach client to keep bladder pressure low.
  High bladder pressure places the client at risk for an irritable bladder, dyssynergia, automatic dysreflexia, and kidney damage (Hammond et al, 1989).

Client/Family Teaching

- Teach techniques for intermittent catheterization including use of clean rather than sterile technique, washing using soap and water or a microwave technique, and reuse of the catheter.
- Teach clients with an indwelling catheter to assess tube for patency, maintain drainage system below level of symphysis pubis, and routinely cleanse the bedside bag.
- Teach clients managed by an indwelling catheter or intermittent catheterization symptoms of a significant urinary infection including hematuria, acute onset incontinence, dysuria, flank pain, or fever.

REFERENCES   Anson C, Gray ML: Secondary complications after spinal cord injury, *Urologic Nurs* 13:107, 1993.

BPH Guideline Panel: *Benign prostatic hyperplasia: diagnosis and treatment,* Rockville, Md, 1994, Agency for Health Care Policy and Research.

Chan H: Noninvasive bladder volume measurement, *J Neurosci Nurs* 25:309, 1993.

Crowe H et al: Randomized study of the effect of midnight removal of urinary catheter, *Urol Nurs* 14:18, 1994.

Gray ML: *Genitourinary disorders,* St Louis, 1992, Mosby.

Hammond Margaret et al, editors: *Yes you can. A guide to self care for persons with spinal cord injury,* 1989, Paralyzed Veterans of America.

Horsley JA, Crane J, Reynolds MA: *Clean intermittent catheterization: conduct and utilization of research in nursing project,* New York, 1982, Grune & Stratton.

Karlowicz KA: *Urologic nursing: principles & practice,* Philadelphia, 1995, WB Saunders.

Lewis NA: Implementing a bladder ultrasound program, *Rehab Nurs* 20:215, 1995.

Maynard FM, Diokno AC: Urinary infection and complications during clean intermittent catheterization following spinal cord injury, *J Urol* 124:392, 1987.

Moore KN, Rayome RG: Problem solving and trouble shooting: the indwelling catheter, *J Wound Ostomy Cont Nurs* 22:242, 1995.

Stickler DJ, Zimakoff J: Complications of urinary tract infections associated with devices used for long term bladder management, *J Hospital Infection* 28:177, 1994.

Urinary Incontinence Guideline Panel: *Urinary incontinence in adults,* Clinical Practice Guideline, Rockville, Md, Agency for Health Care Policy and Research, ed 2, 1996.

White MC, Ragland KE: Urinary catheter—related infections among home care patients, *J Wound Ostomy Cont Nurs* 22:286, 1995.

Williams MP, Wallhagen M, Dowling G: Urinary retention in elderly hospitalized women, *J Gerontol Nurs* 19:7, 1993.

Inability to sustain spontaneous ventilation

Leslie Lysaght

Definition   The state in which a response pattern of decreased energy reserves results in an individual's inability to maintain breathing adequate for supporting life

Defining Characteristics

Major   Dyspnea, increased metabolic rate, increased heart rate, decreased Po_2, increased Pco_2

Minor   Increased restlessness, apprehension, increased use of accessory muscles, decreased tidal volume, decreased cooperation, decreased Sao_2

Related Factors (r/t)

Metabolic factors, respiratory muscle fatigue

Client Outcomes/Goals

- Maintains arterial blood gases within safe parameters
- Remains free of dyspnea or restlessness
- Effectively maintains airway
- Effectively mobilizes secretions

Suggested NIC Interventions

Artificial airway management, mechanical ventilation, respiratory monitoring, resuscitation: neonate, ventilation assistance

Nursing Interventions and Rationales

- Collaborate with client, family, and physician regarding plan and interventions. Ask whether client has advance directive or health care durable power of attorney and integrate those directives into plan of care in conjunction with clinical data regarding overall health and reversibility of medical condition (Campbell, Thill-Baharozian, 1994). *Many clients and their families make decisions about the level of therapy aggressiveness that they desire. Health care providers have a responsibility to allow the client to participate in care decisions.*
- Assess and respond to changes in client's respiratory status. Monitor client for dyspnea, including respiratory rate, use of accessory muscles, intercostal retractions, flaring of nostrils, and subjective complaints. *It is essential to monitor for these signs of impending respiratory failure (McCord, Cronin-Stubbs, 1992).*
- Administer indicated diuretics, analgesics, or antianxiety medications. Facilitate position of comfort, and titrate supplemental oxygen as needed (Grossbach, 1994). *Interventions to decrease heart workload, maintain comfort, minimize anxiety, or increase the available oxygen for gas exchange are necessary interventions in respiratory failure.*
- Recognize that confusion progressing to somnolence may be an ominous sign of respiratory failure with carbon dioxide narcosis.
- If client has unresolved dyspnea, deteriorating arterial blood gases, changes in level of consciousness, or panic, prepare client for intubation and placement on ventilator. *Immediate intervention is necessary for signs and symptoms of acute respiratory failure.*
- Explain intubation intervention to client and family as appropriate and administer sedation for client comfort during procedure per physician order (Kleiber et al, 1994).

Ventilator support

- Stabilize/tape endotracheal tube securely, auscultate breath sounds, and get a chest x-ray to confirm endotracheal tube placement (Kaplow, Bookbinder, 1994). *These interventions are necessary to maintain an adequate airway (Hudak, Gallo, 1992).*
- Suction as needed and hyperoxygenate and hyperventilate per policy. Do not routinely instill normal saline (Raymond, 1995). Note frequency, type, and amount of secretions. Communicate any changes to physician. *These steps ensure adequate oxygenation (Dam, Wild, Baun, 1994).*
- Prevent unplanned extubation by maintaining stability of endotracheal tube, suctioning as indicated, ensuring client comfort, and monitoring client ability to understand and follow directions. Consider relaxation and sedation interventions. Utilize mitts or wrist restraints if less aggressive interventions are inappropriate or unsuccessful (Grap, Glass, Lindamood, 1995). *Endotracheal tube placement must be maintained to ventilate the client.*

- Analyze and respond to arterial blood gas results.
  Ventilatory support must be closely monitored to ensure adequate oxygenation and acid-base balance.
- Support client and family involvement in and awareness of plan of care and treatment goals.
- Assist client in identification and use of an effective alternative communication method, such as using a letter board or paper and pencil or mouthing words.
  Alternative strategies of communication prevent isolation and loss (Menzel, 1994).
- Rotate endotracheal tube from side to side every 24 hours. Assess and document skin condition, and note tube placement at lip line. Provide oral care every 4 hours and prn.
  These steps prevent skin breakdown at the lip line that results from endotracheal tube pressure (Chang, 1995).
- Assess bilateral anterior and posterior breath sounds every 4 hours and prn; respond to any relevant changes.
- Monitor respiratory rate and identify ventilator-assisted and independent respiratory efforts.
  These methods evaluate the client's respiratory efforts.
- Assess tolerance to ventilatory assistance and monitor for dysynchronous chest movement, subjective complaints of breathlessness, and high-pressure alarms. Collaborate with interdisciplinary team in resolving problems with changes in ventilatory settings, sedation, analgesia, relaxation techniques, or neuromuscular blockers.
- Maintain integrity of respiratory circuit. Collaborate with respiratory therapist in response to ventilator alarms; if unable to rapidly locate source of alarm, ambu bag client while waiting for assistance. Common causes of a high-pressure alarm include client resistance or the need for suction. A common cause of a low-pressure alarm is ventilator disconnection.
  Bagging the client with an ambu bag connected to oxygen safely supports ventilation until the mechanical problem can be resolved. Ensure that the ambu bag is available, and maintain competence in its use.
- Collaborate with interdisciplinary team in treating and responding to cause of underlying acute respiratory failure.
  The mechanical ventilator is usually a temporary support until the underlying pathology can be effectively resolved.
- Implement appropriate interventions to maintain client comfort, mobility, nutrition, and skin integrity.
  These interventions prevent functional losses (Gift, Austin, 1992).

Home Care Interventions

- Assess home setting during the discharge process to ensure home can safely accommodate ventilator support (e.g., space, electricity).
- Have family contact the electrical company and place client residence on high risk list in case of power outage (Humphrey, 1994).
  Some home-based care requires special conditions for safe home administration.
- Assess the caregivers for commitment to support a ventilator-dependent client in the home.
  Commitment to care and valuing home as a healing place provide meaning for participating in caregiving and decrease caregiver role strain (Boland, Sims, 1996).
- Be sure that client and family/caregivers are familiar with operation of all ventilation devices and their schedules for cleaning.
  Some home-based care involves specialized technology and require specific skills for administration.

- Assess client and caregiver knowledge of disease and client needs and medications to be administered via ventilation assistive devices. Avoid analgesics. Assess knowledge of how to administer using equipment. Teach as necessary.
  Client receiving ventilation support may not be able to articulate needs. Respiratory medications can have side effects that change the client's respiration or level of consciousness.
- Establish an emergency plan and criteria for use. Identify emergency procedures to be used until medical assistance arrives. Teach and role play emergency care.
  A prepared emergency plan reassures the client and family and ensures client safety.

REFERENCES   Boland D, Sims S: Family caregiving at home as a solitary journey, *Image* 28:1, 1996, Spring.

Campbell M, Thill-Baharozian M: Impact of the DNR therapeutic plan on patient care requirements, *Am J Crit Care* 3:202, 1994.

Campbell R, Branson R: How ventilators provide temporary O_2 enrichment: what happens when you press the 100% suction button? *Respir Care* 37:933, 1992.

Chang V: Protocol for prevention of complications of endotracheal intubation, *Crit Care Nurs* 15:19, 1995.

Dam V, Wild C, Baun B: Effect of oxygen insufflation during endotracheal suctioning on arterial pressure and oxygenation of coronary artery bypass graft patients, *Am J Crit Care* 3:191, 1994.

Gift A, Austin D: The effects of a program of systematic movement of COPD patients, *Rehab Nurs* 17:6, 1992.

Grap M, Glass C, Lindamood M: Factors related to unplanned extubation of endotracheal tubes, *Crit Care Nurs* 15:57, 1995.

Grossbach I: The COPD patient in acute respiratory failure, *Crit Care Nurs* 14:32, 1994.

Hudak C, Gallo B: Management modalities: respiratory system. In *Critical care nursing: a holistic approach,* ed 6, Philadelphia, 1994, Mosby.

Humphrey C: *Home care nursing handbook,* ed 2, Md, 1994, Aspen.

Kaplow R, Bookbinder M: A comparison of four endotracheal tube holders, *Heart Lung* 23:59, 1994.

Kleiber C et al: Emotional responses of family members during a critical care hospitalization, *Am J Crit Care* 3:70, 1994.

McCord M, Cronin-Stubbs D: Operationalizing dyspnea, *Heart Lung* 21:167, 1992.

Menzel L: Need for communication-related research in mechanically ventilated patients, *Am J Crit Care* 3:165, 1994.

Raymond S: Normal saline instillation before suctioning: helpful or harmful? A review of the literature, *Am J Crit Care* 4:267, 1995.

Dysfunctional ventilatory weaning response (DVWR)

Leslie Lysaght

Definition   The state in which a client cannot adjust to lowered levels of mechanical ventilator support, which interrupts and prolongs the weaning process

Defining Characteristics
Mild DVWR

Major   Restlessness, respiratory rate slightly increased above baseline

Minor   Responds to lowered levels of mechanical ventilator support with expressed feelings of increased need for oxygen, breathing discomfort, fatigue, warmth, queries about possible machine malfunction, or an increased concentration on breathing

Moderate DVWR

Major   Responds to lowered levels of mechanical ventilator support with a slight increase above baseline blood pressure (< 20 mm Hg), a slight increase above baseline heart rate (< 20 beats/min), or a baseline increase in respiratory rate (< 5 breaths/min).

| Minor | Hypervigilence to activities, inability to respond to coaching, inability to cooperate, apprehension, diaphoresis, eye widening, decreased air entry on auscultation, color changes (e.g., pale complexion, slight cyanosis), slight respiratory accessory muscle use |

Severe DVWR

| Major | Agitated response to lowered levels of mechanical ventilator support, deterioration in arterial blood gases from current baseline, increase in blood pressure from baseline (> 20 mm Hg), significant increase in respiratory rate from baseline |
| Minor | Profuse diaphoresis, full respiratory accessory muscle use, shallow and gasping breaths, paradoxical abdominal breathing, discoordinated breathing with the ventilator, decreased level of consciousness, adventitious breath sounds, audible airway secretions, cyanosis |

Related Factors (r/t)

Physical	Ineffective airway clearance, sleep pattern disturbance, inadequate nutrition, uncontrolled pain or discomfort
Psychological	Knowledge deficit of the weaning process and patient role, perceived inefficacy about the ability to wean, decreased motivation, decreased self-esteem, moderate or severe anxiety, fear, hopelessness, powerlessness, insufficient trust in nurse
Situational	Uncontrolled episodic energy demands or problems, inappropriate pacing of diminished ventilator support, inadequate social support, adverse environment (e.g., noise, activity, negative events in the room), low nurse-client ratio, extended nurse absence from bedside, unfamiliar nursing staff, history of ventilator dependence (> 1 week); history of multiple unsuccessful weaning attempts

Client Outcomes/Goals

- Remains weaned from ventilator and maintains adequate arterial blood gases
- Maintains blood pressure, pulse, and respiration at baseline
- Remains free of unresolved dyspnea or restlessness
- Effectively clears secretions

Suggested NIC Interventions

Mechanical ventilation, mechanical ventilatory weaning

Nursing Interventions and Rationales

- While client is on ventilator, coach client to increase overall and respiratory muscle strengths. Coach client to strengthen respiratory muscles by differentiating between "independent" and ventilator breaths.
  Prevent functional losses by setting and maintaining realistic activity goals (Gift, Austin, 1992).
- Assess client's readiness for weaning evidenced by the following:
  - Adequate nutritional status with normal serum albumin levels (Grant, 1994)
  - Adequate rest and comfort
  - Resolution of initial medical problem that led to ventilator dependence
  - Stability of any chronic health problems
  - Absence of left ventricular failure
  - Absence of acute hemodynamic event in previous 3 days
  - Psychological readiness, alertness, stable vital signs
  - Adequate respiratory parameters with a negative inspiratory force > 20 cm
  - Ability to clear secretions
  - Fluid balance
  To ensure the best outcome, it is important that the client be in an optimal physiological and psychological state before introducing the stress weaning (Weilitz,

1993). Recognize that weaning is both an art and a science. Controlling for known factors that influence weaning success is essential.

- Identify any reasons for previous unsuccessful weaning attempts, and include that information in development of weaning plan.
  Analyzing client responses after each weaning attempt prevents repeatedly unsuccessful weanings.
- Promote rest and comfort throughout weaning period (comfortable room temperature, small electric fan if indicated, controlled noise level, comfortable positioning in bed or chair, visitors when desired).
  It is important that the client be comfortable during the weaning period.
- Assist client with identifying personal strategies that result in relaxation and comfort (e.g., music, visualization, relaxation techniques, reading, television, family visits). Support implementation of these strategies.
  Personal strategies for relaxation are effective (Gift, Moore, Soeken, 1992; Chlan, 1995).
- Support clients in setting weaning goals; maximize goal achievement within their capabilities.
  Goals promote client rehabilitation (Weaver, Narsagage, 1992).
- Help client identify the desired amount of information about or participation in the weaning plan; help client identify milestones of progress.
  Control of the situation allows clients to participate to their fullest interest and capability.
- Collaborate with an interdisciplinary team (physician, respiratory therapist, and nutritionist) to develop a weaning plan with timeline and goals; revise plan throughout weaning period.
  Effective interdisciplinary collaboration can positively impact patient outcomes (Boggs, 1992).
- Provide a safe and comfortable environment. Make call light button readily available and assure client that needs will be met responsively. Consider timing of other factors in client care environment and impact on ability to provide level of support client may need (e.g., staff off unit, other unit emergencies).
  A client who feels safe and trusts the health care providers can focus on the immediate work of weaning.
- Do not administer narcotics immediately prior to weaning; coordinate any pain management routine to effectively offer analgesia with minimal sedative effects.
- Schedule weaning periods for time of day that client is most rested. Cluster care activities to promote successful weaning. Avoid other procedures during weaning: keep environment quiet and promote restful activities between weaning periods.
  It is important that the client receives adequate rest between weaning periods. The intensive care unit can be a noisy, busy environment. Control of external noises and stimuli can promote restful periods (Cropp et al, 1994).
- Promote normal sleep-wake cycle, allowing uninterrupted periods of night time sleep (Edwards, Schuring, 1993).
- Limit visitors during weaning to close and supportive persons; have visitors leave if they are negatively affecting weaning process.
- During weaning, monitor clients physiological and psychological responses; acknowledge and respond to fears and subjective complaints.
- Monitor subjective and objective data (breath sounds, respiratory pattern, respiratory effort, heart rate, blood pressure, oxygen saturation per oximetry, amount and type of

secretions, anxiety, energy level) throughout weaning to determine client tolerance and responses.

Continued assessment and maintenance of airway clearance throughout weaning supports client comfort, safety, and trust (Carroll, Milkowski, 1996).

- Coach client through episodes of increased anxiety. Remain with client or place a supportive and calm significant other in this role. Give positive reinforcement, and with permission use touch to communicate support and concern.

  It is not unusual for a client with lung disease to experience self-limiting episodes of increased shortness of breath. Supporting and coaching a client through such episodes allows weaning to continue.

- Terminate weaning when client demonstrates predetermined criteria or when signs and symptoms of fatigue or intolerance appear as evidenced by a blood pressure increase or decrease of 20 mm Hg, a pulse rate increase or decrease of 20 beats/min, respirations rate of greater than 25 breaths/min or less than 8 breaths/min, dysrhythmias (especially premature ventricular contractions), decreased oxygen saturation levels, panic, dyspnea, use of accessory muscles, intercostal retraction, flaring of nostrils, changes in level of consciousness, or a subjective inability to continue).

  Immediate response to and intervention in weaning intolerance limits client fatigue and discomfort and promotes the ability for later success.

- If dysfunctional weaning response is severe, consider slowing down weaning to brief increments of time (e.g., 5 minutes). Continue to collaborate with team to determine if an untreated physiological cause for dysfunctional weaning pattern (e.g., diaphragmatic impairment) remains.

- Consider an alternative care setting (subacute, rehabilitation facility, home) for clients with prolonged ventilator dependence as a strategy that can positively affect outcomes (Rudy et al, 1995).

Home Care Interventions

NOTE: Weaning from a ventilator at home should be based on client stability and comfort of client and caregivers under an intermittent care plan. Client and/or family may be more comfortable having client rehospitalized for the process.

- Assess comfort and coping ability of client and/or family to wean at home.

  Compromises in respiratory function are frightening for clients and family who perceive the availability of a high-technology, structured environment as a more appropriate environment for weaning.

- Establish an emergency plan and methods of implementation. Include emergency aeration and reestablishment of the ventilation assistive device.

  Having a prepared emergency plan reassures the client and family and provides for client safety.

- Obtain orders for alternate routes of medication administration when medications have been administered via ventilation device. Instruct client and family in changes.

REFERENCES   Baggs J et al: The association between interdisciplinary collaboration and patient outcomes in a medical intensive care unit, *Heart Lung* 21:18, 1992.

Carroll P, Milikowski K: Getting your patient off a ventilator, *RN* June 1996, p. 42.

Chlan L: Psychophysiologic responses of mechanically ventilated patients to music; a pilot study, *Am J Crit Care* 4:233, 1995.

Clochesy J, Daly B, Monenegro H: Weaning chronically critically ill adults from mechanical ventilatory support, *Am J Crit Care* 4:93, 1995.

Cropp A et al: Name that tone: the proliferation of noise in the intensive care unit, *Chest* 105:1217, 1994.

Edward G, Schuring L: Sleep protocol: a research based practice change, *Crit Care Nurse* 13:84, 1993.

Gift A, Austin D: The effects of a program of systemic movement of COPD patients, *Rehab Nurs* 17:6, 1992.

Gift A, Moore T, Soeken K: Relaxation to reduce dyspnea and anxiety in COPD patients, *Nurs Res* 41:242, 1992.

Grant J: Nutrition care of patients with acute and chronic respiratory failure, *Nutr Clin Prac* 9:11, 1994.

Rudy E et al: Patient outcomes for the chronically critically ill: special care unit vs ICU, *Am J Crit Care* 44:324, 1995.

Weaver T, Narsagage G: Physiological and psychological variables related to functional status in chronic obstructive pulmonary disease, *Nurs Res* 41:286, 1992.

Weilitz P: Weaning a patient from mechanical ventilation, *Crit Care Nurse* 13:33, 1993.

Risk for violence: self-directed or directed at others

Judith S. Rizzo

Definition   The state in which an individual experiences behaviors that can be physically harmful either to the self or others

Risk Factors

Major   Body language (e.g., clenched fists, tense facial expression, rigid posture, tautness indicating effort to control); hostile or threatening verbalizations (e.g., boasting of or prior abuse of others); increased motor activity (e.g., pacing, excitement, irritability, agitation); overt and aggressive acts (e.g., goal-directed destruction of objects in environment); possession of destructive objects (e.g., gun, knife, weapon); rage; self-destructive behavior; active aggressive suicidal acts; suspicion of others; paranoid ideations, delusions, or hallucinations; substance abuse or withdrawal (e.g., verbalized warnings of losing control, increased perspiration, dilated or constricted pupils)

Minor   Increased anxiety levels, fear of self or others, inability to verbalize feelings, repetition of verbalizations (e.g., continued complaints, requests, and demands), anger, provocative behavior (e.g., argumentative, dissatisfied, overreactive, hypersensitive), vulnerable self-esteem, depression (specifically active, aggressive, or suicidal acts), inability to see other options, poor impulse control, low frustration tolerance, poor coping skills

Related Factors (r/t)

Antisocial character, battered woman, catatonic excitement, child abuse, manic excitement, organic brain syndrome, panic states, rage reactions, suicidal behavior, temporal lobe epilepsy, toxic reactions to medications, personality disorder, dyscontrol syndrome

Client Outcomes/Goals

- Does not harm self or others
- Maintains relaxed body language and decreased motor activity
- Displays no aggressive activity
- Demonstrates control or states feelings of control
- Expresses decreased anxiety and control of hallucinations
- Talks about feelings; expresses anger appropriately
- Obtains no access to harmful objects
- Displaces anger to meaningful activities
- Yields access to harmful objects

Suggested NIC Interventions

Environmental management: violence prevention

Nursing Interventions and Rationales

Violence toward others

- Assess for behaviors that indicate impending violence against self or others.
  Knowing, recognizing, and promptly intervening in early precipitating factors prevent violence (Burgess, 1994).
- Attend to early signs of dangerous interactions with clients, respect boundaries, and talk with colleagues about difficult, uncomfortable situations (Vincent, 1994).
  Early and appropriate interventions are important to prevent violence. Early signs are destruction of objects, thoughts of violence, and aggressive behavior (Vincent, 1994). Behavioral warning signs, such as verbal and physical threats, boisterousness, and attacking objects precede violence (Linaker, Bush-Iversen, 1995). Take verbal threats seriously and report them (Linaker, Bush-Iversen, 1995).
- Allow and encourage client to verbalize anger either one-on-one or in a group setting.
  Anger is treatable by short-term, cost-effective, structured group programs (Deffenbacher et al, 1994).
- Teach healthy ways to express anger.
  "Talking replaces action." Talking about anger displaces it and prevents the client from acting on it. Harness anger and use it constructively.
- Help client identify when anger develops. Have client keep an anger diary and discuss alternative responses together.
  Creative coping skills and behavioral techniques are helpful for teaching the client (Linaker, Bush-Iversen, 1995).
- Identify stimuli that initiate violence.
  Studies found that violence was more apt to take place on inpatient units at shift change, in crowded hallways, at medicine time, and in seclusion rooms during transitional activity time. It occurred less often off the unit in offices when escorted (Holbert, 1995).
- Maintain a calm attitude.
  Anxiety is contagious.
- Provide a low level of stimuli in client's environment; place client in a quiet, safe place, and speak slowly and quietly.
  A safe, quiet environment decreases the outside stimuli that may be precipitating violent behavior.
- Redirect possible violent behaviors into physical activities if client is physically able (e.g., punching bags, hitting pillows, walking, jogging).
- Provide sufficient staff if a show of force is necessary to demonstrate control to client.
  When others respond to an escalating or violent situation, it can reassure clients that they will not be allowed to lose control. On the other hand, leave immediately if client becomes violent and you are not trained to handle it.
- Use chemical restraints as ordered. Obtain an order for medication and administer immediately.
  Medications should be offered before restraints or seclusion is considered; the medications used most often are haloperidol (Haldol) and lorazepam (Ativan).
- Use mechanical restraints if ordered and as necessary.
  Physical restraint of children can be therapeutic (Morales, Duphorne, 1995). Clients

externalize why restraining occurred; "beyond my control." Most can verbalize the reason why they were restrained (Outlaw, Lowery, 1994).

- Follow institution's protocol for releasing restraints. Observe client closely, remain calm, and provide positive feedback as client's behavior becomes controlled.
- Know and follow institution's policies and procedures concerning violence.
  Being familiar with and following policies and procedures of the department prevents violence. Policies should be developed and training programs provided in proper use and application of restraints (Daum, 1994).
- Protect other clients in the environment from harm. Follow safety protocols of the department.
  Proper preparation, training, and implementation of strict protocols can save nurse's and others' lives when violence occurs (Burgess, 1994). Others can be injured during a violent outburst, so their safety must be considered.
- Always follow up a violent episode with a debriefing of clients and staff.
  Debriefing afterward will not only evaluate staff effectiveness but will minimize emotional trauma (Poggenpoel, 1995). Nurses can interact with clients experiencing violence by conducting group or individual debriefing (Poggenpoel, 1995). It is good to use staff inservicing and debriefing following violence (Morrison, 1989).

Violence toward self

- Monitor and document client's potential for suicide.
  Traits such as impulsivity, poor social adjustment, and mood disorders are associated with adolescent suicide attempts (Brent et al, 1994).
- Monitor suicidal behaviors or verbalizations (e.g., giving away possessions, stating "I'm going to kill myself" or "My parents won't have to worry about having me around anymore").
  Take verbalizations of suicide seriously until assessment and intervention prove otherwise.
- Monitor seriousness of intent; ask client, "Do you have a plan?" "How will you do it?" and "Do you have the means?"
  Always use a planned intervention model to assess suicide risk and intent.
- Observe client's behavior every 15 minutes; stagger observation times.
  Staggering observations ensures that the client does not memorize a pattern.
- Remove all dangerous objects from client's environment.
- Use suicide precautions if indicated such as one-to-one staffing (constant attendance) and removal of all dangerous objects.
- Make a verbal or written contract with client. Have client state or write, "I will notify staff if I have suicidal or violent thoughts" or "I will not act on my thoughts."
  Written contracts are not legal documents and should be used only as an adjunct to other interventions, never as the primary treatment intervention.
  NOTE: If suicidal client is demonstrating violent behavior, nursing interventions and rationales for **Violence toward others** may be appropriate.

Geriatric
- Monitor for suicidal risk.
  The elderly, who experience multiple losses and have fragile support systems, are at greatest risk for suicide. Assess risk, death wishes, and suicide thoughts. Consider noncompliance with medical treatment a possible means to suicide. Also assess stress, social support, and vulnerability to guide interventions (Valente, 1994).
- Observe for dementia and depression.
- Monitor for paradoxical drug reactions.
  Violent behavior can be stimulated by a medication intended to calm the client.

- Assess for brain insults such as recent falls or injuries, strokes, or transient ischemic attacks.
  Brain injuries, which are related to lowered impulse control and reduced coping, can cause violent reactions to self or others. Brain injury symptoms may be mistaken for mental illness.
- Decrease environmental stimuli if violence is directed at others.
  Removal to a quiet area can lower violent impulses. Use calm voice to "talk down" the client.

Home Care Interventions

- Assess family/caregivers for ability to protect client and themselves.
  Safety of the client between home visits is a nursing priority. Caregivers often need assistance with recognizing or admitting fear of or danger from a loved one.
- Establish an emergency plan including when to use hotlines and 911. Contract with client and family on when to use emergency plan. Role play access to emergency resources with client and caregivers.
  Having an emergency plan and practicing accessing the plan reassures the client and caregivers. Contracting gives guided control to the client and enhances self-esteem.
- Assess home environment for harmful objects. Have family remove or lock objects as able.
  Safety of the client and caregivers is a nursing priority.
- Refer for homemaker services or psychiatric home health aide services for respite and client reassurance.
  Responsibility for a person at high risk for violence creates great caregiver stress. Respite decreases caregiver stress. The presence of caring individuals is reassuring, especially during periods of high client anxiety.
- If client is on psychotropic medications, assess client and family knowledge of medication and its administration and side effects. Teach as necessary.
  Knowledge of the medical regimen supports compliance.
- Evaluate effectiveness and side effects of medications.
  Accurate clinical feedback improves physician ability to prescribe an effective medical regimen specific to client needs.
- If client displays mildly intensifying aggressive behavior, attempt to diffuse anger or violence (e.g., ask for a glass of water to distract client). Later in visit explain that aggressive behavior is not acceptable and present consequences of continued aggressive behavior (i.e., right of agency to discontinue services).
  Mild aggression can be diffused safely. Confronting the client before severe aggression is evident places responsibility on the client and family for respectful partnership in care.
- Document all acts or verbalization of aggression.
  Safety of the staff is a primary responsibility of home health agencies. Law enforcement intervention may be necessary.
- If client verbalizes or displays threatening behavior, notify supervisor and plan to make joint visits with another staff person or a security escort.
  A second person at the visit is a show of power and control used to subdue aggressive behavior.
- Never enter a home or remain in a home if aggression threatens your well-being. Never challenge a show of force such as a gun threat. Leave and notify your supervisor. Document the incident.

Safety of the staff is a primary responsibility of home health agencies. Law enforcement intervention may be necessary.
- If client behaviors intensify, refer for immediate mental health intervention.
  The degree of disturbance and ability to manage care safely at home determines the level of services needed to protect the client.

Client/Family Teaching
- Teach relaxation and exercise as ways to release anger.
- Refer to individual or group therapy.
- Teach family how to recognize client is at increased risk for suicide (changes in behavior and verbal and nonverbal communication, withdrawal, depression, or sudden lifting of depression).
  A client may be at peace because a suicide plan has been made and the client has the energy to carry it out. Therefore when depression lifts, increased vigilance is necessary.
- Teach use of appropriate community resources in emergency situations (e.g., hotline, community mental health agency, emergency room).
- Encourage use of self-help groups in nonemergency situations.
- Inform client and family about medication actions, side effects, target symptoms, and toxic reactions.

REFERENCES   Aguilera D, Messick J: *Crisis intervention: theory and methodology,* ed 7, St Louis, 1994, Mosby.

Bath H: Physical restraint of children: is it therapeutic? *Am J Orthopsychiatry* 64:40, 1994.

Brent D et al: Personality disorder, personality traits, impulsive violence and completed suicide in adolescents, *J Am Acad Child Adolescent Psychiatry* 33:1080, 1994.

Daum A: Disruptive antisocial patient: management strategies, *Nurs Manage* 8:46, 1994.

Deffenbacher J et al: Social skills and cognitive relaxation approaches to general anger reduction, *J Counseling Psychol* 41:386, 1994.

Gates D: Workplace violence, *Am Assoc Occup Health Nurs* 10:536, 1995.

Holbert S: *Staff injuries: patient actions,* Unpublished manuscript, 1995, Canada.

Lehmann L et al: Training personnel in the prevention and management of violent behavior, *Hosp Community Psychiatry* 34:40, 1983.

Linaker O, Bush-Iversen H: Predictors of imminent violence in psychiatric inpatients, *Acta Psychiatr Scand* 92:250, 1995.

McNiel D, Binder R: Clinical assessment of the risk for violence among psychiatric inpatients, *Am J Psychiatry* 10:1317, 1991.

Morales E, Duphorne P: Least restrictive measures: alternatives to four-pt. restraints and seclusion, *J Psychosoc Nurs Ment Health Serv* 33:13, 1995.

Morrison E: Theoretical modeling to predict violence in hospitalized psychiatric patients, *Res Nurs Health* 12:31, 1989.

O'Brien P, Caldwell C, Transwau G: Destroyers: written treatment contracts can help cure self-destructive behaviors of the borderline patient, *J Psychosoc Nurs* 23:19, 1985.

Outlaw F, Lowery B: An attributional study of seclusion and restraint of psychiatric patients, *Arch Psych Nurs* 8:69, 1994.

Pfeiffer C: Suicidal children grow up: ego functions associated with suicide attempts, *J Am Acad Child Adolescent Psychiatry* 34:1310, 1995.

Poggenpoel M: Role and functions of psychiatric-mental health nurse in care and comfort of individuals, families and communities subject to violence, *Holistic Nurs Pract* 9:91, 1995.

Schwartz J, Kettley J, Rizzo J: *Suicide, principles and practice of emergency medicine,* Philadelphia, 1992, Lea & Febiger.

Smith J et al: Validation of the defining characteristics of potential for violence, *Nurs Diagnosis* 5:159, 1994.

Valente S: Suicide and elderly people: assessment and intervention, *J Death Dying* 28:317, 1994.

Vincent M, White K: Patient violence toward a nurse: predictable and preventable, *J Psychosoc Nurs Ment Health Serv* 32:31, 1994.

Worthington K: Taking action against violence in the workplace, *Am Nurse* 6:11,1993.

Appendix A

Nursing diagnoses arranged by Maslow's Hierarchy of Needs*

Because human beings adapt in many ways to establish and maintain the self, health problems are much more than simple physical matters. Maslow's Hierarchy of Needs (see diagram) is a system of classifying human needs. Maslow's hierarchy is based on the idea that lower-level physiological needs must be met before higher-level abstract needs can be met.

For nurses, Maslow's hierarchy has special significance in decision-making and planning for care. By considering need categories as you identify client problems, you will be able to provide more holistic care. For example, a client who demands frequent attention for a seemingly trivial matter may require help with self-esteem needs. Need levels vary from client to client. If a client is short of breath, the client is probably not interested in or capable of discussing spirituality. In addition, a client's need level may change throughout planning and intervention, so you will need to be vigilant in your assessment.

Read the descriptions of each category in the diagram, and see how you would relate them to nursing diagnoses. Compare your evaluation with how the authors categorized the nursing diagnoses according to this hierarchy. Be sure to assess clients for potential problems at all levels of the pyramid, regardless of their initial complaint.

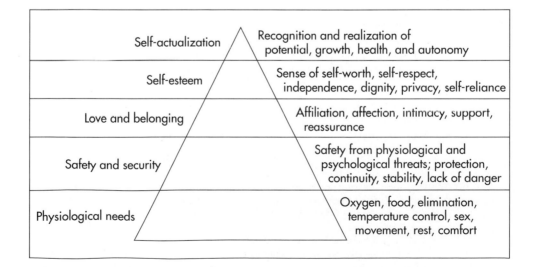

Self-actualization	Recognition and realization of potential, growth, health, and autonomy
Self-esteem	Sense of self-worth, self-respect, independence, dignity, privacy, self-reliance
Love and belonging	Affiliation, affection, intimacy, support, reassurance
Safety and security	Safety from physiological and psychological threats; protection, continuity, stability, lack of danger
Physiological needs	Oxygen, food, elimination, temperature control, sex, movement, rest, comfort

*Modified from Sparks SM, Taylor CM: *Nursing diagnosis reference manual,* Springhouse, Pa, 1991, Springhouse.

Physiological Needs

Activity Intolerance
Activity Intolerance, Risk for
Airway Clearance, Ineffective
Aspiration, Risk for
Breast-feeding, Effective
Breast-feeding, Ineffective
Breast-feeding, Interrupted
Breathing Pattern, Ineffective
Cardiac Output, Decreased
Confusion, Acute
Confusion, Chronic
Constipation
Constipation, Colonic
Constipation, Perceived
Diarrhea
Environmental Interpretation Syndrome,
    Impaired
Fatigue
Fluid Volume Deficit
Fluid Volume Deficit, Risk for
Fluid Volume Excess
Gas Exchange, Impaired
Hyperthermia
Hypothermia
Incontinence, Bowel
Incontinence, Functional
Incontinence, Reflex
Incontinence, Stress
Incontinence, Total
Incontinence, Urge
Infant Behavior, Disorganized
Infant Behavior, Potential for Enhanced Organized
Infant Behavior, Risk for Disorganized
Infant Feeding Pattern, Ineffective
Intracranial, Decreased Adaptive Capacity
Memory, Impaired
Mobility, Impaired Physical
Nutrition, Altered: Less than Body Requirements
Nutrition, Altered: More than Body
    Requirements
Nutrition, Altered: Risk for More than Body
    Requirements
Oral Mucous Membranes, Altered
Pain
Pain, Chronic
Protection, Altered
Self-Care Deficit, Bathing/Hygiene

Self-Care Deficit, Dressing/Grooming
Self-Care Deficit, Feeding
Self-Care Deficit, Toileting
Sensory-Perceptual Alterations (Specify) (Visual,
    Auditory, Kinesthetic, Gustatory, Tactile,
    Olfactory)
Sexual Dysfunction
Sexuality Pattern, Altered
Skin Integrity, Impaired
Skin Integrity, Impaired, Risk for
Sleep Pattern Disturbance
Swallowing Impaired
Temperature, Risk for Altered Body
Thermoregulation, Ineffective
Thought Process, Altered
Tissue Integrity, Impaired
Tissue Perfusion, Altered (Specify) (Renal,
    Cerebral, Cardiopulmonary, Gastrointestinal,
    Peripheral)
Urinary Elimination, Altered
Urinary Retention
Ventilation, Inability to Sustain Spontaneous
Ventilatory Weaning Response, Dysfunctional

Safety and Security Needs

Communication, Impaired Verbal
Disuse Syndrome, Risk for
Dysreflexia
Fear
Grieving, Anticipatory
Grieving, Dysfunctional
Health Maintenance, Altered
Home Maintenance Management, Impaired
Infection, Risk for
Injury, Risk for
Knowledge Deficit
Perioperative Positioning Injury, Risk for
Peripheral Neurovascular Dysfunction, Risk for
Poisoning, Risk for
Suffocation, Risk for
Therapeutic Regimen: Community, Ineffective
    Management of
Therapeutic Regimen: Families, Ineffective
    Management of
Therapeutic Regimen: Individual, Ineffective
    Management of
Trauma, Risk for
Unilateral Neglect

Love and Belonging Needs

Anxiety
Caregiver Role Strain
Caregiver Role Strain, Risk for
Family Coping: Compromised, Ineffective
Family Coping: Disabling, Ineffective
Family Coping: Potential for Growth
Family Processes, Altered
Loneliness, Risk for
Parent/Infant/Child Attachment, Risk for Altered
Parental Role Conflict
Parenting, Altered
Parenting, Altered, Risk for
Relocation Stress Syndrome
Social Interaction, Impaired
Social Isolation

Self-Esteem

Adjustment, Impaired
Alcoholism, Altered Family Process
Body Image Disturbance
Community Coping, Ineffective
Community Coping, Potential for Enhanced
Coping, Defensive
Coping, Ineffective Individual
Decisional Conflict

Denial, Ineffective
Diversional Activity Deficit
Hopelessness
Noncompliance
Personal Identity Disturbance
Post-Trauma Response
Powerlessness
Rape-Trauma Syndrome
Rape-Trauma Syndrome: Compound Reaction
Rape-Trauma Syndrome: Silent Reaction
Role Performance, Altered
Self-Esteem, Chronic Low
Self-Esteem, Situational Low
Self-Esteem Disturbance
Self-Mutilation, Risk for
Violence: Self-Directed or Directed at Others,
    Risk for

Self-Actualization Needs

Effective Management of Therapeutic Regimen:
    Individual
Energy Field Disturbance
Growth and Development, Altered
Health-Seeking Behaviors
Potential for Enhanced Spiritual Well-Being
Spiritual Distress

Appendix B

Nursing diagnoses arranged by Gordon's functional health patterns*

Health-Perception—Health-Management

Health-Seeking Behaviors (Specify)
Altered Health Maintenance
Ineffective Management of Therapeutic
  Regimen
Effective Management of Therapeutic Regimen:
  Individuals
Ineffective Management of Therapeutic
  Regimen: Families
Ineffective Management of Therapeutic
  Regimen: Community
Noncompliance (Specify)
Risk for Infection
Risk for Injury
Risk for Trauma
Risk for Perioperative Positioning Injury
Risk for Poisoning
Risk for Suffocation
Altered Protection
Energy Field Disturbance

Nutritional-Metabolic

Altered Nutrition: More than Body Requirements
Altered Nutrition: Risk for More than Body
  Requirements
Altered Nutrition: Less than Body Requirements
Ineffective Breastfeeding
Interrupted Breastfeeding
Effective Breastfeeding
Ineffective Infant Feeding Pattern
Impaired Swallowing
Risk for Aspiration
Altered Oral Mucous Membranes

Fluid Volume Deficit
Risk for Fluid Volume Deficit
Fluid Volume Excess
Risk for Impaired Skin Integrity
Impaired Skin Integrity
Impaired Tissue Integrity
Risk for Altered Body Temperature
Ineffective Thermoregulation
Hyperthermia
Hypothermia

Elimination

Colonic Constipation
Perceived Constipation
Constipation
Diarrhea
Bowel Incontinence
Altered Urinary Elimination
Functional Incontinence
Reflex Incontinence
Stress Incontinence
Urge Incontinence
Total Incontinence
Urinary Retention

Activity-Exercise

Activity Intolerance
Risk for Activity Intolerance
Fatigue
Impaired Physical Mobility
Risk for Disuse Syndrome
Bathing/Hygienic Self-Care Deficit
Dressing/Grooming Self-Care Deficit

*Modified from Gordon M: *Manual of nursing diagnosis, 1997-1998,* St Louis, 1997, Mosby.

Feeding Self-Care Deficit
Toileting Self-Care Deficit
Diversional Activity Deficit
Impaired Home Maintenance Management
Dysfunctional Ventilatory Weaning Response
Inability to Sustain Spontaneous Ventilation
Ineffective Airway Clearance
Ineffective Breathing Pattern
Impaired Gas Exchange
Decreased Cardiac Output
Altered Tissue Perfusion (Specify Type)
Dysreflexia
Disorganized Infant Behavior
Risk for Disorganized Infant Behavior
Potential for Enhanced Organized Infant
   Behavior
Risk for Peripheral Neurovascular Dysfunction
Altered Growth and Development

Sleep-Rest

Sleep Pattern Disturbance

Cognitive-Perceptual

Pain
Chronic Pain
Sensory/Perceptual Alterations (Specify)
Unilateral Neglect
Knowledge Deficit (Specify)
Altered Thought Processes
Acute Confusion
Chronic Confusion
Impaired Environmental Interpretation
   Syndrome
Impaired Memory
Decisional Conflict (Specify)
Decreased Adaptive Capacity: Intracranial

Self-Perception—Self-Concept

Fear
Anxiety
Risk for Loneliness
Hopelessness
Powerlessness
Self-Esteem Disturbance
Chronic Low Self-Esteem
Situational Low Self-Esteem

Body Image Disturbance
Risk for Self-Mutilation
Personal Identity Disturbance

Role-Relationship

Anticipatory Grieving
Dysfunctional Grieving
Altered Role Performance
Social Isolation or Social Rejection
Social Isolation
Impaired Social Interaction
Relocation Stress Syndrome
Altered Family Processes
Altered Family Processes: Alcoholism
Altered Parenting
Risk for Altered Parenting
Parental Role Conflict
Risk for Altered Parent-Infant/Child Attachment
Caregiver Role Strain
Risk for Caregiver Role Strain
Impaired Verbal Communication
Risk for Violence: Self-Directed or Directed at
   Others

Sexuality-Reproductive

Altered Sexuality Patterns
Sexual Dysfunction
Rape Trauma Syndrome
Rape Trauma Syndrome: Compound Reaction
Rape Trauma Syndrome: Silent Reaction

Coping—Stress-Tolerance

Ineffective Individual Coping
Defensive Coping
Ineffective Denial
Impaired Adjustment
Post-Trauma Response
Family Coping: Potential for Growth
Ineffective Family Coping: Compromised
Ineffective Family Coping: Disabling
Ineffective Community Coping
Potential for Enhanced Community Coping

Value-Belief

Spiritual Distress (Distress of Human Spirit)
Potential for Enhanced Spiritual Well-Being

Appendix C

Nursing diagnoses arranged by NANDA's human response patterns*

Exchanging

Altered Nutrition: More than Body Requirements
Altered Nutrition: Less than Body Requirements
Altered Nutrition: Potential for More than Body
  Requirements
Risk for Infection
Risk for Altered Body Temperature
Hypothermia
Hyperthermia
Ineffective Thermoregulation
Dysreflexia
Constipation
Perceived Constipation
Colonic Constipation
Diarrhea
Bowel Incontinence
Altered Urinary Elimination
Stress Incontinence
Reflex Incontinence
Urge Incontinence
Functional Incontinence
Total Incontinence
Urinary Retention
Altered (Specify Type) Tissue Perfusion (Renal,
  Cerebral, Cardiopulmonary, Gastrointestinal,
  Peripheral)
Fluid Volume Excess
Fluid Volume Deficit
Risk for Fluid Volume Deficit
Decreased Cardiac Output
Impaired Gas Exchange

Ineffective Airway Clearance
Ineffective Breathing Pattern
Inability to Sustain Spontaneous Ventilation
Dysfunctional Ventilatory Weaning Response
  (DVWR)
Risk for Injury
Risk for Suffocation
Risk for Poisoning
Risk for Trauma
Risk for Aspiration
Risk for Disuse Syndrome
Altered Protection
Impaired Tissue Integrity
Altered Oral Mucous Membranes
Impaired Skin Integrity
Risk for Impaired Skin Integrity
Decreased Adaptive Capacity: Intracranial
Energy Field Disturbance

Communicating

Impaired Verbal Communication

Relating

Impaired Social Interaction
Social Isolation
Risk for Loneliness
Altered Role Performance
Altered Parenting
Risk for Altered Parenting
Risk for Altered Parent/Infant/Child Attachment
Sexual Dysfunction

*From North American Nursing Diagnosis Association: *Nursing diagnoses: definitions and classification 1997-1998*, Philadelphia, The Association.

Altered Family Processes
Caregiver Role Strain
Risk for Caregiver Role Strain
Altered Family Process: Alcoholism
Parental Role Conflict
Altered Sexuality Patterns

Valuing

Spiritual Distress (Distress of the Human Spirit)
Potential for Enhanced Spiritual Well Being

Choosing

Ineffective Individual Coping
Impaired Adjustment
Defensive Coping
Ineffective Denial
Ineffective Family Coping: Disabling
Ineffective Family Coping: Compromised
Potential for Enhanced Community Coping
Ineffective Community Coping
Family Coping: Potential for Growth
Ineffective Management of Therapeutic
    Regimen (Individuals)
Noncompliance (Specify)
Ineffective Management of Therapeutic
    Regimen: Families
Ineffective Management of Therapeutic
    Regimen: Community
Effective Management of Therapeutic Regimen:
    Individual
Decisional Conflict (Specify)
Health-Seeking Behaviors (Specify)

Moving

Impaired Physical Mobility
Risk for Peripheral Neurovascular Dysfunction
Risk for Perioperative Positioning Injury
Activity Intolerance
Fatigue
Risk for Activity Intolerance
Sleep Pattern Disturbance
Diversional Activity Deficit
Impaired Home Maintenance Management
Altered Health Maintenance
Feeding Self-Care Deficit
Impaired Swallowing
Ineffective Breast-feeding
Interrupted Breast-feeding

Effective Breast-feeding
Ineffective Infant Feeding Pattern
Bathing/Hygiene Self-Care Deficit
Dressing/Grooming Self-Care Deficit
Toileting Self-Care Deficit
Altered Growth and Development
Relocation Stress Syndrome
Risk for Disorganized Infant Behavior
Disorganized Infant Behavior
Potential for Enhanced Organized Infant
    Behavior

Perceiving

Body Image Disturbance
Self-Esteem Disturbance
Chronic Low Self-Esteem
Situational Low Self-Esteem
Personal Identity Disturbance
Sensory/Perceptual Alterations (Specify) (Visual,
    Auditory, Kinesthetic, Gustatory, Tactile,
    Olfactory)
Unilateral Neglect
Hopelessness
Powerlessness

Knowing

Knowledge Deficit (Specify)
Impaired Environmental Interpretation
    Syndrome
Acute Confusion
Chronic Confusion
Altered Thought Processes
Impaired Memory

Feeling

Pain
Chronic Pain
Dysfunctional Grieving
Anticipatory Grieving
Risk for Violence: Self-Directed or Directed at
    Others
Risk for Self-Mutilation
Post-Trauma Response
Rape-Trauma Syndrome
Rape-Trauma Syndrome: Compound Reaction
Rape-Trauma Syndrome: Silent Reaction
Anxiety
Fear

Appendix D

Pain: assessment guide and equianalgesic chart

Margo McCaffery

Assessment: Use of Pain Rating Scales

Nursing Assessment/Diagnosis of the Pain Sensation. Ask the client about current level of pain if at all possible. The client's self-report of pain is the single most reliable indicator of how much pain the client is experiencing. The rating given by the client is always what is recorded in the client's record.

Basic Measures of Pain. The hierarchy of importance of basic measures of pain are as follows (Agency for Health Care Policy and Research: *Quick Reference on Acute Pain in Childhood,* 1992; Schechter, Altman, Weisman, editors: Report of the Consensus Conference on the Management of Pain in Childhood Cancer, *Pediatrics* 86:813, 1990):

1. Client's self-report
2. Report of parent, family, or others close to client
3. Behaviors (e.g., facial expressions, body movements, crying)
4. Physiological measures, "neither sensitive nor specific as indicators of pain" (Agency for Health Care Policy and Research: *Quick Ref. Acute Pain in Children,* 1992, p. 7)

Client/family teaching

NOTE: When it is obvious that pain is severe (e.g., following trauma or major surgery), a pain rating scale need not be used initially. Give an analgesic and wait until the client is better able to cooperate.

1. Explain the primary purposes of a pain rating scale. Show the client and family the scale.
   a. This step allows quick, consistent communication between client and caregiver/ nurse/physician. Emphasize that the client must volunteer information because caregivers may not know when the client has pain.
   b. This step also helps establish a pain relief goal that is satisfactory to the client.
2. Explain the specific pain rating scale (e.g., 0 to 10; 0 = no pain and 10 = worst possible pain). When a numerical scale is used, verify that the client can count up to the number used. If the client does not understand whatever scale is standard in that clinical setting, select another scale.
3. Discuss the word *pain.* Explain that pain is discomfort that may occur anywhere in the body; may have various characteristics such as aching, hurting, pulling, tightness, burning, or pricking; and may be mild to severe. If the client prefers some other term such as *hurt,* use that word.

4. To verify that clients understand how the word *pain* (or other word preferred by client) is used, ask them to give two examples of pain they have now or have experienced.
5. Ask clients to practice using the pain rating scale by rating their current or past painful experiences.
6. Ask the client what pain rating would be acceptable or satisfactory while at rest and active. This helps set a realistic, initial goal. Zero pain is not always possible. Once the initial goal is achieved, the possibility of better pain relief can be considered. Emphasize to the client that satisfactory pain relief is a level of pain that is noticeable but not distressing and enables the client to sleep, eat, and perform other required or desired physical activities.

0-10 Numerical Descriptive Pain Intensity Scale

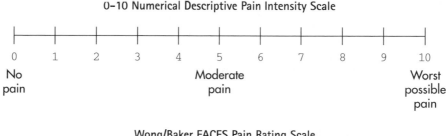

0   1   2   3   4   5   6   7   8   9   10

No
pain

Moderate
pain

Worst
possible
pain

Wong/Baker FACES Pain Rating Scale

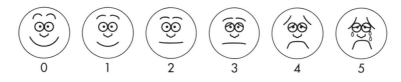

0   1   2   3   4   5

This particular scale is recommended for clients age 3 years and older. Explain to the client that each face is for a person who feels happy because there is no pain (hurt) or sad because there is some or a lot of pain. Face 0 = very happy because there is no hurt at all. Face 1 = hurts just a little bit. Face 2 = hurts a little more. Face 3 = hurts even more. Face 4 = hurts a whole lot. Face 5 = hurts as much as you can imagine, although you don't have to be crying to feel this bad. Ask clients to choose the face that best describes how they are feeling. (From Wong D: *Nursing care of infants and children,* ed 5, 1995, Mosby. The Wong/Baker FACES Pain Scale may be reproduced for clinical use provided the copyright information is retained with the scale. Research reported in Wong D, Baker C: Pain in children: comparison of assessment scales, *Pediatr Nurs* 14:9, 1988.)

Dose equivalents for opioid analgesics in opioid-naive adults and children ≥50 kg body weight[1]

Drug	Approximate equianalgesic dosage		Usual starting dosage for moderate to severe pain	
	Oral	Parenteral	Oral	Parenteral
Opioid agonist[2]				
Morphine[3]	30 mg q3-4h (repeat around-the-clock dosing) 60 mg q3-4h (single dose or intermittent dosing)	10 mg q3-4h	30 mg q3-4h	10 mg q3-4h
Morphine, controlled-release[3,4] (MS Contin, Oramorph)	90-120 mg q12h	N/A	90-120 mg q12h	N/A
Hydromorphone[3] (Dilaudid)	7.5 mg q3-4h	1.5 mg q3-4h	6 mg q3-4h	1.5 mg q3-4h
Levorphanol (Levo-Dromoran)	4 mg q6-8h	2 mg q6-8h	4 mg q6-8h	2 mg q6-8h
Meperidine (Demerol)	300 mg q2-3h	100 mg q3h	N/R	100 mg q3h
Methadone (Dolophine, other)	20 mg q6-8h	10 mg q6-8h	20 mg q6-8h	10 mg q6-8h
Oxymorphone[3] (Numorphan)	N/A	1 mg q3-4h	N/A	1 mg q3-4h
Combination opioid/NSAID preparations[5]				
Codeine[6] (with aspirin or acetaminophen)	180-200 mg q3-4h	130 mg q3-4h	60 mg q3-4h	60 mg q2h (IM/SC)
Hydrocodone (in Lorcet, Lortab, Vicodin, others)	30 mg q3-4h	N/A	10 mg q3-4h	N/A
Oxycodone (Roxicodone, also in Percocet, Percodan, Tylox, others)	30 mg q3-4h	N/A	10 mg q3-4h	N/A

From Jacox H et al: *Management of cancer pain,* Clinical Practice Guideline No 9, Agency for Health Care Policy and Research, Pub No 94-0592, 1994, US Department of Health and Human Services, Public Health Services.

q, Every; *N/A,* not available; *N/R,* not recommended; *IM,* intramuscular; *SQ,* subcutaneous.

[1]Caution: Recommended doses do not apply for adult patients with body weight less than 50 kg.

[2]Caution: Recommended doses do not apply to patients with renal or hepatic insufficiency or other conditions affecting drug metabolism and kinetics.

[3]Caution: For morphine, hydromorphone, and oxymorphone, rectal administration is an alternative route for patients unable to take oral medications. Equianalgesic doses may differ from oral and parenteral doses because of pharmacokinetic differences.

[4]Transdermal fentanyl (Duragesic) is an alternative option. Transdermal fentanyl dosage is not calculated as equianalgesic to a single morphine dose. See the package insert for dosing calculations. Dosages above 25 μg/h should not be used in opioid-naive patients.

[5]Caution: Doses of aspirin and acetaminophen in combination opioid/nonsteroidal antiinflammatory drug (NSAID) preparations must also be adjusted to the patient's body weight. Aspirin is contraindicated in children in the presence of fever or other viral disease because of its association with Reye's syndrome.

[6]Caution: Codeine doses greater than 65 mg often are not appropriate because of diminishing incremental analgesia with increasing doses but continually increasing nausea, constipation, and other side effects.

(NOTE: Published tables vary in the suggested doses that are equianalgesic to morphine. Clinical response is the criterion that must be applied for each patient; titration to clinical responses is necessary. Because there is not complete cross-tolerance among these drugs, it is usually necessary to use a lower than equianalgesic dose when changing drugs and to retitrate to response.)

Appendix E

Nursing interventions classification (NIC) interventions

Abuse Protection
Abuse Protection: Child
Abuse Protection: Elder
Acid-Base Management
Acid-Base Management: Metabolic Acidosis
Acid-Base Management: Metabolic Alkalosis
Acid-Base Management: Respiratory Acidosis
Acid-Base Management: Respiratory Alkalosis
Acid-Base Monitoring
Active Listening
Activity Therapy
Acupressure
Admission Care
Airway Insertion and Stabilization
Airway Management
Airway Suctioning
Allergy Management
Amnioinfusion
Amputation Care
Analgesic Administration
Analgesic Administration: Intraspinal
Anesthesia Administration
Anger Control Assistance
Animal-Assisted Therapy
Anticipatory Guidance
Anxiety Reduction
Area Restriction
Art Therapy
Artificial Airway Management
Aspiration Precautions
Assertiveness Training

Attachment Promotion
Autogenic Training
Autotransfusion
Bathing
Bed Rest Care
Bedside Laboratory Testing
Behavior Management
Behavior Management: Overactivity/Inattention
Behavior Management: Self-Harm
Behavior Management: Sexual
Behavior Modification
Behavior Modification: Social Skills
Bibliotherapy
Biofeedback
Birthing
Bladder Irrigation
Bleeding Precautions
Bleeding Reduction
Bleeding Reduction: Antepartum Uterus
Bleeding Reduction: Gastrointestinal
Bleeding Reduction: Nasal
Bleeding Reduction: Postpartum Uterus
Bleeding Reduction: Wound
Blood Products Administration
Body Image Enhancement
Body Mechanics Promotion
Bottle Feeding
Bowel Incontinence Care
Bowel Incontinence Care: Encopresis
Bowel Irrigation
Bowel Management

From McCloskey JC, Bulechek GM: *Nursing interventions classification (NIC),* ed 2, St Louis, 1996, Mosby.

Bowel Training
Breastfeeding Assistance
Calming Technique
Cardiac Care
Cardiac Care: Acute
Cardiac Care: Rehabilitative
Cardiac Precautions
Caregiver Support
Cast Care: Maintenance
Cast Care: Wet
Cerebral Edema Management
Cerebral Perfusion Promotion
Cesarean Section Care
Chemotherapy Management
Chest Physiotherapy
Childbirth Preparation
Circulatory Care
Circulatory Care: Mechanical Assist Device
Circulatory Precautions
Code Management
Cognitive Restructuring
Cognitive Stimulation
Communication Enhancement: Hearing Deficit
Communication Enhancement: Speech Deficit
Communication Enhancement: Visual Deficit
Complex Relationship Building
Conscious Sedation
Constipation/Impaction Management
Contact Lens Care
Controlled Substance Checking
Coping Enhancement
Cough Enhancement
Counseling
Crisis Intervention
Critical Path Development
Culture Brokerage
Cutaneous Stimulation
Decision-Making Support
Delegation
Delirium Management
Delusion Management
Dementia Management
Developmental Enhancement
Diarrhea Management
Diet Staging
Discharge Planning
Distraction
Documentation

Dressing
Dying Care
Dysreflexia Management
Dysrhythmia Management
Ear Care
Eating Disorders Management
Electrolyte Management
Electrolyte Management: Hypercalcemia
Electrolyte Management: Hyperkalemia
Electrolyte Management: Hypermagnesemia
Electrolyte Management: Hypernatremia
Electrolyte Management: Hyperphosphatemia
Electrolyte Management: Hypocalcemia
Electrolyte Management: Hypokalemia
Electrolyte Management: Hypomagnesemia
Electrolyte Management: Hyponatremia
Electrolyte Management: Hypophosphatemia
Electrolyte Monitoring
Electronic Fetal Monitoring: Antepartum
Electronic Fetal Monitoring: Intrapartum
Elopement Precautions
Embolus Care: Peripheral
Embolus Care: Pulmonary
Embolus Precautions
Emergency Care
Emergency Cart Checking
Emotional Support
Endotracheal Extubation
Energy Management
Enteral Tube Feeding
Environmental Management
Environmental Management: Attachment
    Process
Environmental Management: Comfort
Environmental Management: Community
Environmental Management: Safety
Environmental Management: Violence
    Prevention
Environmental Management: Worker Safety
Examination Assistance
Exercise Promotion
Exercise Promotion: Stretching
Exercise Therapy: Ambulation
Exercise Therapy: Balance
Exercise Therapy: Joint Mobility
Exercise Therapy: Muscle Control
Eye Care
Fall Prevention

Family Integrity Promotion
Family Integrity Promotion: Childbearing Family
Family Involvement
Family Mobilization
Family Planning: Contraception
Family Planning: Infertility
Family Planning: Unplanned Pregnancy
Family Process Maintenance
Family Support
Family Therapy
Feeding
Fertility Preservation
Fever Treatment
Fire-Setting Precautions
First Aid
Flatulence Reduction
Fluid Management
Fluid/Electrolyte Management
Fluid Monitoring
Fluid Resuscitation
Foot Care
Gastrointestinal Intubation
Genetic Counseling
Grief Work Facilitation
Grief Work Facilitation: Perinatal Death
Guilt Work Facilitation
Hair Care
Hallucination Management
Health Care Information Exchange
Health Education
Health Policy Monitoring
Health Screening
Health System Guidance
Heat Exposure Treatment
Heat/Cold Application
Hemodialysis Therapy
Hemodynamic Regulation
Hemorrhage Control
High-Risk Pregnancy Care
Home Maintenance Assistance
Hope Instillation
Humor
Hyperglycemia Management
Hypervolemia Management
Hypnosis
Hypoglycemia Management
Hypothermia Treatment
Hypovolemia Management

Immunization/Vaccination Administration
Impulse Control Training
Incident Reporting
Incision Site Care
Infant Care
Infection Control
Infection Control: Intraoperative
Infection Protection
Insurance Authorization
Intracranial Pressure (ICP) Monitoring
Intrapartal Care
Intrapartal Care: High-Risk Delivery
Intravenous (IV) Insertion
Intravenous (IV) Therapy
Invasive Hemodynamic Monitoring
Kangaroo Care
Labor Induction
Labor Suppression
Laboratory Data Interpretation
Lactation Counseling
Lactation Suppression
Laser Precautions
Latex Precautions
Learning Facilitation
Learning Readiness Enhancement
Leech Therapy
Limit Setting
Malignant Hyperthermia Precautions
Mechanical Ventilation
Mechanical Ventilatory Weaning
Medication Administration
Medication Administration: Enteral
Medication Administration: Interpleural
Medication Administration: Intraosseous
Medication Administration: Oral
Medication Administration: Parenteral
Medication Administration: Topical
Medication Administration: Ventricular Reservoir
Medication Management
Medication Prescribing
Meditation
Memory Training
Milieu Therapy
Mood Management
Multidisciplinary Care Conference
Music Therapy
Mutual Goal Setting
Nail Care

Neurologic Monitoring
Newborn Care
Newborn Monitoring
Nonnutritive Sucking
Normalization Promotion
Nutrition Management
Nutrition Therapy
Nutritional Counseling
Nutritional Monitoring
Oral Health Maintenance
Oral Health Promotion
Oral Health Restoration
Order Transcription
Organ Procurement
Ostomy Care
Oxygen Therapy
Pain Management
Parent Education: Adolescent
Parent Education: Childbearing Family
Parent Education: Childrearing Family
Pass Facilitation
Patient Contracting
Patient-Controlled Analgesia (PCA) Assistance
Patient Rights Protection
Peer Review
Pelvic Floor Exercise
Perineal Care
Peripheral Sensation Management
Peripherally Inserted Central (PIC) Catheter Care
Peritoneal Dialysis Therapy
Phlebotomy: Arterial Blood Sample
Phlebotomy: Blood Unit Acquisition
Phlebotomy: Venous Blood Sample
Phototherapy: Neonate
Physical Restraint
Physician Support
Play Therapy
Pneumatic Tourniquet Precautions
Positioning
Positioning: Intraoperative
Positioning: Neurologic
Positioning: Wheelchair
Postanesthesia Care
Postmortem Care
Postpartal Care
Preceptor: Employee
Preceptor: Student

Preconception Counseling
Pregnancy Termination Care
Prenatal Care
Preoperative Coordination
Preparatory Sensory Information
Presence
Pressure Management
Pressure Ulcer Care
Pressure Ulcer Prevention
Product Evaluation
Progressive Muscle Relaxation
Prosthesis Care
Quality Monitoring
Radiation Therapy Management
Rape-Trauma Treatment
Reality Orientation
Recreation Therapy
Rectal Prolapse Management
Referral
Reminiscence Therapy
Reproductive Technology Management
Research Data Collection
Respiratory Monitoring
Respite Care
Resuscitation
Resuscitation: Fetus
Resuscitation: Neonate
Risk Identification
Risk Identification: Childbearing Family
Role Enhancement
Seclusion
Security Enhancement
Seizure Management
Seizure Precautions
Self-Awareness Enhancement
Self-Care Assistance
Self-Care Assistance: Bathing/Hygiene
Self-Care Assistance: Dressing/Grooming
Self-Care Assistance: Feeding
Self-Care Assistance: Toileting
Self-Esteem Enhancement
Self-Modification Assistance
Self-Responsibility Facilitation
Sexual Counseling
Shift Report
Shock Management
Shock Management: Cardiac

Shock Management: Vasogenic
Shock Management: Volume
Shock Prevention
Sibling Support
Simple Guided Imagery
Simple Massage
Simple Relaxation Therapy
Skin Care: Topical Treatments
Skin Surveillance
Sleep Enhancement
Smoking Cessation Assistance
Socialization Enhancement
Specimen Management
Spiritual Support
Splinting
Staff Supervision
Subarachnoid Hemorrhage Precautions
Substance Use Prevention
Substance Use Treatment
Substance Use Treatment: Alcohol Withdrawal
Substance Use Treatment: Drug Withdrawal
Substance Use Treatment: Overdose
Suicide Prevention
Supply Management
Support Group
Support System Enhancement
Surgical Assistance
Surgical Precautions
Surgical Preparation
Surveillance
Surveillance: Late Pregnancy
Surveillance: Safety
Sustenance Support
Suturing
Swallowing Therapy
Teaching: Disease Process
Teaching: Group
Teaching: Individual
Teaching: Infant Care
Teaching: Preoperative
Teaching: Prescribed Activity/Exercise
Teaching: Prescribed Diet
Teaching: Prescribed Medication
Teaching: Procedure/Treatment

Teaching: Psychomotor Skill
Teaching: Safe Sex
Teaching: Sexuality
Technology Management
Telephone Consultation
Temperature Regulation
Temperature Regulation: Intraoperative
Therapeutic Touch
Therapy Group
Total Parenteral Nutrition (TPN) Administration
Touch
Traction/Immobilization Care
Transcutaneous Electrical Nerve Stimulation (TENS)
Transport
Triage
Truth Telling
Tube Care
Tube Care: Chest
Tube Care: Gastrointestinal
Tube Care: Umbilical Line
Tube Care: Urinary
Tube Care: Ventriculostomy/Lumbar Drain
Ultrasonography: Limited Obstetric
Unilateral Neglect Management
Urinary Bladder Training
Urinary Catheterization
Urinary Catheterization: Intermittent
Urinary Elimination Management
Urinary Habit Training
Urinary Incontinence Care
Urinary Incontinence Care: Enuresis
Urinary Retention Care
Values Clarification
Venous Access Devices (VAD) Maintenance
Ventilation Assistance
Visitation Facilitation
Vital Signs Monitoring
Weight Gain Assistance
Weight Management
Weight Reduction Assistance
Wound Care
Wound Care: Closed Drainage
Wound Irrigation

Index

Entries in **boldface** refer to official NANDA diagnoses; *italics* indicate page numbers in nursing care plans.